Handbook of Psoriatic Arthritis

Handbook of Psoriatic Arthritis

Edited by Robert Jameson

AMERICAN
MEDICAL PUBLISHERS
www.americanmedicalpublishers.com

American Medical Publishers,
41 Flatbush Avenue,
1st Floor, New York,
NY 11217, USA

Visit us on the World Wide Web at:
www.americanmedicalpublishers.com

ISBN: 978-1-63927-395-9

Cataloging-in-Publication Data

Handbook of psoriatic arthritis / edited by Robert Jameson.
p. cm.
Includes bibliographical references and index.
ISBN 978-1-63927-395-9
1. Psoriatic arthritis. 2. Psoriatic arthritis--Diagnosis. 3. Psoriatic arthritis--Treatment.
4. Arthritis. 5. Psoriasis. I. Jameson, Robert.
RC931.P76 P76 2022
616.722 7--dc23

Table of Contents

Preface

Psoriatic arthritis is a chronic inflammatory form of arthritis which occurs in people with psoriasis. It causes swelling of fingers and toes, thickening of nails, depressions in the nail, and detachment of the nail from the nailbed. Certain symptoms are specific to this condition, such as enthesitis and dactylis. Psoriatic arthritis can occur in both children and adults. Genetics, obesity and psoriasis are major risk factors for psoriatic arthritis. There are five different types of disease - oligoarticular, polyarticular, spondyloarthritis, arthritis mutilans and distal interphalangeal predominant. Health history, physical examinations, blood tests and X-rays help in the diagnosis of this condition. Its treatment is directed at the control and reduction of inflammation. Biological response modifiers or disease-modifying antirheumatic drugs are recommended for preventing irreversible joint destruction. NSAIDs are usually effective against milder forms of psoriatic arthritis. This book is compiled in such a manner, that it will provide in-depth knowledge about the symptoms, diagnosis and the care and treatment of psoriatic arthritis. The aim of this book is to present researches that have transformed our understanding of arthritis and aided its advancement. For someone with an interest and eye for detail, this book covers the most significant topics in this domain.

This book is a result of research of several months to collate the most relevant data in the field.

When I was approached with the idea of this book and the proposal to edit it, I was overwhelmed. It gave me an opportunity to reach out to all those who share a common interest with me in this field. I had 3 main parameters for editing this text:

1. Accuracy – The data and information provided in this book should be up-to-date and valuable to the readers.
2. Structure – The data must be presented in a structured format for easy understanding and better grasping of the readers.
3. Universal Approach – This book not only targets students but also experts and innovators in the field, thus my aim was to present topics which are of use to all.

Thus, it took me a couple of months to finish the editing of this book.

I would like to make a special mention of my publisher who considered me worthy of this opportunity and also supported me throughout the editing process. I would also like to thank the editing team at the back-end who extended their help whenever required.

Editor

1

Identification of low-frequency *TRAF3IP2* coding variants in psoriatic arthritis patients and functional characterization

Beate Böhm[1], Harald Burkhardt[1], Steffen Uebe[2], Maria Apel[2], Frank Behrens[1], André Reis[2] and Ulrike Hüffmeier[2*]

Abstract

Introduction: In recent genome-wide association studies for psoriatic arthritis (PsA) and psoriasis vulgaris, common coding variants in the *TRAF3IP2* gene were identified to contribute to susceptibility to both disease entities. The risk allele of p.Asp10Asn (rs33980500) proved to be most significantly associated and to encode a mutant protein with an almost completely disrupted binding property to TRAF6, supporting its impact as a main disease-causing variant and modulator of IL-17 signaling.

Methods: To identify further variants, exons 2-4 encoding both known TNF-receptor-associated factor (TRAF) binding domains were sequenced in 871 PsA patients. Seven missense variants and one three-base-pair insertion were identified in 0.06% to 1.02% of alleles. Five of these variants were also present in 931 control individuals at comparable frequency. Constructs containing full-length wild-type or mutant *TRAF3IP2* were generated and used to analyze functionally all variants for TRAF6-binding in a mammalian two-hybrid assay.

Results: None of the newly found alleles, though, encoded proteins with different binding properties to TRAF6, or to the cytoplasmic tail of the IL-17-receptor α-chain, suggesting that they do not contribute to susceptibility.

Conclusions: Thus, the *TRAF3IP2*-variant p.Asp10Asn is the only susceptibility allele with functional impact on TRAF6 binding, at least in the German population.

Introduction

Recent genome-wide association studies (GWASs) for psoriatic arthritis and psoriasis vulgaris have been quite successful and revealed more than 25 new susceptibility loci [1-7] characterizing psoriatic arthritis (PsA), mainly as an immune-mediated disease that is also affected by barrier proteins. One new PsA and psoriasis-susceptibility gene, *TRAF3IP2*, codes for the adaptor protein ACT1 (nuclear factor-κB activator 1), a regulator of the NF-κB pathway involved in IL-17 signaling. We were able to identify the common coding variant p.Asp10Aspn (rs33980500) as the disease-causing allele with evidence from association findings at single nucleotide polymorphism (SNP) and haplotype levels, as well as binding studies of ACT1 with its interaction partner TRAF6 [2] (Figure 1). However, despite the exponentially increased knowledge of PsA and psoriasis susceptibility, the sum of the currently identified genetic risk factors does not explain the entire genetic contribution to disease.

At the common susceptibility gene *IL23R*, coding for interleukin-23 receptor for Crohn disease, low-frequency variants have been identified as protective factors, and their effects turned out to be larger than those of common variants and accounted for a greater portion of genetic contribution [8]. To find out whether low-frequency coding variants in *TRAF3IP2* contribute to PsA susceptibility, we sequenced exons encoding TRAF-binding domains (Figure 1) [9] and studied their association with PsA as well as the functional consequences of the respective amino acid changes on interaction with TRAF6 and the interleukin-17 receptor α (IL17-RA).

* Correspondence: Ulrike.Hueffmeier@uk-erlangen.de
[2]Institute of Human Genetics, University of Erlangen-Nuremberg, Schwabachanlage 10, 91054 Erlangen, Germany
Full list of author information is available at the end of the article

Materials and methods

Study population

We analyzed a case-control study comprising 871 PsA patients. A subset of 764 patients was described previously

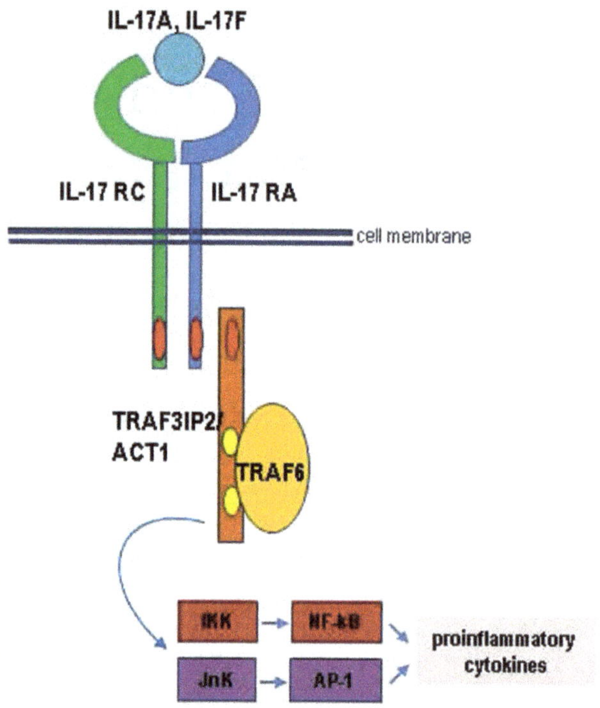

Figure 1 Interleukin (IL)-17A/IL17F binds to the heterodimeric IL-17R and leads to its signaling. Signaling includes recruitment of nuclear factor-κB activator 1 (ACT1) via SEFIR domains (red ovals). Activation of ACT 1 encoded by *TRAF3IP2* allows binding to TRAF6 via TNF receptor-associated factor (TRAF)-binding domains (yellow ovals); this activates NF-κB as well as proinflammatory cytokines.

[2]. All patients fulfilled the recently defined CASPAR (for ClASsification of Psoriatic ARthritis) criteria [10] and were recruited between 2002 and 2011 exclusively by board-certified rheumatologists at five different rheumatology departments in Germany. In comparison to the previously described cohort, clinical characteristics were very similar: the mean (SD) age of onset for PsV was 28.3 ± 13.3 years; 60.8% of the patients were men. For 78% of the patients, the diagnosis of PsA was made ≥ 3 years before recruitment, and 96% of patients had a skin involvement ≥ 3 years before study inclusion. Peripheral joint involvement was detectable in the majority of cases (827 or 94.8%); this was oligoarticular in 183 patients and polyarticular in 644 (21.0% and 73.8% of the entire cohort, respectively). Diagnosis of spinal involvement was based on symptoms of inflammatory back pain, characteristic clinical signs of restricted vertebral movement and/or sacroiliac pain on physical examination, and a subsequent confirmation by radiographic signs of sacroiliitis or spondylitis or both. Spinal involvement was observed in 204 patients, accounting for 23.4% of the PsA cohort. In these patients, sacroiliitis or spondylitis or both were partly associated with concomitant peripheral joint disease.

The 931 German control individuals were healthy blood donors and the same as previously reported [2].

Ethical approvals for all German studies were obtained from the Ethics Committees of the medical faculties of the Universities of Erlangen, Münster, and Frankfurt/Main. All probands gave written informed consent. The investigations were conducted according to the Declaration of Helsinki principles.

Sequencing

All PsA patients were sequenced for exons 2-4 coding for TRAF-binding domains. Mainly intron-based primers for four amplicons were designed with Primer 3 (v.0.4.0) [11]. In general, Sanger sequencing was performed, as described before [12], with the following changes: thermocyclers were Thermo Multiblock (ThermoFisher Scientific, Ulm, Germany); the robotic system for PCR (polymerase chain reaction) clean-up as well as for sequencing reactions was Beckman-Coulter Biomek Nxp (kit for PCR clean-up: Agencourt AMPure; kit for sequencing reactions: CleanSEQ; Beckman-Coulter, Krefeld, Germany). Sequences were analyzed with the Software Sequencher versus 4.10.1 (Gene Codes, Ann Arbor, MI, USA). Genotyping rates of the four amplicons were between 99.8% and 100%. Variants were named according to the usual naming conventions with regard to *TRAF3IP2* reference sequence NM_147686 (coding for 565 amino acids).

Analysis of variants in controls

Control individuals were genotyped for all missense variants as well as the 3bp-insertion with self-designed TaqMan assays (Life Technologies, Carlsbad, CA, USA), as previously described [2]. Missing genotypes or carriers of low-frequency variants were resequenced, resulting in a genotyping rate of 100% for seven variants and 99.8% for the further one.

Statistics

Fisher Exact test, as implemented in R (version 2.13.1) [13], was used for comparison of frequency distributions between cases and controls.

Protein-binding analyses in mammalian two-hybrid system

A mammalian two-hybrid assay (Stratagene) was applied to analyze the interaction of wild-type and mutant protein ACT1 of *TRAF3IP2* with TRAF6 and IL-17RA, as described before [2]. As a change to previous analyses, full-length *TRAF3IP2* mRNA (coding for amino acid residues 1 through 565) was amplified from reverse-transcribed cDNA of the chondrocyte cell line T/C28a4 by using 5'-TGAATTCATGAACCGAAGCATTCCTGTG-3' and 5'-TGCGGCCGCTCACAAGGGAACCACCTGAAG-3'. The cytoplasmic tail of IL-17RA (amino acid residues 343-667, NM_014339) was amplified from reverse-transcribed cDNA of the human macrophage cell line THP-1 by using 5'-AGGATCCATGACCTGGAGGCTAGCTGGGCCTGGAA-3' and 5'-AGCGGCCGCTCAGGTGTGGAGGGGCTGCGGCGCTGGCTGA-3', and cloned into the *Bam*HI/*Not*I site of the pCMV-BD bait vector. HEK 293 cells (1×10^4) were grown in 96-well white tissue-culture plates (Greiner) for 24 hours, and the bait and prey vectors (25 ng each) were co-transfected with a firefly luciferase reporter (250 ng) by using jetPEI reagents according to the supplier's instructions (PeqLab). Transfection efficiency was controlled by co-transfecting a renilla luciferase plasmid (5 ng, pRL-TK vector; Promega). At 48 hours after transfection, luciferase activity of quadruplicate wells was measured by using the Dual Glo Assay System (Promega) on a Mithras LB940 plate reader (Berthold Technologies). Assays were performed ≥ 5 times.

For functional testing of the two common as well as the newly identified rare coding variants of *TRAF3IP2* [2], constructs were generated by site-directed mutagenesis by using the QuickChange site-directed mutagenesis kit (Stratagene). Quality control of all vectors was performed with DNA sequencing. The firefly luciferase values were normalized to the Renilla values. Statistical significance was determined by using an unpaired Student *t* test.

Results

Sanger sequencing in 871 PsA patients revealed eight low-frequency variants: one 3-bp insertion and seven missense variants, one of them being the known SNP rs61756667 (minor allele frequency of 0.10% in the database), as indicated in Table 1. Allele frequencies ranged between 0.06% and 1.03% in PsA cases and 0 to 0.54% in control individuals, respectively. Distributions of allele frequency for single low-frequency variants as well as the sum of the eight variants (P = 0.493) did not show significant differences between cases and controls.

Because our case-control study of ~900 individuals was of limited power to exclude association to very-low-frequency variants (for example, found on one allele of one patient), we investigated the impact of amino acid changes encoded by the new *TRAF3IP2*-variants on functional properties of the ACT1 protein also by mammalian two-hybrid technology. None of the amino acid mutations in the full-length constructs of the new *TRAF3IP2* coding variants exhibited any influence on TRAF6 binding (Figure 2). Also, TRAF6 interaction of the common coding variant rs13190932 (p.Arg74Trp) was comparable to wild-type, in agreement with earlier results obtained in assays using shortened *TRAF3IP2* constructs [2]. In contrast, the analysis of a full-length *TRAF3IP2* construct, containing the earlier described disease-causing variant rs33980500 (p.Asp10Asn), revealed a nearly completely disrupted interaction with TRAF6 (~90%), thereby confirming previous analyses. Moreover, the ability to interact with the cytoplasmic IL-17RA domain did not differ between ACT1 proteins encoded by either wild-type *TRAF3IP2* or by any of its low-frequency variants. In this respect, p.Asp10Asn did not cause different results compared with other *TRAF3IP2* variants.

Table 1 Association analysis of new variants

Coding position	Protein position	Position hg19	Allele	871 PsA patients		931 control individuals		*P* (Fisher Exact)
				n	%	*n*	%	
c.105_106 InsACC	p.Pro35dup	111913185	Ins	2	0.11	3	0.16	1
			WT	1,740	99.89	1,859	99.84	
c.281G > A (rs61756667)	p.Ser94Asn	111913009	A	1	0.06	4	0.21	0.376
			G	1,737	99.94	1,858	99.79	
c.350C > T	p.Ala117Val	111912940	T	1	0.06	0	0	0.483
			C	1,737	99.94	1,858	100.00	
c.649C > A	p.Pro217Thr	111912641	A	18	1.03	10	0.54	0.127
			C	1,724	98.97	1,852	99.46	
c.691C > T	p.Leu231Phe	111912599	T	2	0.11	1	0.05	0.613
			C	1,740	99.89	1,861	99.95	
c.746A > G	p.Gln249Arg	111912544	G	1	0.06	0	0	0.483
			A	1,741	99.94	1,862	100.00	
c.1058G > C	p.Gly353Ala	111896989	C	1	0.06	0	0	0.483
			G	1,741	99.94	1,862	100.00	
c.1184A > G	p.Asn395Ser	111896863	G	3	0.17	7	0.38	0.346
			A	1,739	99.83	1,855	99.62	

WT, wild type. Names, position on chromosome 6, and count/frequency of wild-type alleles/low-frequency alleles of new variants in PsA patients and control individuals are shown, as well as the *P* value of Fisher Exact test.

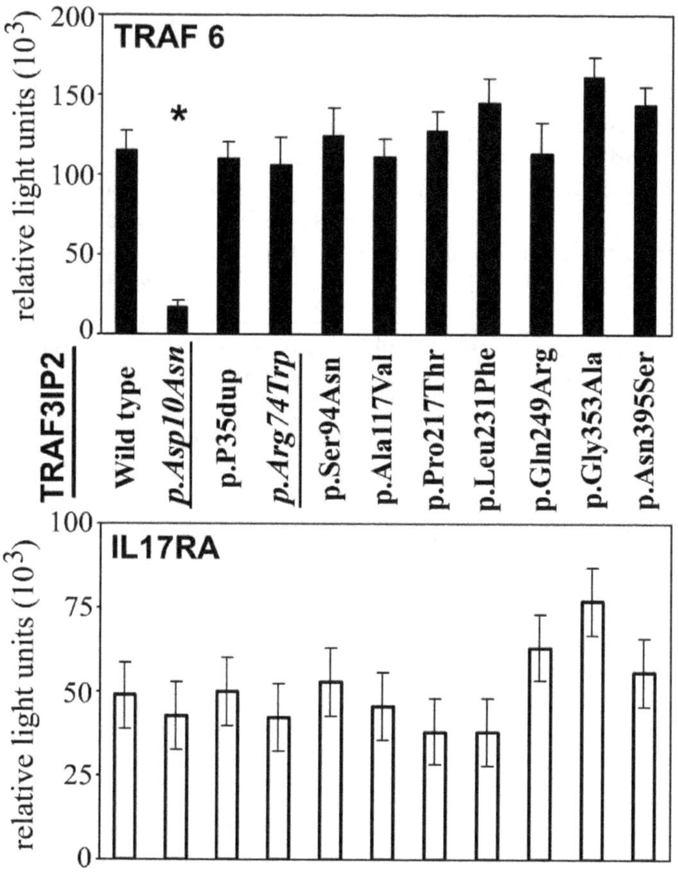

Figure 2 Binding of ACT1 and its mutant variants to TNF receptor-associated factor (TRAF)6 and interleukin (IL)-17RA. Interaction of wild-type *TRAF3IP2*/ACT1 and its mutant variants with either TRAF6, upper panel, or IL-17RA, lower panel, was determined by mammalian two-hybrid system. The *TRAF3IP2* mutant p.Asp10Asn showed a significantly reduced binding to TRAF6. Common coding variants indicated by underlined and italicized letters. *$P < 0.005$, when compared with wild-type *TRAF3IP2*.

Discussion

Our in-depth sequencing of TRAF-binding domains in *TRAF3IP2* revealed a number of new low-frequency variants in PsA patients occurring at a similar frequency in control individuals. This finding is not unexpected, because, for example, newly identified low-frequency variants in most of the susceptibility genes identified in GWAS and sequenced for Crohn disease [8] or type I diabetes [14] were not associated with disease. Further evidence that our newly identified coding variants do not cause disease was derived from functional analyses: none of the variants leading to amino acid changes in the respective ACT1 proteins affected TRAF6 interaction. Reassuringly, we could confirm previous results of a dramatically reduced TRAF6 binding for the ACT1 variant harboring the disease-causing variant p.Asp10Asn under assay conditions analyzing full-length *TRAF3IP2*-transcripts (Figure 2). Binding of ACT1 to the cytoplasmic domain of IL-17RA is mediated via a C-terminal SEFIR domain that remained conserved in wild-type configuration in all investigated *TRAF3IP2* constructs (Figures 1 and 2). Accordingly, a rather limited *a priori* likelihood existed to detect major differences in IL-17RA-binding properties of the investigated mutant *TRAF3IP2* constructs, although an indirect modulatory effect of conformational changes induced by the distantly located mutations in the TRAF-binding domains could not be entirely excluded. However, our studies did not reveal an altered IL-17RA interaction for any of the nine investigated coding variants.

Conclusions

Our data indicate that the common variant rs33980500 (p.Asp10Aspn) is the only risk allele for PsA with functional impact on TRAF6 binding, at least in the German population.

Abbreviations

ACT1: nuclear factor-κB activator 1; CASPAR: ClASsification of Psoriatic Arthritis; GWAS: genome-wide association studies; IL-17RA: interleukin-17 receptor A; NF-κB: nuclear factor-κB; PCR: polymerase chain reaction; PsA:

psoriatic arthritis; PsV: psoriasis vulgaris; SNP: single-nucleotide polymorphism; TRAF: TNF receptor-associated factor; TRAF3: TNF receptor-associated factor 3; TRAF6: TNF receptor-associated factor 6; TRAF3IP2: TRAF3-interacting protein 2.

Acknowledgements
We are grateful to all patients and control probands for participation in this study. We thank Kristin Krause and Petra Badorf for excellent technical assistance.
The work was supported in part by a grant from the Interdisciplinary Centre for Clinical Research (J1; to UH) of the University of Erlangen-Nuremberg, Germany, as well as the German Federal Ministry of Education and Research [Bundesministerium für Bildung und Forschung (BMBF); project ANCYLOSS; to AR and ArthroMark (project 4, 01 EC 1009C); to HB].

Author details
[1]Divisions of Rheumatology, Department of Internal Medicine II, Johann Wolfgang Goethe University, Theodor-Stern-Kai 7, 60590 Frankfurt am Main, Germany. [2]Institute of Human Genetics, University of Erlangen-Nuremberg, Schwabachanlage 10, 91054 Erlangen, Germany.

Authors' contributions
HB, AR, and UH designed the study and worked out its concept. UH planned and performed the genotyping, and SU and UH analyzed genetic data. BB and HB performed functional studies. BB, HB, MA, FB, and UH recruited subjects and collected phenotypic data. UH, BB, and HB wrote a first draft of the manuscript; all authors reviewed and approved the manuscript.

Competing interests
The authors declare that they have no competing interests.

References

1. Ellinghaus E, Ellinghaus D, Stuart PE, Nair RP, Debrus S, Raelson JV, Belouchi M, Fournier H, Reinhard C, Ding J, Li Y, Tejasvi T, Gudjonsson J, Stoll SW, Voorhees JJ, Lambert S, Weidinger S, Eberlein B, Kunz M, Rahman P, Gladman DD, Gieger C, Wichmann HE, Karlsen TH, Mayr G, Albrecht M, Kabelitz D, Mrowietz U, Abecasis GR, Elder JT, *et al*: **Genome-wide association study identifies a psoriasis susceptibility locus at TRAF3IP2.** *Nat Genet* 2010, **42**:991-995.
2. Huffmeier U, Uebe S, Ekici AB, Bowes J, Giardina E, Korendowych E, Juneblad K, Apel M, McManus R, Ho P, Bruce IN, Ryan AW, Behrens F, Lascorz J, Bohm B, Traupe H, Lohmann J, Gieger C, Wichmann HE, Herold C, Steffens M, Klareskog L, Wienker TF, Fitzgerald O, Alenius GM, McHugh NJ, Novelli G, Burkhardt H, Barton A, Reis A: **Common variants at TRAF3IP2 are associated with susceptibility to psoriatic arthritis and psoriasis.** *Nat Genet* 2010, **42**:996-999.
3. Nair RP, Duffin KC, Helms C, Ding J, Stuart PE, Goldgar D, Gudjonsson JE, Li Y, Tejasvi T, Feng BJ, Ruether A, Schreiber S, Weichenthal M, Gladman D, Rahman P, Schrodi SJ, Prahalad S, Guthery SL, Fischer J, Liao W, Kwok PY, Menter A, Lathrop GM, Wise CA, Begovich AB, Voorhees JJ, Elder JT, Krueger GG, Bowcock AM, Abecasis GR: **Genome-wide scan reveals association of psoriasis with IL-23 and NF-kappaB pathways.** *Nat Genet* 2009, **41**:199-204.
4. Zhang XJ, Huang W, Yang S, Sun LD, Zhang FY, Zhu QX, Zhang FR, Zhang C, Du WH, Pu XM, Li H, Xiao FL, Wang ZX, Cui Y, Hao F, Zheng J, Yang XQ, Cheng H, He CD, Liu XM, Xu LM, Zheng HF, Zhang SM, Zhang JZ, Wang HY, Cheng YL, Ji BH, Fang QY, Li YZ, Zhou FS, *et al*: **Psoriasis genome-wide association study identifies susceptibility variants within LCE gene cluster at 1q21.** *Nat Genet* 2009, **41**:205-210.
5. Strange A, Capon F, Spencer CC, Knight J, Weale ME, Allen MH, Barton A, Band G, Bellenguez C, Bergboer JG, Blackwell JM, Bramon E, Bumpstead SJ, Casas JP, Cork MJ, Corvin A, Deloukas P, Dilthey A, Duncanson A, Edkins S, Estivill X, Fitzgerald O, Freeman C, Giardina E, Gray E, Hofer A, Huffmeier U, Hunt SE, Irvine AD, Jankowski J, *et al*: **A genome-wide association study identifies new psoriasis susceptibility loci and an interaction between HLA-C and ERAP1.** *Nat Genet* 2010, **42**:985-990.
6. Stuart PE, Nair RP, Ellinghaus E, Ding J, Tejasvi T, Gudjonsson JE, Li Y, Weidinger S, Eberlein B, Gieger C, Wichmann HE, Kunz M, Ike R, Krueger GG, Bowcock AM, Mrowietz U, Lim HW, Voorhees JJ, Abecasis GR, Weichenthal M, Franke A, Rahman P, Gladman DD, Elder JT: **Genome-wide association analysis identifies three psoriasis susceptibility loci.** *Nat Genet* 2010, **42**:1000-1004.
7. Sun LD, Cheng H, Wang ZX, Zhang AP, Wang PG, Xu JH, Zhu QX, Zhou HS, Ellinghaus E, Zhang FR, Pu XM, Yang XQ, Zhang JZ, Xu AE, Wu RN, Xu LM, Peng L, Helms CA, Ren YQ, Zhang C, Zhang SM, Nair RP, Wang HY, Lin GS, Stuart PE, Fan X, Chen G, Tejasvi T, Li P, Zhu J, *et al*: **Association analyses identify six new psoriasis susceptibility loci in the Chinese population.** *Nat Genet* 2010, **42**:1005-1009.
8. Momozawa Y, Mni M, Nakamura K, Coppieters W, Almer S, Amininejad L, Cleynen I, Colombel JF, de Rijk P, Dewit O, Finkel Y, Gassull MA, Goossens D, Laukens D, Lemann M, Libioulle C, O'Morain C, Reenaers C, Rutgeerts P, Tysk C, Zelenika D, Lathrop M, Del-Favero J, Hugot JP, de Vos M, Franchimont D, Vermeire S, Louis E, Georges M: **Resequencing of positional candidates identifies low frequency IL23R coding variants protecting against inflammatory bowel disease.** *Nat Genet* 2011, **43**:43-47.
9. Hunter CA: **Act1-ivating IL-17 inflammation.** *Nature Immunol* 2007, **8**:232-234.
10. Taylor W, Gladman D, Helliwell P, Marchesoni A, Mease P, Mielants H: **Classification criteria for psoriatic arthritis: development of new criteria from a large international study.** *Arthritis Rheum* 2006, **54**:2665-2673.
11. **Primer 3 vs. 0.4.0, Pick primers from a DNA sequence.** [http://frodo.wi.mit.edu/].
12. Huffmeier U, Lascorz J, Traupe H, Bohm B, Schurmeier-Horst F, Stander M, Kelsch R, Baumann C, Kuster W, Burkhardt H, Reis A: **Systematic linkage disequilibrium analysis of SLC12A8 at PSORS5 confirms a role in susceptibility to psoriasis vulgaris.** *J Invest Dermatol* 2005, **125**:906-912.
13. **R = language and environment for statistical computing and graphics.** [http://www.r-project.org/].
14. Nejentsev S, Walker N, Riches D, Egholm M, Todd JA: **Rare variants of IFIH1, a gene implicated in antiviral responses, protect against type 1 diabetes.** *Science* 2009, **324**:387-389.

2

Hepatic steatosis, carotid plaques and achieving MDA in psoriatic arthritis patients starting TNF-α blockers treatment

Matteo Nicola Dario Di Minno[1*], Rosario Peluso[2], Salvatore Iervolino[3], Roberta Lupoli[1], Anna Russolillo[1], Giovanni Tarantino[1] and Raffaele Scarpa[2]

Abstract

Introduction: We prospectively evaluated whether hepatic steatosis (HS) and the presence of carotid plaques (CPs) impacts on achieving minimal disease activity (MDA) in psoriatic arthritis (PsA) patients starting tumor necrosis factor (TNF)-α blockers treatment.

Methods: Before starting treatment with TNF-α blockers, consecutive PsA subjects with an active disease were evaluated for the presence of the metabolic syndrome (MetS), HS and CPs. The incidence of MDA was evaluated 12 and 24 months later.

Results: Among 270 PsA subjects, 91 (33.7%) exhibited the MetS, 58 (21.5%) CPs and 76 (28.1%) HS. At the 12-month follow-up, 98 (36.3%) individuals achieved MDA. Compared with those who did, a higher prevalence of the MetS, HS and CPs was found in subjects who did not achieve the MDA (P always < 0.001). After adjusting for the MetS and for all the other demographic/clinical characteristics analyzed, the presence of HS and CPs at baseline independently predicted the risk of not achieving MDA (Hazard Ratio: 1.91, 95% confidence interval (CI): 1.04 to 3.38, $P = 0.035$ and Hazard Ratio: 3.21, 95%CI: 1.64 to 6.29, $P = 0.001$, respectively). Separate Kaplan-Meier survival models confirmed this (Log-Rank: 12.894, $P < 0.001$ and Log-Rank: 12.849, $P < 0.001$, respectively). Compared with those without, progressively increasing Hazard Ratios of not achieving MDA were found in those with HS, CPs or HS + CPs at baseline. Moreover, the presence of HS and/or CPs predicted the risk of relapse during the additional 12-month follow-up (Hazard Ratio: 2.85, 95%CI: 1.27 to 6.37, $P = 0.011$ and Hazard Ratio: 3.17, 95%CI: 1.57 to 6.41, $P = 0.001$ respectively).

Conclusions: HS and/or CPs at baseline are negative predictors of achieving and maintaining MDA.

Introduction

Psoriatic arthritis (PsA) is a chronic arthropathy associated with psoriasis, marked by an axial and/or peripheral joint involvement [1]. In addition to joint manifestations, subjects with PsA exhibit an abnormally high cardiovascular (CV) risk and, in turn, risk of the metabolic syndrome (MetS), one of its major vascular risk factors (VRFs) [2,3]. Accordingly, as compared with healthy controls, PsA patients exhibit a higher than normal platelet reactivity [4] and a higher than normal prevalence of hepatic steatosis (HS) [5] and of carotid plaques (CPs) [6]. All these conditions are well known markers of atherosclerosis and of CV risk [7,8].

Chronic inflammation may interact with VRFs, leading to a further increase of the CV risk in PsA patients [9,10]. In addition to being involved in the inflammatory process, most cytokines (TNF-α, IL-1, IL-6) play a role in the genesis and in the progression of atherosclerosis [11]. Both HS and CPs are strongly influenced by the severity of chronic inflammation [12-15] and are directly correlated with the MetS and its features.

Compared with those with minimal disease activity (MDA), PsA subjects with an active disease show an exaggerated worsening of HS degree [16] and an increased

* Correspondence: dario.diminno@hotmail.it
[1]Department of Clinical and Experimental Medicine, Reference Centre for Coagulation Disorders, Federico II University, Via Sergio Pansini 5, Naples, 80129 Italy
Full list of author information is available at the end of the article

prevalence of CPs [17]. Thus, in addition to being associated with a cardio-metabolic impairment, CPs and/or HS may be markers of the severity of the inflammatory process in PsA subjects [12-15].

In view of this, we prospectively evaluated whether, regardless of the presence of MetS, the presence of HS and/or CPs at baseline impacts *per se* on the achieving of MDA in subjects with PsA who start a treatment with TNF-α blockers.

Materials and methods

During a three-year period (January 2007 to January 2010), all patients with a diagnosis of PsA (according to the Classification Criteria for Psoriatic Arthritis (CASPAR) criteria) [1] who were non-responders to traditional disease modifying anti-rheumatic drugs (DMARDs) and who were referred to the Regional Reference Center for the treatment of spondyloarthropathies of the Federico II University of Naples to start treatment with TNF-α blockers, were evaluated for enrollment in this study. For all enrolled subjects, exclusion criteria were: lack of informed consent signature, age < 18 years, previous treatment with TNF-α blockers, adequate clinical response to traditional DMARDs treatment, malignancy, hematologic diseases, autoimmune diseases other than PsA, unstable medical conditions, ongoing pregnancy, history of venous and/or arterial thrombosis and of alcohol abuse. After approval of the study by the local Ethics Committee and after informed consent signature, data about age, gender, height, weight, disease duration, disease activity, previous and/or current treatments and vascular risk factors were collected from all patients as previously described [13]. All PsA subjects had clinically active disease at the time of enrollment and were classified into different clinical subsets (Moll and Wright criteria) [18]. Briefly, PsA patients were classified as having axial disease if they had at least grade 2 unilateral sacroiliitis in the presence of a combination of inflammatory back pain plus back stiffness. The PsA patients were classified as pure axial if they had no peripheral joint involvement, mixed if they had both peripheral joint arthritis and axial disease, or as having only peripheral joint involvement. The rare mutilans form was diagnosed in the presence of distal interphalangeal joint bone resorption (osteolysis), 'pencil-in-cup' radiographic findings or telescoping motion of the digit. According to the National Cholesterol Education Program (NCEP) criteria [19], abdominal obesity was defined as a waist circumference ≥102 cm for men and ≥88 cm for women; hypertriglyceridemia, as triglyceride levels ≥150 mg/dL; hypercholesterolemia with low-HDL cholesterol as a total cholesterol ≥200 mg/dL with HDL-cholesterol < 40 mg/dL for men and < 50 mg/dL for women; hypertension as a blood pressure ≥130 and/or 85 mmHg; and impaired fasting glucose (IFG) as a fasting glucose ≥100 mg/dL. Patients were defined as having the MetS if three or more of these VRFs were present. In addition, the presence of CPs and the presence/severity of HS were evaluated in each PsA subject according to previously validated scanning protocols [13,16]. All the carotid artery ultrasound examinations were performed by the same operator. After a five minute rest in the supine position, the subjects underwent a bilateral carotid ultrasonography (US) with a 7.5 to 12 MHz linear-array transducer and a duplex scanner (ESAOTE MyLab 25Gold, Genoa, Italy). The ultrasound evaluation was performed longitudinally and transversally by using gray-scale and color-Doppler US imaging. The scan protocol requires the full-length visualization of the near and far wall of the right and left common carotid artery (CCA) and of the bulb in three different projections (anterior, lateral and posterior). The intima-media thickness (IMT) was measured in each of the three projections in the CCA and bulb and the presence of CPs was defined for IMT ≥1.3 mm. The reproducibility of the vascular measurement was evaluated in 20 subjects within 1 week from the first ultrasonographic examination. The overall Pearson's r value for the IMT measurements was 0.89 ($P < 0.001$). The presence of HS was assessed with a US diagnostic system (Logiq P5, General Electric, Milan, Italy) with a 3.5-MHz convex probe. All the US determinations were made by the same trained operator. The intra-operator variability, as evaluated in 20 subjects within 1 week from the first ultrasonographic examination, showed an overall r value of 0.92 ($P < 0.001$). As previously validated [16], the presence/severity of HS was defined by comparing the echogenicity of the liver and of the kidney cortex: Grade 0 (absent): iso-echogenicity; Grade 1 (mild): diffuse and homogeneous hyper-echogenicity; Grade 2 (moderate): attenuation of the ultrasonic beam rear; Grade 3 (severe): lack of diaphragm profile visualization. The presence of CPs and of a moderate/severe ($2^{nd}/3^{rd}$ degree) HS were recorded in all subjects at baseline (T0). At T0 as well as every three months after having started the treatment with TNF-α blockers, all PsA subjects underwent a complete clinical rheumatologic and laboratory evaluation that included: tender joint count (TJC, n = 78), swollen joint count (SJC, n = 76), tender entheseal count (according to the Maastricht Ankylosing Spondylitis Enthesitis Score), psoriasis area severity index (PASI), health assessment questionnaire (HAQ), visual analog scale for pain (VAS), patient global disease activity VAS score, erythrocyte sedimentation rate (ESR) and C-reactive protein (CRP). The data obtained at 12 months were recorded as (T1). During the first 12 months of follow-up (from T0 to T1), PsA subjects were classified as having achieved MDA when fulfilling 5 or more of the following 7 outcome measures at T1: TJC ≤1; SJC ≤1; PASI ≤1 or body surface area ≤3; VAS for pain ≤15; patient global disease activity VAS score of ≤20; HAQ ≤0.5 and tender entheseal points ≤1 [20]. Otherwise, they were considered as not having achieved MDA (non-MDA). To test the achieving of sustained-MDA (s-MDA), those who had achieved MDA, were re-evaluated every 3 months thereafter during the additional 12-months (T2). s-MDA was defined as fulfilling the same criteria employed for MDA in all the visits carried out between T1 and T2.

The present study protocol has been approved by the Federico II University Local Ethic Committee.

Statistical analysis

Statistical analysis was performed with the SPSS 16 system (SPSS Inc., Chicago, IL, USA). Continuous data were expressed as means ± SD; categorical variables were expressed as percent. The t-test was performed to compare continuous variables; the chi-square test was employed to analyze categorical data. When the minimum expected value was < 5, the Fisher's exact test was used.

A Kaplan-Meier survival model (with the Log-Rank test) was adopted to evaluate the cumulative achieving MDA according to the presence of HS or CPs. To adjust for all the other variables (with emphasis on the presence of the MetS) and to evaluate the achieving of MDA (or of s-MDA), separate COX regression analyses (stepwise method) were adopted, with the achieving MDA (or s-MDA) as the dependent variable and the MetS, CPs, HS, number of CV risk markers, obesity, hypertension, hypercholesterolemia, hypertriglyceridemia, impaired fasting glucose, smoking habit, TJC, SJC, tender entheseal count, PASI, HAQ, VAS for pain, patient global VAS, ESR, CRP, concomitant treatment with methotrexate, gender, age and disease duration as independent variables. Multi-collinearity effect in multivariable regression models was excluded by a stepwise approach with each variable included for $P < 0.05$ and excluded for $P > 0.1$. A tolerance test was employed to exclude models in which the sum of the values exceeded the sum of the variances for all variables. All the results are presented as two-tailed values with statistical significance if P values < 0.05.

As to the sample size calculation, to plan a study with a minimal pre-defined Hazard Ratio (HR) ≥1.4, an accrual interval of 3 years, and a follow-up period of 24 months, at least 222 subjects are needed to achieve a > 80% power with an 5% α error. With an expected drop-out of 25% during the follow-up, 280 subjects were enrolled in the study.

Results

After excluding those already under treatment with TNF-α blockers (n = 224) and those with adequate clinical response to traditional DMARDs treatment (n = 545), 280 PsA subjects were enrolled in this study. Of these, 10 were missed during the follow-up (because of missing baseline data, missing follow-up visits, premature withdrawal of treatment with TNF-α blockers). Thus, 270 PsA subjects, completing their follow-up, were included in the analysis. Their clinical and demographic characteristics are reported in Table 1.

As to the use of TNF-α blockers, adalimumab (40 mg/every 2 weeks) was employed in 80 subjects (29.6%); etanercept (50 mg/week) in 111 (41.1%) and infliximab (5 mg/kg every 8 weeks) in 79 subjects (29.3%). A MetS was diagnosed in 84 (31.1%) subjects. The presence of CPs and of HS was found in 36 (13.3%) and 71 (26.3%) subjects, respectively. On the other hand, 163 (60.4%) PsA subjects did not have CPs or HS; 80 (29.6%) had either one of the two, and 27 (10%) had both. A direct correlation was found between CRP and ESR with the IMT values (r = 0.531, $P < 0.001$ and r = 0.476, $P < 0.001$). Whereas no difference in the prevalence of HS was found

Table 1 Clinical and demographic characteristics of the study population

Variable	PsA subjects (number = 270)
Male gender	124 (45.9%)
Age (years)	51.73 ± 11.49
Disease subset	
Axial + peripheral	95 (35.2%)
Peripheral	95 (35.2%)
Axial	64 (23.7%)
Mutilans	16 (5.9%)
MetS	91 (33.7%)
HS	76 (28.1%)
CPs	58 (21.5%)
Concomitant MTX	111 (41.1%)
Disease duration (years)	4.87 ± 2.94
ESR (mm/h)	18.05 ± 13.19
CRP (mg/L)	2.64 ± 2.93
SJC	3.77 ± 4.08
TJC	11.93 ± 5.48
PASI	1.48 ± 0.71
HAQ	2.47 ± 1.45
VAS	76.7 ± 20.12
Patient global VAS	74.25 ± 22.38
Tender entheseal count	10.97 ± 5.40
Hypercholesterolemia	139 (51.5%)
Hypertriglyceridemia	92 (34.1%)
Impaired fasting glucose	20 (7.4%)
Hypertension	57 (21.1%)
Smoking habit	65 (24.1%)
Obesity	111 (41.1%)

CPs, presence of carotid plaques (carotid intima-media thickness > 1.3 mm); CRP, C-reactive protein; ESR, erythrocyte sedimentation rate; HAQ, Health Assessment Questionnaire; HS, hepatic steatosis; MetS, metabolic syndrome; MTX: Methotrexate; PASI, Psoriasis Area Severity Index; SJC, swollen joint count; TJC, tender joint count; VAS, Visual Analogue Scale for pain.

based on stratification according to different clinical subsets (Pearson's χ^2 for inter-groups independence P = 0.516), the presence of CPs was found in 10.5% of subjects with peripheral subset; 14.1% of those with axial subset, 26.3% in the axial + peripheral subset and in 87.5% of those with the mutilans subset (Pearson's χ^2 for inter-groups independence $P < 0.001$).

Twelve-month follow-up (T0-T1)

During the follow-up, no changes in treatment schedules and/or in VRFs prevalence were reported in the study population. As a whole, 98/270 (36.3%) PsA individuals, achieving 5 or more of the minimal disease activity criteria [20], were classified in MDA.

MDA was achieved in 33 (41.8%) subjects receiving infliximab, in 41 (36.9%) of those receiving etanercept and in 24 (30%) of those receiving adalimumab (Pearson's χ^2 for inter-groups independence P = 0.299). As reported in Table 2 the prevalence of different clinical subsets did not differ among those who achieved MDA and those who did not. Overall, the rate of achieving MDA did not differ according to PsA clinical subsets (Pearson's χ^2 for inter-groups independence P = 0.092).

Those who had achieved MDA were more often men (P = 0.001) and had a younger age (P = 0.042), a longer disease duration (P = 0.004), a higher ESR ($P < 0.001$) and CRP ($P < 0.001$), and a lower TJC ($P < 0.001$) and tender entheseal counts (P = 0.003) than those who did not (Table 2). Conversely, the MetS, CPs and HS (P always < 0.001) were more frequent in those who did not achieve MDA as compared with those who did. As to the features of the MetS, the prevalence of obesity and of hypercholesterolemia was higher in those who did not achieve MDA.

Separate Kaplan-Meier survival models (Figure 1) showed a significant difference in those achieving MDA whether or not HS (Log-Rank: 12.894, $P < 0.001$) and CPs (Log-Rank: 12.849, $P < 0.001$) were present. After adjusting for the presence of the MetS as well as for all the other demographic characteristics and for rheumatologic and cardiovascular variables, HS and CPs independently predicted the risk of not achieving MDA (HR: 1.91, 95%CI: 1.04 to 3.38, P = 0.035 and HR: 3.21, 95%CI: 1.64 to 6.29, P = 0.001, respectively).

MDA was achieved by 76 (46.6%) subjects with neither HS nor CPs, by 20 (25.0%) of those with HS or CPs and by 2 (7.4%) of those with both HS and CPs (Pearson's χ^2 for inter-groups independence $P < 0.001$). As compared with those with neither HS nor CPs, a progressively increasing HR of not achieving MDA was found in those with HS or CPs and in those with both HS and CPs (Figure 2).

In addition to HS and CPs, male gender (HR: 2.25, 95% CI: 1.47 to 3.43, $P < 0.001$), a low TJC (HR: 1.15, 95%CI: 1.08 to 1.23, $P < 0.001$), and a high CRP (HR: 1.18, 95%CI: 1.07 to 1.30, $P < 0.001$) independently predicted achieving MDA in this regression model.

Table 2 Clinical and demographic characteristics of the population at baseline.

Variable	Non-MDA patients Number = 172	MDA patients Number = 98	*P*
Age (years)	52.66 ± 10.60	50.08 ± 8.81	0.042
Male gender	65 (37.8%)	59 (60.2%)	0.001
Clinical subset			
Axial + Peripheral	63 (36.6%)	32(32.7%)	0.596
Peripheral	59 (34.3%)	36 (36.7%)	0.693
Axial	41 (23.8%)	23 (23.5%)	1.000
Mutilans	9(5.2%)	7(7.1%)	0.595
MetS	73(42.4%)	18(18.4%)	< 0.001
HS	62(36.0%)	14(14.3%)	< 0.001
CPs	48(27.9%)	10(10.2%)	0.001
Disease duration (months)	101.72 ± 74.01	126.93 ± 58.83	0.004
ESR (mm/h)	14.35 ± 11.06	20.16 ± 13.86	< 0.001
CRP (mg/L)	1.66 ± 1.83	3.20 ± 3.28	< 0.001
SJC	3.75 ± 4.30	3.80 ± 3.68	0.929
TJC	12.99 ± 5.62	10.06 ± 4.71	< 0.001
PASI	1.49 ± 0.68	1.45 ± 0.76	0.700
HAQ	2.39 ± 1.41	2.61 ± 1.52	0.230
VAS	77.50 ± 17.30	75.30 ± 24.33	0.390
Patient global VAS	74.24 ± 21.08	74.28 ± 24.62	0.988
Tender entheseal count	11.71 ± 5.45	9.66 ± 5.06	0.003
Hypercholesterolemia	103(59.9%)	36(36.7%)	< 0.001
Hypertriglyceridemia	60(34.9%)	32(32.7%)	0.790
Impaired fasting glucose	11(6.4%)	9(9.2%)	0.470
Hypertension	39(22.7%)	18(18.4%)	0.441
Smoking habit	36(20.9)	29(29.6)	0.138
Obesity	88(51.2%)	23(23.5%)	< 0.001

Stratification according to the achieving of MDA at 12-month follow-up. CPs, presence of carotid plaques (carotid intima-media thickness > 1.3 mm); CRP, C-reactive protein; ESR, erythrocyte sedimentation rate; HAQ, Health Assessment Questionnaire; HS, hepatic steatosis; MetS, metabolic syndrome; PASI, Psoriasis Area Severity Index; SJC, swollen joint count; TJC, tender joint count; VAS, Visual Analogue Scale for pain.

Twenty-four-month follow-up (T1-T2)

Among the 98 subjects who had achieved MDA during the first 12 months of follow-up, 17 (17.3%) relapsed and 81 (82.7%) maintained their MDA during the additional 12-months of follow-up (T2). In a regression model in which only the 98 subjects who had achieved

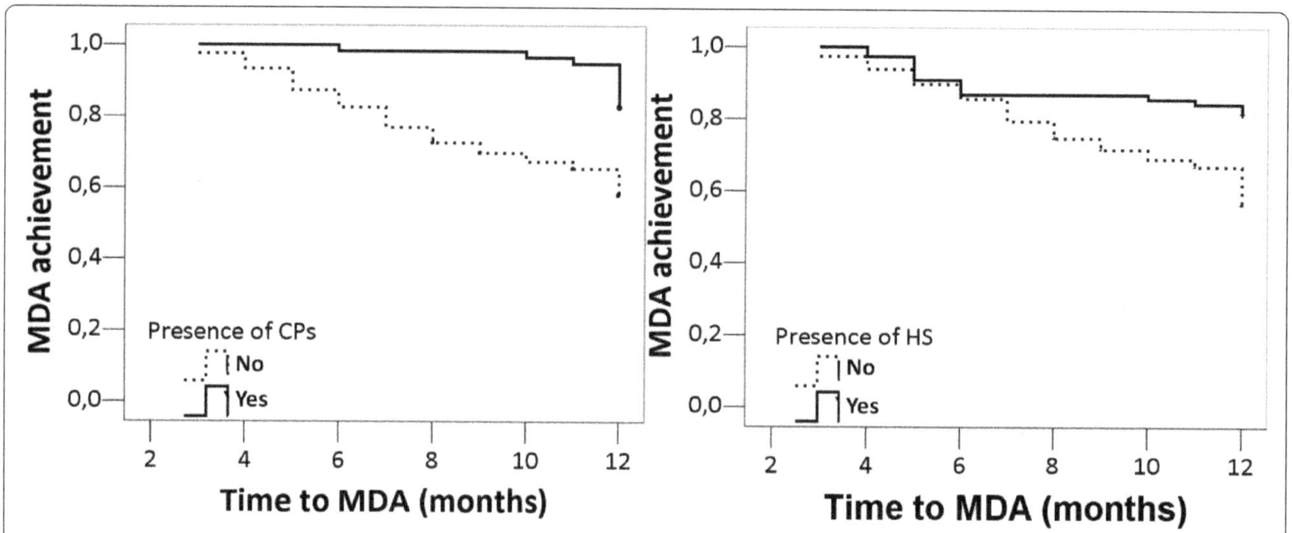

Figure 1 Kaplan-Meier survival model for achieving minimal disease activity (MDA) according to the presence of CPs and HS. CPs, presence of carotid plaques (carotid intima-media thickness > 1.3 mm); HS, hepatic steatosis; MDA, minimal disease activity.

MDA during the first 12-month follow-up were evaluated, the presence of HS or CPs was associated with a high risk of disease relapsing during the additional 12-months of follow-up (HR:2.85, 95%CI:1.27 to 6.37, P = 0.011 and HR: 3.17,95%CI:1.57 to 6.41, P = 0.001, respectively). Compared with subjects with neither HS nor CPs, the HR of PsA relapse was higher in those with HS or CPs (HR: 3.05, 95%CI:1.67 to 5.55, P < 0.001) and in those with both HS and CPs (HR: 8.93, 95%CI:1.21 to 66.66, P = 0.032).

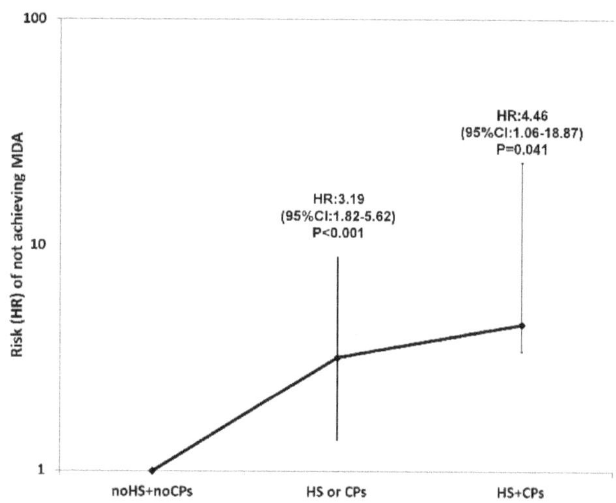

Figure 2 Risk of not achieving minimal disease activity (MDA) at 12-month follow-up according to the presence of HS and/or CPs. 95%CI, 95% confidence interval; CPs, presence of carotid plaques (carotid intima-media thickness > 1.3 mm); HR, hazard ratio; HS, hepatic steatosis; MDA, minimal disease activity.

Discussion

In the setting of PsA subjects, several clinical and laboratory predictors of six-month and three-month response to TNF-α blockers have been identified [21,22]. In PsA subjects starting treatment with TNF-α blockers, this prospective study shows that HS or CPs at baseline are associated *per se* with a high risk of not achieving MDA.

A variety of variables (CRP, complement C3, IL-6 and TNF-α) implicated in the regulation of the inflammatory process [23] and, in turn, in the pathophysiology of arthritides [24], are relevant in the etiology and the development of atherosclerosis [25-27]. Major markers of atherosclerosis (HS and CPs) that assess the global damage due to metabolic and inflammatory determinants [14] are affected in PsA subjects [9,13,16]. Accordingly, subjects who exhibit a high prevalence of HS and of CPs are likely to have experienced a more severe inflammatory state [12-15].

Among the 98/270 PsA patients who achieved MDA at 12 months, the prevalence of HS and of CPs was significantly lower than in those who did not. Accordingly, the presence of one of these atherosclerosis markers was associated with a high risk of not achieving MDA. Moreover, the presence of HS or of CPs was associated with a poor probability of sustained MDA at the 24-month follow-up. However, because of the relatively small number of patients included in this sub-analysis, the evaluation of the impact of CPs and/or HS on achieving sustained MDA, although statistically significant, should be considered only as a proof of concept.

The combined data lend credence to the possibility that the presence of CPs and/or HS is a negative predictor of achieving and maintaining MDA.

By evaluating such a large number of consecutive PsA patients (270 PsA subjects), the MetS was diagnosed in 33.7%, HS was found in 28.1% and CPs in 21.5% of subjects. These data are in line with previous literature data obtained on smaller size samples [3,5,6]. Further strengthening the link between cardiometabolic variables and inflammation, in a previous analysis on the present population, we have found that obesity (defined as a Body Mass Index > 30) is associated with a statistically significant increase in the risk of a poor treatment response in PsA subjects receiving TNF-α blockers [28]. At variance with the already published data, in this study the presence of obesity is defined according to the waist circumference measurement (which is a major NCEP criterion for the diagnosis of the MetS) [19]. However, as highlighted in Table 2 also in this case, the prevalence of obesity is higher in those not achieving MDA. Moreover, since obesity is a major feature of the MetS, and being known to impact on HS and CPs presence, a multivariate regression analysis was performed to adjust all the results of this study for the presence of MetS and of its features and to exclude collinearity in the prediction of achieving MDA. In this respect, we are confident to have excluded some important bias in this study.

In addition to CPs and HS, other demographic (male gender) and rheumatologic (CRP and TJC) variables predicted the achieving of MDA. The relevance of CPs and HS as MDA predictors has been adjusted (regression model) for the large majority of clinical and laboratory variables known to predict the achieving of MDA [22].

All the carotid and liver ultrasound evaluations were performed only at the study baseline evaluation. A prospective evaluation of changes in these parameters during the treatment with TNF-α blockers could have further clarified the interrelation between IMT, HS and PsA disease activity. Although some literature data [29] suggest that treatment with 'biologic agents' is associated with the lowering of the IMT as well as of the degree of liver steatosis, further *ad hoc* designed studies are needed to address this important issue.

The link between inflammation and atherosclerosis is strongly supported by the finding of a direct correlation between CRP and ESR with the IMT in the present setting. All these inflammatory reactants have been included in the regression model to adjust for their values. The finding that the achieving of MDA is directly associated with a high CRP level and negatively associated with HS and CPs might sound like a contrasting result. However, these findings are in line with the possibility that HS and the presence of CPs are atherosclerosis markers influenced both by inflammation and by other variables (that is, obesity, aging) known to negatively impact on the achieving of MDA [22,28]. Although further studies are needed to describe better the underlying pathophysiologic mechanisms, this finding suggests that the presence of HS and CPs can be reliable markers of a cumulative (inflammatory + metabolic) damage.

A noteworthy finding is that the presence of CPs was found in 87.5% of those with the mutilans PsA subset. Because of the rarity of this clinical subset, the number of subjects evaluated was extremely low and no statistical inferences are possible from these data. However, that the CPs prevalence is maximal in the most severe PsA subset needs to be further evaluated in properly designed studies.

A series of markers is involved in the interrelation between inflammation and atherosclerosis [9,27]. In addition to ESR and CRP, the evaluation of TNF-α and IL-6 levels could have been of interest in the present setting. However, these measurements were not available in all cases.

Among PsA subjects enrolled in the present setting, the prevalence of an axial involvement is high (23.7%). At variance with most data in the literature, we have enrolled subjects experiencing a failure of treatment with traditional DMARDs and with the indication to start treatment with TNF-α blockers. Because of its high rate of refractoriness to DMARDs, the presence of an axial subset has been recognized as a major criterion to start treatment with TNF-α blockers [30]. The selection criteria used could have caused such a high prevalence of the axial subset in our study population. However (Table 2), there was no significant difference in the achieving of MDA after stratifying the population according to the different PsA clinical subsets.

Most previous studies in PsA subjects employed different criteria to define a good clinical response. We have chosen the criteria of achieving MDA proven to be appropriate in providing an outcome measure for clinical trials [21]. As to clinical and demographic variables known to predict MDA, the hazard ratios found in the present study are in line with those of previous reports [22].

In addition to their obvious pathophysiological significance, these data may have pharmaco-economic implications [31]. Because of their high cost and their side effects (that is, a higher than normal risk of infections and of malignancies) [32], the identification of predictors of the success of TNF-α blockers is mandatory. By stratifying the achieving of a good clinical response, a risk/benefit evaluation may be performed in each case and for each patient. This, in turn, would hinder the use of TNF-α blockers in subjects with a low probability of success. Further studies with higher numbers of subjects are needed to address this important issue.

Conclusions

The presence of HS and/or CPs is a negative predictor of achieving and maintaining MDA during treatment with TNF-α blockers.

Abbreviations

CCA: common carotid artery; CPs: carotid plaques; CRP: C-reactive protein; CV: cardiovascular; DMARDs: disease modifying anti-rheumatic drugs; ESR: erythrocyte sedimentation rate; HAQ: health assessment questionnaire; HR: hazard ratio; HS: hepatic steatosis; IFG: impaired fasting glucose; IL: interleukin; IMT: intima-media thickness; MDA: minimal disease activity; MetS: metabolic syndrome; MTX: Methotrexate; NCEP: National Cholesterol Education Program; Non-MDA: subjects not achieving MDA; PASI: psoriasis area severity index; PsA: psoriatic arthritis; SJC: swollen joint count; s-MDA: sustained MDA; TJC: tender joint count; SD: standard deviation; TNF-α: tumor necrosis factor-α; US: ultrasonography; VAS: visual analog scale for pain; VRFs: vascular risk factors.

Author details

[1]Department of Clinical and Experimental Medicine, Reference Centre for Coagulation Disorders, Federico II University, Via Sergio Pansini 5, Naples, 80129 Italy. [2]Department of Clinical and Experimental Medicine, Rheumatology Research Unit, Psoriatic Arthritis Clinic, Federico II University, Via Sergio Pansini 5, Naples, 80129 Italy. [3]Rheumatology and Rehabilitation Research Unit, I.R.C.C.S. "Salvatore Maugeri" Via Bagni Vecchi 1, Telese Terme (BN), 82037 Italy.

Authors' contributions

MNDDM conceived and designed the study, performed statistical analyses, interpreted results and drafted the manuscript; RP designed the study and interpreted results; SI designed the study and acquired clinical data; RL and AR acquired clinical data and drafted the manuscript; GT and RS interpreted results and performed critical revision of the manuscript. All authors read and approved the final manuscript.

Competing interests

The authors declare that they have no competing interests.

References

1. Taylor W, Gladman D, Helliwell P, Marchesoni A, Mease P, Mielants H, CASPAR study group: **Classification criteria for psoriatic arthritis: development of new criteria from a large international study.** *Arthritis Rheum* 2006, **54**:2665-2673.
2. Tyrrell PN, Beyene J, Feldman BM, McCrindle BW, Silverman ED, Bradley TJ: **Rheumatic disease and carotid intima-media thickness: a systematic review and meta-analysis.** *Arterioscler Thromb Vasc Biol* 2010, **30**:1014-1026.
3. Mok CC, Ko GT, Ho LY, Yu KL, Chan PT, To CH: **Prevalence of atherosclerotic risk factors and the metabolic syndrome in patients with chronic inflammatory arthritis.** *Arthritis Care Res (Hoboken)* 2011, **63**:195-202.
4. Di Minno MN, Iervolino S, Peluso R, Scarpa R, Di Minno G: **Platelet reactivity and disease activity in subjects with psoriatic arthritis.** *J Rheumatol* 2012, **39**:334-336.
5. Seitz M, Reichenbach S, Möller B, Zwahlen M, Villiger PM, Dufour JF: **Hepatoprotective effect of tumour necrosis factor alpha blockade in psoriatic arthritis: a cross-sectional study.** *Ann Rheum Dis* 2010, **69**:1148-1150.
6. Gonzalez-Juanatey C, Llorca J, Amigo-Diaz E, Dierssen T, Martin J, Gonzalez-Gay MA: **High prevalence of subclinical atherosclerosis in psoriatic arthritis patients without clinically evident cardiovascular disease or classic atherosclerosis risk factors.** *Arthritis Rheum* 2007, **57**:1074-1080.
7. Targher G, Day CP, Bonora E: **Risk of cardiovascular disease in patients with nonalcoholic fatty liver disease.** *N Engl J Med* 2010, **363**:1341-1350.
8. Lorenz MW, Markus HS, Bots ML, Rosvall M, Sitzer M: **Prediction of clinical cardiovascular events with carotid intima-media thickness: a systematic review and meta-analysis.** *Circulation* 2007, **115**:459-467.
9. Sattar N, McCarey DW, Capell H, McInnes IB: **Explaining how "high-grade" systemic inflammation accelerates vascular risk in rheumatoid arthritis.** *Circulation* 2003, **108**:2957-2963.
10. Del Rincon ID, Williams K, Stern MP, Freeman GL, Escalante A: **High incidence of cardiovascular events in a rheumatoid arthritis cohort not explained by traditional cardiac risk factors.** *Arthritis Rheum* 2001, **44**:2737-2745.
11. Di Minno MND, Iervolino S, Lupoli R, Russolillo A, Peluso R, Coppola A, Scarpa R, Di Minno G: **Cardiovascular risk in rheumatic patients: the link between inflammation and atherosclerosis.** *Semin Thromb Hemost* 2012, **38**:497-505.
12. Tarantino G, Savastano S, Colao A: **Hepatic steatosis, low-grade chronic inflammation and hormone/growth factor/adipokine imbalance.** *World J Gastroenterol* 2010, **16**:4773-4783.
13. Di Minno MND, Iervolino S, Peluso R, Scarpa R, Di Minno G: **Carotid intima-media thickness in psoriatic arthritis. Differences between tumor necrosis factor-alpha-blockers and traditional disease modifying anti-rheumatic drugs.** *Arterioscler Thromb Vasc Biol* 2011, **31**:705-712.
14. Di Minno MN, Iervolino S, Peluso R, Scarpa R, Di Minno G: **TNF-α blockers and carotid intima-media thickness: an emerging issue in the treatment of psoriatic arthritis.** *Intern Emerg Med* 2012, **7(Suppl 2)**:97-98.
15. Shoenfeld Y, Gerli R, Doria A, Matsuura E, Cerinic MM, Ronda N, Jara LJ, Abu-Shakra M, Meroni PL, Sherer Y: **Accelerated atherosclerosis in autoimmune rheumatic diseases.** *Circulation* 2005, **112**:3337-3347.
16. Di Minno MN, Iervolino S, Peluso R, Russolillo A, Lupoli R, Scarpa R, Di Minno G, Tarantino G, CaRRDS Study Group: **Hepatic steatosis and disease activity in subjects with psoriatic arthritis on TNF-α blockers.** *J Rheumatol* 2012, **39**:1042-1046.
17. Eder L, Zisman D, Barzilai M, Laor A, Rahat M, Rozenbaum M, Bitterman H, Feld J, Rimar D, Rosner I: **Subclinical atherosclerosis in psoriatic arthritis: a case-control study.** *J Rheumatol* 2008, **35**:877-882.
18. Moll JM, Wright V: **Psoriatic arthritis.** *Semin Arthritis Rheum* 1973, **3**:55-78.
19. Di Minno MN, Tufano A, Guida A, Di Capua M, De Gregorio AM, Cerbone AM, Tarantino G, Di Minno G: **Abnormally high prevalence of major components of the metabolic syndrome in subjects with early-onset idiopathic venous thromboembolism.** *Thromb Res* 2011, **127**:193-197.
20. Coates LC, Helliwell PS: **Validation of minimal disease activity criteria for psoriatic arthritis using interventional trial data.** *Arthritis Care Res (Hoboken)* 2010, **62**:965-969.
21. Coates LC, Cook R, Lee K, Chandran V, Gladman DD: **Frequency, predictors, and prognosis of sustained minimal disease activity in an observational psoriatic arthritis cohort.** *Arthritis Care Res (Hoboken)* 2010, **62**:970-976.
22. Iervolino S, Di Minno MN, Peluso R, Lofrano M, Russolillo A, Di Minno G, Scarpa R: **Predictors of early minimal disease activity in patients with psoriatic arthritis treated with tumor necrosis factor-α blockers.** *J Rheumatol* 2012, **39**:568-573.
23. Rocha VZ, Libby P: **The multiple facets of the fat tissue.** *Thyroid* 2008, **18**:175-183.
24. van Kuijk AW, Reinders-Blankert P, Smeets TJ, Dijkmans BA, Tak PP: **Detailed analysis of the cell infiltrate and the expression of mediators of synovial inflammation and joint destruction in the synovium of patients with psoriatic arthritis: implications for treatment.** *Ann Rheum Dis* 2006, **65**:1551-1557.
25. Dixon WG, Symmons DP: **What effects might anti-TNF-alpha treatment be expected to have on cardiovascular morbidity and mortality in rheumatoid arthritis? A review of the role of TNF-alpha in cardiovascular pathophysiology.** *Ann Rheum Dis* 2007, **66**:1132-1136.
26. Popa C, van den Hoogen FH, Radstake TR, Netea MG, Eijsbouts AE, den Heijer M, van der Meer JW, van Riel PL, Stalenhoef AF, Barrera P: **Modulation of lipoprotein plasma concentrations during long-term anti-TNF therapy in patients with active rheumatoid arthritis.** *Ann Rheum Dis* 2007, **66**:1503-1507.
27. Libby P: **Changing concepts of atherogenesis.** *J Intern Med* 2000, **247**:349-358.
28. Di Minno MN, Peluso R, Iervolino S, Lupoli R, Russolillo A, Scarpa R, Di Minno G: **Obesity and the prediction of minimal disease activity. A prospective study in psoriatic arthritis.** *Arthritis Care Res (Hoboken)* 2012, doi: 10.1002/acr.21711.
29. Tam LS, Li EK, Shang Q, Tomlinson B, Li M, Leung YY, Kuan WP, Kwok LW, Li TK, Zhu Y, Kun EW, Yip G, Yu CM: **Tumour necrosis factor alpha blockade is associated with sustained regression of carotid intima-media**

thickness for patients with active psoriatic arthritis: a 2-year pilot study. *Ann Rheum Dis* 2011, **70**:705-706.

30. van der Heijde D, Sieper J, Maksymowych WP, Dougados M, Burgos-Vargas R, Landewé R, Rudwaleit M, Braun J, Assessment of SpondyloArthritis international Society: **2010 update of the international ASAS recommendations for the use of anti-TNF agents in patients with axial spondyloarthritis.** *Ann Rheum Dis* 2011, **70**:905-908.
31. Olivieri I, Mantovani LG, D'Angelo S, Padula A, de Portu S: **Psoriatic arthritis: pharmacoeconomic considerations.** *Curr Rheumatol Rep* 2009, **11**:263-269.
32. Bongartz T, Sutton AJ, Sweeting MJ, Buchan I, Matteson EL, Montori V: **Anti-TNF antibody therapy in rheumatoid arthritis and the risk of serious infections and malignancies: systematic review and meta-analysis of rare harmful effects in randomized controlled trials.** *JAMA* 2006, **295**:2275-2285.

3

Expression of IL-20 in synovium and lesional skin of patients with psoriatic arthritis: differential response to alefacept treatment

Maria C Lebre[1,2*†], Christina L Jonckheere[1†], Maarten C Kraan[1,3], Arno WR van Kuijk[1], Jan D Bos[4], Menno de Rie[4,5], Danielle M Gerlag[1] and Paul P Tak[1,6]

Abstract

Introduction: Psoriatic arthritis (PsA) is an inflammatory joint disease associated with psoriasis. Alefacept (a lymphocyte function-associated antigen (LFA)-3 Ig fusion protein that binds to CD2 and functions as an antagonist to T-cell activation) has been shown to result in improvement in psoriasis but has limited effectiveness in PsA. Interleukin-20 (IL-20) is a key proinflammatory cytokine involved in the pathogenesis of psoriasis. The effects of alefacept treatment on IL-20 expression in the synovium of patients with psoriasis and PsA are currently unknown.

Methods: Eleven patients with active PsA and chronic plaque psoriasis were treated with alefacept (7.5 mg per week for 12 weeks) in an open-label study. Skin biopsies were taken before and after 1 and 6 weeks, whereas synovial biopsies were obtained before and 4 and 12 weeks after treatment. Synovial biopsies from patients with rheumatoid arthritis (RA) (n = 10) were used as disease controls. Immunohistochemical analysis was performed to detect IL-20 expression, and stained synovial tissue sections were evaluated with digital image analysis. Double staining was performed with IL-20 and CD68 (macrophages), and conversely with CD55 (fibroblast-like synoviocytes, FLSs) to determine the phenotype of IL-20-positive cells in PsA synovium. IL-20 expression in skin sections (n = 6) was analyzed semiquantitatively.

Results: IL-20 was abundantly expressed in both PsA and RA synovial tissues. In inflamed PsA synovium, $CD68^+$ macrophages and $CD55^+$ FLSs coexpressed IL-20, and its expression correlated with the numbers of FLSs. IL-20 expression in lesional skin of PsA patients decreased significantly (P = 0.04) 6 weeks after treatment and correlated positively with the Psoriasis Area and Severity Index (PASI). IL-20 expression in PsA synovium was not affected by alefacept.

Conclusions: Conceivably, the relatively limited effectiveness of alefacept in PsA patients (compared with anti-tumor necrosis factor (TNF) therapy) might be explained in part by persistent FLS-derived IL-20 expression.

Introduction

Psoriatic arthritis (PsA) is an inflammatory joint disease associated with psoriasis, characterized by a heterogeneous clinical presentation including spinal involvement, peripheral synovitis, and enthesitis. Cellular infiltration plays an important role in the induction of inflammation in joint tissues, as well as in psoriatic skin [1].

* Correspondence: c.lebre@amc.uva.nl
† Contributed equally
[1]Division of Clinical Immunology and Rheumatology, Academic Medical Center/University of Amsterdam, Amsterdam, The Netherlands
Full list of author information is available at the end of the article

Alefacept is a lymphocyte function-associated antigen (LFA)-3 immunoglobulin (Ig) fusion protein that binds to CD2 and functions as an antagonist to T-cell activation. Alefacept was the first of the biologic agents to be approved in the United States for the treatment of adult patients with moderate-to-severe chronic plaque psoriasis who are candidates for systemic therapy or phototherapy. This fully human fusion protein inhibits activation of memory T cells ($CD45RO^+$), a subpopulation of lymphocytes that plays a critical role in the pathogenesis of psoriasis [2]. This therapy has been shown to be effective in patients with psoriasis

[3], and it also has some efficacy in PsA [4,5] compared with anti-TNF therapy. Clinical response, as determined by the American College of Rheumatology 20 (ACR20) response at week 24, was achieved by a significantly greater proportion of patients receiving alefacept plus methotrexate (54%) compared with those receiving placebo plus methotrexate (23%), but proportions of patients achieving ACR50 and ACR70 responses at week 24 were not significantly different in a randomized, double-blind, placebo-controlled study in 185 PsA patients [5].

Interleukin-20 (IL-20) belongs to the IL-10 cytokine family. IL-20 receptor (IL-20R) and IL-20 are expressed in several normal tissue types, including the lungs, skin, and kidney [6,7]. Moreover, IL-20 has been implicated to play an important role in several autoimmune diseases that include rheumatoid arthritis (RA), lupus nephritis, and Crohn disease (reviewed in [8]). Recent reports have shown that IL-20 functions as a proinflammatory cytokine in several inflammatory diseases, of which psoriasis has been the most extensively studied [9,10]. *IL-20* gene and protein expression was elevated in lesional psoriatic skin compared with normal and nonlesional skin [11-13]. Interestingly, its expression in PsA has as yet not been investigated. IL-20 is expressed mainly by activated monocytes [14]. Other sources of IL-20 are keratinocytes (KCs) [14,15], maturing dendritic cells (DCs) [16], synovial fibroblasts [17], endothelial cells [18,19], and renal mesangial cells [20]. IL-20 signals through two alternative receptor complexes: type I, which is composed of IL-20R1/IL-20R2 chains, and type II, which consists of an IL-22R/IL-20R2 heterodimer [21]. IL-20R1, IL-20R2, and IL-22R chains are coexpressed at high levels in the skin [7,22]. In addition, KCs [23,24], rheumatoid synovium (fibroblasts and synovial fluid cells) [17,24,25], and endothelial cells [17] express IL-20R chains. The interaction between IL-20 and its receptors leads to various biologic effects that include hyperproliferation of KCs [7], production of inflammatory cytokines and chemokines by synovial fibroblasts [17] and KCs [7], neutrophil chemotaxis, and angiogenesis [17]. Recently, a role for IL-20 in osteoclast differentiation was reported [26].

Decreased expression of IL-20 in the skin has been observed after effective treatment with calcipitriol, cyclosporine [22], and infliximab [27]. Of interest, reduced IL-20 expression has also been demonstrated in the skin of patients after alefacept treatment [13], but only in those who responded clinically (12 responders versus eight nonresponders). Thus, these initial data suggest that IL-20 might serve as a biomarker associated with efficacy in patients with psoriasis. Here, we extend the findings for the skin of patients with psoriasis and demonstrate for the first time the effects of alefacept treatment on IL-20 expression in the synovium of patients with PsA. Moreover, in view of these data, it is clear that IL-20 is a key proinflammatory cytokine for both skin and synovium. The unique use of paired skin and synovium from patients with PsA (with active psoriasis) allowed us to address the question whether alefacept treatment leads to a specific tissue-response mechanism.

Methods

Patients and tissue samples

Skin and synovial biopsy specimens were obtained from patients with chronic plaque psoriasis and PsA (n = 11 synovial biopsies; n = 6 skin biopsies) in a prospective open-label clinical trial, as previously described [4]. Clinical characteristics have been previously reported [4]. Patients received a weekly dose of alefacept (LFA-3TIP, anti-CD2; Amevive, Biogen, San Diego, CA, USA; 7.5 mg, intravenously) for 12 weeks. In brief, skin biopsies were taken before and after 1 and after 6 weeks, whereas synovial biopsies were taken before and 4 and 12 weeks after treatment. Synovial biopsy specimens from active RA patients (Table 1; n = 10) served as disease control group for IL-20 expression at baseline. Patient's disease activity score (DAS28), visual analogue scale (VAS) for global disease activity (scale, 0 to 100 mm), swollen-joint count (SJC), tender-joint count (TJC), erythrocyte sedimentation rate (ESR), and serum levels of C-reactive protein (CRP) were used to evaluate disease activity. The study was conducted according to International Conference of Harmonization (ICH)/Declaration of Helsinki, approved by the Medical Ethics Committee of Academic Medical Center (AMC)/University of Amsterdam, and all patients gave written informed consent. Psoriasis area and severity index (PASI) was assessed as previously described [28].

Synovial and skin biopsy immunohistochemical staining

All samples were, immediately after collection, embedded *en bloc* in Tissue Tec OCT (Miles, Elkhart, IN, USA) and subsequently snap frozen. The frozen blocks were stored in liquid nitrogen until processed.

Table 1 Demographic and clinical characteristics of RA patients at baseline

	RA patients
Sex, female/male (n)	8/2 (10)
Age in years, mean (range)	55.5 (44-64)
DAS28	4.9 (2.9-6.5)
SJC, mean (range)	11.7 (6-18)
TJC, mean (range)	9.8 (1-16)
VAS, mean (range)	22 (10-32)
CRP (mg/l), mean (range)	21 (3-52)
ESR mm/h, mean (range)	23.9 (3-74)

Shortly before staining, 5-μm sections were cut and mounted on glass slides (Star Frost; Knittelgläser, Braunschweig, Germany). The glass slides were sealed and stored at -80°C until immunohistochemical analysis was performed.

In brief, after fixation with acetone, endogenous peroxidase activity was inhibited by using 0.1% sodium azide and 0.3% hydrogen peroxide in phosphate-buffered saline (PBS). The primary antibody against human IL-20 (Zymogenetics, Seattle, WA, USA) was incubated overnight at 4°C followed by secondary antibody affinity-purified horseradish peroxidase (HRP)-conjugated goat anti-mouse (Dako Cytomation, Glostrup, Denmark) for 30 minutes, followed by subsequent incubation with biotinylated tyramide (Perkin Elmer, Boston, MA, USA) for 30 minutes and HRP-conjugated streptavidin for 30 minutes. HRP activity was detected by using hydrogen peroxide as substrate and amino ethylcarbazole (AEC; SK-4200; Vector Laboratories, Burlingame, CA, USA) as dye. With this procedure, IL-20-positive cells stained red. Slides were counterstained with Mayer hematoxylin (Merck, Darmstadt, Germany) and, after washing with distilled water, mounted in Kayser glycerol gelatin (Merck).

To identify IL-20-expressing cells in PsA synovial tissue, double staining was performed by using anti-IL-20 antibody together with FITC-labeled anti-CD55 (M2192; Sanquin Reagents, Amsterdam, The Netherlands) or FITC-labeled anti-CD68 (clone KP1; Dakocytomation). Fixation and blocking endogenous peroxidase activity was performed as stated earlier. The primary antibody against human IL-20 (Zymogenetics) was incubated overnight at 4°C followed by secondary antibody affinity-purified horseradish peroxidase (HRP)-conjugated goat anti-mouse (Dako Cytomation) for 30 minutes, and subsequent incubation with biotinylated tyramide (Perkin Elmer) for 30 minutes and HRP-conjugated streptavidin for 30 minutes. After a blocking step of 15 minutes with 10% mouse serum (Sanquin Reagents), FITC-labeled anti-CD55 or FITC-labeled anti-CD68 was added to the sections and incubated for 1 hour at room temperature. Then the sections were incubated for 30 minutes with rabbit anti-FITC followed by alkaline phosphatase-conjugated swine anti-rabbit secondary antibodies (both from Dako Cytomation). HRP activity was detected as stated earlier. Alkaline phosphatase activity was detected by using the Alkaline Phosphatase Substrate III kit (SK-5300; Vector Laboratories). With this procedure, IL-20-positive cells stained red, CD55- or CD68-positive cells stained blue, and double-positive cells stained purple.

Quantification of IL-20-expressing cells in skin and synovium

Skin biopsy specimens were scored semiquantitatively for IL-20 expression on a 5-point scale by two independent observers who were not aware of the clinical data. The scoring methods were described previously [29]. In brief, a score of 0 represented minimal staining, whereas a score of 4 represented widespread expression of IL-20 in this case. Individual readings were identical or differed by only 1 point. Minor differences between the observers were resolved by mutual agreement.

Quantification of IL-20-expressing cells in PsA and RA synovial tissues was performed with computer-assisted image analysis, as previously described [30]. The same holds true for CD68 and CD55 quantification. In brief, after immunohistochemical staining, all coded sections (one section per patient per time point) were randomly analyzed (18 high-power fields from different parts of the section were analyzed; for example, the mean of the 18 high-power fields was calculated). The images of the high-power fields were analyzed by using the Qwin analysis system (Leica, Cambridge, UK). Positive staining of CD68 and CD55 was expressed as positive cells/mm^2. Positive staining for IL-20 was expressed as integrated optical density (IOD/mm^2).

Statistical analysis

SPSS version 15.0 for Windows (SPSS, Chicago, IL, USA) was used for statistical analysis. The Wilcoxon signed ranks test was used for comparison of nonparametric variables in related samples, and the Mann-Whitney *U* test was used for comparison of nonparametric variables in independent samples. Correlations between synovial IL-20 expression and disease activity score 28 (DAS28), synovial CD4, CD8, CD68, and CD55 were analyzed with Spearman rank correlation. Correlations between skin IL-20 and PASI were analyzed with Spearman rank correlation.

Results

Expression of IL-20 in PsA and RA synovia

First we analyzed whether IL-20 expression in PsA and RA synovia differ from each other. IL-20 was expressed in the intimal lining layer, in the synovial sublining, and on endothelium in both PsA and RA patients (Figure 1A). Digital image analysis of synovial tissue demonstrated clear IL-20 expression with comparable overall scores in both patient groups (median Integrated Optical Density (IOD) (range)): PsA, 60,064 (1,588 to 567,696); RA, 68,554 (1,171 to 530,218) (Figure 1B). Double staining of inflamed PsA synovium showed that CD68$^+$ macrophages and CD55$^+$ FLS coexpress IL-20 (Figure 1C).

Alefacept treatment does not affect IL-20 expression in PsA synovium

As previously described, alefacept treatment resulted in clinical improvement and in a reduction of CD4$^+$ T cells and CD68$^+$ macrophages in the synovial infiltrate [4]. Despite the clinical improvement and change in cellular

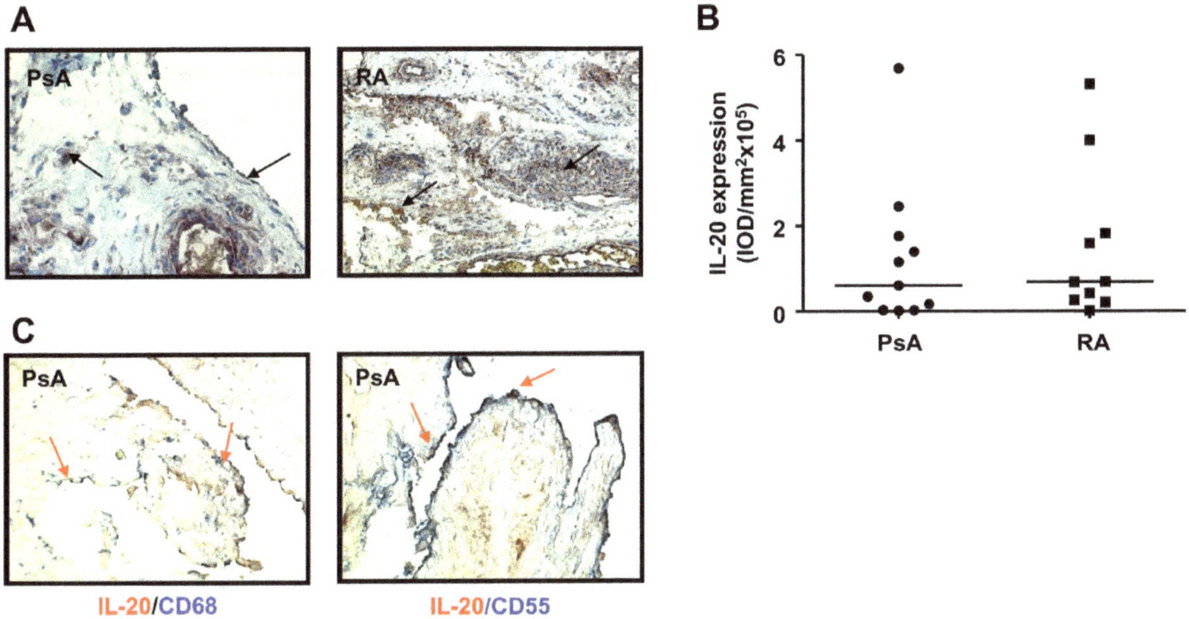

Figure 1 IL-20 is expressed in PsA and RA synovial tissues. (A) Representative immunohistochemical staining of baseline IL-20 expression in synovial tissue from PsA and RA patients. Arrows indicate expression of IL-20 in both lining and sublining. **(B)** Quantification of IL-20 expression in RA and PsA synovial tissues. Results are shown as median IOD (integrated optical density)/mm^2 × 10^5 of 10 patients with RA and 11 patients with PsA. **(C)** Double-immunohistochemistry stainings of IL-20 (red) and CD68$^+$ macrophages (blue) and CD55$^+$ FLS (blue) in PsA synovium. A representative double immunostaining of PsA synovium from one patient is shown. Arrows indicate double-positive cells. Original magnification, ×200. CRP, C-reactive protein; DAS28, disease activity score; ESR, erythrocyte sedimentation rate; SJC, swollen-joint count; TJC, tender-joint count; VAS, visual analogue scale (100 mm).

infiltrate [4], no change was found in IL-20 expression in the synovium before and after treatment (Figure 2A and 2B). As CD68$^+$ macrophages and CD55$^+$ FLSs express IL-20, we investigated whether the levels of synovial IL-20 were associated with the numbers of these cells present in synovial tissue. Although no correlation was present between the levels of IL-20 and the numbers of both total CD68$^+$ and sublining CD68$^+$ macrophages (data not shown), the levels of IL-20 were positively correlated with the numbers of CD55$^+$ FLSs (r = 0.4238; P = 0.0196). In addition, the levels of synovial IL-20 expression were not correlated with disease-activity parameters: DAS28, C-reactive protein (CRP), and erythrocyte sedimentation rate (ESR) (data not shown).

Decreased IL-20 expression in PsA skin lesions after alefacept treatment

In contrast to findings in the synovium, IL-20 expression in PsA lesional skin was significantly decreased (P = 0.04) 6 weeks after alefacept treatment (Figure 3A and 3B). IL-20 expression in PsA lesional skin was positively correlated with disease activity (PASI score): r = 0.5062; P = 0.031 (Figure 3C).

Discussion

Here we show that IL-20 is expressed in PsA synovium, similar to the levels in RA synovium. In PsA inflamed synovium, both CD68$^+$ macrophages and CD55$^+$ FLSs coexpress IL-20. This study is the first to investigate the effects of alefacept treatment on IL-20 expression in paired synovial tissue and psoriatic lesional skin of patients with both PsA and psoriasis. Whereas IL-20 expression in PsA synovium was not affected by alefacept treatment, its expression in lesional skin was significantly decreased after this treatment. In addition, in psoriatic lesional skin, IL-20 expression was positively correlated with disease activity (PASI) at baseline and after treatment. In contrast, synovial IL-20 expression was not correlated with disease-activity parameters (DAS28, CRP, ESR; data not shown). The observed expression of IL-20 in both PsA and RA synovial tissues is consistent with previous observations showing comparable levels of this proinflammatory cytokine in synovial fluid of patients with RA compared with those with spondyloarthritides, including PsA [24]. These data suggest that synovial IL-20 expression is a feature of various inflammatory rheumatic diseases.

As reported for RA [17,24], we found that both macrophages and FLSs are a source of IL-20 in the synovium of PsA patients. The exact biologic effects of synovial IL-20 have yet to be determined, but it is tempting to speculate that this cytokine might affect cells present in inflamed synovium. Consistent with this notion, it was reported that IL-20 induced the production of IL-6 and IL-8 and

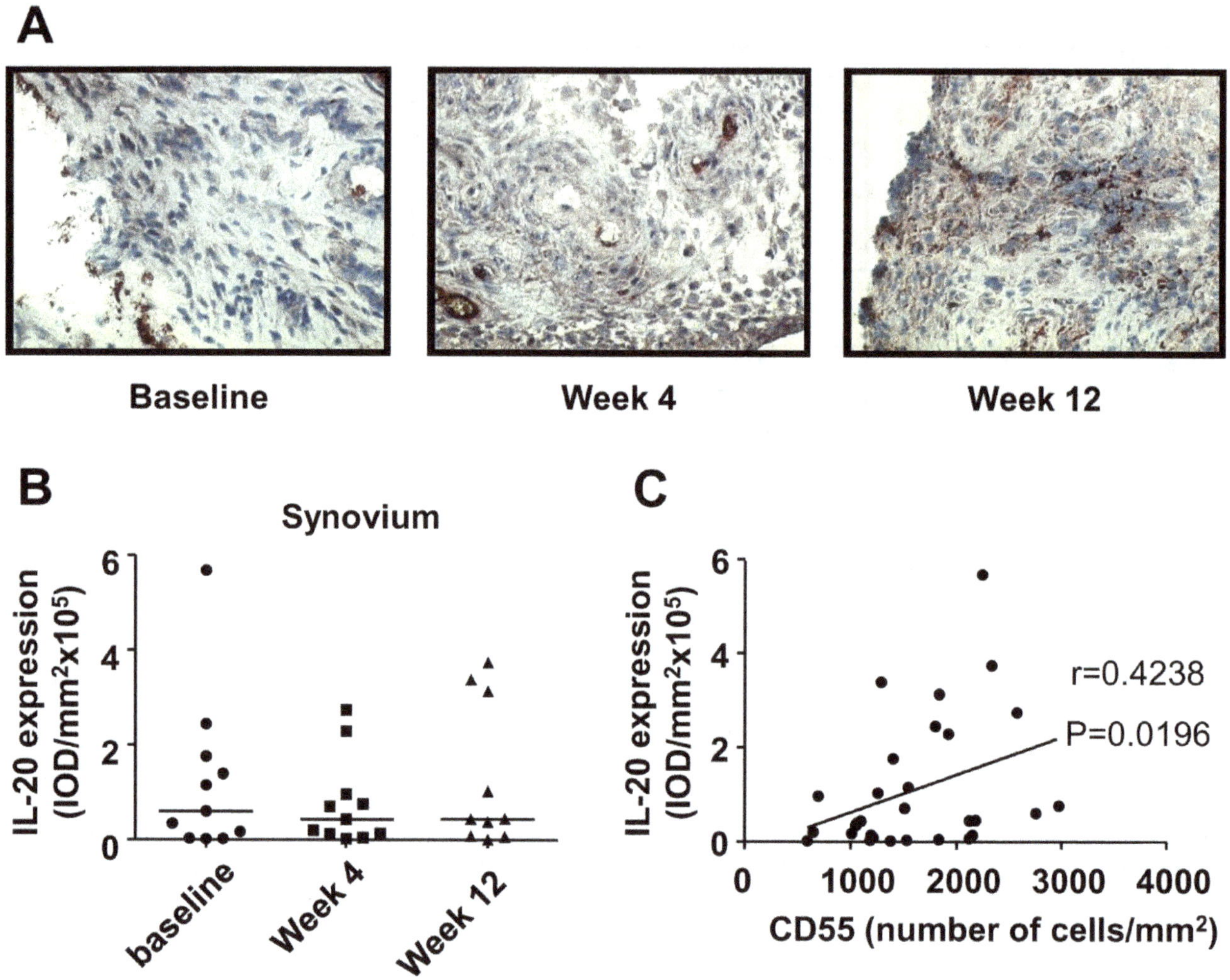

Figure 2 Alefacept treatment does not affect IL-20 expression in PsA synovium. **(A)** Representative immunohistochemical staining of IL-20 in the synovium of a PsA patient. **(B)** Quantification of IL-20 expression in PsA synovium. Results are shown as median IOD (integrated optical density)/mm^2 × 10^5 of 11 patients with PsA. **(C)** Correlation between the expression of IL-20 and the number of CD55$^+$ FLSs in PsA synovium. Original magnification, ×200. Each dot represents the mean of the 18 high-power fields per patient per time point. CRP, C-reactive protein; DAS28, disease activity score; ESR, erythrocyte sedimentation rate; SJC, swollen-joint count; TJC, tender-joint count; VAS, visual analogue scale (100 mm).

monocyte chemoattractant protein 1 by FLSs [17]. A considerable amount of evidence suggests that FLSs are key cells that contribute to RA pathogenesis. In this way, IL-20 could play a role in perpetuating the inflammatory process by promoting the release of inflammatory cytokines and chemokines at the site of inflammation [17].

Alefacept treatment resulted in changes in synovial inflammation in PsA patients that included a significant reduction in CD4$^+$ lymphocytes, CD8$^+$ lymphocytes, and CD68$^+$ sublining macrophages [4], supporting the hypothesis that T cells orchestrate synovial inflammation in PsA. However, the expression of synovial IL-20 was not affected by alefacept treatment, in contrast to the findings in the skin. This may be explained by the fact that alefacept treatment did not affect the numbers of intimal macrophages or the CD55$^+$ FLSs [4]; both cell types are sources of IL-20, but only the numbers of CD55$^+$ FLSs were positively correlated with the levels of synovial IL-20. Together, the data show that alefacept treatment does not affect the major cellular source of IL-20 in the synovium (FLSs), in contrast to the findings in the skin. Of note, alefacept treatment has been abandoned as a treatment of PsA, consistent with its limited clinical efficacy compared with TNF-α-targeted therapies [31-33]. As discussed, alefacept treatment was associated with decreased IL-20 expression in lesional psoriatic skin. As alefacept targets T cells, it is tempting to speculate that in the skin, T cells are involved in the proximal regulation of IL-20. It is well established that in psoriasis skin, cross-talk between infiltrating T cells and resident KCs is

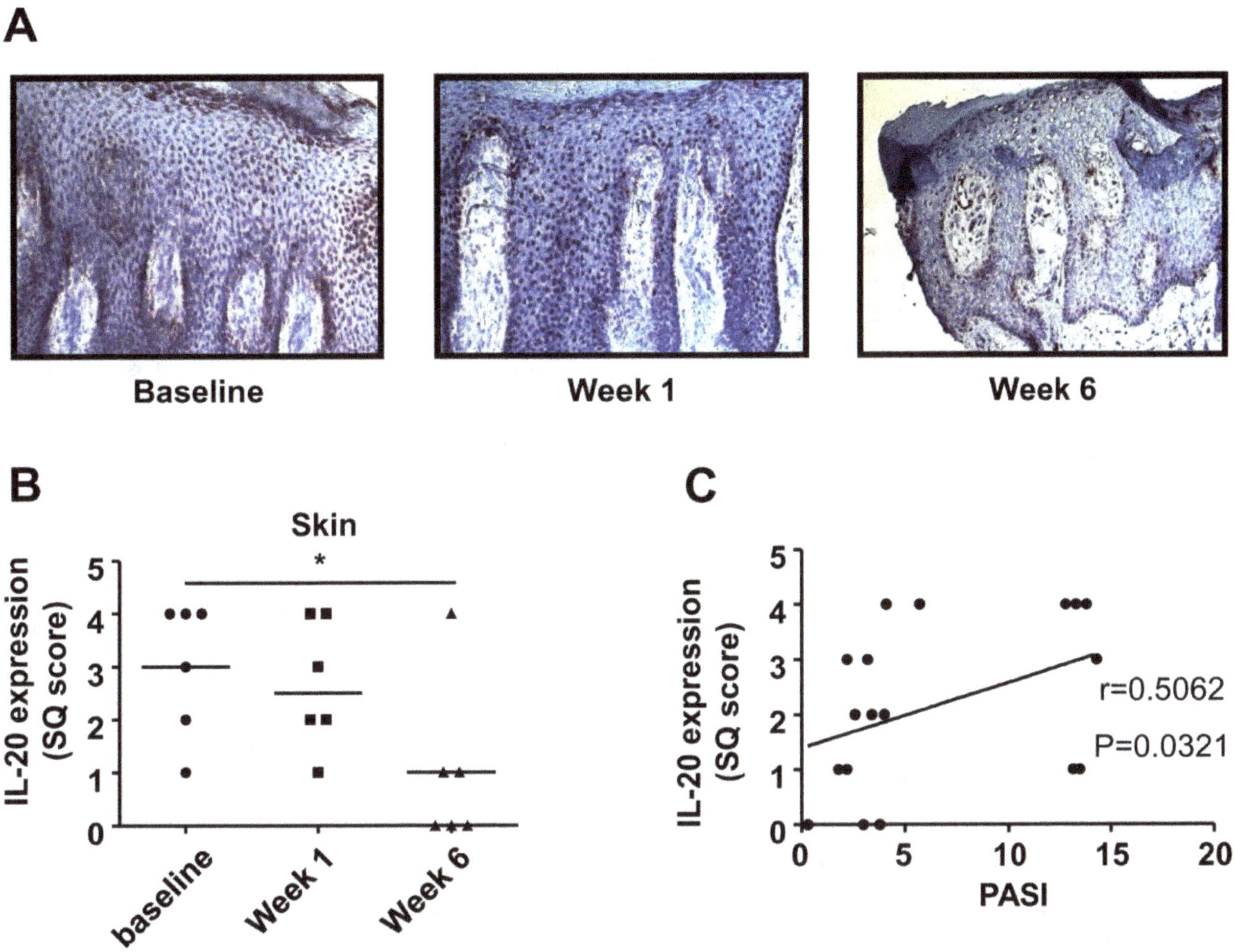

Figure 3 Decreased IL-20 expression in PsA skin lesions after alefacept treatment. **(A)** Representative immunohistochemical staining of IL-20 expression in the lesional skin of a PsA patient. **(B)** Quantification of IL-20 expression in PsA lesional skin. Results are shown as median of semiquantitative score (SQ) of six patients with PsA. **(C)** IL-20 expression in PsA lesional skin is correlated with disease activity (PASI). All time points are depicted (each dot represents one patient per time point). *Statistical significance, $P = 0.04$. Original magnification, ×200. CRP, C-reactive protein; DAS28, disease activity score; ESR, erythrocyte sedimentation rate; SJC, swollen-joint count; TJC, tender-joint count; VAS, visual analogue scale (100 mm).

involved in disease pathogenesis [34]. In addition, it was recently reported that T cell-derived cytokines (IL-17 and IL-22) mediate IL-20 production by KCs [35]. Thus, in psoriatic skin of PsA patients, alefacept may affect KC-derived IL-20 by decreasing the number of infiltrating T cells that interact with KCs.

Conclusions

IL-20 has been implicated in several inflammatory diseases. The results presented here show that IL-20 is expressed in psoriatic skin lesions and synovial tissue from patients with both psoriasis and PsA. It remains to be established whether the observed effects of alefacept are specific for IL-20 or also are seen with other members of the IL-10 subfamily (IL-19 and IL-24). Conceivably, the limited effectiveness of alefacept in PsA patients compared with anti-TNF therapy [31-33] might be explained in part by persistent IL-20 production by sublining macrophages and FLSs in the synovium.

Abbreviations

ACR: American College of Rheumatology; AMC: Academic Medical Center; CRP: C-reactive protein; DAS28: disease activity score; DC: dendritic cell; ESR: erythrocyte sedimentation rate; FLS: fibroblast-like synoviocyte; HRP: horseradish peroxidase; ICH: International Conference of Harmonization; IL-20: interleukin-20; IL-20R: IL-20 receptor; IOD: integrated optical density; KC: keratinocytes; LFA-3: lymphocyte function-associated antigen-3; PASI: Psoriasis Area and Severity Index; PsA: psoriatic arthritis; RA: rheumatoid arthritis; SJC: swollen-joint count; TJC: tender-joint count; TNF: tumor necrosis factor; VAS: visual analogue scale.

Acknowledgements

The authors thank G. Appel (Academic Medical Centre/University of Amsterdam, Department of Dermatology, Amsterdam, The Netherlands) and Man-Wai Tang (Academic Medical Centre/University of Amsterdam, Division of Clinical Immunology & Rheumatology, Amsterdam, The Netherlands) for helping with collection of patient demographics and Dr. T. Smeets (Academic Medical Centre/University of Amsterdam, Division of Clinical Immunology & Rheumatology, Amsterdam, The Netherlands) for performing synovial immunohistochemistry staining.

Author details

[1]Division of Clinical Immunology and Rheumatology, Academic Medical Center/University of Amsterdam, Amsterdam, The Netherlands. [2]Department of Experimental Immunology, Academic Medical Center/University of Amsterdam, Amsterdam, The Netherlands. [3]AstraZeneca, Mölndal, Sweden. [4]Department of Dermatology, Academic Medical Center/University of Amsterdam, Amsterdam, The Netherlands. [5]Department of Dermatology, Erasmus Medical Center, Rotterdam, The Netherlands. [6]Academic Medical Center/University of Amsterdam and GlaxoSmithKline, Stevenage, UK.

Authors' contributions

All authors meet the criteria for authorship and more specifically for contributorship statement: MCL and CLJ analyzed and interpreted the data and wrote the article under the close supervision of PPT and thereby take responsibility for this work. MCK, AWvK, JDB, MdR, DMG, and PPT conceived the study and participated in its design and coordination. MCK and AWvK collected and supplied the data. All authors agreed to publish this work and critically reviewed the article. Conception and design of this work were discussed with all authors.

Competing interests

The authors declare that they have no competing interests.

References

1. Kaltwasser JP: **Leflunomide in psoriatic arthritis.** *Autoimmun Rev* 2007, **6**:511-514.
2. Heffernan MP, Leonardi CL: **Alefacept for psoriasis.** *Semin Cutan Med Surg* 2010, **29**:53-55.
3. Krueger GG, Papp KA, Stough DB, Loven KH, Gulliver WP, Ellis CN: **A randomized, double-blind, placebo-controlled phase III study evaluating efficacy and tolerability of 2 courses of alefacept in patients with chronic plaque psoriasis.** *J Am Acad Dermatol* 2002, **47**:821-833.
4. Kraan MC, van Kuijk AW, Dinant HJ, Goedkoop AY, Smeets TJ, de Rie MA, Dijkmans BA, Vaishnaw AK, Bos JD, Tak PP: **Alefacept treatment in psoriatic arthritis: reduction of the effector T cell population in peripheral blood and synovial tissue is associated with improvement of clinical signs of arthritis.** *Arthritis Rheum* 2002, **46**:2776-2784.
5. Mease PJ, Reich K: **Alefacept with methotrexate for treatment of psoriatic arthritis: open-label extension of a randomized, double-blind, placebo-controlled study.** *J Am Acad Dermatol* 2009, **60**:402-411.
6. Wei CC, Hsu YH, Li HH, Wang YC, Hsieh MY, Chen WY, Hsing CH, Chang MS: **IL-20: biological functions and clinical implications.** *J Biomed Sci* 2006, **13**:601-612.
7. Blumberg H, Conklin D, Xu WF, Grossmann A, Brender T, Carollo S, Eagan M, Foster D, Haldeman BA, Hammond A, Haugen H, Jelinek L, Kelly JD, Madden K, Maurer MF, Parrish-Novak J, Prunkard D, Sexson S, Sprecher C, Waggie K, West J, Whitmore TE, Yao L, Kuechle MK, Dale BA, Chandrasekher YA: **Interleukin 20: discovery, receptor identification, and role in epidermal function.** *Cell* 2001, **104**:9-19.
8. Leng RX: **IL-19, IL-20 and IL-24: potential therapeutic targets for autoimmune diseases.** *Expert Opin Ther Targets* 2011, **15**:119-126.
9. Stenderup K, Rosada C, Worsaae A, Clausen JT, Norman DT: **Interleukin-20 as a target in psoriasis treatment.** *Ann N Y Acad Sci* 2007, **1110**:368-381.
10. Stenderup K, Rosada C, Worsaae A, Gnaes-Hansen F, Steiniche T, Hasselager E, Iversen LF, Zahn S, Woldike H, Holmberg HL, Romer J, Kragballe K, Clausen JT, Dam TN: **Interleukin-20 plays a critical role in maintenance and development of psoriasis in the human xenograft transplantation model.** *Br J Dermatol* 2009, **160**:284-296.
11. Wei CC, Chen WY, Wang YC, Chen PJ, Lee JY, Wong TW, Chen WC, Wu JC, Chen GY, Chang MS, Lin YC: **Detection of IL-20 and its receptors on psoriatic skin.** *Clin Immunol* 2005, **117**:65-72.
12. Otkjaer K, Kragballe K, Funding AT, Clausen JT, Noerby PL, Steiniche T, Iversen L: **The dynamics of gene expression of interleukin-19 and interleukin-20 and their receptors in psoriasis.** *Br J Dermatol* 2005, **153**:911-918.
13. Wang F, Lee E, Lowes MA, Haider AS, Fuentes-Duculan J, Abello MV, Chamian F, Cardinale I, Krueger JG: **Prominent production of IL-20 by CD68+/CD11c+ myeloid-derived cells in psoriasis: gene regulation and cellular effects.** *J Invest Dermatol* 2006, **126**:1590-1599.
14. Wolk K, Kunz S, Asadullah K, Sabat R: **Immune cells as sources and targets of the IL-10 family members?** *J Immunol* 2002, **168**:5397-5402.
15. Sabat R, Wolk K: **Research in practice: IL-22 and IL-20: significance for epithelial homeostasis and psoriasis pathogenesis.** *J Dtsch Dermatol Ges* 2011, **9**:518-523.
16. Wolk K, Witte K, Witte E, Proesch S, Schulze-Tanzil G, Nasilowska K, Thilo J, Asadullah K, Sterry W, Volk HD, Sabat R: **Maturing dendritic cells are an important source of IL-29 and IL-20 that may cooperatively increase the innate immunity of keratinocytes.** *J Leukoc Biol* 2008, **83**:1181-1193.
17. Hsu YH, Li HH, Hsieh MY, Liu MF, Huang KY, Chin LS, Chen PC, Cheng HH, Chang MS: **Function of interleukin-20 as a proinflammatory molecule in rheumatoid and experimental arthritis.** *Arthritis Rheum* 2006, **54**:2722-2733.
18. Hammer T, Tritsaris K, Hubschmann MV, Gibson J, Nisato RE, Pepper MS, Dissing S: **IL-20 activates human lymphatic endothelial cells causing cell signalling and tube formation.** *Microvasc Res* 2009, **78**:25-32.
19. Hsieh MY, Chen WY, Jiang MJ, Cheng BC, Huang TY, Chang MS: **Interleukin-20 promotes angiogenesis in a direct and indirect manner.** *Genes Immun* 2006, **7**:234-242.
20. Li HH, Chen HH, Sun KH, Wei CC, Li CF, Chen WC, Wu WM, Chang MS: **Interleukin-20 targets renal mesangial cells and is associated with lupus nephritis.** *Clin Immunol* 2008, **129**:277-285.
21. Wegenka UM: **IL-20: biological functions mediated through two types of receptor complexes.** *Cytokine Growth Factor Rev* 2010, **21**:353-363.
22. Romer J, Hasselager E, Norby PL, Steiniche T, Thorn CJ, Kragballe K: **Epidermal overexpression of interleukin-19 and -20 mRNA in psoriatic skin disappears after short-term treatment with cyclosporine a or calcipotriol.** *J Invest Dermatol* 2003, **121**:1306-1311.
23. Sa SM, Valdez PA, Wu J, Jung K, Zhong F, Hall L, Kasman I, Winer J, Modrusan Z, Danilenko DM, Ouyang W: **The effects of IL-20 subfamily cytokines on reconstituted human epidermis suggest potential roles in cutaneous innate defense and pathogenic adaptive immunity in psoriasis.** *J Immunol* 2007, **178**:2229-2240.
24. Kragstrup TW, Otkjaer K, Holm C, Jorgensen A, Hokland M, Iversen L, Deleuran B: **The expression of IL-20 and IL-24 and their shared receptors are increased in rheumatoid arthritis and spondyloarthropathy.** *Cytokine* 2008, **41**:16-23.
25. Sakurai N, Kuroiwa T, Ikeuchi H, Hiramatsu N, Maeshima A, Kaneko Y, Hiromura K, Nojima Y: **Expression of IL-19 and its receptors in RA: potential role for synovial hyperplasia formation.** *Rheumatology (Oxford)* 2008, **47**:815-820.
26. Hsu YH, Chen WY, Chan CH, Wu CH, Sun ZJ, Chang MS: **Anti-IL-20 monoclonal antibody inhibits the differentiation of osteoclasts and protects against osteoporotic bone loss.** *J Exp Med* 2011, **208**:1849-1861.
27. Ogilvie AL, Luftl M, Antoni C, Schuler G, Kalden JR, Lorenz HM: **Leukocyte infiltration and mRNA expression of IL-20, IL-8 and TNF-R P60 in psoriatic skin is driven by TNF-alpha.** *Int J Immunopathol Pharmacol* 2006, **19**:271-278.
28. Heydendael VM, Spuls PI, Opmeer BC, de Borgie CA, Reitsma JB, Goldschmidt WF, Bossuyt PM, Bos JD, de Rie MA: **Methotrexate versus cyclosporine in moderate-to-severe chronic plaque psoriasis.** *N Engl J Med* 2003, **349**:658-665.
29. Tak PP, Thurkow EW, Daha MR, Kluin PM, Smeets TJ, Meinders AE, Breedveld FC: **Expression of adhesion molecules in early rheumatoid synovial tissue.** *Clin Immunol Immunopathol* 1995, **77**:236-242.
30. Haringman JJ, Vinkenoog M, Gerlag DM, Smeets TJ, Zwinderman AH, Tak PP: **Reliability of computerized image analysis for the evaluation of serial synovial biopsies in randomized controlled trials in rheumatoid arthritis.** *Arthritis Res Ther* 2005, **7**:R862-R867.
31. Antoni CE, Kavanaugh A, Kirkham B, Tutuncu Z, Burmester GR, Schneider U, Furst DE, Molitor J, Keystone E, Gladman D, Manger B, Wassenberg S, Weier R, Wallace DJ, Weisman MH, Kalden JR, Smolen J: **Sustained benefits of infliximab therapy for dermatologic and articular manifestations of**

psoriatic arthritis: results from the Infliximab Multinational Psoriatic Arthritis Controlled Trial (IMPACT). *Arthritis Rheum* 2005, **52**:1227-1236.

32. Mease PJ, Kivitz AJ, Burch FX, Siegel EL, Cohen SB, Ory P, Salonen D, Rubenstein J, Sharp JT, Tsuji W: **Etanercept treatment of psoriatic arthritis: safety, efficacy, and effect on disease progression.** *Arthritis Rheum* 2004, **50**:2264-2272.
33. Mease PJ, Gladman DD, Ritchlin CT, Ruderman EM, Steinfeld SD, Choy EH, Sharp JT, Ory PA, Perdok RJ, Weinberg MA: **Adalimumab for the treatment of patients with moderately to severely active psoriatic arthritis: results of a double-blind, randomized, placebo-controlled trial.** *Arthritis Rheum* 2005, **52**:3279-3289.
34. Rebholz B, Haase I, Eckelt B, Paxian S, Flaig MJ, Ghoreschi K, Nedospasov SA, Mailhammer R, Debey-Pascher S, Schultze JL, Weindl G, Forster I, Huss R, Stratis A, Ruzicka T, Rocken M, Pfeffer K, Schmid RM, Rupec RA: **Crosstalk between keratinocytes and adaptive immune cells in an IkappaBalpha protein-mediated inflammatory disease of the skin.** *Immunity* 2007, **27**:296-307.
35. Tohyama M, Hanakawa Y, Shirakata Y, Dai X, Yang L, Hirakawa S, Okazaki H, Sayama K, Hashimoto K: **The Th17 cytokine IL-22 induces IL-20 production in keratinocytes: a novel immunological cascade with potential relevance in psoriasis.** *Eur J Immunol* 2009, **39**:2779-2788.

4

Synovial cytokine expression in psoriatic arthritis and associations with lymphoid neogenesis and clinical features

Raquel Celis[1], Núria Planell[2], José L Fernández-Sueiro[3], Raimon Sanmartí[1], Julio Ramírez[1], Isidoro González-Álvaro[4], José L Pablos[5] and Juan D Cañete[1*]

Abstract

Introduction: Psoriatic arthritis (PsA) is an autoantibody-negative immune-mediated disease in which synovial lymphoid neogenesis (LN) occurs. We determined whether LN is associated with specific patterns of inflammatory cytokine expression in paired synovial tissue (ST) and fluid (SF) samples and their potential correlation with the clinical characteristics of PsA.

Methods: ST and paired SF samples were obtained from the inflamed knee of PsA patients. ST samples were immunostained with CD3 (T cell), CD20 (B cell), and MECA-79 (high endothelial vessels). Total ST mRNA was extracted, and the gene expression of 21 T-cell-derived and proinflammatory cytokines were measured with quantitative real-time PCR. SF concentrations of Th1, Th2, Th17, and proinflammatory cytokines were determined with the Quantibody Human Th17 Array. Clinical and biologic data were collected at inclusion and after a median of 27 months of follow-up.

Results: Twenty (43.5%) of 46 patients had LN. Only two genes showed differences (Wilcoxon test, $P < 0.06$) in ST between LN-positive and LN-negative patients: interleukin-23A (*IL-23A*) ($P = 0.058$) and transforming growth factor-beta (*TGF-β1*) ($P = 0.050$). IL-23A expression was higher, and TGF-β1 expression was lower in LN-positive patients. ST IL-15 mRNA showed a nonsignificant trend toward higher expression in LN-positive patients, and SF IL-15 protein levels were significantly higher in LN-positive patients ($P = 0.002$). In all PsA patients, IL-23A mRNA expression correlated with C-reactive protein (CRP) ($r = 0.471$; $P = 0.001$) and swollen-joint count (SJC) ($r = 0.350$; $P = 0.018$), whereas SF levels of IL-6 and CC chemokine-ligand 20 (CCL-20) correlated with CRP levels ($r = 0.377$; $P = 0.014$ and $r = 0.501$; $P < 0.0001$, respectively).

Conclusions: These findings suggest differences in the cytokine profile of PsA patients with LN, with a higher expression of IL-23A and IL-15 and a lower expression of TGF-β1. In the entire group of patients, IL-23 ST expression and CCL20 SF levels strongly correlated with markers of disease activity. This cytokine pattern was not accompanied by gross clinical or biologic differences between LN-positive and -negative patients. Taken together, these results suggest a role of the IL-17/IL-23 cytokine axis in synovial LN in PsA.

Introduction

Psoriatic arthritis (PsA) is a chronic, inflammatory, musculoskeletal disease associated with skin psoriasis that is mediated by the immune system and can lead to significant bone and cartilage destruction, functional impairment, and reduced quality of life [1].

Histopathologic analyses of PsA versus rheumatoid arthritis (RA) synovial tissues have revealed differential characteristics that may be of potential value in the diagnostic classification of patients with undifferentiated arthritis, although they share basic features [2]. Of these, ectopic lymphoid neogenesis (LN) has been observed in similar proportions in patients with RA and PsA [3-5]. LN results from the organized aggregation of T and B cells around specialized vessels known as high endothelial venules (HEVs), and correlates with the ectopic

* Correspondence: jcanete@clinic.ub.es
[1]Arthritis Unit, Rheumatology Department, Hospital Clinic de Barcelona and IDIBAPS, c/Villarroel, 170, 08036 Barcelona, Spain
Full list of author information is available at the end of the article

expression of a restricted set of homing chemokines, which are physiologically involved in the traffic and tissue compartmentalization of T and B cells in secondary lymphoid organs [6].

A previous study of patients with PsA and LN by our group suggested that LN is a stable feature in these patients that is reversed only after therapeutic remission [3]. However, its pathogenetic and clinical significance in RA and PsA patients remains unclear.

LN in PsA patients remains intriguing because no specific autoantibodies have been described, and because rheumatoid factor (RF) and anti-citrullinated protein/peptide antibodies (ACPAs) are detected in low titers in only a small proportion of PsA patients [7]. However, B cells and LN structures could drive antibody-independent synovial inflammation through the development of specific T-cell responses or by enhancing cytokine production [8]. This might result in differences in the disease phenotype between patients with and without synovial LN, which might have prognostic interest.

To determine whether synovial LN is associated with differential patterns of cytokine expression, we quantified T-cell polarization (Th1/Th2; Th17/IL-23) and proinflammatory cytokines in paired synovial tissue (ST) and fluid (SF) samples of patients with PsA with and without synovial LN. We also analyzed the potential association between these mediators and markers of disease activity.

Methods

Patients and synovial tissues

Synovial biopsy specimens were obtained with needle arthroscopy from patients of Hospital Clinic (Barcelona, Spain) and Complejo Hospitalario Universitario, (La Coruña, Spain) meeting the CASPAR criteria for PsA [9], selected according to the presence of active knee synovitis (pain and inflammatory synovial fluid). Paired synovial fluid samples were also obtained at the same time from 42 of these patients. All patients gave informed consent, and the study was approved by the Ethics Committee of the Hospital Clinic of Barcelona, Barcelona, Spain.

Arthroscopy was performed under diagnostic and/or therapeutic (lavage) conditions with a 2.7-mm arthroscope (Storz, Tullingen, Germany). Eight synovial tissue samples were obtained from the suprapatellar pouch and the medial and lateral gutter in each patient [3]. Four samples were fixed in 4% formaldehyde and embedded in paraffin wax for immunohistochemistry, and the remaining four, collected on RLT lysis buffer (Qiagen, Crawley, West Sussex, UK for RNA extraction.

Patients were evaluated every 3 to 4 months, and the treatment was changed if the disease remained active (that is, DAS28 > 3.2 or ≥ 2 swollen and tender joints). Therapy with methotrexate was initiated (up to 20 mg/week if tolerated), and if no response occurred or adverse events were noted, patients were switched to anti-TNF-α or to combined therapy, according to their rheumatologist's judgment. Clinical and biologic data (joint pattern, DAS28, C-reactive protein (CRP) and erythrocyte sedimentation rate (ESR), disease-modifying antirheumatic drugs (DMARDs), and biologic therapy administered) were collected at study inclusion and the last clinical control. Psoriasis severity at inclusion was evaluated by Physician Global Assessment [10].

Immunohistochemistry

Sequential sections of PsA synovial tissues were analyzed for the presence of lymphoid aggregates and the expression of the following markers by peroxidase immunohistochemical analysis. T cells were labeled with polyclonal rabbit anti-human CD3 (A0452; DAKO, Cambridge, UK); B cells, with mouse anti-human CD20 (clone L26, DAKO); and HEV, with rat anti-human PNAd (clone MECA-79; PharMingen, Oxford, UK). Antigen retrieval, which was required for most antibodies, was performed with microwave heating in 1 m*M* EDTA for 15 minutes.

Primary antibodies were developed with appropriate secondary biotinylated antibodies according to a biotin peroxidase-based method (ABC; Vector Laboratories, Burlingame, CA, USA), by using diaminobenzidine as chromogen. Sections were counterstained in Gill hematoxylin.

Analysis of lymphoid aggregates

The highest grade of lymphoid aggregation within each synovial tissue sample was determined according to a previously described scoring method [11] based on the number of radial cell counts: grade 1, two to five radial cell counts; grade 2, six to 10 radial cell counts; and grade 3, more than 10 radial cell counts. The presence of T/B cell segregation and PNAd+ HEV within lymphoid aggregates was analyzed.

Real-time quantitative PCR

Total RNA was extracted from ST samples of 46 PsA patients by using the RNeasy FFPE Kit (Qiagen) according to the manufacturer's recommendations. cDNA was synthesized by using a high-capacity cDNA archive kit (Applied Biosystems, Warrington, UK). The primers for *CCR7, IFN-γ, IL-1β, IL-2, IL-6, IL-7, IL-8, IL-10, IL-12A, IL-13, IL-15, IL-17A, IL-18, IL-21, IL-22, IL-23A, IL-28, IL-33, TGF-β1, TNF- α*, and lymphotoxin (*LTβ*), were purchased from Applied Biosystems, and gene expression was measured with duplicate quantitative real-time PCR by using the TaqMan Gene Expression Assay (Applied Biosystems).

The expression of 23 target genes and one housekeeping gene (*GAPDH*) was measured with qPCR. To quantify transcript levels, target-gene Ct values were normalized by using the DeltaCt method (ΔCt = Ct reference gene - Ct target gene). Fold changes were calculated by using the differences of medians of the two groups, and a nonparametric Mann-Whitney-Wilcoxon test was used to examine statistically different expression patterns between groups. A P value of ≤ 0.05 was considered statistically significant. Ct values were calculated by using the SDS 2.4 and RQ Manager software (Applied Biosystems).

Quantification of cytokines in synovial fluid

SF cytokines were analyzed by using Quantibody Human TH17 Array 1 (GM-CSF, IL-1β, IL-2, IL-4, IL-5, IL-6, IL-10, IL-12p70, IL-13, IL-17A, IL-17F, IL-21, IL-22, IL-23, IFN-γ, CCL20, TGF-β1, TNF-α, and TNF-β) (RayBiotech, Norcross, GA, USA), according to the manufacturer's specifications. Each sample was prepared in quadruplicate. An Axon scanner 4000B with GenePix software was used to collect fluorescence intensities. Detection limits for cytokines are displayed on the manufacture's website [12].

IL-15 levels in synovial fluid supernatants were measured with enzyme-linked immunoassay (ELISA), as previously described [13].

Statistical analysis

Numeric variables were described as median and interquartile range (IQR), and categoric variables, as frequencies and percentages. The Wilcoxon Rank Sum test or Kruskal-Wallis test was used to compare the distribution of numeric variables between groups.

The Fisher Exact test was used to compare categoric variables. Correlation between numeric variables was expressed by Spearman correlation coefficient, and the null hypothesis was tested (coefficient = zero).

Correlation between two categoric variables or between one numeric and one categoric variable was assessed by using the Fisher Exact test and the Wilcoxon Rank Sum test or Kruskal-Wallis test. Univariate and multivariate logistic regression models were performed to evaluate association with LN, and the area under the curve (AUC) of the receiver operating characteristic (ROC) curve was used to assess the performance of prediction models. Classifiers with an AUC > 0.5 have at least some ability to discriminate between groups. All analyses were performed by using R statistical environment, version 2.12.1 [14].

Results

Clinical and demographic data

Forty-six PsA patients (57% male), aged (median; IQR) 50 (37; 61) years were included; disease duration at inclusion was 7.5 years (3.7; 13), and follow-up time after inclusion was 27 months (9; 52). Twenty-three (50%) patients had oligoarthritis, 18 (39%), polyarthritis, and five (11%), mixed-pattern (peripheral arthritis with axial involvement. PGA was 21 (46%) clear, 22 (48%) mild, and three (6%) moderate.

C-reactive protein (CRP) was 0.7 (0.3; 2) mg/dl; TJC, 1 (1; 2); SJC, 1 (1; 2); and DAS28, 3.3 (3; 4.2). Three patients were RF positive at low titers (< 80 U/mL), and no patient was ACPA positive (> 25 U/mL) (Table 1).

Twenty-eight (60.3%) patients were treated during the follow-up: 23 with methotrexate, three of them combined with TNF-blockers, and five with TNF-blockers in monotherapy. In this cohort, the main target of treatment was arthritis. LN-negative patients were treated with significantly more TNF-blockers than were LN-positive patients, but this finding could reflect differences in the rheumatologist criteria (Table 1).

Twelve (26%) patients had erosive disease at the end of follow-up, without differences between LN-positive and -negative patients.

Of the 28 patients treated during follow-up, 71% achieved a EULAR response (46% good and 25% moderate), without differences between LN-positive and -negative patients (Table 1).

Synovial cytokine expression in the entire group of PsA patients

All 21 cytokine genes studied were expressed in ST in most patients, although some were expressed in fewer than 50% of patients (*IL-13, IL-17A, IL-21, IL-22*, and *IL-28A*). In SF, IL-12 and IL-28A were not detected at all, and some cytokines were detected in only a small percentage of patients in comparison with mRNA expression. The exceptions were SF IL-6, IL-15, and CCL20, which were detected in either ST or SF in > 80% of patients (Tables 2 and 3). No correlation was found between the two compartments for any cytokine, probably because of the dissociation of cytokine expression between ST and SF.

Correlation of cytokines with markers of disease activity

IL-23 A mRNA expression was correlated with CRP (r = 0.471; P = 0.001) and SJC (r = 0.350; P = 0.018), whereas SF levels of IL-6 and CCL-20 correlated with CRP levels (r = 0.377; P = 0.014; and r = 0.501; P < 0.0001, respectively).

Synovial cytokines and lymphoid neogenesis

Twenty (43.5%) patients had synovial LN (follicular aggregates grade ≥ 2 with T/B cell segregation and HEV). Previous studies in RA showed a good correlation between LN and the expression of cytokines *IL-7* and *LTβ* and several homing chemokines and their receptors [15]. In our PsA cohort, a modest, nonsignificant increase in CCR7, IL-7, and LTβ mRNA expression was detected in LN-positive patients (Table 2 and Figure 1). Differences between

Table 1 Clinical and biologic characteristics of patients stratified by lymphoid neogenesis

Demographic	All (*n* = 46)	LN+ (*n* = 20)	LN- (*n* = 26)	*P*
Age (years)	50 (37; 61)	48 (36; 59)	54 (38.5; 63)	NS
Male (%)	26 (57)	13 (65)	13 (50)	NS
Disease duration (years)	7.5 (3.75; 13)	6 (2; 14)	8 (4.5; 12.5)	NS
Follow-up (months)	27 (9; 52)	21 (8; 50)	27 (12; 55)	NS
Clinical status				
TJC	1 (1; 2)	1 (1; 2)	1 (1; 2)	NS
SJC	1 (1; 2)	1 (1; 2)	1 (1; 2)	NS
Articular pattern, *n* (%)				
Oligoarthritis	23 (50)	13 (57)	10 (43)	NS
Poliarthritis	18 (39)	7 (39)	11 (61)	
Mixed (peripheral plus axial)	5 (11)	2 (40)	3 (60)	
ESR (mm/h)	19 (10; 30)	20 (9; 31)	18 (12; 25)	NS
CRP (mg/dl)	0.72 (0.32; 2.01)	1.00 (0.51; 1.83)	0.44 (0.29; 2.32)	NS
DAS28	3.31 (3.01; 4.2)	3.31 (2.94; 4.14)	3.34 (3.01; 4.28)	NS
Erosive disease, *n* (%)	12 (26)	7 (35)	5 (19)	NS
Treatment				
DMARDs taken, *n* (%)	23 (50)	12 (60)	11 (42)	NS
TNF-blockers, *n* (%)	8 (17)	1 (5)	7 (27)	**0.041**
EULAR response	Treated (*n* = 28)	LN+ (*n* = 11)	LN- (*n* = 17)	*P*
No response, *n* (%)	8 (29)	3 (27)	5 (29)	0.541
Moderate, *n* (%)	7 (25)	4 (36)	3 (18)	
Good, *n* (%)	13 (46)	4 (36)	9 (53)	

Data are expressed as median (IQR) or as percentage.

Table 2 RT-PCR of 21 cytokine genes expressed as Delta Ct value and stratified by LN

	n (%) of positive patients	All *n* = 46	LN+ *n* = 20 (43.5%)	LN- *n* = 26 (52.4%)	Wilcoxon *P* value
CCR7	45 (98%)	8 (-10; -7)	-8 (-9; -7)	-8 (-10; -7)	0.465
IFN-γ	35 (76%)	-10 (-12; -9)	-10 (-11; -9)	-11 (-12; -8)	0.656
IL-10	45 (98%)	-7 (-8; -6)	-7 (-8; -7)	-7 (-8; -6)	0.312
IL-12A	41 (89%)	-9 (-10; -8)	-9 (-10; -8)	-10 (-11; -8)	0.188
IL-13	11 (24%)	-14 (-15; -13)	-15 (-16; -15)	-13 (-14; -11)	0.109
IL-15	42 (91%)	**-9 (-9; -8)**	**-8 (-9; -8)**	**-9 (-10; -8)**	**0.104**
IL-17A	15 (33%)	-11 (-13; -9)	-13 (-14; -11)	-11 (-11; -9)	0.121
IL-18	46 (100%)	-6 (-7; -6)	-7 (-7; -6)	-6 (-7; -5)	0.418
IL-1β	43 (94%)	-8 (-9; -7)	-9 (-9; -8)	-8 (-9; -7)	0.517
IL-2	29 (59%)	-12 (-14; -11)	-13 (-14; -11)	-12 (-14; -12)	0.846
IL-21	20 (43%)	-13 (-14; -12)	-13 (-14; -12)	-13 (-14; -12)	0.909
IL-22	7 (15%)	-12 (-14; -11)	-13 (-15; -12)	-11 (-13; -11)	0.629
IL-23A	45 (98%)	**-5 (-6; -5)**	**-5 (-6; -4)**	**-6 (-8; -5)**	**0.058**
IL-28A	21 (46%)	-10 (-12; -9)	-10 (-12; -8)	-11 (-11; -10)	0.622
IL-33	41 (89%)	-11 (-12; -9)	-11 (-12; -9)	-11 (-12; -9)	0.646
IL-6	44 (96%)	-8 (-10; -6)	-8 (-9; -7)	-8 (-10; -5)	0.706
IL-7	44 (96%)	-6 (-7; -6)	-6 (-7; -5)	-7 (-7; -6)	0.608
IL-8	46 (100%)	-4 (-6; -2)	-4 (-5; -3)	-3 (-6; -2)	0.877
LTβ	44 (96%)	-6 (-8; -5)	-6 (-7; -5)	-6 (-8; -6)	0.443
TGF-β1	46 (100%)	**-3 (-4; -2)**	**-3 (-4; -3)**	**-3 (-3; -2)**	**0.050**
TNF-α	46 (100%)	-7 (-8; -6)	-7 (-8; -6)	-7 (-8; -6)	0.816

Table 3 Cytokine levels (pg/mL) in patients with PsA stratified by LN

	n (%) of positive patients	All *n* = 42	LN+ *n* = 20 (47.6%)	LN- *n* = 22 (52.4%)	Wilcoxon *P* value
GM.CSF	4 (10%)	0 (0; 0)	0 (0; 0)	0 (0; 0)	0.051
IFN-γ	6 (14%)	0 (0; 0)	0 (0; 0)	0 (0; 0)	0.444
IL-1β	7 (7%)	0 (0; 0)	0 (0; 0)	0 (0; 0)	0.632
IL-2	21 (50%)	42 (0; 133)	0 (0; 151)	83 (0; 119)	0.851
IL-4	2 (2%)	0 (0; 0)	0 (0; 0)	0 (0; 0)	0.365
IL-5	19 (19%)	0 (0; 0)	0 (0; 0)	0 (0; 0)	0.440
IL-6	41 (98%)	1241 (503; 1,544)	1324 (764; 1,496)	1093 (258; 1,720)	0.462
IL-10	22 (52%)	4 (0; 13)	4.4 (0; 12)	0 (0; 14)	0.926
IL-12p70	0	0 (0; 0)	0 (0; 0)	0 (0; 0)	NA
IL-13	4 (10%)	0 (0; 0)	0 (0; 0)	0 (0; 0)	0.348
IL-15	38 (91%)	**114 (47; 197)**	**180 (109; 261)**	**62 (23; 115)**	**0.002**
IL-17	11 26%)	0 (0; 20)	0 (0; 7)	0 (0; 26)	0.757
IL-17F	12 (29%)	0 (0; 12)	0 (0; 6)	0 (0; 12)	0.728
IL-21	19 (45%)	0 (0; 817)	0 (0; 773)	0 (0; 958)	0.591
IL-22	1 (2%)	0 (0; 0)	0 (0; 0)	0 (0; 0)	0.317
IL-23	15 (36%)	0 (0; 212)	0 (0; 190)	0 (0; 262)	0.758
IL-28A	0	0 (0; 0)	0 (0; 0)	0 (0; 0)	NA
CCL20	34 (81%)	37 (6; 497)	23 (7; 284)	40 (1; 624)	0.752
TGF-β1	8 (19%)	0 (0; 0)	0 (0; 0)	0 (0; 446)	0.157
TNF-α	4 (10%)	0 (0; 0)	0 (0; 0)	0 (0; 0)	0.323
TNF-β	7 (17%)	0 (0; 0)	0 (0; 0)	0 (0; 0)	0.684

Data are expressed as median (IQR). NA, not applicable.

LN-positive and -negative patients (Wilcoxon $P < 0.06$) were found in ST in only two genes: *IL-23A* ($P = 0.058$) and *TGF-β1* ($P = 0.05$). The expression of *IL-23A* was higher in LN-positive patients, and that of *TGF-β1* was higher in LN-negative patients (Table 2 and Figure 2). The combination of *IL-23A* and *TGF-β1* in a multivariate logistic regression model of factors influencing LN confirmed these genes as predictors of LN [AUC, 0.736; 95% CI, 0.5897 to 0.8823; *IL-23 A*, OR, 1.62 (1.06 to 2.48); $P = 0.027$; *TGF-β1*, OR, 0.72 (0.05 to 1.03), $P = 0.075$)].

However, TGF-β1 mRNA expression correlated with the number of B-cell grade 3 aggregates ($r = 0.363$; $P = 0.046$) and with the percentage of B cells in synovial samples ($r = 0.508$; $P = 0.005$). Although not significantly higher in LN-positive patients, IL-21 mRNA expression strongly correlated with the number of B-cell grade 3 aggregates ($r = 0.686$; $P = 0.0048$).

ST IL-15 mRNA was higher in LN-positive patients, with only a trend to significance (Wilcoxon $P = 0.104$) (Table 2). In SF, only IL-15 levels were significantly higher in LN-positive patients (Wilcoxon $P = 0.0023$; Table 2). Accordingly, SF IL-15 levels correctly classified patients as LN positive or negative (AUC, 0.791; 95% CI, 0.64 to 0.941; Table 3).

Discussion

It has been suggested that ectopic LN might play a role in the pathogenesis of chronic inflammatory conditions by driving T-cell responses and producing proinflammatory cytokines [16]. The proportion of our PsA patients showing LN features is similar to that described previously and also to that of studies in RA [3,4]. The clinical significance of ectopic LN has recently been analyzed in RA, in which several studies point to more-refractory disease [4], greater inflammation [17], and more-erosive disease in this subset of patients [18].

Our study provides the first approach to this issue in PsA. Because PsA is not associated with B-cell responses, it represents a good model to explore whether T-cell polarization can be modified by LN, independent of B-cell responses. Our results show that PsA patients with synovial LN have a higher expression of *IL-23A* and a lower expression of *TGF-β1* in synovial tissue compared with LN-negative patients. The combination of these two genes in a multivariable logistic regression model confirmed that they were associated with LN. Additional differences of lower magnitude in IL-15 and IL-21 mRNA expression also pointed to subtle differences in the cytokine profile of this PsA subset.

An unexpected finding of our study is the weaker correlation between molecular markers of LN, such as CCR7, IL-7, and LTβ, and LN, as defined by T-/B-cell aggregates, T/B compartmentalization, and MECA-79 epitope expression. The expression of these factors has been associated with synovial LN in RA patients and experimental animal models [6,19-21]. It is possible that

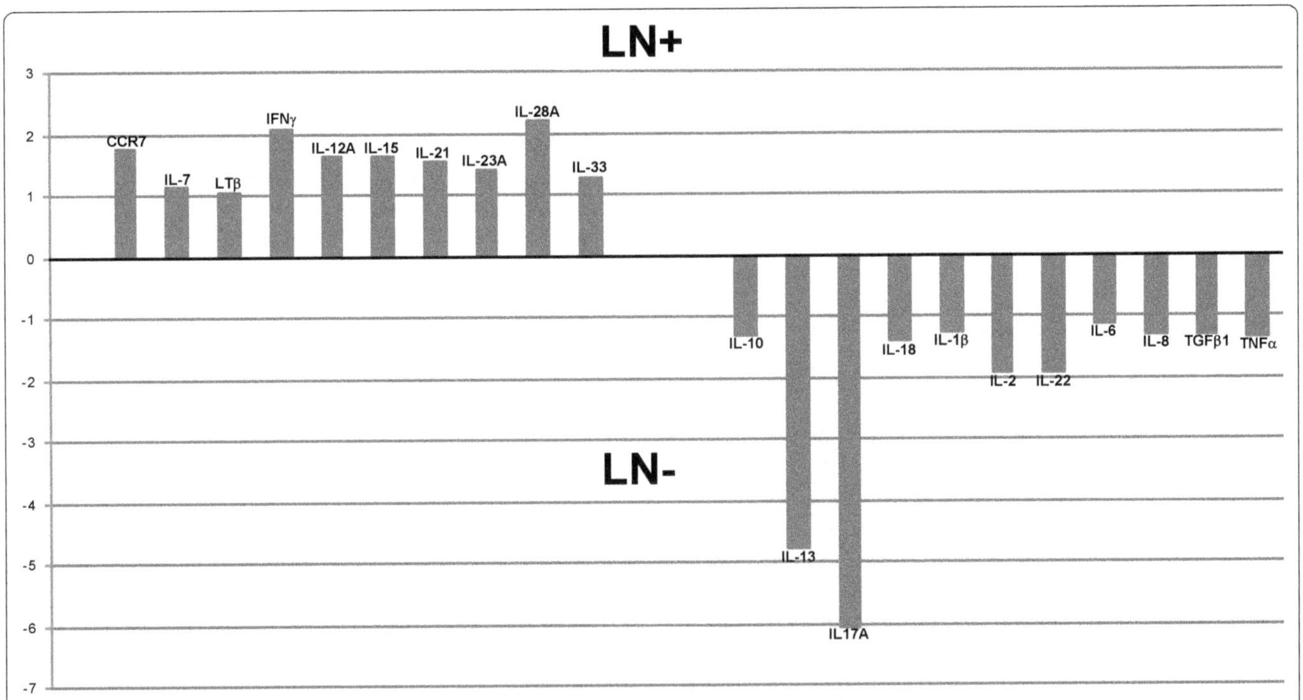

Figure 1 Distribution of mRNA of all cytokines studied according their higher relative expression (fold change) as lymphoid neogenesis (LN) positive (+) or negative (-).

the wide variation in the extension of lymphoid aggregates in different tissues, and the different histologic criteria used to identify LN may explain the variable associations of LN with molecular markers and disease severity found in different studies analyzing lymphocyte aggregation and organization [22]. This could lead to contradictory findings, as is the case with ST TGF-β1 mRNA expression, which was higher in LN-negative patients, but paradoxically, it correlated with B-cell aggregates grade 3 and strongly with the percentage of B cells in ST. Supporting this hypothesis, we specifically find a strong correlation between mature B-cell aggregates and IL-21 mRNA expression, but no significant differences according to LN classification.

We found an association between higher IL-23A mRNA expression and LN. Furthermore, IL-23A mRNA expression significantly correlated with SJC and CRP, and we noted a strong trend to correlate with DAS28. This finding did not correlate with the level of IL-23 in the SF, in which only a third of these patients had detectable IL-23.

IL-23 is expressed mainly by macrophages and dendritic cells and plays a key role in the differentiation and

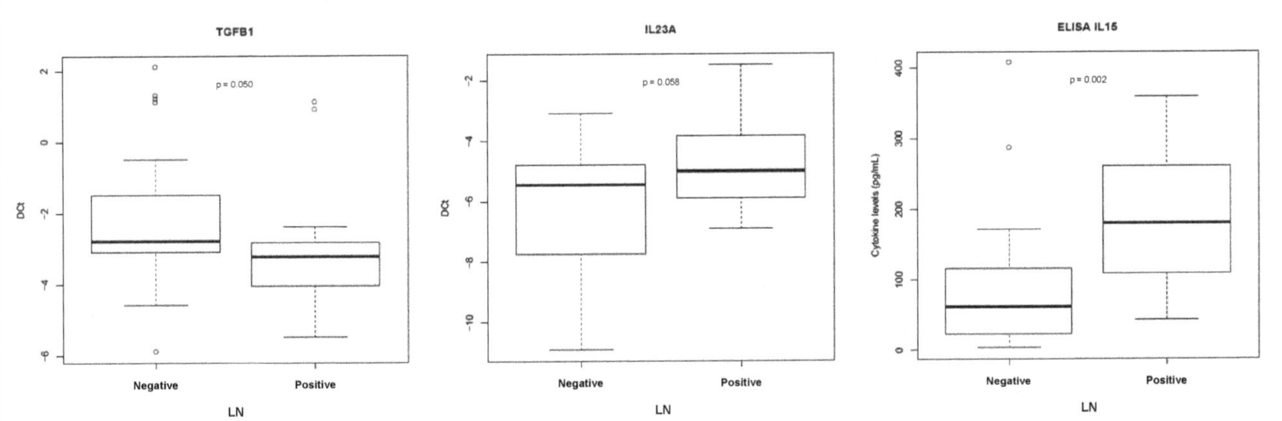

Figure 2 Differential expression of TGF-β1 and IL-23A mRNA in synovial tissue, and IL-15 levels in synovial fluid, according to lymphoid neogenesis (LN) status.

survival of Th17 cells and in IL-17 production by non-T cells [23]. IL-23 acts as an end-stage effector cytokine through direct action on macrophages [24], the main producers of proinflammatory cytokines in synovium. This mechanism of action is in line with our finding of a positive correlation between IL-23A ST expression and systemic markers of inflammation. However, a correlation between (serum) IL-23 levels and disease activity has previously been reported only in patients with RA [25,26].

The role of IL-23 in the pathogenesis of PsA is less clear. Genetic studies have confirmed the association of *IL-23A* and *IL-23R* genes with PsA susceptibility, underlining its potential pathogenetic relevance [27,28]. In addition, ustekinumab, an anti-IL-12/IL-23 antibody, has shown efficacy in PsA patients [29]. In ankylosing spondylitis, a disease grouped together with PsA in the concept of spondyloarthritis, a potential role for IL-23 has also been proposed [30]. Further research may better define the pathways through which IL-23 is produced and exerts its actions in PsA.

In this series, IL-15 mRNA was expressed in grossly 90% of paired ST and SF samples. Previous studies also detected IL-15 in PsA ST [31,32]. IL-15 stimulates the production of IL-17 in synovial monocytes and synergizes with IL-23 to increase IL-17 production. Additional effects on T- and B-cell survival and monocytes, mast cells, and neutrophils activation might also contribute to PsA pathogenesis [33,34]. In RA, IL-15 serum levels correlated with disease activity and may predict a severe disease course [35]. Our data show higher IL-15 expression in LN-positive patients, supporting its potential pathogenetic role. Overall, IL-15 and IL-23 expression would point to a link between LN and the Th17/IL-23 axis. However, the expression of Th17-related cytokines was moderate (IL-17A and IL-21) or very low (IL-22) in ST and SF, which may be in line with the low abundance of Th17 cells in PsA or SpA ST, in which the majority of IL-17-producing cells are non-T cells [36].

Regarding other factors potentially implicated in T-cell traffic and differentiation, in our study, SF CCL20 levels correlated with markers of inflammation. Previously a correlation was reported between SF CCL20 levels and the number of SF PMNs in PsA, but not with markers of disease activity [25]. CCL20 is a chemokine that attracts several types of cells, predominantly Th17 cells expressing the CCR6 receptor. In addition, it has been reported that IL-17F induces CCL20 production [37]. Upregulation of IL-23 and CCL20 in PsA supports the role of the IL-17/IL-23 axis disturbance in this disease. As expected, SF IL-6 levels correlated with CRP levels [38].

TGF-β1 is a multifaceted cytokine participating in many biologic processes: inflammation, fibrosis, lymphocyte recruitment, and lymphocyte-effector differentiation (Treg and Th17) [39]. Given that no previous reports exist of TGF-β1 in PsA, it is difficult to ascertain the clinical significance of the lower expression of these cytokines in LN in this disease.

Although these data suggest that synovial LN might be associated with a distinctive cytokine profile with a more-inflammatory phenotype, we found no clinical differences between LN-positive and -negative patients.

Our study has some limitations. First, all samples of ST and SF are from knee arthritis, which may not be representative of other inflamed joints in the same patient. However, previous studies in RA patients suggested that ST from an active joint is a good representation of other active joints in the same patient [40]. Another limitation is that this is a retrospective study, with established disease in the majority of patients, when the ideal scenario for evaluating the clinical significance of LN might be early untreated PsA patients [22]. Nevertheless, our exploratory study identifies some differences in the cytokine profile that support the existence of pathogenetic differences in the LN-positive PsA subset.

Conclusion

The results of this study suggest differences in the cytokine profile of PsA patients with LN, with a higher expression of *IL-23A* and IL-15 and a lower expression of *TGF-β1*. This cytokine pattern was not accompanied by gross clinical or biologic differences between LN-positive and -negative patients. In the entire group of patients, *IL-23A* ST expression and CCL20 SF levels strongly correlated with markers of disease activity. Taken together, these results suggest a role of the IL-17/IL-23 axis in synovial LN in PsA.

Abbreviations

CCL20: CC-Chemokine Ligand 20; CCR7: CC-Chemokine Receptor type 7; CRP: C-reactive protein; DAS28: 28-joint Disease Activity Score; DMARDs: disease-modifying antirheumatic drugs; ESR: erythrocyte sedimentation rate; IFN-γ: interferon gamma; IL: interleukin; LT-β: lymphotoxin β; TGF-β1: transforming growth factor β1; TJC: tender-joint count; SJC: swollen-joint count; TNF-α: tumor necrosis factor-α; TNF-β: tumor necrosis factor-β.

Acknowledgements

We thank Juan Jose Lozano, Plataforma Bioinformática de Barcelona, CIBERehd, Barcelona, Spain, for his advice on statistical analysis.
JDC was supported by a grant from Fondo de Investigación Sanitaria, Ministerio de Sanidad de España, PI080206, and by Red de Investigación en Inflamación y Enfermedades Reumáticas (RIER), Instituto Carlos III, RD008/0075/0006. Cofinanciado por FEDER, Unión Europea. JLFS is supported by a grant from Fondo de Investigación Sanitaria, Ministerio de Sanidad de España, PI11/00390.

Author details

[1]Arthritis Unit, Rheumatology Department, Hospital Clinic de Barcelona and IDIBAPS, c/Villarroel, 170, 08036 Barcelona, Spain. [2]Plataforma de Bioinformática, Centro de Investigación Biomédica en Red de Enfermedades Hepáticas y Digestivas (CIBERehd), c/Córcega 180, 08036 Barcelona, Spain. [3]Rheumatology Division, Complejo Hospitalario Universitario, c/Xubias, 84,

15006 La Coruña, Spain. [4]Rheumatology Department, Hospital Universitario de la Princesa, IIS Princesa. c/Diego de León, 62, 28006 Madrid, Spain. [5]Instituto de Investigación, Hospital 12 de Octubre (I+12), Avda Córdoba s/n° 28041 Madrid, Spain.

Authors' contributions
JDC had full access to all the data in the study and takes responsibility for the integrity of the data and the accuracy of data analysis. JDC and JLP were responsible for the study design. RC, NP, JLFS, RS, JR, IGA, JLP, and JDC performed data acquisition, analysis, interpretation, and final approval of the manuscript. NP performed statistical analysis. Manuscript preparation was by JDC, JLP, and RC. All authors read and approved the final manuscript.

Competing interests
The authors declare that they have no competing interests.

References

1. Fitzgerald O, Winchester R: **Psoriatic arthritis: from pathogenesis to therapy.** *Arthritis Res Ther* 2009, **11**:214.
2. Kruithof E, Baeten D, De Rycke L, Vandooren B, Foell D, Roth J, Cañete JD, Boots AM, Veys EM, De Keyser F: **Synovial histopathology of psoriatic arthritis, both oligo- and polyarticular, resembles spondyloarthropathy more than it does rheumatoid arthritis.** *Arthritis Res Ther* 2005, **7**: R569-R580.
3. Cañete JD, Santiago B, Cantaert T, Sanmartí R, Palacin A, Celis R, Graell E, Gil-Torregrosa B, Baeten D, Pablos JL: **Ectopic lymphoid neogenesis in psoriatic arthritis.** *Ann Rheum Dis* 2007, **66**:720-726.
4. Cañete JD, Celis R, Moll C, Izquierdo E, Marsal S, Sanmartí R, Palacín A, Lora D, de la Cruz J, Pablos JL: **Clinical significance of synovial lymphoid neogenesis and its reversal after anti-tumour necrosis factor alpha therapy in rheumatoid arthritis.** *Ann Rheum Dis* 2009, **68**:751-756.
5. Cantaert T, Kolln J, Timmer T, van der Pouw Kraan TC, Vandooren B, Thurlings RM, Cañete JD, Catrina AI, Out T, Verweij CL, Zhang Y, Tak PP, Baeten D: **B lymphocyte autoimmunity in rheumatoid synovitis is independent of ectopic lymphoid neogenesis.** *J Immunol* 2008, **181**:785-794.
6. Weyand CM, Kurtin PJ, Goronzy JJ: **Ectopic lymphoid organogenesis: a fast track for autoimmunity.** *Am J Pathol* 2001, **159**:787-793.
7. Vander Cruyssen B, Hoffman IE, Zmierczak H, Van den Berghe M, Kruithof E, De Rycke L, Mielants H, Veys EM, Baeten D, De Keyser F: **Anti-citrullinated peptide antibodies may occur in patients with psoriatic arthritis.** *Ann Rheum Dis* 2005, **64**:1145-1149.
8. Takemura S, Klimiuk PA, Braun A, Goronzy JJ, Weyand CM: **T cell activation in rheumatoid synovium is B cell dependent.** *J Immunol* 2001, **167**:4710-4718.
9. Taylor W, Gladman D, Helliwell P, Marchesoni A, Mease P, Mielants H, The CASPAR Study Group: **Classification criteria for psoriatic arthritis: development of new criteria from a large international study.** *Arthritis Rheum* 2006, **54**:2665-2673.
10. Robinson A, Kardos M, Kimball AB: **Physician Global Assessment (PGA) and Psoriasis Area and Severity Index (PASI): Why do both? A systematic analysis of randomized controlled trials of biologic agents for moderate to severe plaque psoriasis.** *J Am Acad Dermatol* 2012, **66**:369-375.
11. Manzo A, Paoletti S, Carulli M, Blades MC, Barone F, Yanni G, Fitzgerald O, Bresnihan B, Caporali R, Montecucco C, Uguccioni M, Pitzalis C: **Systematic microanatomical analysis of CXCL13 and CCL21 in situ production and progressive lymphoid organization in rheumatoid synovitis.** *Eur J Immunol* 2005, **35**:1347-1359.
12. **RayBiotech.** [http://www.raybiotech.com].
13. Ortiz AM, Laffon A, Gonzalez-Alvaro I: **CD69 expression on lymphocytes and interleukin-15 levels in synovial fluids from different inflammatory arthropathies.** *Rheumatol Int* 2002, **21**:182-188.
14. R Development Core Team: **R: A Language and Environment For Statistical Computing. R Foundation for Statistical Computing, Vienna, Austria.** 2010 [http://www.R-project.org], ISBN 3-900051-07-0.
15. Timmer TC, Baltus B, Vondenhoff M, Huizinga TW, Tak PP, Verweij CL, Mebius RE, van der Pouw Kraan TC: **Inflammation and ectopic lymphoid structures in rheumatoid arthritis synovial tissues dissected by genomics technology: identification of the interleukin-7 signaling pathway in tissues with lymphoid neogenesis.** *Arthritis Rheum* 2007, **56**:2492-2502.
16. Weyand CM, Kang YM, Kurtin PJ, Goronzy JJ: **The power of the third dimension: tissue architecture and autoimmunity in rheumatoid arthritis.** *Curr Opin Rheumatol* 2003, **15**:259-266.
17. Thurlings RM, Wijbrandts CA, Mebius RE, Cantaert T, Dinant HJ, van der Pouw-Kraan TC, Verweij CL, Baeten D, Tak PP: **Synovial lymphoid neogenesis does not define a specific clinical rheumatoid arthritis phenotype.** *Arthritis Rheum* 2008, **58**:1582-1589.
18. Bugatti S, Manzo A, Vitolo B, Fusetti C, Caporali R, Pitzalis C, Montecucco C: **Clinical, radiographic and biomolecular features of B cell synovitis in rheumatoid arthritis [Abstract].** *Arthritis Rheum* 2011, **62**:S110.
19. Takemura S, Braun A, Crowson C, Kurtin PJ, Cofield RH, O'Fallon WM, Goronzy JJ, Weyand CM: **Lymphoid neogenesis in rheumatoid synovitis.** *J Immunol* 2001, **167**:1072-1080.
20. Braun A, Takemura S, Vallejo AN, Goronzy JJ, Weyand CM: **Lymphotoxin beta-mediated stimulation of synoviocytes in rheumatoid arthritis.** *Arthritis Rheum* 2004, **50**:2140-2150.
21. Wengner AM, Höpken UE, Petrow PK, Hartmann S, Schurigt U, Bräuer R, Lipp M: **CXCR5- and CCR7-dependent lymphoid neogenesis in a murine model of chronic antigen-induced arthritis.** *Arthritis Rheum* 2007, **56**:3271-3283.
22. Bugatti S, Manzo A, Bombardieri M, Vitolo B, Humby F, Kelly S, Montecucco C, Pitzalis C: **Synovial tissue heterogeneity and peripheral blood biomarkers.** *Curr Rheumatol Rep* 2011, **13**:440-448.
23. Tang C, Chen S, Qian H, Huang W: **Interleukin-23 as a target drug for autoimmune inflammatory diseases.** *Immunology* 2011, **135**:112-124.
24. Cua DJ, Sherlock J, Chen Y, Murphy CA, Joyce B, Seymour B, Lucian L, To W, Kwan S, Churakova T, Zurawski S, Wiekowski M, Lira SA, Gorman D, Kastelein RA, Sedgwick JD: **Interleukin-23 rather than interleukin-12 is the critical cytokine for autoimmune inflammation of the brain.** *Nature* 2003, **421**:744-748.
25. Melis L, Vandooren B, Kruithof E, Jacques P, De Vos M, Mielants H, Verbruggen G, De Keyser F, Elewaut D: **Systemic levels of IL-23 are strongly associated with disease activity in rheumatoid arthritis but not spondyloarthritis.** *Ann Rheum Dis* 2010, **69**:618-623.
26. Rasmussen TK, Andersen T, Hvid M, Hetland ML, Hørslev-Petersen K, Stengaard-Pedersen K, Holm CK, Deleuran B: **Increased interleukin 21 (IL-21) and IL-23 are associated with increased disease activity and with radiographic status in patients with early rheumatoid arthritis.** *J Rheumatol* 2010, **37**:2014-2020.
27. Filer C, Ho P, Smith RL, Griffiths C, Young HS, Worthington J, Bruce IN, Barton A: **Investigation of association of the *IL12B* and *IL23R* genes with psoriatic arthritis.** *Arthritis Rheum* 2008, **58**:3705-3709.
28. Bowes J, Orozco G, Flynn E, Ho P, Brier R, Marzo-Ortega H, Coates L, McManus R, Ryan AW, Kane D, Korendowych E, McHugh N, FitzGerald O, Packham J, Morgan AW, Bruce IN, Barton A: **Confirmation of *TNIP1* and *IL23A* as susceptibility loci for psoriatic arthritis.** *Ann Rheum Dis* 2011, **70**:1641-1644.
29. Gottlieb A, Menter A, Mendelsohn A, Shen YK, Li S, Guzzo C, Fretzin S, Kunynetz R, Kavanaugh A: **Ustekinumab, a human interleukin 12/23 monoclonal antibody, for psoriatic arthritis: randomised, double-blind, placebo-controlled, crossover trial.** *Lancet* 2009, **373**:633-640.
30. Gaston JS, Goodall JC, Baeten D: **Interleukin-23: a central cytokine in the pathogenesis of spondyloarthritis.** *Arthritis Rheum* 2011, **63**:3668-3671.
31. Danning CL, Illei GG, Hitchon C, Greer MR, Boumpas DT, McInnes IB: **Macrophage-derived cytokine and nuclear factor kappaB p65 expression in synovial membrane and skin of patients with psoriatic arthritis.** *Arthritis Rheum* 2000, **43**:1244-1256.
32. Kane D, Gogarty M, O'Leary J, Silva I, Bermingham N, Bresnihan B, Fitzgerald O: **Reduction of synovial sublining layer inflammation and proinflammatory cytokine expression in psoriatic arthritis treated with methotrexate.** *Arthritis Rheum* 2004, **50**:3286-3295.
33. McInnes IB, Liew FY: **Interleukin 15: a proinflammatory role in rheumatoid arthritis synovitis.** *Immunol Today* 1998, **19**:75-79.
34. Noordenbos T, Yeremenko N, Gofita I, van de Sande M, Tak PP, Cañete JD, Baeten D: **Interleukin-17-positive mast cells contribute to synovial inflammation in spondylarthritis.** *Arthritis Rheum* 2012, **64**:99-109.
35. González-Álvaro I, Ortiz AM, Alvaro-Gracia JM, Castañeda S, Díaz-Sánchez B, Carvajal I, García-Vadillo JA, Humbría A, López-Bote JP, Patiño E, Tomero EG, Vicente EF, Sabando P, García-Vicuña R: **Interleukin 15 levels in serum may**

predict a severe disease course in patients with early arthritis. *PLoS One* 2011, **6**:e29492.

36. Yeremenko N, Baeten D: **IL-17 in spondyloarthritis: is the T-party over?** *Arthritis Res Ther* 2011, **13**:115.
37. Nozato K, Fujita J, Kawaguchi M, Ohara G, Morishima Y, Ishii Y, Huang SK, Kokubu F, Satoh H, Hizawa N: **IL-17F induces CCL20 in bronchial epithelial cells.** *J Allergy (Cairo)* 2011, **2011**:587204.
38. Alenius GM, Eriksson C, Rantapää Dahlqvist S: **Interleukin-6 and soluble interleukin-2 receptor alpha-markers of inflammation in patients with psoriatic arthritis?** *Clin Exp Rheumatol* 2009, **27**:120-123.
39. Wahl SM, Orenstein JM, Chen W: **TGF-beta influences the life and death decisions of T lymphocytes.** *Cytokine Growth Factor Rev* 2000, **11**:71-79.
40. Kraan MC, Reece RJ, Smeets TJ, Veale DJ, Emery P, Tak PP: **Comparison of synovial tissues from the knee joints and the small joints of rheumatoid arthritis patients: implication for pathogenesis and evaluation of treatment.** *Arthritis Rheum* 2002, **46**:2034-2038.

5

Secukinumab provides sustained PASDAS-defined remission in psoriatic arthritis and improves health-related quality of life in patients achieving remission: 2-year results from the phase III FUTURE 2 study

L. C. Coates[1*], D. D. Gladman[2], P. Nash[3], O. FitzGerald[4], A. Kavanaugh[5], T. K. Kvien[6], L. Gossec[7,8], V. Strand[9], L. Rasouliyan[10], L. Pricop[11], K. Ding[11], S. M. Jugl[12], C. Gaillez[12] and on behalf of the FUTURE 2 study group

Abstract

Background: Secukinumab has demonstrated sustained improvement in the signs and symptoms of psoriatic arthritis (PsA) over 2 years in the FUTURE 2 study (NCT01752634). This post hoc analysis assessed the ability of secukinumab to achieve Psoriatic Arthritis Disease Activity Score (PASDAS)-based remission or low disease activity (LDA) through 2 years among patients with PsA in the FUTURE 2 study.

Methods: PASDAS (cut-off scores: remission ≤ 1.9; LDA > 1.9 and < 3.2; Moderate Disease Activity ≥ 3.2 and < 5.4; and high disease activity [HDA] ≥ 5.4) was assessed in the overall population (tumour necrosis factor inhibitor [TNFi]-naïve and TNFi-experienced), in patients stratified by prior TNFi use and by disease duration at weeks 16, 52 and 104. The impact of secukinumab on individual PASDAS core components and on the relationship between PASDAS states and patient-reported outcomes (PROs), including physical function, health-related quality of life (HRQoL) and work productivity, were also assessed. Data for the approved doses of secukinumab (300 and 150 mg) are reported. PASDAS scores and core components were reported as observed, and PROs were analysed using mixed models for repeated measures.

Results: In the overall population, PASDAS remission and LDA were achieved in 15.6% and 22.9%, respectively, of patients treated with secukinumab 300 mg and in 15.2% and 19.2%, respectively, in the secukinumab 150 mg group versus 2.3% and 13.8%, respectively, with placebo at week 16. In the TNFi-naïve group, a higher proportion of patients achieved remission + LDA at week 16 with secukinumab 300 and 150 mg (46.2% and 42.9%, respectively) versus placebo (17.5%), with corresponding responses in TNFi-experienced patients being 22.6% and 19.4% versus 13.3%. Remission/LDA responses with secukinumab were sustained through 2 years. Patients achieving remission/LDA reported greater improvements in PROs than patients in HDA through 2 years.

(Continued on next page)

* Correspondence: laura.coates@ndorms.ox.ac.uk
[1]Nuffield Department of Orthopaedics, Rheumatology and Musculoskeletal Sciences, University of Oxford, Botnar Research Centre, Windmill Road, Oxford OX3 7LD, UK
Full list of author information is available at the end of the article

(Continued from previous page)

Conclusions: Secukinumab-treated patients achieved higher PASDAS-defined remissions or LDA compared with placebo at week 16, which were sustained through 2 years. Remission/LDA was achieved by both TNFi-naïve and TNFi-experienced patients treated with secukinumab, with higher rates in TNFi-naïve patients. Secukinumab-treated patients achieving remission/LDA reported significantly greater improvements in PROs, including physical function and different dimensions of health-related quality of life and work, than patients in HDA.

Keywords: Psoriatic arthritis, Secukinumab, PASDAS, Remission, Interleukin-17A, FUTURE 2 study

Introduction

Psoriatic arthritis (PsA) is an inflammatory musculoskeletal disease comprising several domains, including peripheral arthritis, axial disease, enthesitis, dactylitis, and skin and nail disease [1, 2]. Different tools, such as Disease Activity Score (DAS) and American College of Rheumatology (ACR) response criteria, which primarily focus on peripheral joint manifestations and were validated in patients with rheumatoid arthritis, have been used for measuring joint responses in PsA. However, outcome measures borrowed from rheumatoid arthritis, such as ACR response criteria and DAS28-CRP, do not reflect the variety of disease manifestations [3, 4]. One of the overarching principles of the treat-to-target recommendations for patients with PsA by international task forces [5], the Group for Research and Assessment of Psoriasis and Psoriatic Arthritis (GRAPPA) [6], and the European League Against Rheumatism (EULAR) [7] is to achieve the lowest possible level of disease activity across all domains of disease. Disease remission and low/minimal disease activity are defined by the minimal disease activity (MDA), which measures all domains of the disease, or Disease Activity Index for Psoriatic Arthritis (DAPSA), which measures peripheral arthritis and acute-phase reactants [4, 8, 9].

Another measure, the Psoriatic Arthritis Disease Activity Score (PASDAS), was developed by the GRAPPA Composite Exercise Project and provides different validated thresholds to identify remission, low disease activity (LDA), moderate disease activity (MoDA) and high disease activity (HDA) [10]. PASDAS assesses multiple manifestations of PsA, distinguishes treatment effects, performs better than traditional joint-only indices, and can be used as a treatment target in PsA randomized controlled trials (RCTs) [10–12].

Secukinumab, a fully human IgG1 monoclonal antibody that selectively neutralizes IL-17A, has substantial efficacy in the treatment of moderate to severe psoriasis, PsA and ankylosing spondylitis, demonstrating rapid onset of action and sustained responses with a favourable safety profile [13–19]. In the placebo-controlled, double-blind, phase III FUTURE 2 trial (NCT01752634), secukinumab treatment resulted in significant improvements in key clinical domains of PsA compared with placebo, and these improvements were sustained through week 104 [15, 16].

In the present study, we explored the ability of secukinumab-treated patients to achieve remission or LDA using PASDAS scores at weeks 16, 52 and 104 in the FUTURE 2 study. This post hoc analysis also determined the impact of secukinumab on individual components of PASDAS and the relationship of PASDAS states with patient-reported outcomes (PROs), including health related-quality of life (HRQoL), physical function, work productivity and activity impairments.

Methods

Study design and patients

FUTURE 2 is a phase III multicentre RCT designed to evaluate the efficacy and safety of subcutaneous secukinumab treatment in patients with active PsA. Details of the study design, inclusion and exclusion criteria, and 104-week efficacy and safety results have been reported previously [15, 16]. Briefly, patients were randomized (1:1:1:1) to receive subcutaneous (s.c.) secukinumab 300, 150 or 75 mg or placebo at baseline; weeks 1, 2, 3 and 4; and every 4 weeks thereafter. Placebo-treated patients were re-randomized to receive secukinumab 300 or 150 mg at either week 16 or week 24, based on clinical responses [15]. Data only with the approved doses of secukinumab (i.e., 300 and 150 mg) and placebo are reported herein.

The study was conducted in accordance with the principles of the Declaration of Helsinki, the International Conference on Harmonisation good clinical practice guidelines, and all applicable laws and regulations. All centres received approval from independent ethics committees or institutional review boards (IRBs). Patients provided written informed consent before starting the study-related procedures. The details of the study were mentioned in the earlier FUTURE 2 publications [15, 16].

Outcomes

PASDAS is a composite score that includes physician and patient global assessment of skin and joint disease by visual analogue scale (VAS), the physical component summary score of the Medical Outcomes Study Short Form Health Survey (SF-36 PCS), swollen joint count based on 66 joints (SJC66), tender joint count based on 68 joints (TJC68), Leeds Enthesitis Index enthesitis count, tender dactylitis count and CRP level [6, 11]. The continuous PASDAS score [11] was calculated for each patient with evaluable data at each point of interest. Disease activity states are defined as follows:

- Remission: PASDAS score ≤ 1.9
- LDA: 1.9 < PASDAS score < 3.2
- MoDA: 3.2 ≤ PASDAS score < 5.4
- HDA: PASDAS score ≥ 5.4

The proportions of patients in remission, LDA, MoDA and HDA were assessed at weeks 16, 52 and 104 in the overall population, and patients stratified by prior TNF inhibitor treatment (TNFi-naïve or TNFi-experienced) or by time since diagnosis (≤ 2 versus > 2 years). Shifts in disease activity in patients in each PASDAS state at week 16 were evaluated for secukinumab 300 and 150 mg treatment to assess sustainability of responses at weeks 52 and 104.

PASDAS states and individual core components

The impact of secukinumab treatment on individual PASDAS components was calculated among patients categorized in each disease activity state at weeks 16, 52 and 104.

PASDAS states and patient-reported outcomes

The relationship between PASDAS disease activity and PROs was assessed at weeks 16, 52 and 104 using data pooled across the treatment groups. HRQoL was assessed using SF-36 PCS (a component of the PASDAS score) and SF-36 MCS scores, Psoriatic Arthritis Quality of Life questionnaire (PsAQoL), Dermatology Life Quality Index (DLQI), physical function by Health Assessment Questionnaire Disability Index (HAQ-DI), fatigue by Functional Assessment of Chronic Illness Therapy–Fatigue (FACIT-Fatigue) and work productivity by the Work Productivity and Activity Impairment (WPAI) questionnaire.

Statistical analysis

The percentages of patients in each PASDAS disease activity state in the overall population (TNFi-naïve and TNFi-experienced) and by prior TNFi treatment status and disease duration at baseline were reported using mutually exclusive categories at the group level according to as-observed analyses, including shifts in disease activity states from week 16 to weeks 52/104.

Median, first (Q1) and third quartiles (Q3) were computed for each of the individual core PASDAS components at weeks 16, 52 and 104 for each disease activity state in patients with data at weeks 16/52 and 16/104.

Additionally, SF-36 PCS and MCS scores, PsAQoL, DLQI, HAQ-DI, FACIT-Fatigue and WPAI were assessed at weeks 16, 52 and 104 using mixed models for repeated measures (MMRM) analyses with analysis visit, PASDAS disease activity state at the analysis visit (remission, LDA, MoDA and HDA), and randomization stratum (TNFi-naïve or TNFi-experienced) as factors and weight and baseline score as continuous covariates. PASDAS disease activity state and baseline score by analysis visit were included as interaction terms. An unstructured covariance structure was used for MMRM analysis. Least-squares mean (LSM) estimates and SEs along with *P* values were provided at each assessment for patients in each disease activity state. Analysis data were pooled across treatment arms (secukinumab + placebo) pertaining to relationship between PASDAS disease activity states and PROs. All statistical analyses were performed using SAS version 9.4 or higher software (SAS Institute, Cary, NC, USA).

Results

Patients

Demographic and baseline characteristics were well balanced across treatment groups in FUTURE 2 [15]; the parameters relevant to PASDAS are shown in Table 1. Mean (SD) PASDAS scores at baseline were 5.9 (0.9), 6.0 (1.0) and 5.8 (1.0) in the secukinumab 300 mg, secukinumab 150 mg and placebo groups, respectively. At baseline, > 60% of patients were TNFi-naïve across the groups (Table 1). Retention rates of enrolled patients at week 104 were 86% (86/100) and 76% (76/100) with secukinumab 300 and 150 mg, respectively. Discontinuations due to lack of efficacy at week 104 were 3% (3/100) and 7% (7/100) in the secukinumab 300 and 150 mg groups, respectively [16].

PASDAS states

In the overall population, a higher proportion of secukinumab 300 mg (38.5% [37/96]) and 150 mg (34.3% [34/99])-treated patients achieved PASDAS remission + LDA at week 16 versus placebo (16.1% [14/87]). At week 104, 22.9% (19/83) and 14.3% (11/77) patients achieved remission, and 36.1% (30/83) and 35.1% (27/77) patients reached LDA with secukinumab 300 and 150 mg, respectively. The proportions of patients in PASDAS remission, LDA, MoDA and HDA at weeks 16, 52 and 104 are depicted in Fig. 1a. The shift analysis from weeks 16 to 104 showed that the majority of secukinumab 300 mg-treated patients who achieved remission at week 16 maintained remission (60%) or were in LDA (40%) at week 104, and 79% of patients in LDA at week 16 maintained or improved their status to remission at week

Table 1 Demographics and baseline disease characteristics relevant to Psoriatic Arthritis Disease Activity Score

Characteristic mean (SD) unless otherwise stated	Secukinumab 300 mg s.c. (*N* = 100)	Secukinumab 150 mg s.c. (*N* = 100)	Placebo (*N* = 98)
Age, years	46.9 (12.6)	46.5 (11.7)	49.9 (12.5)
Female, *n* (%)	49 (49.0)	45 (45.0)	59 (60.2)
Time since diagnosis of PsA in years	7.4 (7.5)	6.5 (8.2)	7.3 (7.8)
TNFi-naïve, *n* (%)	67 (67.0)	63 (63.0)	63 (64.3)
Psoriasis ≥ 3% of BSA, *n* (%)	41 (41.0)	58 (58.0)	43 (43.9)
Physician's global VAS	55.0 (14.7)	56.7 (16.6)	55.0 (16.0)
Patient's global VAS	60.7 (18.9)	62.0 (19.5)	57.6 (19.8)
SF-36 PCS	36.9 (8.0)	36.2 (8.1)	37.4 (8.8)
Dactylitis count[a]	3.6 (3.5)	4.5 (5.1)	2.7 (2.2)
Enthesitis count[b]	2.8 (1.7)	3.2 (16)	3.1 (1.7)
TJC (78 joints)	20.2 (13.3)	24.1 (19.4)	23.4 (19.0)
SJC (76 joints)	11.2 (7.8)	11.9 (10.1)	12.1 (10.7)
PASDAS score	5.9 (0.9); n = 98	6.0 (1.0); *n* = 99	5.8 (1.0); *n* = 98

Abbreviations: BSA Body surface area, *SJC* Swollen joint count, *TJC* Tender joint count, *VAS* Visual analogue scale
n, number of patients in each treatment group providing data; N, number of randomized patient
[a]The dactylitis count is the number of fingers and toes with dactylitis, with a range of 0–20 and if dactylitis is present with any finger or toe, the patient is counted as a patient with dactylitis
[b]Enthesitis was evaluated by Leeds Enthesitis Index, a validated enthesitis index. If enthesitis is present in any of the 6 sites (lateral epicondyle humerus L + R, proximal Achilles L + R and medial condyle femur L + R), the patient is counted as a patient with enthesitis

104; all patients in MoDA at week 16 either maintained or improved their status. In contrast, patients treated with secukinumab 150 mg who achieved remission at week 16 maintained remission (35.7%) or were in LDA (42.9%) or MoDA (22%) at week 104, patients in LDA at week 16 maintained or improved their status (60%) or lost their status (40%), and 97% of patients in MoDA maintained or improved their status at week 104 (Fig. 1b).

A higher proportion of TNFi-naïve and TNF-experienced patients achieved remission or LDA at week 16 versus placebo with generally higher response rates in the TNFi-naïve subgroup. In TNFi-naïve patients, remission + LDA was achieved by 46.2% (30/65) patients with secukinumab 300 mg and 42.9% (27/63) with 150 mg versus placebo (17.5% [10/57]), with responses in TNFi-experienced patients being 22.6% (7/31) for secukinumab 300 mg and 19.4% (7/36) for 150 mg versus 13.3% (4/30) for placebo. These response rates were sustained at weeks 52 and 104 in both TNFi-naïve and TNFi-experienced subgroups (Fig. 2a). Regardless of time since PsA diagnosis (≤ 2 years versus > 2 years), a higher proportion of secukinumab-treated patients achieved PASDAS remission or LDA than placebo at week 16. This proportion of patients achieving remission/LDA increased further at weeks 52 and 104, regardless of time since PsA diagnosis (Fig. 2b).

PASDAS states and core components

The median (Q1, Q3) scores of PASDAS core components in each PASDAS state at weeks 16, 52 and 104 are shown in Fig. 3. The most improved individual components in patients achieving PASDAS remission and LDA were dactylitis, enthesitis, SF-36 PCS, physician global VAS and SJC at weeks 16, 52 and 104. For dactylitis and enthesitis core components, median improvements were numerically similar in patients reaching PASDAS remission and LDA.

PASDAS states and PROs

At week 16, LSM changes from baseline in SF-36 PCS and MCS, PsAQoL, DLQI, HAQ-DI and FACIT-Fatigue scores were significantly higher ($P < 0.0001$) among patients reaching PASDAS remission and LDA than those in HDA (Fig. 4). Similarly, higher LSM changes in these PROs were reported by patients in PASDAS remission and LDA versus those in HDA at weeks 52 and 104 (Fig. 4).

As shown in Fig. 5, a decrease ($P < 0.0001$) from baseline to week 16 in the percentage of activity impairment due to health, overall work impairment due to health, and impairment while working due to health were reported by patients in PASDAS remission and LDA compared with those in HDA. Similar reductions in percentage of activity impairment due to health ($P < 0.0001$) and impairment while working due to health ($P < 0.05$) were reported by patients in PASDAS remission and LDA than HDA at weeks 52 and 104; percentage of overall work impairment due to health was reduced ($P < 0.0001$) at week 52. The percentage of work time missed due to health decreased ($P < 0.01$)

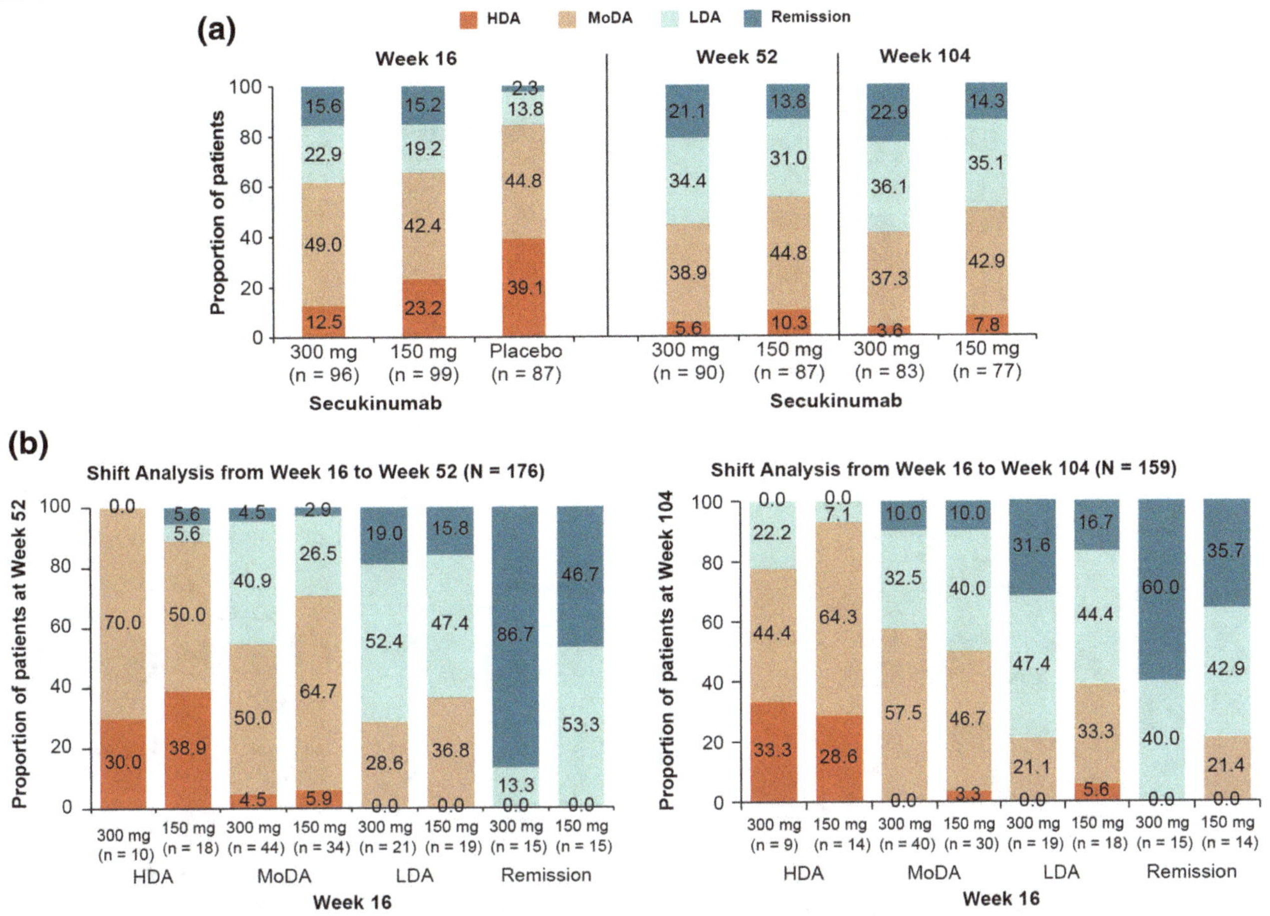

Fig. 1 a Proportion of patients achieving Psoriatic Arthritis Disease Activity Score (PASDAS) remission, LDA, MoDA and HDA at weeks 16, 52 and 104 in overall population. Data were reported using mutually exclusive categories at group level and as observed analysis. LDA: 1.9 < PASDAS score < 3.2; remission: PASDAS score ≤ 1.9. Secukinumab 300 and 150 mg data are reported (approved doses). *n* = number of patients in the treatment group with evaluation. **b** Shift analysis of PASDAS disease activity states from week 16 to week 52 or 104. Data were reported using mutually exclusive categories at group level and as observed analysis. *n* = number of patients in each PASDAS state at week 16; *N* = total number of patients with non-missing PASDAS scores at week 16 and weeks 52/104. *HDA* High disease activity, *LDA* Low disease activity, *MoDA* Moderate disease activity

from baseline to week 52 among patients in remission and LDA compared with HDA at week 52.

Discussion

PASDAS is a novel composite index which assesses multiple facets of PsA, including tender and swollen joints, dactylitis, enthesitis, and HRQoL, and offers both a treatment target and a disease activity state assessment across important clinical domains with validated cut points. PASDAS distinguishes treatment effect, performs better than traditional joint-only indices, and could be used as a treatment target in RCTs and longitudinal observational studies in PsA. There are limited data available on PASDAS in two TNFi clinical trials and in two ixekizumab trials. A study on a golimumab data set (GO-REVEAL trial) showed that PASDAS was able to distinguish treatment effect, having larger effect size at week 24 [20]. Another study using data on certolizumab pegol (RAPID-PsA trial) also showed that PASDAS demonstrated good responsiveness and discriminative ability at week 12, supporting further exploration of its use in PsA clinical trials [21]. Assessment of PASDAS-defined LDA and very low disease activity (VLDA) was also reported with ixekizumab data from SPIRIT-P1 and SPIRIT-P2 trials [22] and showed that the proportions of patients achieving PASDAS LDA and PASDAS VLDA were greater with ixekizumab than with placebo [22], further confirming the validity of PASDAS as a measure that can differentiate treatment effect. Therefore, in the present study, the ability of secukinumab to reach PASDAS-related remission or LDA was evaluated using data from the FUTURE 2 trial. To the best of our knowledge FUTURE 2 is the first trial to report detailed PASDAS-based analysis in a mixed TNFi-naïve and

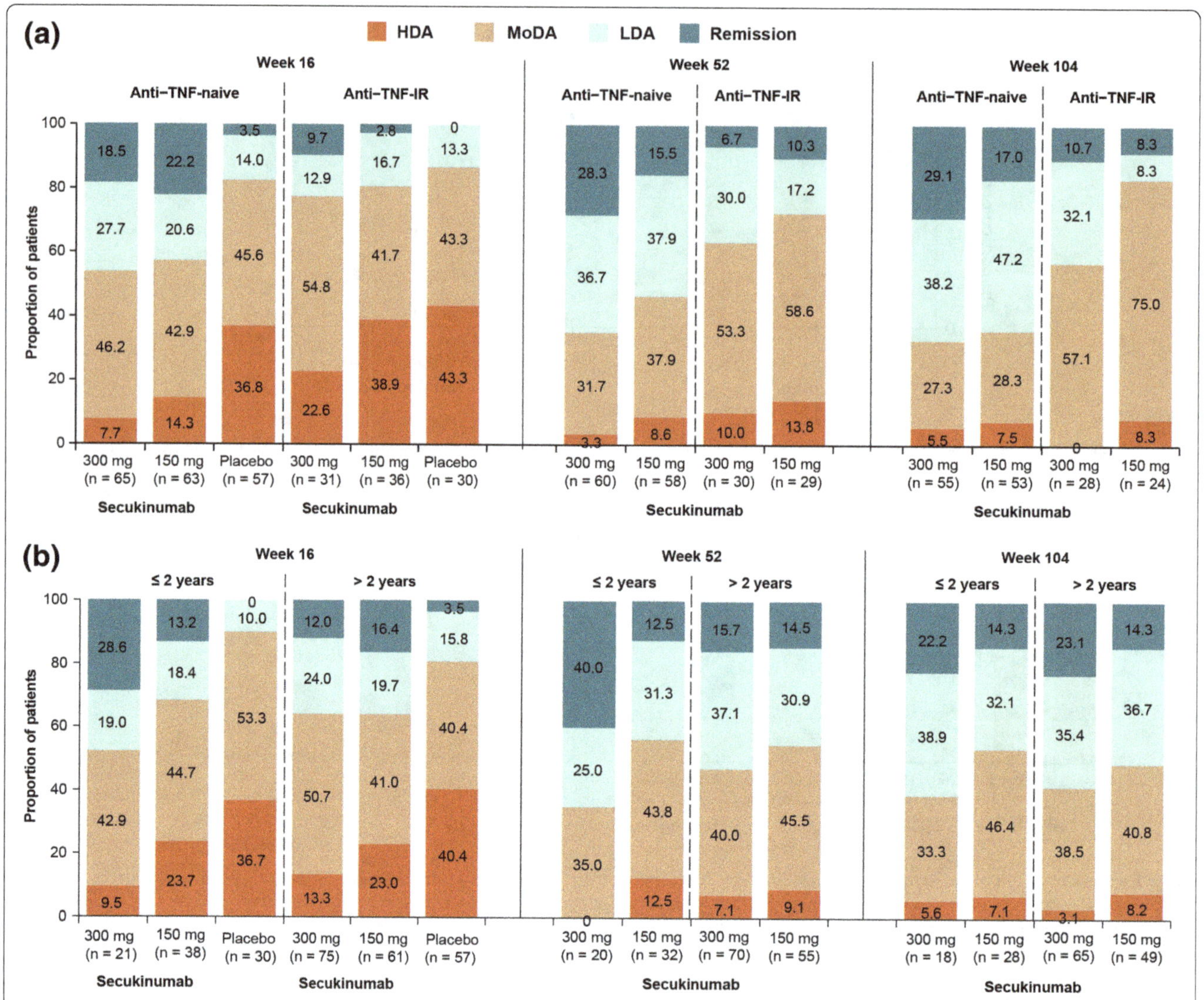

Fig. 2 Proportion of patients achieving Psoriatic Arthritis Disease Activity Score (PASDAS) remission, LDA, MoDA and HDA at weeks 16, 52 and 104 by (**a**) Tumour necrosis factor inhibitor (TNFi) status and (**b**) time since psoriatic arthritis diagnosis. *HDA* High disease activity, *LDA* Low disease activity, *MoDA* Moderate disease activity. *n* = number of patients in the treatment group with evaluation

TNFi-experienced PsA population treated with an IL-17A inhibitor.

Sustained clinical benefit with secukinumab was previously demonstrated through 104 weeks in the treatment of moderate to severe PsA in the phase III FUTURE 2 trial [15, 16], which included the more stringent clinical end points such as ACR70 responses, PASI 90 response, resolution of enthesitis and dactylitis, and high retention rate as a surrogate marker [15, 16, 23]. Results of this post hoc analysis using PASDAS scores showed that higher proportions of patients treated with secukinumab 300 and 150 mg achieved PASDAS remission or LDA at week 16 than those who received placebo in the overall population at a group level with responses sustained through week 104. Shift analysis of PASDAS states from weeks 16 to 52 and from weeks 16 to 104 confirmed that at an individual level, a majority of patients meeting either PASDAS remission or LDA either maintained or improved their status over time. These data illustrate that secukinumab can meet more stringent treatment goals in line with EULAR and GRAPPA recommendations [6, 7]. Results of this post hoc analysis complement and extend previous reports from the FUTURE 2 trial which have shown that patients treated with secukinumab achieved and sustained remission or LDA defined by other composite indices such as MDA/VLDA and DAPSA up to 2 years [24, 25]. At week 16, in the overall population, the proportions of patients treated with secukinumab 300/150 mg achieving remission were 14%/10% (DAPSA-REM) and 8%/6% (VLDA), respectively, and in those achieving LDA the proportions were 42%/44% (DAPSA REM/LDA) and 28%/23% (MDA) [24, 25], respectively. These results were sustained through week 104.

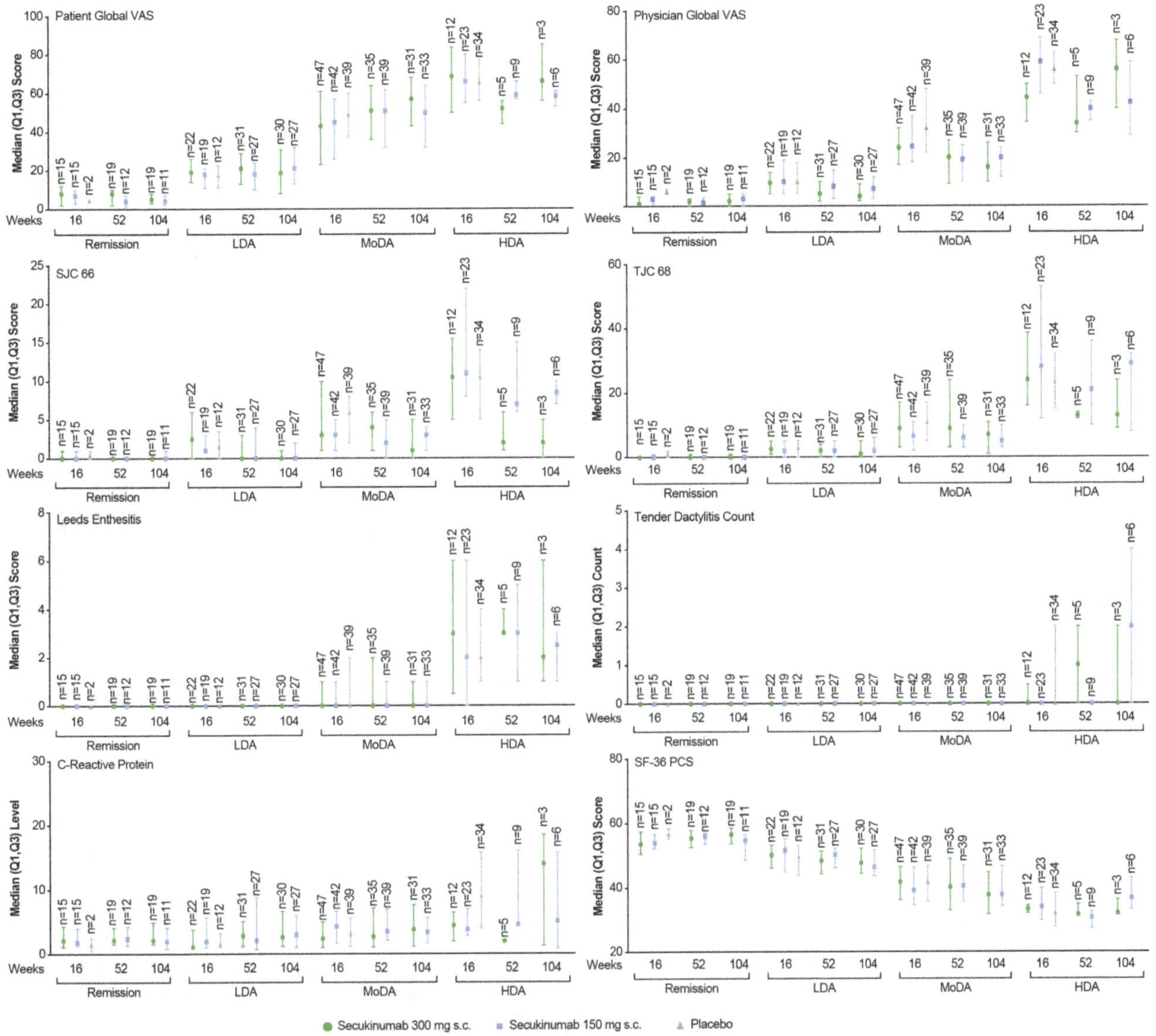

Fig. 3 Scores of Psoriatic Arthritis Disease Activity Score (PASDAS) components at weeks 16, 52 and 104. The median value is denoted by symbol in the figure, and the upper and lower error bars represent third (Q3) and first (Q1) quartiles, respectively. *n* = number of patients in respective disease states at assessment. *HDA* High disease activity, *LDA* Low disease activity, *MoDA* Moderate disease activity, *SF-36 MCS* Short Form Health Survey Mental Component Summary, *SJC* Swollen joint count, *TJC* Tender joint count, *VAS* Visual analogue scale

Secukinumab (300 and 150 mg)-treated patients achieving remission and LDA had improved median scores across all PASDAS core components relating to physician and patient global VAS, SF-36 PCS, SJC 66, TJC 68, dactylitis and enthesitis in contrast to PASDAS HDA. Among these, physician and patient global VAS, TJC 68, SJC 66, dactylitis and enthesitis were most improved.

In the subgroup analysis by previous TNFi use, the proportion of secukinumab-treated patients achieving remission and LDA at week 16 was higher in both TNFi-naïve and TNFi-experienced patients than in patients receiving placebo, with responses in secukinumab groups sustained or increased at weeks 52 and 104. The proportion of secukinumab-treated patients achieving remission and LDA was generally greater in the TNFi-naïve subgroup than in the TNFi-experienced subgroup through week 104. In a recent cross-sectional analysis of a longitudinal cohort, of 79 patients with PsA receiving their first biologic DMARD (32: etanercept, 24: adalimumab, 18: golimumab, and 5: ustekinumab) for at least 6 months, 12.6% achieved remission (PASDAS ≤ 1.9) and 41.8% were in PASDAS LDA [26]. Our study showed in 128 TNFi-naïve patients treated with secukinumab (300 or 150 mg) that 16–28% of patients achieved remission and 37–38% achieved LDA at week 52.

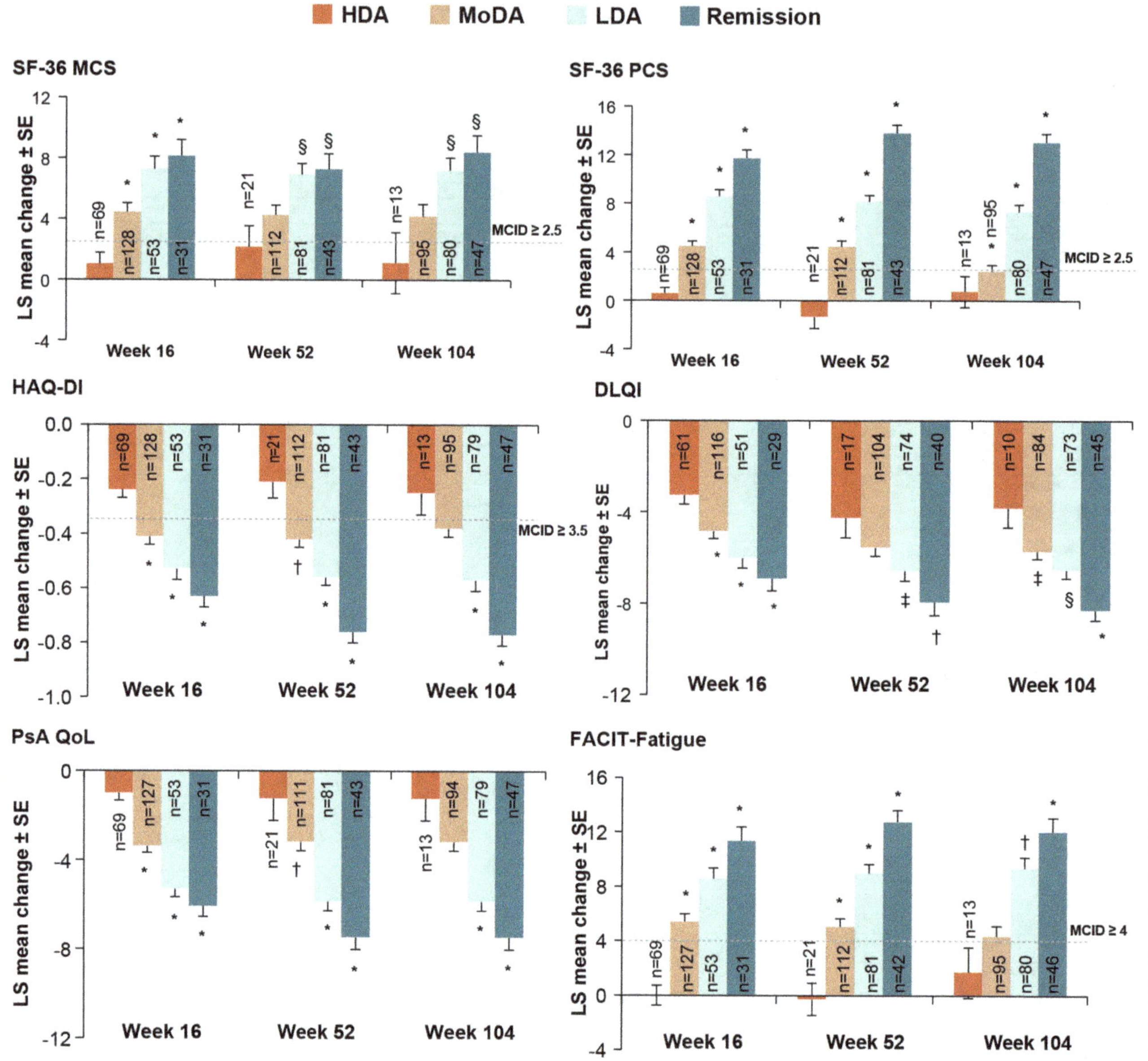

Fig. 4 Mean change in patient-reported outcome scores by Psoriatic Arthritis Disease Activity Score (PASDAS) states at weeks 16, 52 and 104. Data are from mixed model for repeated measures analysis. *$P < 0.0001$; †$P < 0.001$; §$P < 0.01$; ‡$P < 0.05$ versus HDA. n = number of patients with measurements at baseline and post-baseline visits; N = number of patients in each group of the specified analysis set. *DLQI* Dermatology Life Quality Index, *FACIT-Fatigue* Functional Assessment of Chronic Illness Therapy–Fatigue, *HAQ-DI* Health Assessment Questionnaire Disability Index, *HDA* High disease activity, *LDA* Low disease activity, *LS* Least squares, *PsAQoL* Psoriatic arthritis-specific quality of life, *SF-36 MCS* Short Form Health Survey Mental Component Summary, *SF-36 PCS* Short Form Health Survey Physical Component Summary. Week 16: $N = 32$ (remission), $N = 53$ (LDA), $N = 128$ (MoDA) and $N = 69$ (HDA); week 52: $N = 44$ (remission), $N = 81$ (LDA), $N = 112$ (MoDA) and $N = 21$ (HDA); week 104: $N = 47$ (remission), N = 81 (LDA), $N = 95$ (MoDA) and $N = 13$ (HDA). Analytic data were pooled across treatment arms

At week 16, a higher proportion of patients treated with secukinumab achieved PASDAS remission or LDA versus placebo, regardless of time since PsA diagnosis (≤ 2 years versus > 2 years). A numerically higher proportion of secukinumab-treated patients reached PASDAS remission or LDA at weeks 52 and 104 than at week 16, regardless of time since PsA diagnosis. Although PASDAS includes SF-36 PCS as one of its core components, patients achieving PASDAS remission and LDA also reported greater improvements in other PROs (HRQoL, mental health, physical function, fatigue and work productivity) through week 104, confirming that these stringent goals translate into improved patient quality of life and function as well as for society owing to higher workforce productivity.

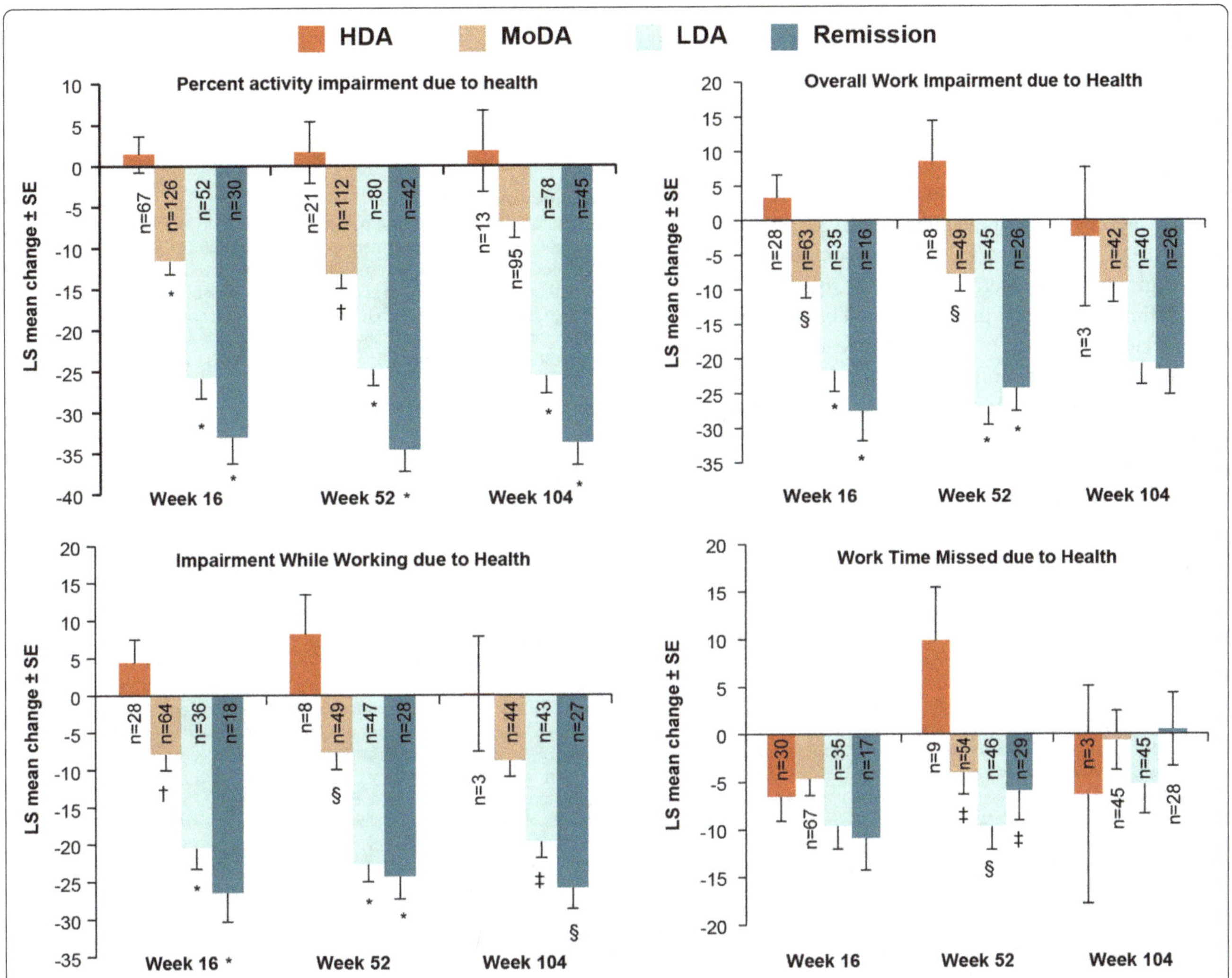

Fig. 5 Mean change in work productivity and activity impairment outcome measures by Psoriatic Arthritis Disease Activity Score (PASDAS) states at weeks 16, 52 and 104. Data are from mixed model for repeated measures analysis. *$P < 0.0001$; †$P < 0.001$; §$P < 0.01$ and ‡$P < 0.05$ versus HDA. n = number of patients with measurements at both baseline and post-baseline visits; N = number of patients in each group of the specified analysis set. *HDA* High disease activity, *LDA* Low disease activity, *LS* Least squares, *MoDA* Moderate disease activity. Week 16: $N = 32$ (remission), $N = 53$ (LDA), $N = 128$ (MoDA) and $N = 69$ (HDA); week 52: $N = 44$ (remission), $N = 81$ (LDA), $N = 112$ (MoDA) and $N = 21$ (HDA); week 104: $N = 47$ (remission), $N = 81$ (LDA), $N = 95$ (MoDA) and $N = 13$ (HDA). Analytic data were pooled across treatment arms

The PASDAS has certain limitations in that, being a complex composite index, it requires complex mathematical calculations, which are time-consuming, although this has been overcome with an application allowing for an easy calculation. PASDAS thus may be more appropriately used in RCTs [10]. It does not include a measure for axial involvement and patient pain, both important manifestations of PsA. Moreover, PASDAS-based publications on RCT data are sparse to place it in context with other composite indices used in PsA. Another limitation of this study was that patients in HDA were not specifically treated to reach the preferable REM/LDA states. Furthermore, while PASDAS change from baseline was an exploratory end point in the FUTURE 2 study, the cut points related to the different disease activity states were recently validated, and this post hoc analysis was generated following the more recently validated cut-offs. These data will require confirmation in new RCTs. Also, there is a lack of assessment in relation to structural outcomes as per the FUTURE 2 study protocol. Further, while we appreciate the fact that SF-36 PCS is one of the core components of PASDAS and therefore a question of circularity in looking at the relationship of PASDAS states and PROs could be raised, we still think it is relevant to do this analysis and see how PASDAS states translate to patient well-being and thus outcomes reported by them.

Conclusions

In summary, this post hoc analysis of FUTURE 2 data showed that secukinumab treatment resulted in PASDAS remission or LDA at week 16 with responses sustained or further improved through week 104 at the group and individual levels. Improvement or sustainability of MoDA, LDA and remission states were more frequently achieved with secukinumab 300 mg than 150 mg. PASDAS remission/LDA was associated with significantly greater improvements in HRQoL, physical function, fatigue and work productivity. These results extend the previous findings of maintenance of other stringent clinical efficacy end points, including VLDA and MDA, in the FUTURE 2 trial, demonstrating that secukinumab treatment can result in sustained PASDAS-defined remission or LDA, thus demonstrating the potential utility of PASDAS as an outcome measure in RCTs in PsA.

Abbreviations

ACR: American College of Rheumatology; CPDAI: Composite Psoriatic Disease Activity Index; CRP: C-reactive protein; DAPSA: Disease Activity Index for Psoriatic Arthritis; DAS: Disease Activity Score; DAS-28 CRP: 28-joint Disease Activity Score based on C-reactive protein; DLQI: Dermatology Life Quality Index; DMARD: Disease-modifying anti-rheumatic drug; EULAR: European League Against Rheumatism; FACIT: Functional Assessment of Chronic Illness Therapy; GRAPPA: Group for Research and Assessment of Psoriasis and Psoriatic Arthritis; HAQ-DI: Health Assessment Questionnaire Disability Index; HDA: High disease activity; HRQoL: Health-related quality of life; IL: Interleukin; IRB: Institutional review board; LDA: Low disease activity; LS: Least squares; MoDA: Moderate disease activity; NSAID: Non-steroidal anti-inflammatory drug; PASDAS: Psoriatic Arthritis Disease Activity Score; PASI: Psoriasis Area Severity Index; PRO: Patient-reported outcome; PsA: Psoriatic arthritis; PsAQoL: Psoriatic Arthritis Quality of Life questionnaire; Q: Quartile; RCT: Randomized controlled trial; REM: Remission; s.c.: Subcutaneous; SF-36 MCS: Short Form Health Survey Mental Component Summary; SF-36 PCS: Short Form Health Survey Physical Component Summary; SJC: Swollen joint count; TJC: Tender joint count; TNF: Tumour necrosis factor; VAS: Visual analogue scale; WPAI: Work Productivity and Activity Impairment questionnaire

Acknowledgements

The authors thank the patients who participated in this study; the study investigators; and John Gallagher, medical consultant for Novartis Pharma AG, Basel, Switzerland. Scientific review support was provided by Neeta Pillai, Novartis Healthcare Pvt. Ltd., Hyderabad, India. Manuscript writing support was provided by Santoshkumar Tota, Novartis Healthcare Pvt. Ltd., Hyderabad, India.

Funding

Novartis Pharma AG (Basel, Switzerland).

Availability of data and materials

Novartis is committed to sharing with qualified external researchers access to patient-level data and supporting clinical documents from eligible studies. These requests are reviewed and approved by an independent review panel on the basis of scientific merit. All data provided are anonymized to respect the privacy of patients who have participated in the trial, in line with applicable laws and regulations. The trial data availability is according to the criteria and process described at www.clinicalstudydatarequest.com.
Trial details are available at https://www.clinicaltrialsregister.eu/ctr-search/search?query=2012-004439-22 and https://clinicaltrials.gov/ct2/show/NCT01752634.

Study sponsor statement

This study was sponsored by Novartis Pharma AG, Basel, Switzerland, and was designed by the scientific steering committee and Novartis personnel. Medical writing support was funded by Novartis.

Authors' contributions

All authors had access to the data, contributed to its interpretation and collaborated in the development of the manuscript. The initial draft of the manuscript was written by a medical writer employed by the study sponsor. All authors critically reviewed and provided feedback on subsequent versions. All authors made the decision to submit the manuscript for publication and vouch for the accuracy and completeness of the data and fidelity of this report to the study protocol. All authors read and approved the final manuscript.

Consent for publication

Patients provided written informed consent before starting the study-related procedures.

Competing interests

LCC is funded by a National Institute for Health Research Clinician Scientist award. The present research was supported by the National Institute for Health Research (NIHR) Oxford Biomedical Research Centre (BRC). The views expressed are those of the author(s) and not necessarily those of the NHS, the NIHR or the Department of Health. LCC has received grant/research support from AbbVie, Janssen, Lilly, Novartis and Pfizer and has served as a consultant for AbbVie, Amgen, Bristol-Myers Squibb, Celgene, Pfizer, UCB, MSD, Boehringer Ingelheim, Novartis, Lilly, Janssen, Sun Pharma, Prothena and Galapagos. DDG has received grants and/or personal fees from Amgen, AbbVie, Bristol-Myers Squibb, Celgene, Eli Lilly, Janssen, Novartis, Pfizer and UCB. PN has received research grants for clinical trials and honoraria for lectures and advice from Novartis, AbbVie, Roche, Pfizer, Bristol-Myers Squibb, Janssen and Celgene. OF has received fees for speaking or consulting from Bristol-Myers Squibb, AbbVie, Pfizer Inc., UCB Pharma Ltd., Lilly, Novartis, Celgene and Janssen Research. OF has received grants from Bristol-Myers Squibb, AbbVie, Novartis and Pfizer Inc. AK has served as a consultant for Novartis. TKK has received fees for speaking and/or consulting from AbbVie, Biogen, Bristol-Myers Squibb, Boehringer Ingelheim, Celltrion, Eli Lilly, Epirus, Janssen, Merck-Serono, MSD, Mundipharma, Novartis, Oktal, Orion Pharma, Hospira/Pfizer, Roche, Sandoz and UCB. LG has received research grants from AbbVie, Bristol-Myers Squibb, Celgene, Janssen, Novartis, MSD, Roche and UCB. VS has served as a consultant for AbbVie, Amgen, Bristol-Myers Squibb, Celgene, Celltrion, CORRONA, Genentech/Roche, GSK, Janssen, Lilly, Merck, Novartis, Pfizer, Regeneron, Sanofi and UCB. LR has served as a consultant for Novartis through employment at RTI Health Solutions and is an employee of RTI Health Solutions. LP is a shareholder of Novartis and an employee of Novartis. KD is a shareholder of Novartis and an employee of Novartis. SMJ is an employee of Novartis. CG is a shareholder of Novartis and Bristol-Myers Squibb and is an employee of Novartis.

Author details

[1]Nuffield Department of Orthopaedics, Rheumatology and Musculoskeletal Sciences, University of Oxford, Botnar Research Centre, Windmill Road, Oxford OX3 7LD, UK. [2]Department of Medicine, Rheumatology, University of Toronto, Toronto Western Hospital, Toronto, Ontario, Canada. [3]Department of Medicine, University of Queensland, Brisbane, Australia. [4]Department of Rheumatology, St Vincent's University Hospital and Conway Institute for Biomolecular Research, University College Dublin, Dublin, Ireland. [5]UC San Diego School of Medicine, La Jolla, CA, USA. [6]Department of Rheumatology, Diakonhjemmet Hospital, Oslo, Norway. [7]Sorbonne Universités, UPMC

Université Paris 06, Paris, France. [8]Rheumatology Department, Hôpital Pitié Salpêtrière, AP-HP, Paris, France. [9]Division of Immunology/Rheumatology, Stanford University School of Medicine, Palo Alto, CA, USA. [10]RTI Health Solutions, Barcelona, Spain. [11]Novartis Pharmaceuticals Corporation, East Hanover, NJ, USA. [12]Novartis Pharma AG, Basel, Switzerland.

References

1. Gladman DD, Antoni C, Mease P, Clegg DO, Nash P. Psoriatic arthritis: epidemiology, clinical features, course, and outcome. Ann Rheum Dis. 2005; 64(Suppl 2):ii14–7.
2. Rosen CF, Mussani F, Chandran V, Eder L, Thavaneswaran A, Gladman DD. Patients with psoriatic arthritis have worse quality of life than those with psoriasis alone. Rheumatology (Oxford). 2012;51:571–6.
3. Her M, Kavanaugh A. A review of disease activity measures for psoriatic arthritis: what is the best approach? Expert Rev Clin Immunol. 2014;10: 1241–54.
4. Lubrano E, Perrotta FM, Kavanaugh A. An overview of low disease activity and remission in psoriatic arthritis. Clin Exp Rheumatol. 2015;33(5 Suppl 93):S51–4.
5. Smolen JS, Schöls M, Braun J, Dougados M, FitzGerald O, Gladman DD, et al. Treating axial spondyloarthritis and peripheral spondyloarthritis, especially psoriatic arthritis, to target: 2017 update of recommendations by an international task force. Ann Rheum Dis. 2018;77(1):3–17.
6. Coates LC, Kavanaugh A, Mease PJ, Soriano ER, Laura Acosta-Felquer M, Armstrong AW, et al. Group for Research and Assessment of Psoriasis and Psoriatic Arthritis 2015 treatment recommendations for psoriatic arthritis. Arthritis Rheumatol. 2016;68:1060–71.
7. Gossec L, Smolen JS, Ramiro S, de Wit M, Cutolo M, Dougados M, et al. European League Against Rheumatism (EULAR) recommendations for the management of psoriatic arthritis with pharmacological therapies: 2015 update. Ann Rheum Dis. 2016;75:499–510.
8. Chandran V, Maharaj AB. Assessing disease activity in psoriasis and psoriatic arthritis: impact on management and therapy. Expert Rev Clin Immunol. 2016;12:573–82.
9. Smolen JS, Schoels M, Aletaha D. Disease activity and response assessment in psoriatic arthritis using the Disease Activity index for Psoriatic Arthritis (DAPSA): a brief review. Clin Exp Rheumatol. 2015;33(5 Suppl 93):S48–50.
10. Helliwell PS, FitzGerald O, Fransen J, Gladman DD, Kreuger GG, Callis-Duffin K, et al. The development of candidate composite disease activity and responder indices for psoriatic arthritis (GRACE project). Ann Rheum Dis. 2013;72:986–91.
11. Coates LC, Helliwell PS. Defining low disease activity states in psoriatic arthritis using novel composite disease instruments. J Rheumatol. 2016; 43:371–5.
12. Helliwell PS, Waxman R. Modification of the Psoriatic Arthritis Disease Activity Score (PASDAS). Ann Rheum Dis. 2018;77:467–8.
13. Langley RG, Elewski BE, Lebwohl M, Reich K, Griffiths CE, Papp K, et al. Secukinumab in plaque psoriasis--results of two phase 3 trials. N Engl J Med. 2014;371:326–38.
14. Mease PJ, McInnes IB, Kirkham B, Kavanaugh A, Rahman P, van der Heijde D, et al. Secukinumab inhibition of interleukin-17a in patients with psoriatic arthritis. N Engl J Med. 2015;373(14):1329–39.
15. McInnes IB, Mease PJ, Kirkham B, Kavanaugh A, Ritchlin CT, Rahman P, et al. Secukinumab, a human anti-interleukin-17A monoclonal antibody, in patients with psoriatic arthritis (FUTURE 2): a randomised, double-blind, placebo-controlled, phase 3 trial. Lancet. 2015;386:1137–46.
16. McInnes IB, Mease PJ, Ritchlin CT, Rahman P, Gottlieb AB, Kirkham B, et al. Secukinumab sustains improvement in signs and symptoms of psoriatic arthritis: 2 year results from the phase 3 FUTURE 2 study. Rheumatology (Oxford). 2017;56:1993–2003.
17. Nash P, Mease PJ, McInnes IB, Rahman P, Ritchlin CT, Blanco R, et al. Efficacy and safety of secukinumab administration by autoinjector in patients with psoriatic arthritis: results from a randomized, placebo-controlled trial (FUTURE 3). Arthritis Res Ther. 2018;20:47.
18. Baeten D, Sieper J, Braun J, Baraliakos X, Dougados M, Emery P, et al. Secukinumab, an interleukin-17a inhibitor, in ankylosing spondylitis. N Engl J Med. 2015;373:2534–48.
19. Baraliakos X, Kivitz AJ, Deodhar AA, Braun J, Wei JC, Delicha EM, et al. Long-term effects of interleukin-17A inhibition with secukinumab in active ankylosing spondylitis: 3-year efficacy and safety results from an extension of the phase 3 MEASURE 1 trial. Clin Exp Rheumatol. 2018;36:50–5.
20. Helliwell PS, Kavanaugh A. Comparison of composite measures of disease activity in psoriatic arthritis using data from an interventional study with golimumab. Arthritis Care Res (Hoboken). 2014;66:749–56.
21. Helliwell P, Mease PJ, Nurminen T, FitzGerald O. Further analysis of Psoriatic Arthritis Disease Activity Score (PASDAS) and Composite Psoriatic Disease Activity Index (CPDAI) using data from a placebo-controlled trial of certolizumab pegol in psoriatic arthritis. Ann Rheum Dis. 2014;73:740.
22. Coates LC, Husni ME, Lespessailles E, Kerr L, Gallo G. Ixekizumab makes very low disease activity and remission with psoriatic arthritis disease activity score possible in active psoriatic arthritis patients for up to 1 year: SPIRIT-P1 AND SPIRIT-P2 trials. Ann Rheum Dis. 2018;77:375.
23. Mease PJ, Kavanaugh A, Reimold A, Tahir H, Rech J, Hall S, et al. Secukinumab provides sustained improvements in the signs and symptoms of active psoriatic arthritis through 3 years: efficacy and safety results from a phase 3 trial [abstract 961]. Arthritis Rheumatol. 2016;68(suppl 10).
24. Coates LC, Mease PJ, Gossec L, Kirkham B, Sherif B, Gaillez C, et al. Minimal Disease Activity among Active Psoriatic Arthritis Patients Treated with Secukinumab: 2-year Results from the FUTURE 2 Study. Arthritis Care Res (Hoboken). 2018;70:1529–35.
25. Coates LC, Nash P, Kvien T, Gossec L, Mease PJ, Rasouliyan L, et al. Secukinumab Provides Sustained Minimal Disease Activity (MDA) and Remission Related to Disease Activity Index for Psoriatic Arthritis (DAPSA): 2-Year Results from a Phase 3 Study [abstract 622]. Arthritis Rheumatol. 2017; 69(suppl 10).
26. Lubrano E, De Socio A, Perrotta FM. Comparison of composite indices tailored for psoriatic arthritis treated with csDMARD and bDMARD: a cross-sectional analysis of a longitudinal cohort. J Rheumatol. 2017;44:1159–64.

6

Improved patient-reported outcomes in patients with psoriatic arthritis treated with abatacept

Vibeke Strand[1], Evo Alemao[2*], Thomas Lehman[2], Alyssa Johnsen[2], Subhashis Banerjee[2], Harris A. Ahmad[2] and Philip J. Mease[3]

Abstract

Background: To explore the effect of abatacept treatment on patient-reported outcomes (PROs) in psoriatic arthritis (PsA).

Methods: Patients with PsA were randomised (1:1) to subcutaneous abatacept 125 mg weekly/placebo for 24 weeks with early escape (EE) to open-label abatacept (week 16). Adjusted mean changes from baseline to weeks 16 (all patients) and 24 (non-EE responders) in Health Assessment Questionnaire-Disability Index (HAQ-DI), Short Form-36 (SF-36; physical and mental component summary and domains), Dermatology Life Quality Index and Functional Assessment of Chronic Illness Therapy-Fatigue (FACIT-F) were evaluated. Subpopulations were analysed by baseline C-reactive protein (CRP) level (> vs ≤ upper limit of normal [ULN]) and prior tumour necrosis factor inhibitor (TNFi) exposure. Proportions of patients reporting improvements ≥ minimal clinically important differences (MCIDs) and ≥ normative values (NVs) in HAQ-DI, SF-36 and FACIT-F (week 16 before EE) were analysed.

Results: In total population, numerically higher improvements in most PROs were reported with abatacept ($n = 213$) versus placebo ($n = 211$) at both time points ($P > 0.05$). Higher proportions of abatacept versus placebo patients reported PRO improvements ≥ MCID and ≥ NV at week 16. At week 16, all PRO improvements were numerically greater ($P > 0.05$) in patients with baseline CRP > ULN versus CRP ≤ ULN (all significant [95% confidence interval] for abatacept vs placebo); improvements in SF-36 component summaries and FACIT-F were greater in TNFi-naïve versus TNFi-exposed patients (abatacept > placebo). Week 24 subgroup data were difficult to interpret due to low patient numbers.

Conclusions: Abatacept treatment improved PROs in patients with PsA versus placebo, with better results in elevated baseline CRP and TNFi-naïve subpopulations.

Keywords: DMARDs (biologic), Outcomes research, Patient perspective, Psoriatic arthritis

* Correspondence: evo.alemao@bms.com
[2]Bristol-Myers Squibb, Princeton, NJ, USA
Full list of author information is available at the end of the article

Background

Psoriatic arthritis (PsA) is a chronic inflammatory autoimmune disease with a range of clinical manifestations affecting skin and musculoskeletal systems [1]. Health-related quality of life (HRQoL) can vary greatly according to a patient's specific symptoms; hence, assessing treatment effects using patient-reported outcomes (PROs) is particularly important in PsA [2–6]. Several PRO instruments have been validated in PsA, including the Health Assessment Questionnaire-Disability Index (HAQ-DI) [4, 7] and Short Form-36 (SF-36) [5, 6].

Abatacept, a selective T-cell co-stimulation modulator [8], has a distinct mechanism of action upstream of currently available agents, and is approved for treatment of rheumatoid arthritis and juvenile idiopathic arthritis, and recently for active PsA in adults [9]. In the phase 3 Active pSoriaTic aRthritis rAndomizEd triAl (ASTRAEA, NCT01860976), subcutaneous (SC) abatacept 125 mg weekly significantly increased the proportion of patients achieving ≥ 20% improvement in the American College of Rheumatology criteria (ACR20) compared with placebo at week 24 (primary endpoint: 39.4% vs 22.3%; $P < 0.001$) and was well tolerated in patients with active PsA [10]. A numerically higher proportion of patients with HAQ-DI responses (reductions from baseline ≥ 0.35) was evident with abatacept versus placebo ($P > 0.05$). Abatacept treatment also reduced progression of structural damage with an overall beneficial effect on musculoskeletal symptoms. However, due to the hierarchical testing procedure employed, it was not possible to attribute significance to endpoints ranked below HAQ-DI responses in the hierarchical testing [10].

The effect of factors associated with poor prognosis and treatment resistance, such as elevated C-reactive protein (CRP) levels and prior exposure to tumour necrosis factor inhibitors (TNFi) [11], was also evaluated in ASTRAEA. Higher ACR20 responses were observed with abatacept versus placebo in both TNFi-naïve and TNFi-exposed subpopulations at week 24, with the largest treatment differences seen in TNFi-naïve patients [10]. Moreover, patients with baseline CRP ≥ upper limits of normal (ULN) had the highest ACR20 responses at week 24 with abatacept versus placebo [10].

The goal of the analyses reported here was to examine the impact of abatacept versus placebo treatment on PROs in ASTRAEA for the overall population and in subgroups by baseline CRP levels and previous TNFi exposure.

Methods

Study design and treatment

The design, eligibility criteria, and main efficacy and safety endpoints of this phase 3, randomised, double-blind, placebo-controlled, multicentre trial have been reported in detail previously [10]. Patients were randomised (1:1) to receive SC abatacept 125 mg weekly or placebo for 24 weeks, after which all patients were transitioned to receive open-label SC abatacept weekly for 28 weeks (total study period of 52 weeks). Patients without ≥ 20% improvement in tender and swollen joint counts at week 16 were switched to open-label abatacept for 28 weeks (early escape [EE], total study period of 44 weeks). Key eligibility criteria included age ≥ 18 years, PsA per the Classification Criteria for PsA (CASPAR) [12], active arthritis (defined as ≥ 3 tender and ≥ 3 swollen joints), active plaque psoriasis with ≥ 1 qualifying target lesion ≥ 2 cm in diameter and inadequate response or intolerance to ≥ 1 non-biologic disease-modifying anti-rheumatic drug (DMARD). Both TNFi-naïve and TNFi-exposed patients were included.

Patient-reported outcomes

HAQ-DI [4, 7], SF-36 physical component summary (PCS), mental component summary (MCS) and individual domain scores [5, 6], Functional Assessment of Chronic Illness Therapy-Fatigue scale (FACIT-F) [3] and Dermatology Life Quality Index (DLQI) [2] scores were assessed at weeks 16 and 24 in the overall population (prespecified) and in patient subpopulations (post hoc) by baseline CRP (> or ≤ ULN, defined as 3 mg/L) and prior TNFi use. The hierarchical order of the secondary and exploratory PRO endpoints [10] was predefined as: proportions of patients reporting HAQ-DI responses ≥ minimal clinically important differences (MCIDs) and mean changes from baseline in SF-36 PCS and MCS scores (summary and domain scores).

Here, in the overall population, the proportions of patients reporting improvements from baseline in HAQ-DI, SF-36 (summary and domain) and FACIT-F scores ≥ MCID (expressed as a value established for each instrument, and defined as the smallest change in score perceived by a patient to be clinically important) [13] and ≥ normative values (defined based on age/gender-matched population) were analysed (post hoc) at week 16 prior to confounding due to EE to open-label abatacept treatment. Defined MCIDs were: HAQ-DI ≥ – 0.35 [14], SF-36 PCS ≥ 2.5 [13, 15–17], SF-36 MCS ≥ 2.5 [13, 15, 17], SF-36 domains ≥5.0 [13, 15, 17], and FACIT-F ≥ – 4.0 [3]. Normative values were: HAQ-DI < 0.5 [7, 18, 19], SF-36 PCS ≥ 50 [17, 20], SF-36 MCS ≥ 50 [20] and FACIT-F ≥ 40.1 [21].

Statistical analyses

All efficacy analyses included all randomised patients who received at least one dose of study medication (intent-to-treat population). Week 16, prior to EE, was the last time point at which all patients were analysed. For week 24 analyses, EE patient data were set to missing. As previously reported, the effect of abatacept on the first key secondary endpoint in the statistical hierarchy (HAQ-DI responses) did not reach significance; therefore, only nominal *P* values were generated for subsequent outcomes, which were ranked lower in the hierarchy. The significance of the treatment effect cannot be definitively attributed for these outcomes as they were not adjusted for multiplicity (however, 95% confidence intervals [CIs] were not overlapping) [10]. Nonetheless, these lower-ranking outcomes still provide a measure of clinical meaningfulness. Adjusted mean changes from baseline in PROs including SF-36 domain scores were evaluated, and corresponding adjusted mean differences (95% CI) between the abatacept and placebo groups were calculated using a longitudinal repeated measures model. This model included the fixed categorical effects of treatment, day, prior TNFi use, methotrexate (MTX) use, body surface area (BSA), day-by-treatment interaction, prior TNFi-use-by-day interaction, MTX-use-by-day interaction, BSA-use-by-day interaction and the continuous fixed covariate of baseline score and baseline score-by-day interaction. The estimate of difference (95% CI) between abatacept and placebo groups for MCID and normative values was calculated using a two-sided Cochran–Mantel–Haenszel chi-square test adjusted for stratification criteria.

Patient consent and ethics approval

All patients or their legal representatives gave written, informed consent prior to study entry. The study was conducted in accordance with the Declaration of Helsinki, International Conference on Harmonisation Guidelines for Good Clinical Practice and local regulations. Schulman Associates Institutional Review Board or Independent Ethics Committees approved the protocol, consent form and any other written information provided to patients or their legal representatives.

Results

Patients

Of 424 patients randomised, 213 received abatacept and 211 placebo; 76 (35.7%) and 89 (42.2%), respectively, met criteria for EE [10]. Baseline demographic and disease characteristics were similar between treatment groups and were reported in detail previously [10].

Overall population analysis

Changes from baseline at weeks 16 and 24

In the total population, greater improvements from baseline in most PROs were reported with abatacept versus placebo at both week 16, which comprised all patients,

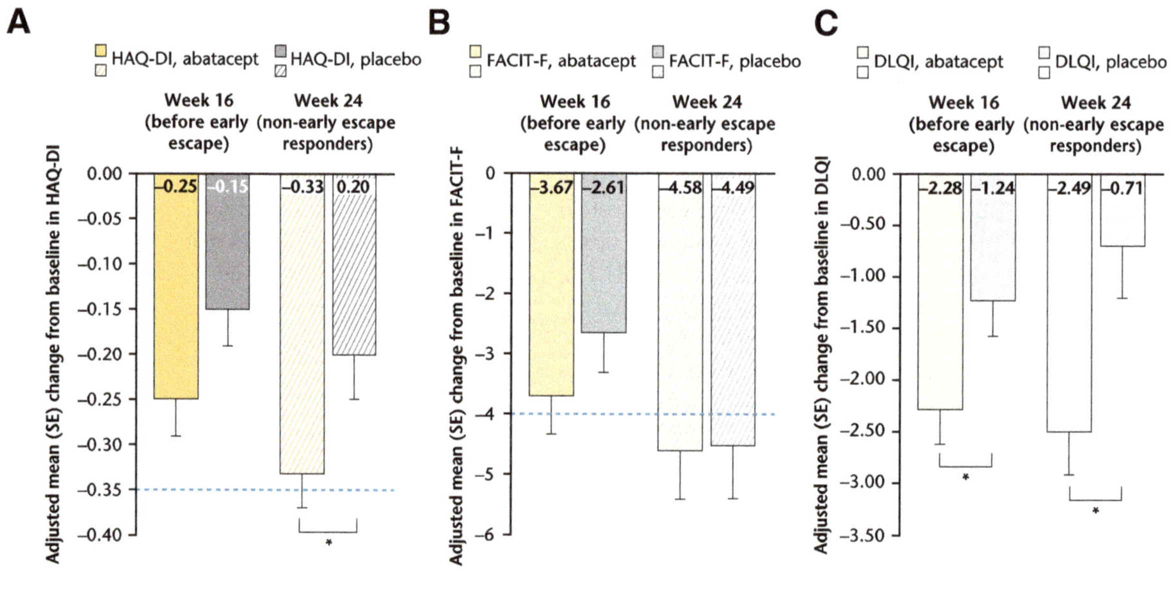

	HAQ-DI Week 16	HAQ-DI Week 24	FACIT-F Week 16	FACIT-F Week 24	DLQI Week 16	DLQI Week 24
Adjusted mean difference from placebo (95% CI)	−0.11 (−0.21, 0.00)	−0.13 (−0.25, −0.01)	NA	NA	−1.04 (−1.93, −0.14)	−1.78 (−2.94, −0.63)
Abatacept, n	202	124	202	126	212	126
Placebo, n	187	98	189	99	189	98

Fig. 1 HAQ-DI (**a**), FACIT-F (**b**), DLQI (**c**) change from baseline (weeks 16 and 24, overall population). *Statistically significant difference. *Dotted lines* represent MCID (HAQ-DI: ≥ − 0.35; FACIT-F: ≥ − 4.0). *CI* confidence interval, *DLQI* Dermatology Life Quality Index, *FACIT-F* Functional Assessment of Chronic Illness Therapy-Fatigue scale, *HAQ-DI* Health Assessment Questionnaire-Disability Index, *MCID* minimal clinically important difference, *NA* not applicable, *SE* standard error

and week 24, which included only patients showing a response to either treatment (response defined as 20% improvement in tender and swollen joint counts; Figs. 1, 2 and 3a). Statistically significant (95% CI of difference vs placebo not crossing 0) improvements from baseline with abatacept versus placebo were reported in HAQ-DI scores in the week 24 responder group (Fig. 1a), in SF-36 PCS (Fig. 2), SF-36 physical functioning (PF), bodily pain (BP) and vitality (VT) domains (adjusted mean difference [95% CI], respectively: 4.44 [0.39 to 8.49], 5.36 [1.40 to 9.33] and 4.07 [0.67 to 7.47]), and in DLQI (Fig. 1c) scores at weeks 16 and 24.

Changes from baseline in SF-36 MCS scores were not statistically significant, but were numerically greater with abatacept versus placebo at week 16 (adjusted mean change from baseline [standard error (SE)]: 2.42 [0.70] vs 1.15 [0.73], adjusted mean difference [95% CI]: 1.28 [− 0.58 to 3.13]; $P > 0.05$), but were not meaningfully different for the responder-only analysis at week 24 (adjusted change from baseline [SE]: 2.56 [0.83] vs 2.62 [0.92], adjusted mean difference [95% CI]: −0.06 [− 2.32 to 2.20]). All SF-36 domains showed nonsignificant trends towards greater improvements from baseline with abatacept than placebo at week 16; improvements from baseline in all domains increased in both abatacept and placebo groups among responders at week 24 (Fig. 3a; see Additional file 1: Table S1).

Minimal clinically important differences and normative values

A statistically significant benefit at week 16 with abatacept versus placebo was evident in SF-36 PCS and MCS scores, and PF, BP and role–emotional (RE) domains (Fig. 4a; see Additional file 2: Table S2). The proportions of patients reporting scores ≥ normative values at week 16 were significantly greater (estimate of difference [95% CI]) with abatacept versus placebo in FACIT-F (10.4 [0.4 to 20.3]) and SF-36 RE domain (10.3 [3.4 to 17.1]) scores.

A numerically greater proportion of patients reported improvements ≥ MCID with abatacept versus placebo at week 16 in HAQ-DI scores, but the difference did not reach statistical significance (Fig. 4a). At week 16, the proportion of patients reporting improvements ≥ MCID in FACIT-F scores (Fig. 4a) and SF-36 role–physical (RP), general health (GH), VT, social function and mental health (MH) domain scores (see Additional file 2: Table S2) were numerically higher with abatacept versus placebo. In the abatacept treatment group, changes from baseline exceeded MCID in six of eight SF-36 domains, the exceptions being GH and MH; whereas in the placebo group, mean changes exceeded MCID in the RP and BP domains only.

The proportions of patients who reported scores ≥ normative values at week 16, although not statistically significant, were numerically higher with abatacept than

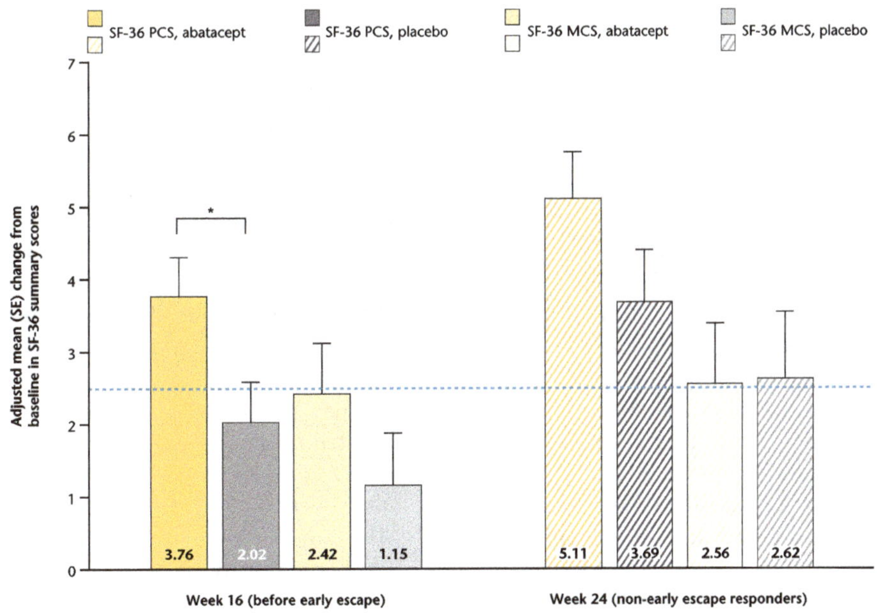

	Week 16 PCS	Week 16 MCS	Week 24 PCS	Week 24 MCS
Adjusted mean difference from placebo (95% CI)	1.74 (0.30, 3.19)	1.28 (−0.58, 3.13)	1.42 (−0.32, 3.15)	−0.06 (−2.32, 2.20)
Abatacept, n	202	202	124	124
Placebo, n	186	186	97	97

Fig. 2 SF-36 PCS and MCS change from baseline (weeks 16 and 24, overall population). *Statistically significant difference. *Dotted line* represents MCID (≥ 2.5). *CI* confidence interval, *MCID* minimal clinically important difference, *MCS* mental component summary, *PCS* physical component summary, *SE* standard error, *SF-36* Short Form-36

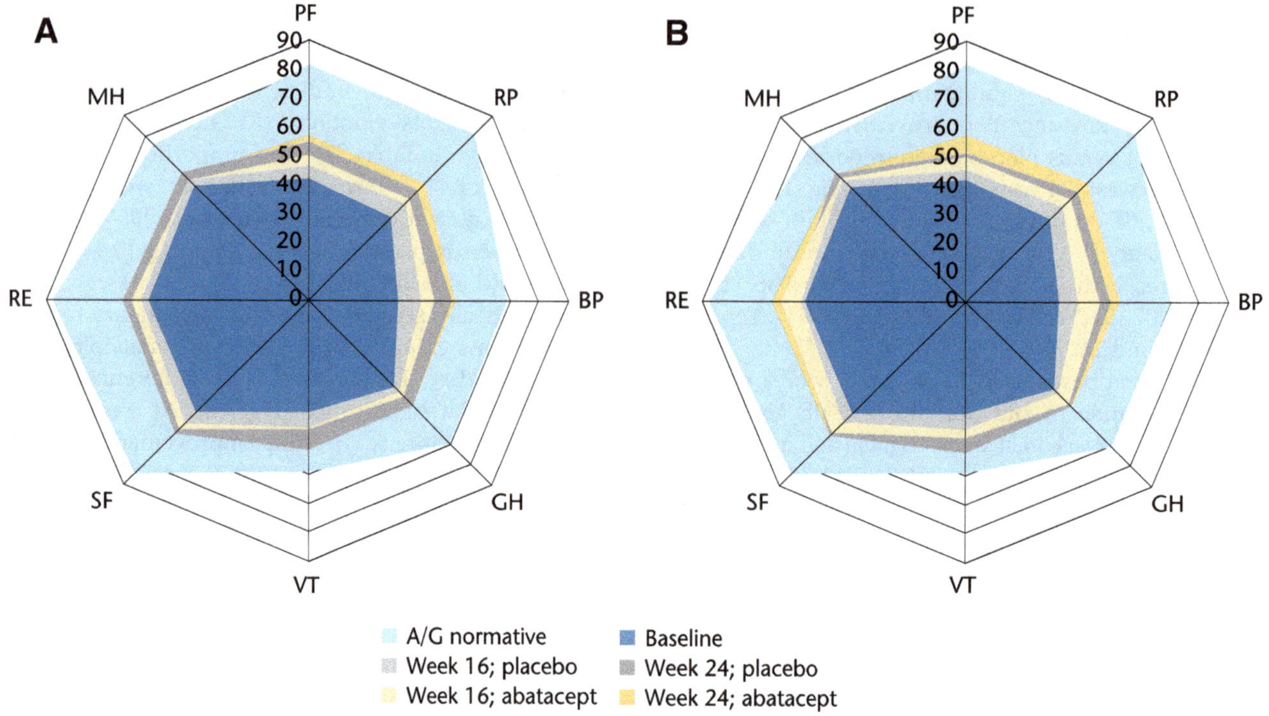

Fig. 3 Abatacept/placebo SF-36 domain scores (baseline, weeks 16, 24) versus normative population (**a**, overall; **b**, CRP > ULN). Normative values for SF-36 individual domains were defined based on matching the age/gender distribution of this protocol population to US 1999 norms in patients without chronic disease or arthritis [20, 34]: PF and RP 81.9, BP 69.7, GH 70.4, VT 59.3, SF 84.4, RE 87.8, MH 75.6. *A/G* age/gender, *BP* bodily pain, *CRP* C-reactive protein, *GH* general health, *MH* mental health, *PF* physical function, *RE* role-emotional, *RP* role-physical, *SF* social function, *SF-36* Short-Form 36, *ULN* upper limit of normal, *VT* vitality

placebo in HAQ-DI, SF-36 PCS and MCS, and FACIT-F (Fig. 4b) scores and all SF-36 domains (see Additional file 3: Table S3) ($P > 0.05$).

Subpopulation analyses

Changes from baseline at weeks 16 and 24

Across all PROs, improvements from baseline to week 16, although not statistically significant, were numerically greater in patients with baseline CRP > ULN versus those with CRP ≤ ULN in both abatacept and placebo groups ($P > 0.05$; Table 1). In the CRP > ULN subpopulation, improvements with abatacept versus placebo were significantly greater in HAQ-DI, SF-36 PCS, MCS, FACIT-F and DLQI scores (Table 1). Across all SF-36 domains, with the exception of MH, statistically significantly greater improvements were reported at week 16 with abatacept versus placebo in patients with baseline CRP > ULN (Fig. 3b and Fig. 5). Statistically significant improvements (adjusted mean difference [95% CI]) in DLQI (– 2.32 [– 3.80 to – 0.83]; Table 1) and SF-36 PF (8.57 [2.15 to 14.99]) and BP (6.62 [0.15 to 13.09]) (Fig. 5b) domain scores were reported in the baseline CRP > ULN subpopulation with abatacept versus placebo at week 24; however, data should be interpreted with caution due to low patient numbers. In the CRP ≤ ULN subpopulation, no significant improvements with abatacept versus placebo were evident at week 16 (Table 1).

A statistically significant benefit for abatacept versus placebo was reported by TNFi-naïve patients at week 16 in SF-36 MCS (Table 1) scores. Among abatacept-treated TNFi-naïve patients at baseline, numerically, although not statistically significant, greater improvements in SF-36 PCS, MCS and FACIT-F scores at week 16 were reported versus TNFi-exposed patients ($P > 0.05$; Table 1). In the TNFi-naïve abatacept-treated subpopulation, adjusted mean changes from baseline at week 16 exceeded MCID in SF-36 PCS, MCS and FACIT- F scores (Table 1), and seven of eight SF-36 domains with exception of MH (data not shown). In TNFi-exposed abatacept-treated patients, improvements exceeded MCID in SF-36 PCS scores (Table 1).

Discussion

These analyses demonstrated that abatacept treatment generally improved PROs in patients with active PsA in the phase 3 ASTRAEA trial, particularly in those who were TNFi-naïve and/or with elevated CRP at baseline. In the overall population at week 16, prior to EE,

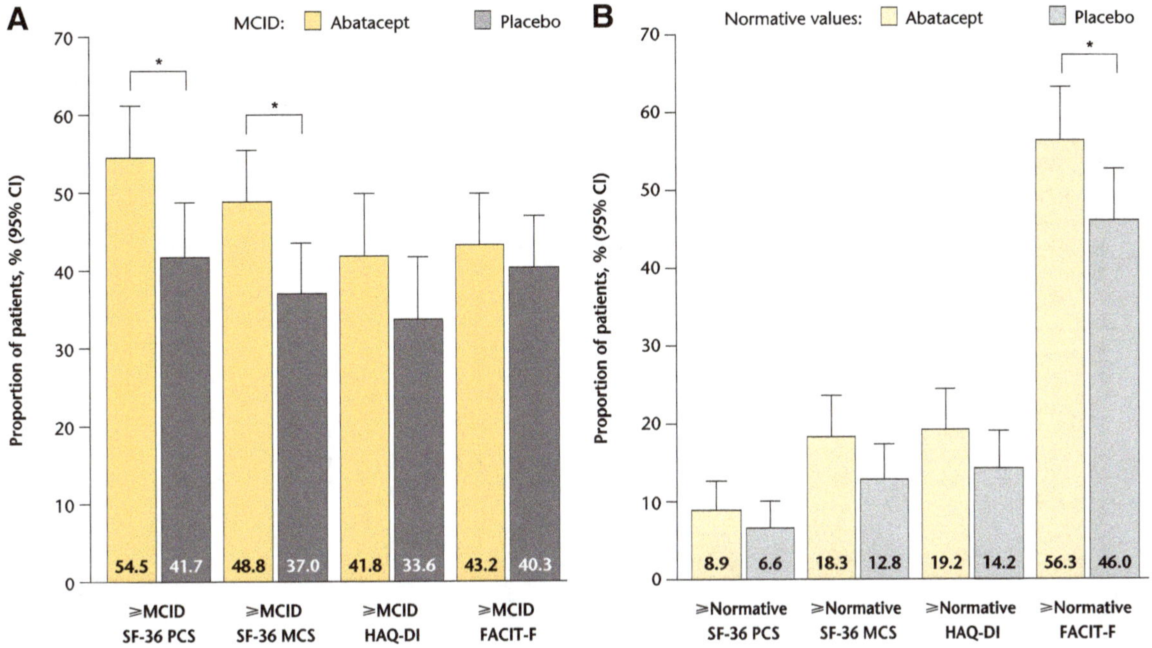

	≥MCID SF-36 PCS	≥MCID SF-36 MCS	≥MCID HAQ-DI	≥MCID FACIT-F	≥Normative SF-36 PCS	≥Normative SF-36 MCS	≥Normative HAQ-DI	≥Normative FACIT-F
Estimate of difference from placebo (95% CI)	12.8 (2.8, 22.7)	11.9 (2.0, 21.7)	7.1 (−2.7, 17.0)	2.9 (−6.9, 12.8)	2.3 (−3.3, 7.8)	5.5 (−1.8, 12.9)	5.0 (−2.5, 12.6)	10.4 (0.4, 20.3)

Fig. 4 Rates of PRO improvements ≥ MCID (**a**) or ≥ normative values (**b**) at week 16 (overall population). *Statistically significant difference. MCID values: HAQ-DI ≥ − 0.35, SF-36 PCS ≥ 2.5, SF-36 MCS ≥ 2.5, FACIT-F ≥ − 4.0 and SF-36 domains ≥5.0. Normative values: HAQ-DI ≥ 0.5, SF-36 PCS ≥ 50, SF-36 MCS ≥ 50 and FACIT-F ≥ 40.1. *CI* confidence interval, *FACIT-F* Functional Assessment of Chronic Illness Therapy-Fatigue scale, *HAQ-DI* Health Assessment Questionnaire-Disability Index, *MCID* minimal clinically important difference, *MCS* mental component summary, *PCS* physical component summary, *PRO* patient-reported outcome, *SF-36* Short Form-36

abatacept administration was associated with improved PROs compared with placebo; significant improvements with abatacept versus placebo were reported in SF-36 PCS, PF, BP and VT domain scores as well as DLQI, reflecting those areas of HRQoL most impacted by PsA. At week 24 in the non-EE responder analysis, a potential benefit of abatacept treatment was evident compared with placebo, with significantly greater improvements reported in physical function (by HAQ-DI) and dermatological manifestations (by DLQI). The proportion of patients with clinically meaningful HAQ-DI responses (reductions from baseline score ≥ 0.35) at week 24 was numerically higher with abatacept versus placebo: 31.0% versus 23.7%; however, as this did not reach statistical significance, it was not possible to definitively attribute significance to lower-ranking secondary endpoints in the hierarchical testing (nominal *P* values only were generated; 95% CIs were not overlapping) [10]. Notably, significant improvements in DLQI, the only PRO investigated here that directly measures the skin domain in PsA, were reported by those patients with a background of an overall modest skin response (by Psoriatic Area and Severity Index) in ASTRAEA at week 24 [10]. Nevertheless, as the week 24 analysis included only non-EE responders, the placebo arm comprised patients who reported responses to placebo. Therefore, it may be expected that differences between treatment groups would be less obvious at week 24 than week 16. In addition, the number of patients analysed at this time point was lower than at week 16.

Comparisons of the proportion of patients reporting improvements ≥ MCID is considered a clinically meaningful estimate of therapy effects [22]. Overall, the proportion of abatacept-treated patients reporting improvements ≥ MCID in PROs exceeded the proportion of placebo-treated patients: at week 16, 41.8–58.2% of abatacept-treated patients across different PROs reported clinically meaningful improvements in HAQ-DI, SF-36 PCS and MCS, individual SF-36 domains and FACIT-F scores compared with 33.6–47.9% of those treated with placebo.

In addition to the overall population analysis, PROs were analysed in subpopulations of patients by baseline CRP, as elevated CRP is an identified poor prognostic factor [11]. There was a non-statistically significant trend towards improved PROs in patients with elevated baseline CRP regardless of treatment arm at week 16. However, among patients with elevated CRP, those receiving abatacept reported greater improvements compared with placebo. Similarly, in the main ASTRAEA study, the highest

Table 1 Adjusted mean change from baseline in PROs at weeks 16 (all patients) and 24 (non-EE responder analysis) in patients treated with abatacept or placebo and stratified by baseline CRP level or prior TNFi use

Subpopulation	Week 16 (before EE)			Week 24 (non-EE responders)		
CRP > ULN	Abatacept	Placebo	Adjusted mean difference (95% CI)	Abatacept	Placebo	Adjusted mean difference (95% CI)
HAQ-DI	−0.34 (0.05),* $n = 139$	−0.19 (0.05), $n = 115$	−0.15 (−0.28 to −0.02)	−0.41 (0.07), n = 86	−0.23 (0.08), $n = 59$	−0.18 (−0.37 to 0.01)
SF-36 PCS	4.97 (0.70),* $n = 139$	2.50 (0.75), $n = 112$	2.47 (0.63 to 4.31)	6.41 (0.83), $n = 86$	4.04 (0.95), $n = 58$	2.37 (0.13 to 4.61)
SF-36 MCS	4.54 (0.86),* $n = 139$	1.39 (0.94), $n = 112$	3.14 (0.85 to 5.44)	4.05 (1.05), $n = 86$	2.71 (1.24), $n = 58$	1.34 (−1.54 to 4.22)
FACIT-F	−5.19 (0.83),* $n = 139$	−2.81 (0.88), $n = 116$	−2.38 (−4.57 to −0.19)	−6.44 (1.03), $n = 87$	−5.44 (1.21), $n = 60$	−1.00 (−3.81 to 1.80)
DLQI	−2.72 (0.42),* $n = 141$	−1.48 (0.45), $n = 116$	−1.24 (−2.35 to −0.13)	−2.74 (0.55),* $n = 87$	−0.42 (0.64), $n = 60$	−2.32 (−3.80 to −0.83)
CRP ≤ ULN	Abatacept	Placebo	Adjusted mean difference (95% CI)	Abatacept	Placebo	Adjusted mean difference (95% CI)
HAQ-DI	−0.08 (0.06), $n = 62$	−0.08 (0.06), $n = 70$	0.01 (−0.14 to 0.15)	−0.12 (0.08), $n = 37$	−0.08 (0.08), $n = 39$	−0.04 (−0.26 to 0.19)
SF-36 PCS	1.33 (0.91), $n = 62$	1.56 (0.88), $n = 72$	−0.23 (−2.63 to 2.18)	3.04 (1.03), $n = 37$	3.10 (1.04), $n = 39$	−0.06 (−2.88 to 2.77)
SF-36 MCS	−1.95 (1.20), $n = 62$	0.85 (1.17), $n = 72$	−2.80 (−6.00 to 0.40)	−0.69 (1.29), $n = 37$	1.67 (1.31), $n = 39$	−2.37 (−5.94 to 1.21)
FACIT-F	−0.58 (1.03), $n = 66$	−2.47 (1.02), $n = 78$	1.89 (−0.86 to 4.63)	−0.77 (1.24), $n = 38$	−3.22 (1.28), $n = 39$	2.45 (−0.99 to 5.89)
DLQI	−1.28 (0.57), $n = 63$	−1.04 (0.56), $n = 71$	−0.24 (−1.77 to 1.28)	−1.60 (0.72), $n = 38$	−0.92 (0.75), $n = 38$	−0.69 (−2.70 to 1.33)
TNFi-naïve	Abatacept	Placebo	Adjusted mean difference (95% CI)	Abatacept	Placebo	Adjusted mean difference (95% CI)
HAQ-DI	−0.24 (0.06), $n = 80$	−0.15 (0.06), $n = 75$	−0.08 (−0.25 to 0.08)	−0.29 (0.06), $n = 50$	−0.17 (0.07), $n = 35$	−0.12 (−0.30 to 0.06)
SF-36 PCS	3.63 (0.89), $n = 82$	2.05 (0.91), $n = 78$	1.58 (−0.79 to 3.95)	4.70 (0.97), $n = 49$	2.92 (1.08), $n = 34$	1.78 (−0.91 to 4.46)
SF-36 MCS	2.98 (1.06),* $n = 82$	−0.02 (1.08), $n = 78$	3.00 (0.19 to 5.81)	2.54 (1.17), $n = 49$	2.79 (1.38), $n = 34$	−0.25 (−3.60 to 3.10)
FACIT-F	−4.08 (1.01), $n = 81$	−2.17 (1.02), $n = 79$	−1.91 (−4.57 to 0.76)	−4.14 (1.21), $n = 51$	−4.65 (1.41), $n = 35$	0.51 (−0.29 to 3.93)
DLQI	−1.87 (0.51), $n = 83$	−0.92 (0.52), $n = 79$	−0.95 (−2.31 to 0.41)	−1.52 (0.67), $n = 51$	−0.23 (0.75), $n = 34$	−1.29 (−3.16 to 0.57)
TNFi-exposed†	Abatacept‡	Placebo§	Adjusted mean difference (95% CI)	Abatacept‡	Placebo§	Adjusted mean difference (95% CI)
HAQ-DI	−0.25 (0.05), $n = 122$	−0.13 (0.05), $n = 112$	−0.12 (−0.25 to 0.01)	−0.35 (0.06), $n = 74$	−0.18 (0.07), $n = 63$	−0.16 (−0.33 to 0.00)
SF-36 PCS	3.50 (0.70), $n = 120$	1.68 (0.74), $n = 108$	1.82 (−0.02 to 3.66)	5.02 (0.86), $n = 75$	3.70 (0.93), $n = 63$	1.32 (−0.95 to 3.59)
SF-36 MCS	2.03 (0.94), $n = 120$	1.97 (0.99), $n = 108$	0.06 (−2.41 to 2.53)	2.46 (1.16), $n = 75$	2.37 (1.24), $n = 63$	0.09 (−2.95 to 3.13)
FACIT-F	−3.34 (0.86), $n = 121$	−2.96 (0.89), $n = 110$	−0.39 (−2.64 to 1.86)	−4.61 (1.09), $n = 75$	−4.13 (1.16), $n = 64$	−0.48 (−3.34 to 2.38)
DLQI	−2.68 (0.45), $n = 122$	−1.61 (0.48), $n = 110$	−1.07 (−2.27 to 0.12)	−2.76 (0.59),* $n = 75$	−0.71 (0.63), $n = 64$	−2.04 (−3.59 to −0.49)

Data are adjusted mean change (SE) unless otherwise indicated. A positive change in SF-36 PCS and SF-36 MCS and a negative change in FACIT-F, HAQ-DI and DLQI corresponded to an improvement
CI confidence interval, *CRP* C-reactive protein, *DLQI* Dermatology Life Quality Index, *EE* early escape, *FACIT-F* Functional Assessment of Chronic Illness Therapy-Fatigue scale, *HAQ-DI* Health Assessment Questionnaire-Disability Index, *MCS* mental component summary, *PCS* physical component summary, *PRO* patient-reported outcome, *SE* standard error, *SF-36* Short Form-36, *TNFi* tumour necrosis factor inhibitor, *ULN* upper limit of normal

*95% CI of difference versus placebo did not cross 0

†At least 70% of the TNFi-exposed subpopulation were TNFi failures

‡Prior TNFi use, *n* (%): 1 TNFi, 94 (44.1); 2 TNFi, 31 (14.6); ≥ 3 TNFi, 4 (1.9)

§Prior TNFi use, *n* (%): 1 TNFi, 92 (43.6); 2 TNFi, 36 (17.1); ≥ 3 TNFi, 2 (0.9)

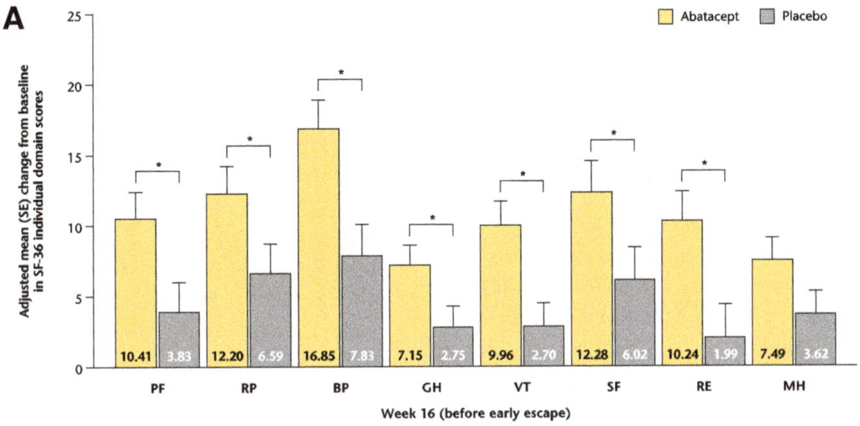

	PF	RP	BP	GH	VT	SF	RE	MH
Adjusted mean difference from placebo (95% CI)	6.58 (1.45, 11.70)	5.61 (0.57, 10.65)	9.02 (3.91, 14.14)	4.40 (0.79, 8.02)	7.26 (2.90, 11.63)	6.26 (0.59, 11.93)	8.25 (2.60, 13.89)	3.87 (−0.16, 7.90)
Abatacept, n	140	140	139	140	140	140	140	140
Placebo, n	113	113	113	113	112	113	113	112

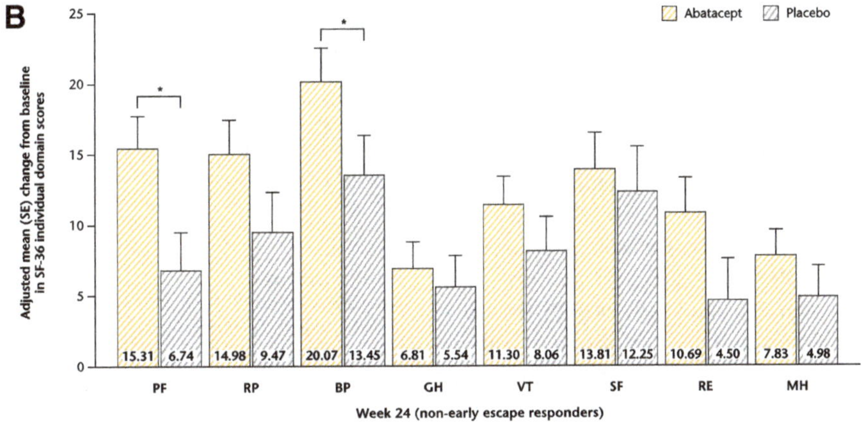

	PF	RP	BP	GH	VT	SF	RE	MH
Adjusted mean difference from placebo (95% CI)	8.57 (2.15, 14.99)	5.51 (−1.04, 12.06)	6.62 (0.15, 13.09)	1.27 (−3.99, 6.53)	3.24 (−2.40, 8.89)	1.56 (−5.76, 8.88)	6.19 (−0.79, 13.18)	2.85 (−2.25, 7.95)
Abatacept, n	87	87	87	87	86	87	87	86
Placebo, n	58	58	58	58	58	58	58	58

Fig. 5 SF-36 domain score changes from baseline for CRP > ULN population: weeks 16 (**a**) and 24 (**b**). *Statistically significant difference. *BP* bodily pain, *CI* confidence interval, *CRP* C-reactive protein, *GH* general health, *MH* mental health, *PF* physical function, RE role–emotional, *RP* role–physical, *SE* standard error, *SF* social function, *SF-36* Short Form-36, *VT* vitality

ACR20 responses with abatacept versus placebo were seen in patients with CRP > ULN at baseline [10], suggesting that these patients may be particularly responsive to abatacept. Our results suggest that baseline CRP should be taken into consideration when evaluating the clinical efficacy of different treatments. PROs were also analysed in subpopulations by previous exposure to TNFi treatment. At week 16, improvements were greater with abatacept than with placebo in both TNFi-naïve and TNFi-exposed subpopulations. However, in abatacept-treated patients, reported improvements in PROs were generally larger in the TNFi-naïve versus TNFi-exposed subpopulations. Indeed, greater efficacy would be expected in TNFi-naïve than in TNFi-exposed patients [23]. These findings are in line with clinical outcomes observed with abatacept in this trial, which were generally better in patients with elevated CRP at baseline and TNFi-naïve patients [10]. The PRO data reported here support previous results that abatacept may be particularly effective in certain subpopulations of patients.

The effects of other DMARDs, including TNFi agents, on PROs in patients with active PsA have been investigated previously, with most studies assessing effects over 24 or 48 weeks. Statistically and clinically meaningful improvements in SF-36 PCS and MCS and all individual domain scores from baseline to week 24 have been reported with etanercept [24]; clinically meaningful improvements in PROs including HAQ-DI and SF-36 PCS scores have also been reported over 48 weeks of treatment [25]. Similarly, adalimumab has been shown to improve HRQoL, based on SF-36 PCS, HAQ-DI, FACIT-F and DLQI scores, after 48 weeks of treatment [26]. The effects of the newer interleukin inhibitors on PROs have also been studied. Ustekinumab, an anti-interleukin-12 and -23 agent, improved physical function (by SF-36 PCS and HAQ-DI) and dermatological manifestations (by DLQI) at week 24 [27, 28]. Beneficial effects on PROs have also been reported after 24 weeks with the anti-interleukin-17A agent secukinumab [29, 30]. Furthermore, apremilast, a phosphodiesterase 4 inhibitor, was shown to significantly improve HAQ-DI scores by week 16 compared with placebo in a 24-week trial in which < 10% of patients had previously failed a biologic therapy [31]. In the current study, improvements in PROs achieved with abatacept appeared less marked than that reported with other biologic DMARDs (bDMARDs) in earlier studies; however, differences in trial design and patient populations preclude comparisons of efficacy between abatacept and other bDMARDs based on currently available evidence.

The therapeutic options for PsA have greatly increased over the past 10 years and, as more new treatments are introduced, assessing responses to therapy including PROs will become increasingly important, aiding treatment choices. A recent literature review provided an evidence-based overview of 44 instruments per core PsA outcome domain to ascertain applicability and best instrument for each domain of the many available PROs [32]. However, further research is warranted to develop and validate specific PRO measures that better capture the impact of all PsA symptoms [33]. In the meantime, using a combination of instruments and/or the best available instrument per domain, as in this trial, provides a more complete picture [33].

A number of study limitations should be considered. First, subpopulation comparisons and ascertainment of scores ≥ MCID and ≥ normative values were post hoc in nature. Second, owing to the particular trial design, a high proportion of patients were subject to EE at week 16; as such, week 24 analyses included a limited number of patients who were still receiving blinded treatment in either arm of the trial. Only nominal *P* values were provided for endpoints that ranked lower in the statistical hierarchy than the first secondary endpoint, which did not reach statistical significance at the 5% level. For other endpoints, only 95% CIs of differences between abatacept and placebo arms were generated, without associated *P* values. In addition, due to the low patient numbers, the reported data for subpopulations were difficult to interpret, particularly at week 24. Finally, certain PROs may improve less rapidly over time and thus the week 16 time point may have not allowed maximal effects of abatacept treatment to be observed. In addition, although some statistically significant improvements were noted with abatacept, these may not necessarily be clinically important.

Conclusions

In conclusion, abatacept treatment improved PROs at week 16 in patients with active PsA, with evidence of some effects sustained at week 24. Furthermore, PRO improvements were greater in TNFi-naïve patients and those with elevated CRP. These results demonstrate that clinical improvements in PsA signs and symptoms previously reported with abatacept treatment [10] also result in clinically meaningful improvements in PROs.

Additional files

Additional file 1: Table S1. Adjusted mean change from baseline in SF-36 individual domains at weeks 16 (all patients) and 24 (non-EE responder analysis) in patients treated with abatacept or placebo (overall population).

Additional file 2: Table S2. Proportion of patients (95% CI) treated with abatacept or placebo reporting improvements ≥MCID in SF-36 individual domains at week 16 (all patients) in the overall population.

Additional file 3: Table S3. Proportion of patients (95% CI) treated with abatacept or placebo reporting improvements ≥normative values in SF-36 individual domains at week 16 (all patients) in the overall population.

Abbreviations

ACR20: American College of Rheumatology criteria; ASTRAEA: Active pSoriaTic aRthritis rAndomizEd triAl; bDMARDS: Biologic disease-modifying anti-rheumatic drugs; BP: Bodily pain; BSA: Body surface area; CASPAR: Classification Criteria for Psoriatic Arthritis; CI: Confidence interval; CRP: C-reactive protein; DLQI: Dermatology Life Quality Index; DMARD: Disease-modifying antirheumatic drug; EE: Early escape; FACIT-F: Functional Assessment of Chronic Illness Therapy-Fatigue; GH: General health; HAQ-DI: Health Assessment Questionnaire-Disability Index; HRQoL: Health-related quality of life; MCID: Minimal clinically important difference; MCS: Mental component summary; MH: Mental health; MTX: Methotrexate; NV: Normative values; PCS: Physical component summary; PF: Physical functioning; PRO: Patient-reported outcome; PsA: Psoriatic arthritis; RE: Role–emotional; RP: Role–physical; SC: Subcutaneous; SE: Standard error; SF-36: Short Form-36; TNFi: Tumour necrosis factor inhibitor; ULN: Upper limit of normal; VT: Vitality

Acknowledgements

Under the direction of the authors, Katerina Kumpan, PhD, of Caudex, Oxford, UK (funded by Bristol-Myers Squibb), provided medical writing assistance for the development of this manuscript. Sandra Overfield, Protocol Manager, Bristol-Myers Squibb, assisted in initial design and operational aspects of the study.

Funding

This study was funded by Bristol-Myers Squibb.

Consent to participate

All patients or their legal representatives gave written, informed consent prior to study entry.

Patient consent

All patients or their legal representatives gave written, informed consent prior to study entry.

Authors' contributions

VS, PM and SB were responsible for the conception and design of the study, and the acquisition, analysis and interpretation of data. All authors had full access to the study data, critically reviewed the manuscript, approved the final version prior to submission, and take responsibility for the integrity and accuracy of the reported data.

Competing interests

VS reports receiving consulting fees from AbbVie, Amgen Corporation, AstraZeneca, Biogen, Bristol-Myers Squibb, Boehringer Ingelheim, Celgene, Celltrion, Corrona, Crescendo/Myriad Genetics, EMD Serono, Genentech/Roche, GlaxoSmithKline, Janssen, Lilly, Merck, Novartis, Pfizer, Regeneron, Samsung, Sandoz, Sanofi and UCB. EA, TL, AJ, SB and HAA are employees of Bristol-Myers Squibb and report holding stock in Bristol-Myers Squibb. PJM reports receiving consulting fees from AbbVie, Amgen, Bristol-Myers Squibb, Celgene, Corrona, Janssen, Lilly, Merck, Novartis, Pfizer, Sun, UCB and Zynerba; and speaker fees from AbbVie, Amgen, Bristol-Myers Squibb, Celgene, Genentech, Janssen, Novartis, Pfizer and UCB.

Author details

[1]Division of Immunology/Rheumatology, Stanford University School of Medicine, Palo Alto, CA, USA. [2]Bristol-Myers Squibb, Princeton, NJ, USA. [3]Swedish Medical Center and University of Washington, Seattle, WA, USA.

References

1. Gladman DD, Antoni C, Mease P, Clegg DO, Nash P. Psoriatic arthritis: epidemiology, clinical features, course, and outcome. Ann Rheum Dis. 2005; 64(Suppl 2):ii14–7.
2. Finlay AY, Khan GK. Dermatology Life Quality Index (DLQI)--a simple practical measure for routine clinical use. Clin Exp Dermatol. 1994;19(3):210–6.
3. Hewlett S, Dures E, Almeida C. Measures of fatigue: Bristol Rheumatoid Arthritis Fatigue Multi-Dimensional Questionnaire (BRAF MDQ), Bristol Rheumatoid Arthritis Fatigue Numerical Rating Scales (BRAF NRS) for severity, effect, and coping, Chalder Fatigue Questionnaire (CFQ), Checklist Individual Strength (CIS20R and CIS8R), Fatigue Severity Scale (FSS), Functional Assessment Chronic Illness Therapy (Fatigue) (FACIT-F), Multi-Dimensional Assessment of Fatigue (MAF), Multi-Dimensional Fatigue Inventory (MFI), Pediatric Quality Of Life (PedsQL) Multi-Dimensional Fatigue Scale, Profile of Fatigue (ProF), Short Form 36 Vitality Subscale (SF-36 VT), and Visual Analog Scales (VAS). Arthritis Care Res (Hoboken). 2011;63(Suppl 11):S263–S86.
4. Husted JA, Gladman DD, Long JA, Farewell VT. A modified version of the Health Assessment Questionnaire (HAQ) for psoriatic arthritis. Clin Exp Rheumatol. 1995;13(4):439–43.
5. Husted JA, Gladman DD, Farewell VT, Long JA, Cook RJ. Validating the SF-36 health survey questionnaire in patients with psoriatic arthritis. J Rheumatol. 1997;24(3):511–7.
6. Mease PJ. Measures of psoriatic arthritis: Tender and Swollen Joint Assessment, Psoriasis Area and Severity Index (PASI), Nail Psoriasis Severity Index (NAPSI), Modified Nail Psoriasis Severity Index (mNAPSI), Mander/Newcastle Enthesitis Index (MEI), Leeds Enthesitis Index (LEI), Spondyloarthritis Research Consortium of Canada (SPARCC), Maastricht Ankylosing Spondylitis Enthesis Score (MASES), Leeds Dactylitis Index (LDI), Patient Global for Psoriatic Arthritis, Dermatology Life Quality Index (DLQI), Psoriatic Arthritis Quality of Life (PsAQOL), Functional Assessment of Chronic Illness Therapy-Fatigue (FACIT-F), Psoriatic Arthritis Response Criteria (PsARC), Psoriatic Arthritis Joint Activity Index (PsAJAI), Disease Activity in Psoriatic Arthritis (DAPSA), and Composite Psoriatic Disease Activity Index (CPDAI). Arthritis Care Res (Hoboken). 2011;63(Suppl 11):S64–85.
7. Bruce B, Fries JF. The Stanford Health Assessment Questionnaire: dimensions and practical applications. Health Qual Life Outcomes. 2003;1:20.
8. Cutolo M, Nadler S. Advances in CTLA-4-Ig-mediated modulation of inflammatory cell and immune response activation in rheumatoid arthritis. Autoimmun Rev. 2013;12(7):758–67.
9. Orencia Prescribing Information 2017 February 2, 2018. Available from: http://packageinserts.bms.com/pi/pi_orencia.pdf. Accessed 2 Feb 2018.
10. Mease PJ, Gottlieb AB, van der Heijde D, FitzGerald O, Johnsen A, Nys M, et al. Efficacy and safety of abatacept, a T-cell modulator, in a randomised, double-blind, placebo-controlled, phase III study in psoriatic arthritis. Ann Rheum Dis. 2017;76:1550–8.
11. Gossec L, Smolen JS, Ramiro S, de Wit M, Cutolo M, Dougados M, et al. European League Against Rheumatism (EULAR) recommendations for the management of psoriatic arthritis with pharmacological therapies: 2015 update. Ann Rheum Dis. 2016;75(3):499–510.
12. Taylor W, Gladman D, Helliwell P, Marchesoni A, Mease P, Mielants H. Classification criteria for psoriatic arthritis: development of new criteria from a large international study. Arthritis Rheum. 2006;54(8):2665–73.
13. Gladman DD, Mease PJ, Cifaldi MA, Perdok RJ, Sasso E, Medich J. Adalimumab improves joint-related and skin-related functional impairment in patients with psoriatic arthritis: patient-reported outcomes of the Adalimumab Effectiveness in Psoriatic Arthritis Trial. Ann Rheum Dis. 2007;66(2):163–8.
14. Mease PJ, Woolley JM, Bitman B, Wang BC, Globe DR, Singh A. Minimally important difference of Health Assessment Questionnaire in psoriatic arthritis: relating thresholds of improvement in functional ability to patient-rated importance and satisfaction. J Rheumatol. 2011;38(11):2461–5.
15. Kosinski M, Zhao SZ, Dedhiya S, Osterhaus JT, Ware JE Jr. Determining minimally important changes in generic and disease-specific health-related quality of life questionnaires in clinical trials of rheumatoid arthritis. Arthritis Rheum. 2000;43(7):1478–87.
16. Shikiar R, Willian MK, Okun MM, Thompson CS, Revicki DA. The validity and responsiveness of three quality of life measures in the assessment of psoriasis patients: results of a phase II study. Health Qual Life Outcomes. 2006;4(1):71.
17. Strand V, Mease P, Burmester GR, Nikaï E, Coteur G, van Vollenhoven R, et al. Rapid and sustained improvements in health-related quality of life, fatigue, and other patient-reported outcomes in rheumatoid arthritis patients treated with certolizumab pegol plus methotrexate over 1 year: results from the RAPID 1 randomized controlled trial. Arthritis Res Ther. 2009;11(6):R170.
18. Krishnan E, Sokka T, Häkkinen A, Hubert H, Hannonen P. Normative values for the Health Assessment Questionnaire disability index: benchmarking disability in the general population. Arthritis Rheum. 2004;50(3):953–60.
19. Strand V, Rentz AM, Cifaldi MA, Chen N, Roy S, Revicki D. Health-related quality of life outcomes of adalimumab for patients with early rheumatoid arthritis: results from a randomized multicenter study. J Rheumatol. 2012;39(1):63–72.
20. Revicki DA, Menter A, Feldman S, Kimel M, Harnam N, Willian MK. Adalimumab improves health-related quality of life in patients with moderate to severe plaque psoriasis compared with the United States general population norms: results from a randomized, controlled Phase III study. Health Qual Life Outcomes. 2008;6(1):75.
21. Webster K, Cella D, Yost K. The Functional Assessment of Chronic Illness Therapy (FACIT) Measurement System: properties, applications, and interpretation. Health Qual Life Outcomes. 2003;1:79.
22. Strand V, Boers M, Idzerda L, Kirwan JR, Kvien TK, Tugwell PS, et al. It's good to feel better but it's better to feel good and even better to feel good as soon as possible for as long as possible. Response criteria and the importance of change at OMERACT 10. J Rheumatol. 2011;38(8):1720–7.
23. Mease P, van der Heijde D, Landewé R, et al. Secukinumab improves active psoriatic arthritis symptoms and inhibits radiographic progression: primary results from the randomised, double-blind, phase III FUTURE 5 study. Ann Rheum Dis. 2018;77:890–7.
24. Strand V, Sharp V, Koenig AS, Park G, Shi Y, Wang B, et al. Comparison of health-related quality of life in rheumatoid arthritis, psoriatic arthritis and psoriasis and effects of etanercept treatment. Ann Rheum Dis. 2012;71(7):1143–50.
25. Mease PJ, Woolley JM, Singh A, Tsuji W, Dunn M, Chiou CF. Patient-reported outcomes in a randomized trial of etanercept in psoriatic arthritis. J Rheumatol. 2010;37(6):1221–7.
26. Fleischmann R, Weinblatt ME, Schiff M, Khanna D, Maldonado MA, Nadkarni A, et al. Patient-reported outcomes from a two-year head-to-head comparison of subcutaneous abatacept versus adalimumab for rheumatoid arthritis. Arthritis Care Res (Hoboken). 2015;68(7):907–13.
27. Rahman P, Puig L, Gottlieb AB, Kavanaugh A, McInnes I, Ritchlin C, et al. SAT0264 ustekinumab improves physical function, quality of life and work productivity of patients with active psoriatic arthritis who were naïve to

MTX, despite MTX therapy or previously treated with anti-TNF: results from Psummit I and Psummit II. Ann Rheum Dis. 2013;72(Suppl 3):A671–A2.

28. Ritchlin C, Rahman P, Kavanaugh A, McInnes IB, Puig L, Li S, et al. Efficacy and safety of the anti-IL-12/23 p40 monoclonal antibody, ustekinumab, in patients with active psoriatic arthritis despite conventional non-biological and biological anti-tumour necrosis factor therapy: 6-month and 1-year results of the phase 3, multicentre, double-blind, placebo-controlled, randomised PSUMMIT 2 trial. Ann Rheum Dis. 2014;73(6):990–9.
29. McInnes IB, Mease PJ, Kirkham B, Kavanaugh A, Ritchlin CT, Rahman P, et al. Secukinumab, a human anti-interleukin-17A monoclonal antibody, in patients with psoriatic arthritis (FUTURE 2): a randomised, double-blind, placebo-controlled, phase 3 trial. Lancet. 2015;386(9999):1137–46.
30. Strand V, Mease P, Gossec L, Elkayam O, Van den Bosch F, Zuazo J, et al. Secukinumab improves patient-reported outcomes in subjects with active psoriatic arthritis: results from a randomised phase III trial (FUTURE 1). Ann Rheum Dis. 2017;76(1):203–7.
31. Kavanaugh A, Mease PJ, Gomez-Reino JJ, Adebajo AO, Wollenhaupt J, Gladman DD, et al. Treatment of psoriatic arthritis in a phase 3 randomised, placebo-controlled trial with apremilast, an oral phosphodiesterase 4 inhibitor. Ann Rheum Dis. 2014;73(6):1020–6.
32. Højgaard PKL, Orbai AM, Holmsted K, Bartels EM, Leung YY, Goel N, de Wit M, Gladman DD, Mease P, Dreyer L, Kristensen LE, FitzGerald O, Tillett W, Gossec L, Helliwell P, Strand V, Ogdie A, Terwee CB, Christensen R. A systematic review of measurement properties of patient reported outcome measures in psoriatic arthritis: A GRAPPA-OMERACT initiative. Semin Arthritis Rheum. 2018;47(5):654–65.
33. Mease P, Strand V, Gladman D. Functional impairment measurement in psoriatic arthritis: Importance and challenges. Semin Arthritis Rheum. 2018. https://doi.org/10.1016/j.semarthrit.2018.05.010.
34. Ware JE, Kosinski M. In: 2nd, editor. SF-36 Physical & Mental Health Summary Scales: A Manual for Users of Version 1. Lincoln: QualityMetric Incorporated; 2001.

7

Calprotectin strongly and independently predicts relapse in rheumatoid arthritis and polyarticular psoriatic arthritis patients treated with tumor necrosis factor inhibitors

José Inciarte-Mundo[1], Julio Ramirez[1], Maria Victoria Hernández[1], Virginia Ruiz-Esquide[1], Andrea Cuervo[1], Sonia Raquel Cabrera-Villalba[1], Mariona Pascal[2], Jordi Yagüe[2], Juan D. Cañete[1] and Raimon Sanmarti[1*]

Abstract

Background: Calprotectin is a biomarker of disease activity in rheumatoid arthritis (RA) and psoriatic arthritis (PsA) and predicts relapse in juvenile idiopathic arthritis. Higher drug trough serum levels are associated with a good response in patients treated with tumor necrosis factor inhibitors (TNFi). Power Doppler ultrasound synovitis is predictive of relapse and structural damage progression in patients in clinical remission. The purpose of this study was to analyze the accuracy of serum calprotectin levels, drug trough serum levels (TSL), and power Doppler (PD) activity as predictors of relapse in RA and PsA patients in remission or with low disease activity receiving TNFi.

Methods: This was a longitudinal, prospective, 1-year single-center study of 103 patients (47 RA, 56 PsA) receiving TNFi in remission or with low disease activity (28-joint Disease Activity Score (DAS28) $\leq$ 3.2). The predictive value of serum calprotectin, TNFi TSL, and PD were assessed using receiver operating characteristic (ROC) analyses. To illustrate the predictive performance of calprotectin, TNFi TSL, and PD score, Kaplan-Meier curves were constructed from baseline to relapse. Associations between baseline factors and relapse were determined using Cox regression models. Multivariate models were constructed to analyze the effect of covariates and to fully adjust the association between calprotectin, TNFi TSL, and PD score with relapse. A generalized estimating equation model with an identity link for longitudinal continuous outcomes was used to assess the effect of covariates on TNFi TSL.

(Continued on next page)

* Correspondence: sanmarti@clinic.cat
[1]Department of Rheumatology, Hospital Clinic, University of Barcelona, Carrer Villarroel 170, 08036 Barcelona, Spain
Full list of author information is available at the end of the article

(Continued from previous page)

Results: Ninety-five patients completed 1 year of follow-up, of whom 12 experienced a relapse. At baseline, relapsers had higher calprotectin levels, lower TNFi TSL, and higher PD activity than nonrelapsers. ROC analysis showed calprotectin fully predicted relapse (area under the curve (AUC) = 1.00). TNFi TSL and PD had an AUC of 0.790 (95% confidence interval (CI) 0.691–0.889) and 0.877 (95% CI 0.772–0.981), respectively. Survival analyses and log rank tests showed significant differences between groups according to calprotectin serum levels ($p < 0.001$), TNFi TSL ($p = 0.004$), and PD score ($p < 0.001$). Univariate Cox regression models showed that time-to-remission/low disease activity (hazard ratio (HR) = 1.17, $p < 0.001$), calprotectin levels (HR = 2.38, $p < 0.001$), TNFi TSL (HR = 0.47, $p = 0.018$), and PD score (HR = 1.31, $p < 0.001$) were significantly associated with disease relapse. In the multivariate analysis, only baseline calprotectin levels independently predicted disease relapse (HR = 2.41, $p = 0.002$). The generalized estimating equation analysis showed that only disease activity by DAS28-erythrocyte sedimentation rate (ESR) was significantly associated with longitudinal changes in TNFi TSL (regression coefficient 0.26 (0.0676 to 0.0036), $p = 0.001$).

Conclusion: Time-to-remission/low disease activity, calprotectin serum levels, TNFi TSL, and PD score were significantly associated with disease relapse. However, only baseline calprotectin serum levels independently predicted disease relapse in RA and PsA patients under TNFi therapy.

Keywords: Calprotectin, TNFi serum trough levels, Ultrasound, Relapse, Biomarkers, Predictors, Rheumatoid arthritis, Psoriatic arthritis

Background

Biological therapies have dramatically improved the management and prognosis of rheumatoid arthritis (RA) and psoriatic arthritis (PsA). Remission or low disease activity is possible in an increasing number of patients. Nevertheless, persistent remission is more difficult to achieve since disease relapses are common. In patients classified as in clinical remission, low-grade inflammatory activity may persist but remain undetectable by routine tests. Subclinical disease activity may result in disease relapse. Musculoskeletal ultrasound (MSUS) has shown that a significant proportion of patients classified as in remission exhibit a power Doppler (PD) signal [1] which is associated with short-term relapse in RA patients [2, 3].

Calprotectin, a member of the S100 protein family, is an important proinflammatory factor of innate immunity, acting as an endogenous damage-associated molecular pattern molecule via Toll-like receptor 4 activation. Higher calprotectin levels have been found in serum from RA and PsA patients [4, 5]. Calprotectin serum levels correlate with disease activity and are independently associated with radiographic progression in RA [6, 7]. Moreover, calprotectin levels predict the response to biologic therapy in RA and PsA patients [8, 9]. Our research group has demonstrated that serum calprotectin stratifies disease activity more accurately than C-reactive protein (CRP) or the erythrocyte sedimentation rate (ESR) in patients receiving tumor necrosis factor inhibitors (TNFi) [10] or tocilizumab [11], and strongly correlates with power Doppler ultrasound synovitis (PDUS) in RA and PsA patients with low disease activity [12]. In other rheumatic diseases, such as juvenile idiopathic arthritis, calprotectin more accurately predicted relapse in patients in remission [13]; therefore, calprotectin might be useful in predicting relapse in RA and PsA patients with low disease activity.

Recent studies have found a significant dose-response relationship between the extent of clinical improvement and TNFi trough serum levels in RA and spondyloarthritis (SpA) patients [14, 15]. Higher TNFi trough serum levels have been associated with good therapeutic responses [16].Therefore, patients with low TNFi trough serum levels might be more prone to relapse.

The aim of this study was to determine the accuracy of baseline calprotectin, TNFi trough serum levels, and power Doppler (PD) score in predicting disease relapse in RA and PsA patients in remission or with low disease activity. In addition, we examined other baseline factors related to relapse, the performance of calprotectin and TNFi trough serum levels during relapse, and factors associated with longitudinal changes in TNFi trough serum levels.

Patients and methods

This longitudinal prospective observational single-center study included 103 consecutive RA patients (according to American College of Rheumatology (ACR) 1987 criteria) and polyarticular PsA patients (according to the Classification of Psoriatic Arthritis (CASPAR)) from our Arthritis Unit. Patients were enrolled between March 2013 and September 2014, with follow-up ending in September 2015. All patients were in remission (28-joint Disease Activity Score (DAS28)-ESR ≤ 2.6) or had low disease activity (DAS28-ESR ≤ 3.2) in two consecutive visits at least 3 months apart and were currently receiving adalimumab (ADA), etanercept (ETN), or infliximab (IFX). Exclusion criteria included patients with higher levels of disease activity (DAS28 > 3.2) or PsA patients with axial or entheseal involvement, or an oligoarticular peripheral pattern. Details on demographic data, disease duration, autoantibody status, radiological data, concomitant conventional synthetic disease-modifying antirheumatic drug (csDMARD) therapy, and dose and duration of biological therapy were collected. Some patients received a reduced dose of biologic therapy due to persistent remission/low disease activity. A reduced dose was defined as treatment with a lower amount of the drug or longer intervals of administration than recommended in each product package insert.

Definition of disease relapse

A disease relapse was defined using the revised European League Against Rheumatism (EULAR) response criteria [17]. The criterion for disease relapse was current DAS28 > 3.2 and an increase in DAS28 > 0.6 compared with baseline. Patients were encouraged to contact investigators if they had a disease relapse between two visits. Patients fulfilling this criterion were classified as relapsers, while patients remaining stable during follow-up were classified as nonrelapsers.

Measurement of clinical disease activity

All patients underwent clinical assessment at baseline and at 4, 8, and 12 months, including 28-joint swollen and tender joint counts (28-SJC and 28-TJC, respectively), physician and patient global assessment with visual analogue scales (0–100 mm), ESR (mm), and CRP (mg/dL). Three composite disease activity indices were subsequently calculated: DAS28-ESR [18], Clinical Disease Activity Index (CDAI) [19], and Simple Disease Activity Index (SDAI) [20].

Serum biomarkers: calprotectin and TNFi trough levels

Calprotectin serum levels, TNFi trough serum levels, and antidrug antibodies were determined at baseline (visit 0) and during disease relapse using an enzyme-linked immunosorbent assay (ELISA) test kit (Calprolab™ calprotectin ELISA (ALP), Calpro AS, Oslo, Norway, and Promonitor®, Progenika SA, Spain, respectively) according to the manufacturers' protocol as previously described [10]. These ELISA kits are validated and show adequate correlation for the measurement of drug levels and antidrug antibodies [21]. To reduce variations in calprotectin determinations, the whole procedure was performed in a Triturus® autoanalyzer. Additionally, serum samples were collected at 4, 8, and 12 months of follow-up to assess longitudinal changes in drug trough serum levels.

Imaging Biomarkers: power Doppler score

A sonographic assessment was made at baseline (visit 0) using high-sensitivity ultrasound equipment (MyLab Twice®, Esaote, Italy) as previously described [12]. Joint MSUS findings were defined according to published Outcome Measures in Rheumatology (OMERACT) definitions [22]. One experienced sonographer (JR) who was blinded to the results of the clinical joint examination evaluated 11 joints and tendons of each hand (including the proximal interphalangeal joints, metacarpophalangeal joints, and wrists) for synovial hypertrophy (SH) and intra-articular PD signal according to EULAR guidelines [23]. SH and the PD signals were graded according to the methodology of Szkudlarek et al. [24]. Intra-rater agreement on the MSUS assessment, calculated as previously described [25], was 0.83 for SH and 0.90 for PD. We made a double ultrasound assessment in the first 10 patients included in the study. The two evaluations were separated by between 24 and 72 h. The same sonographer made both ultrasound explorations and noted the results. This index was calculated as the percentage of agreement between these scores at two time points. The following cut-off values, analogous to kappa coefficients, were defined for intra-rater reliability: < 0.0 = none, 0 to 0.20 = poor, 0.21 to 0.40 = modest, 0.41 to 0.60 = fair, 0.61 to 0.80 = good, and 0.81 to 1.00 = excellent.

By summing the scores for elementary lesions in each joint, we calculated the PD score (range 0–66), the SH score (range 0–66), and the global score (which is the sum of the PD and SH scores; range 0–132). PDUS was defined as a PD signal in synovial tissue [26]. A more-stringent definition of active synovitis (ultrasound-defined active synovitis (UdAS)) developed by our group (SH grade ≥ 2 plus PDUS signal) was also recorded [25].

This study was conducted in accordance with the Declaration of Helsinki and was approved by the Clinical Research Ethics Committee of the Hospital Clínic of Barcelona (Reg. 2013/8382). Signed informed consent was obtained from all patients before study enrolment.

Statistical analysis

Continuous data are presented as medians and interquartile ranges (IQR) and categorical variables as absolute frequencies and percentages. Relapsers versus nonrelapsers were compared using the Student's t test or Mann-Whitney test when appropriate. The predictive value of calprotectin, TNFi trough serum levels, and PD score for the risk of relapse was assessed using the receiver operating characteristic (ROC), and the most sensitive and specific cut-off was identified; they were then dichotomized, applying an optimal cut-off as per ROC analysis. The predictive values, accuracy, positive likelihood ratio, and maximum Youden index were calculated. The area under the curve (AUC) was estimated using Hanley's corrected confidence intervals (CIs). To illustrate the predictive performance of calprotectin, TNF serum levels, and PD score, Kaplan-Meier curves were constructed from baseline to

Table 1 Baseline characteristics of patients with disease relapse ("relapsers") or stable disease activity ("nonrelapsers") during 1 year of follow-up

Characteristic	Total ($n = 95$)	Nonrelapsers ($n = 83$)	Relapsers ($n = 12$)	p value
Age (years)	57 (50–66)	57 (50–66)	57 (48–63.5)	0.614
Female, *n* (%)	61 (64.2%)	53 (63.9%)	8 (66.7%)	1.000
Disease duration (years)	15 (9–21)	15 (9–21)	14.5 (7.5–24.5)	0.831
Diagnosis, *n* (%)				0.215
Psoriatic arthritis	51 (53,7%)	47 (56.6%)	4 (33.3%)	
Rheumatoid arthritis	44 (46.3%)	36 (43,4%)	8 (66.7%)	
Time to csDMARD (months)	25.6 (5.1–62.2)	24.4 (5.5–62.2)	32.6 (5.1–92.3)	0.911
Time to bDMARD (months)	98.5 (36.9–165.9)	98.5 (38.8–160.9)	95.9 (33.6225.9)	0.823
Time-to-remission/LDA (months)	3.27 (2.13–4.3)	3.07 (1.9–3.97)	20.4 (16.8–24.3)	**< 0.001**
Time-in-remission/LDA (months)	58.7 (26.7–86.6)	60.1 (27.6–88.0)	25.0 (9.4–59.3)	**0.027**
Calprotectin (μg/mL)	1.66 (0.69–2.68)	1.44 (0.62–2.34)	6.01 (5.01–6.44)	**< 0.001**
CRP (mg/dL)	0.10 (0.04–0.26)	0.09 (0.03–0.22)	0.17 (0.04–0.52)	0.388
ESR (mm)	10 (7–18)	10 (7–16)	14.5 (8–21.5)	0.225
Albumin (g/L)	42 (31–48)	43 (31–48)	31 (31–47)	0.210
Biologic treatment, *n* (%)				0.843
Adalimumab	34 (35.8%)	30 (36.1%)	4 (33.3%)	
Etanercept	44 (46.3%)	39 (47.0%)	5 (41.7%)	
Infliximab	17 (17.9%)	14 (16.9%)	3 (25.0%)	
Biological treatment duration (months)	61.6 (30.8–91.4)	63.2 (31.8–92.7)	39.9 (25.1–61.2)	0.136
Reduced dose of biologics[a], *n* (%)	45 (47.4%)	40 (48.2%)	5 (41.7%)	0.672
Monotherapy, *n* (%)	45 (47.4%)	42 (50.6%)	3 (25.0%)	0.127
Concomitant steroids, *n* (%)	18 (18.9%)	13 (15.7%)	5 (41.7%)	**0.047**
Global TNFi trough serum levels (μg/mL)	2.20 (1.07–6.26)	2.70 (1.18–6.83)	1.14 (0.73–1.52)	**0.001**
Adalimumab (μg/mL)	7.04 (2.69–9.40)	7.19 (5.78–9.88)	1.28 (0.73–1.59)	**0.009**
Etanercept (μg/mL)	1.45 (1.00–2.25)	1.52 (0.92–2.32)	1.24 (1.20–1.54)	0.698
Infliximab (μg/mL)	2.94 (0.86–3.26)	3.16 (1.92–4.84)	0 (0–1.05)	**0.023**
DAS28-ESR	2.03 (1.68–2.6)	1.99 (1.67–2.52)	2.43 (1.89–2.74)	0.145
Remission, *n* (%)	72 (75.8%)	65 (78.3%)	7 (58.3%)	0.175
Low disease activity, *n* (%)	23 (24.2%)	18 (21.7%)	5 (41.7%)	0.127
SDAI	6.03 (2.2–6.26)	6.02 (2.11–6.22)	6.18 (4.53–6.96)	0.087
CDAI	6 (2–6)	6 (2–6)	6 (4–6.5)	0.220
Global ultrasound score	8 (3–13)	8 (3–13)	17.5 (9.5–31)	**0.041**
PD score	1 (0–2)	1 (0–2)	5.5 (2.5–10)	**< 0.001**
SH score	7 (3–11)	6 (3–10)	8.5 (5–12)	0.210
PDUS, *n* (%)	50 (52.6%)	38 (45.8%)	8 (66.6%)	**< 0.001**
Number of joints with PDUS	1 (0–2)	1 (0–2)	3.5 (2.5–5)	**< 0.001**
UdAS, *n* (%)	29 (30.5%)	17 (20.5%)	7 (58.3%)	**< 0.001**

Values are shown as median (interquartile range) unless otherwise stated
Significant *p* values are shown in bold typeface
bDMARD biologic disease-modifying antirheumatic drug, *CDAI* Clinical Disease Activity Index, *CRP* C-reactive protein, *csDMARD* conventional synthetic disease-modifying antirheumatic drug, *DAS28* 28-joint Disease Activity Score, *ESR* erythrocyte sedimentation rate, *LDA* low disease activity, *PD* power Doppler, *PDUS* power Doppler ultrasound synovitis, *SH* synovial hypertrophy, *SDAI* Simplified Disease Activity Index, *TNFi* tumor necrosis factor inhibitors, *UdAS* ultrasound-defined active synovitis
[a]Treatment regimen with a lower amount of the drug or longer intervals of administration than those recommended in the package insert for each product

relapse. Associations between baseline factors and disease relapse were assessed using Cox proportional hazards regression models. Crude odds ratios (ORs) with 95% CIs were calculated. Multivariate models were constructed to analyze the effect of covariates and to fully adjust the association between calprotectin, TNFi trough serum levels, and PD score with relapse. Models were fitted separately and compared using Akaike Information Criterion (AIC) and the Bayesian Information Criterion (BIC). The generalized estimating equation (GEE) model with an identity link for longitudinal continuous outcomes was used to assess the effect of covariates on TNFi trough serum levels at 0, 4, 8, and 12 months. The analysis was made using STATA version 11 (STATA Corp., College Station, TX, USA).

Results

Baseline characteristics

Of the 103 consecutive enrolled patients (47 RA, 56 PsA), eight were lost to follow-up, and 95 patients completed a 1-year follow-up (44 RA, 51 PsA). Table 1 shows the clinical characteristics at baseline. Patients included were mostly women with established disease on prolonged biological treatment: 44 patients were treated with ETN, 34 with ADA, and 17 with IFX, and 45 patients had received a reduced dose of biologics and 45 were on monotherapy. Seventy-two (75.8%) and 23 patients (24.2%) fulfilled the DAS28 remission and low disease activity criteria, respectively. Fifty (52.6%) patients had PDUS, and the median number of joints with PDUS was 1. Twenty-nine (30.5%) patients fulfilled UdAS criteria.

Baseline serum calprotectin, TNFi trough serum levels, and PDUS, and association with disease relapse

Eighty-three patients remained in remission/low disease activity over 1 year, and 12 (eight RA, four PsA) relapsed (six patients at 4 months, four at 8 months, and two at 12 months). No differences in disease duration, biological treatment duration, reduced dose, or monotherapy were observed between relapsers and nonrelapsers (Table 1).

Clinically, relapsers had a longer time-to-remission/low disease activity, shorter time-in-remission/low disease activity, and were more often on steroid treatment compared with nonrelapsers. No differences in time to csDMARD or biological DMARD were observed (Table 1).

At baseline, relapsers had higher calprotectin levels and lower mean TNFi trough serum levels, even when analyzed according to biological agent in the ADA and IFX group. No differences in CRP or ESR were observed (Table 1).

Relapsers showed higher PD activity, with more patients with PDUS, more joints with a PD signal, and a higher global score and PD score than nonrelapsers. In addition, more relapsers fulfilled UdAS criteria. Similar results were obtained when patients were analyzed according to diagnosis (Table 1).

Calprotectin had greater discriminatory capacity to predict relapse than TNFi trough serum levels and the PD score

The cut-off levels determined by ROC analysis for the optimal prediction of relapse for calprotectin, TNFi serum levels, and PD score were 3.7 μg/mL, 1.61 μg/mL, and 4, respectively, and the Youden index was 0.99, 0.51, and 0.64, respectively. ROC analyses showed that calprotectin (AUC = 1, 95% CI 1.00–1.00) had greater discriminatory capacity than TNFi trough serum levels and PD score in predicting relapse. Table 2 shows further diagnostic statistics of the dichotomized biomarkers. This calprotectin cut-off level had a sensitivity of 100% and a specificity of 98.8% for the diagnosis of a relapse (positive likelihood ratio 83, negative likelihood ratio 0).

Predictive performance of calprotectin, TNFi trough serum levels, and PD score for disease relapse

Kaplan-Meier curves were constructed from baseline to disease relapse to illustrate the predictive performance of calprotectin, TNF serum levels, and PD score. Biomarkers were dichotomized into high versus low according to cut-off levels for optimal prediction of relapse previously calculated by ROC analysis. Survival analyses by log rank tests showed significant differences between groups according to calprotectin serum levels ($p < 0.001$), TNFi trough serum levels ($p = 0.004$), and PD score ($p < 0.001$) (Fig. 1).

Table 2 Diagnostic statistics of dichotomized biomarkers

	Calprotectin	TNFi trough serum levels	Power Doppler score
Cut-off level to predict relapse	≥ 3.7 μg/mL	< 1.61 μg/mL	≥ 4
Area under the curve	1.000 (1.000–1.000)	0.790 (0.691–0.889)	0.877 (0.772–0.981)
Sensitivity	100%	68.7%	75.0%
Specificity	98.8%	83.3%	89.2%
Positive likelihood ratio	83.0	4.12	6.92
Negative likelihood ratio	0.00	0.37	0.28
Correctly classified	98.9%	70.5%	87.4%
Youden index	0.99	0.51	0.64

TNFi tumor necrosis factor inhibitors

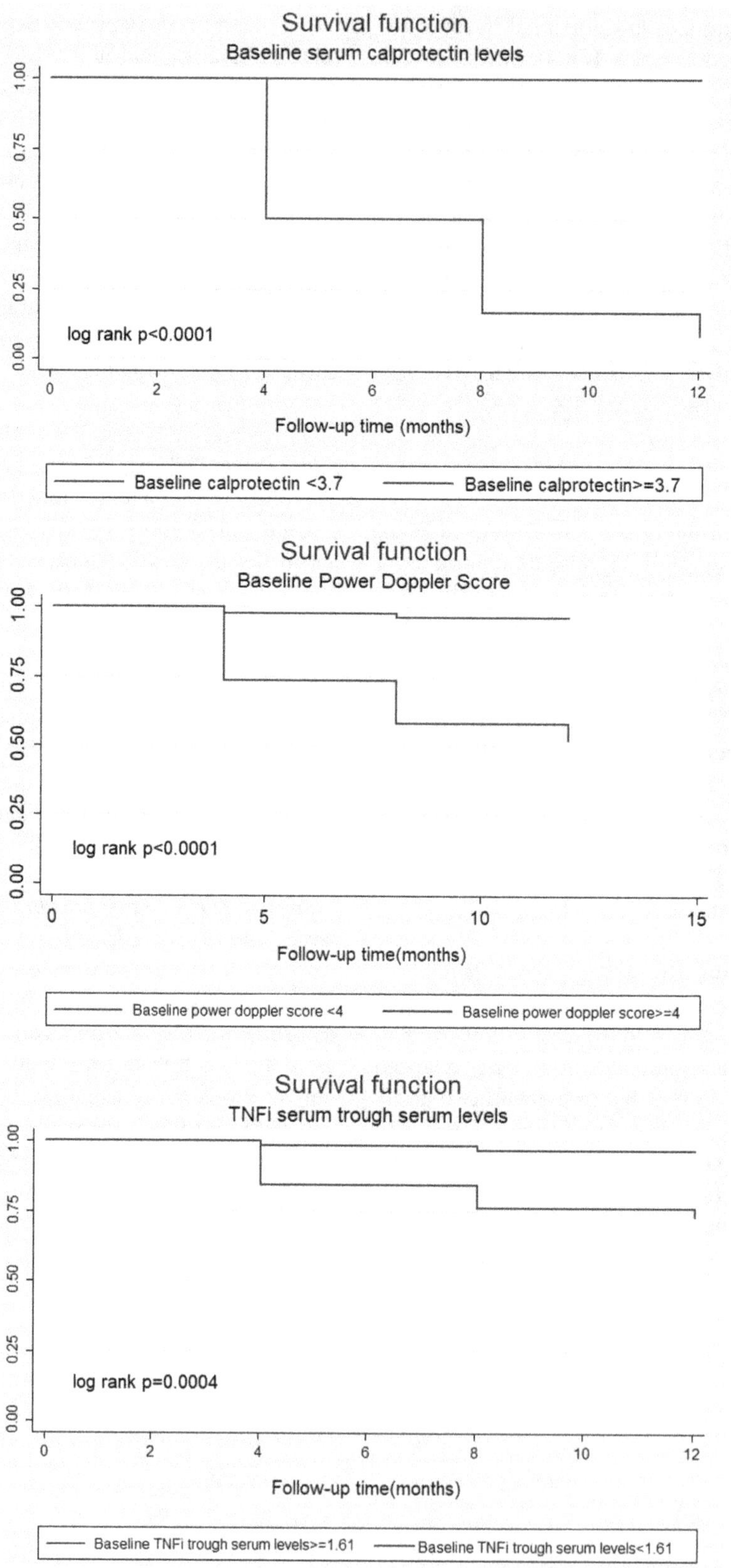

Fig. 1 Kaplan-Meier curves of biomarkers from the time of inclusion to disease relapse. **a** Calprotectin serum levels. **b** Power Doppler score. **c** Tumor necrosis factor inhibitors (TNFi) trough serum levels

Factors associated with disease relapse

Univariate Cox regression analyses showed time-to-remission/low disease activity (hazard ratio (HR) = 1.17, $p < 0.001$) was the only clinical variable associated with an increased risk of relapse. In addition, steroid use, calprotectin, TNFi trough serum levels, and PD score were significantly associated with disease relapse. In the multivariate regression, only baseline calprotectin levels were independently associated with disease relapse (HR = 2.74, $p < 0.0001$). No significant interaction terms were detected (Table 3).

Calprotectin and TNFi trough serum levels during relapse

Serum samples from the 12 relapsers were analyzed during relapse. A significant increase in calprotectin levels was observed in 10 patients, while TNFi trough serum levels decreased in all relapsers compared with baseline values (Fig. 2).

After 1 year, antidrug antibodies were detected in four patients, who all had a relapse (ADA in two out of four relapsers and IFX in two out of three relapsers). All patients with detectable antidrug antibodies had undetectable TNFi trough serum levels.

Longitudinal changes in TNFi trough serum levels

Multivariate GEE analysis showed that only disease activity by DAS28-ESR was significantly associated with longitudinal changes in TNFi trough serum levels (regression coefficient 0.26 (0.068 to 0.004), $p = 0.001$). This effect was independent of other factors analyzed, such as diagnosis, monotherapy, steroids, and reduced dose of biologics (Table 4).

Discussion

The results of our study show that TNFi trough serum levels, PD score, and time-to-remission/low disease activity were significantly associated with disease relapse. However, only baseline calprotectin levels independently predicted disease relapse in RA and PsA patients treated with TNFi after a 1-year follow-up.

The innate immune system plays a central role in local inflammation in RA and PsA patients, as demonstrated by the massive infiltration of macrophages into the synovial tissue [27–29]. Most biologics, including TNFi and anti-interleukin (IL)-6, specifically target cytokines related to this cell type, and thus it is not surprising that changes in the number of synovial sublining macrophages correlate with clinical improvement in RA patients [30]. Calprotectin is released by innate immune cells, particularly neutrophils and macrophages, and calprotectin levels provide reliable information about neutrophil activation associated with disease activity in RA and PsA patients [4, 25, 31–33].

In our cohort, calprotectin performed particularly well because all relapsers showed a baseline calprotectin level > 3.7 μg/mL; this high accuracy in predicting disease relapses is not completely unexpected. In other inflammatory conditions, such as juvenile idiopathic arthritis (JIA) [13], systemic-onset juvenile idiopathic arthritis (SoJIA) [34], ANCA-associated vasculitis [35], or inflammatory bowel disease (IBD) [36], calprotectin has been shown to be a more sensitive indicator of disease activity and, in consequence, more accurately predicts relapse [34, 37–40].

We have previously demonstrated that RA patients in remission with a PD signal had significantly greater macrophage infiltration in the synovial tissue, comparable

Table 3 Baseline factors associated with disease relapse using Cox proportional hazards regression models

Baseline characteristics	Univariate HR (95% CI; *p* value)	Multivariate HR (95% CI; *p* value)
Calprotectin (μg/mL)	**2.38 (1.79–3.16; < 0.0001)**	**2.74 (1.71–4.41; < 0.0001)**
Power Doppler score, 0–66	**1.31 (1.18–1.45; < 0.0001)**	
TNFi trough serum levels (μg/mL)	**0.47 (0.26–0.88; 0.018)**	0.36 (0.10–1.30; 0.120)
DAS-ESR	2.10 (0.72–6.18; 0.175)	
Time-to-remission (months)	**1.17 (1.11–1.23; < 0.0001)**	
Time-in-remission (months)	0.98 (0.97–1.00; 0.087)	
Female gender	1.25 (0.38–4.15; 0.716)	
Disease duration (months)	1.02 (0.96–1.08; 0.510)	
Diagnosis, RA/PsA	2.39 (0.72–7.93; 0.155)	0.80 (0.10–6.30; 0.832)
Age (years)	0.98 (0.94–1.03; 0.535)	
Monotherapy	0.36 (0.10–1.33; 0.125)	0.51 (0.08–3.35; 0.484)
Steroids	**3.12 (1.02–10.1; 0.046)**	0.22 (0.04–1.21; 0.082)

Significant values are shown in bold typeface
CI confidence interval, *DAS-ESR* Disease Activity Score-erythrocyte sedimentation rate, *HR* hazard ratio, *PsA* psoriatic arthritis, *RA* rheumatoid arthritis, *TNFi* tumor necrosis factor inhibitors

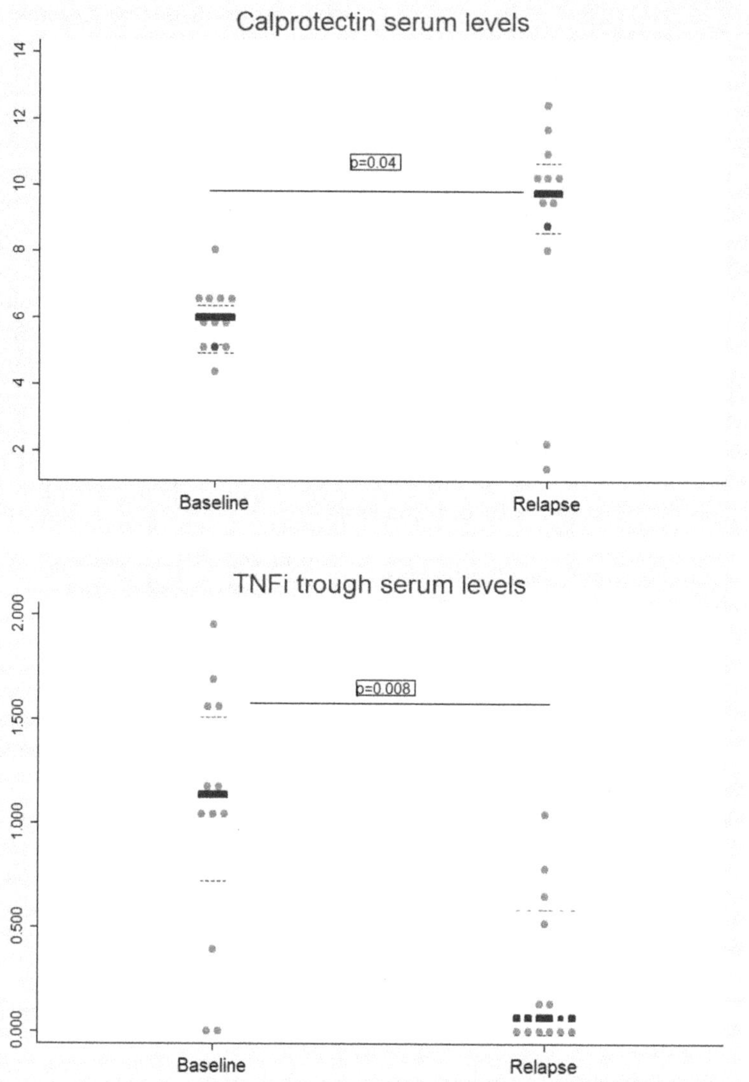

Fig. 2 Biomarkers levels during relapse. **a** Calprotectin serum levels during relapse. **b** TNFi trough serum levels during relapse

to clinically active patients [25], which may explain why these patients had threefold higher calprotectin serum levels compared with healthy blood donors [10]. As expected, relapsers showed a significant increase in calprotectin serum levels during the disease relapse, reflecting local ongoing inflammation. Thus, calprotectin serum levels may identify residual inflammatory activity in patients with low disease activity and are a strong predictor of disease relapse.

Nonrelapsers had higher drug trough serum levels than relapsers, even according to the biologic agent, and these significantly decreased during relapse, supporting a previous report on the relationship between inflammation and TNFi pharmacokinetics in RA. In patients with substantial inflammation, IFX serum levels were decreased due to its capture by TNFα [41]. Our results support the emerging role of TNFi trough serum levels as a relevant factor associated with disease activity in RA and PsA patients receiving biological therapy [14–16, 42].

In accordance with previous reports [1], 52.6% of our patients in clinical remission or with low disease activity (65.9% RA, 41.1% PsA) showed PD activity in at least one joint, which has been associated with a higher risk of disease relapse in RA [2, 3]. Although there are no data available for polyarticular PsA, logistic regression analyses showed that the PD score, regardless of diagnosis, was associated with relapse, which is a relevant contribution of our study. Remission is not equivalent to the

Table 4 Factors associated with longitudinal changes in TNFi trough serum levels over 1 year of follow-up using GEE multivariate models

Variable	TNFi trough serum levels β coefficient (95% CI)	*p* value
DAS28-ESR	**0.26 (0.068–0.004)**	**0.001**
Reduced dose (yes/no)	0.022 (0.168–0.012)	0.271
Diagnosis (RA/PsA)	0.005 (0.058–0.144)	0.662
Monotherapy (yes/no)	0.0004 (0.090–0.062)	0.863
Follow-up		
Baseline	1	
4-month visit	0.012 (0.044–0.0004)	0.023
8-month visit	0.004 (0.032–0.002)	0.280
12-month visit	0.002 (0.005–0.032)	0.409
Steroids	0.020 (0.325–0.090)	0.538
Constant	**4.45 (2.99 to 6.25)**	**< 0.0001**

Significant values are shown in bold typeface
CI confidence interval, *DAS28-ESR* 28-joint Disease Activity Score-erythrocyte sedimentation rate, *GEE* generalized estimating equation, *PsA* psoriatic arthritis, *RA* rheumatoid arthritis, *TNFi* tumor necrosis factor inhibitors

absence of inflammation. Persistence of the PD signal could explain the radiographic damage progression observed in RA and PsA patients in clinical remission [1, 43].

As in previous reports, the only clinical factor associated with relapse identified in our study was time-to-remission/low disease activity. Sustained remission was only determined by time-to-remission in a cohort of early RA patients; the probability of sustained remission increased significantly with decreasing time-to-remission, independently of the DMARD type or strategy [44].

Accurately predicting relapses could avoid delays and related costs [45]. Calprotectin [46] and TNFi trough levels [47] have been included in guidelines on monitoring the therapeutic response in IBD patients. In RA, there are some proposals for decision algorithms which have included calprotectin [48] and TNFi trough levels [49].

The small sample size and low percentage of relapsing patients (12.6%) could be a limitation. However, we were able to detect statically significant differences between relapsers and nonrelapsers, which is a strength of our study. We presumed that the use of DAS28 ≤ 3.2 as the inclusion criteria could limit the interpretation of our results, since this composite index allows residual tender and/or swollen joints in patients classified as being in remission. However, it is the most widely used composite articular index, and therefore our results would be clinically applicable, contributing to the strengths of this study. Although developed to assess disease activity in RA, studies support the use of DAS28 in PsA patients receiving biological therapy [50]. A single rheumatologist performed the US assessment in both hands, and therefore inter-observer reliability could not be calculated, and there is a known significant variability between observers in the assessment of synovitis using US. Also, US assessment focused on the hand could be insufficient to capture inflammatory activity of systemic diseases, such as RA and PsA. However, US examination of hands only could be sufficient to detect > 90% of RA patients in the clinic with subclinical inflammation [51].

Considering these limitations, we have demonstrated a high accuracy of baseline calprotectin serum levels in predicting relapse in patients with low levels of disease activity.

Conclusions

In RA and PsA patients with low levels of disease activity, time-to-remission/low disease activity, calprotectin serum levels, TNFi trough serum levels, and PD score were significantly associated with disease relapse. However, only baseline calprotectin levels were independently associated with disease relapse. Calprotectin may be used to stratify disease activity more accurately in patients with low disease activity, guiding therapeutic decisions towards safer and more cost-effective strategies.

Abbreviations

ACR: American College of Rheumatology; ADA: Adalimumab; AIC: Akaike Information Criterion; AUC: Area under the curve; BIC: Bayesian Information Criterion; CASPAR: Classification of Psoriatic Arthritis; CDAI: Clinical Disease Activity Index; CI: Confidence interval; CRP: C-reactive protein; csDMARD: Conventional synthetic disease-modifying antirheumatic drug; DAS28: 28-Joint Disease Activity Score; ESR: Erythrocyte sedimentation rate; ETN: Etanercept; EULAR: European League Against Rheumatism; GEE: Generalized estimating equation; HR: Hazard ratio; IFX: Infliximab; MSUS: Musculoskeletal ultrasound; OMERACT: Outcome Measures in Rheumatology; OR: Odds ratio; PD: Power Doppler; PDUS: Power Doppler ultrasound synovitis; PsA: Psoriatic arthritis; RA: Rheumatoid arthritis; ROC: Receiver operating characteristic; SDAI: Simple Disease Activity Index; SH: Synovial hypertrophy; TNFi: Tumor necrosis factor inhibitors; UdAS: Ultrasound-defined active synovitis

Acknowledgements

The authors acknowledge the statistical assistance provided by Dr. Loreto Carmona and Dr. María Jesús García de Yébenes y Prous, the technical advice of David Buss, and the Spanish Rheumatology Society.

Funding

This study was financially supported by research grants from the Hospital Clinic of Barcelona "Emili Letang 2013", Investigator Initiated Research (IIR) from Pfizer (WS2392358), and the Catalan Society of Rheumatology.

Authors' contributions

All authors were involved in drafting the article or revising it critically for important intellectual content, and all authors approved the final version to be published. Study conception and design: RS, JI-M, JR, and JY. Acquisition of data: RS, JI-M, JR, MVH, SRC-V, and VR-E. Analysis and interpretation of data: RS, JI-M, JR, VR-E, JDC, MP, SRC-V, and MVH.

Competing interests

The authors declare that they have no competing interests.

Author details
[1]Department of Rheumatology, Hospital Clinic, University of Barcelona, Carrer Villarroel 170, 08036 Barcelona, Spain. [2]Department of Immunology, Hospital Clinic, University of Barcelona, Barcelona, Spain.

References

1. Brown AK, Quinn MA, Karim Z, Conaghan PG, Peterfy CG, Hensor E, et al. Presence of significant synovitis in rheumatoid arthritis patients with disease-modifying antirheumatic drug-induced clinical remission: evidence from an imaging study may explain structural progression. Arthritis Rheum. 2006;54:3761–73.
2. Scirè CA, Montecucco C, Codullo V, Epis O, Todoerti M, Caporali R. Ultrasonographic evaluation of joint involvement in early rheumatoid arthritis in clinical remission: power Doppler signal predicts short-term relapse. Rheumatology. 2009;48:1092–7.
3. Saleem B, Brown AK, Quinn M, Karim Z, Hensor EM, Conaghan P, et al. Can flare be predicted in DMARD treated RA patients in remission, and is it important? A cohort study. Ann Rheum Dis. 2012;71:1316–21.
4. Berntzen HB, Munthe E, Fagerhol MK. A longitudinal study of the leukocyte protein L1 as an indicator of disease activity in patients with rheumatoid arthritis. J Rheumatol. 1989;16:1416–20.
5. Hansson C, Eriksson C, Alenius G-M. S-calprotectin (S100A8/S100A9): a potential marker of inflammation in patients with psoriatic arthritis. J Immunol Res. 2014;2014:696415.
6. Hammer HB, Odegard S, Fagerhol MK, Landewé R, van der Heijde D, Uhlig T, et al. Calprotectin (a major leucocyte protein) is strongly and independently correlated with joint inflammation and damage in rheumatoid arthritis. Ann Rheum Dis. 2007;66:1093–7.
7. Hammer HB, Ødegård S, Syversen SW, Landewé R, van der Heijde D, Uhlig T, et al. Calprotectin (a major S100 leucocyte protein) predicts 10-year radiographic progression in patients with rheumatoid arthritis. Ann Rheum Dis. 2010;69:150–4.
8. Choi IY, Gerlag DM, Herenius MJ, Thurlings RM, Wijbrandts CA, Foell D, et al. MRP8/14 serum levels as a strong predictor of response to biological treatments in patients with rheumatoid arthritis. Ann Rheum Dis. 2015;74: 499–505.
9. Ademowo OS, Hernandez B, Collins E, Rooney C, Fearon U, van Kuijk AW, et al. Discovery and confirmation of a protein biomarker panel with potential to predict response to biological therapy in psoriatic arthritis. Ann Rheum Dis. 2016;75:234–41.
10. Inciarte-Mundo J, Victoria Hernández M, Ruiz-Esquide V, Raquel Cabrera-Villalba S, Ramirez J, Cuervo A, et al. Serum calprotectin versus acute-phase reactants in the discrimination of inflammatory disease activity in rheumatoid arthritis patients receiving tumor necrosis factor inhibitors. Arthritis Care Res. 2016;68:899–906.
11. Inciarte-Mundo J, Ruiz-Esquide V, Hernández MV, Cañete JD, Cabrera-Villalba SR, Ramirez J, et al. Calprotectin more accurately discriminates the disease status of rheumatoid arthritis patients receiving tocilizumab than acute phase reactants. Rheumatology. 2015;54:2239–43.
12. Inciarte-Mundo J, Ramirez J, Hernández MV, Ruiz-Esquide V, Cuervo A, Cabrera-Villalba SR, et al. Calprotectin and TNF trough serum levels identify power Doppler ultrasound synovitis in rheumatoid arthritis and psoriatic arthritis patients in remission or with low disease activity. Arthritis Res Ther. 2016;18:160.
13. Gerss J, Roth J, Holzinger D, Ruperto N, Wittkowski H, Frosch M, et al. Phagocyte-specific S100 proteins and high-sensitivity C reactive protein as biomarkers for a risk-adapted treatment to maintain remission in juvenile idiopathic arthritis: a comparative study. Ann Rheum Dis. 2012;71:1991–7.
14. Bartelds GM, Krieckaert CL, Nurmohamed MT, van Schouwenburg PA, Lems WF, Twisk JW, et al. Development of antidrug antibodies against adalimumab and association. JAMA Intern Med. 2011;305:1460–8.
15. de Vries MK, Wolbink GJ, Stapel SO, de Vrieze H, van Denderen JC, Dijkmans BA, et al. Decreased clinical response to infliximab in ankylosing spondylitis is correlated with anti-infliximab formation. Ann Rheum Dis. 2007;66:1252–4.
16. Chen DY, Chen YM, Tsai WC, Tseng JC, Chen YH, Hsieh CW, et al. Significant associations of antidrug antibody levels with serum drug trough levels and therapeutic response of adalimumab and etanercept treatment in rheumatoid arthritis. Ann Rheum Dis. 2015;74:e16.
17. Van Gestel AM, Haagsma CJ, Van Riel PLCM. Validation of rheumatoid arthritis improvement criteria that include simplified joint counts. Arthritis Rheum. 1998;41:1845–50.
18. Prevoo ML, van't Hof MA, Kuper HH, van Leeuwen MA, van de Putte LB, van Riel PL. Modified disease activity scores that include twenty-eight-joint counts: development and validation in a prospective longitudinal study of patients with rheumatoid arthritis. Arthritis Rheum. 1995;38:44–8.
19. Aletaha D, Nell V, Stamm T, Uffmann M, Pflugbeil S, Machold K, et al. Acute phase reactants add little to composite disease activity indices for rheumatoid arthritis: validation of a clinical activity score. Arthritis Res Ther. 2005;7:R796–806.
20. S Smolen JS, Breedveld FC, Schiff MH, Kalden JR, Emery P, Eberl G, et al. A simplified disease activity index for rheumatoid arthritis for use in clinical practice. Rheumatology. 2003;42:244–57.
21. Valor L, Hernández-Flórez D, de la Torre I, Llinares F, Rosas J, Yagüe J, et al. Agreement in assessment of infliximab and adalimumab levels in rheumatoid arthritis: interlaboratory and interassay comparison. Clin Exp Rheumatol. 2015;33:617–23.
22. Wakefield RJ, Balint PV, Szkudlarek M, Filippucci E, Backhaus M, D'Agostino MA, et al. Musculoskeletal ultrasound including definitions for ultrasonographic pathology. J Rheumatol. 2005;32:2485–7.
23. Backhaus M, Burmester GR, Gerber T, Grassi W, Machold KP, Swen WA, et al. Guidelines for musculoskeletal ultrasound in rheumatology. Ann Rheum Dis. 2001;60:641–9.
24. Szkudlarek M, Court-Payen M, Jacobsen S, Klarlund M, Thomsen HS, Østergaard M. Interobserver agreement in ultrasonography of the finger and toe joints in rheumatoid arthritis. Arthritis Rheum. 2003;48:955–62.
25. Ramírez J, Celis R, Usategui A, Ruiz-Esquide V, Faré R, Cuervo A, et al. Immunopathologic characterization of ultrasound-defined synovitis in rheumatoid arthritis patients in clinical remission. Arthritis Res Ther. 2016;18:74.
26. Naredo E, Collado P, Cruz A, Palop MJ, Cabero F, Richi P, et al. Longitudinal power Doppler ultrasonographic assessment of joint inflammatory activity in early rheumatoid arthritis: predictive value in disease activity and radiologic progression. Arthritis Care Res. 2007;57:116–24.
27. Youssef PP, Smeets TJ, Bresnihan B, Cunnane G, Fitzgerald O, Breedveld F, et al. Microscopic measurement of cellular infiltration in the rheumatoid arthritis synovial membrane: a comparison of semiquantitative and quantitative analysis. Br J Rheumatol. 1998;37:1003–7.
28. Taccari E, Fattorossi A, Moretti S, Riccieri V, Fasani M, Zoppini A. Phenotypic profile of major synovial cell populations in longstanding psoriatic arthritis. J Rheumatol. 1987;14:525–30.
29. Veale D, Yanni G, Rogers S, Barnes L, Bresnihan B, Fitzgerald O. Reduced synovial membrane macrophage numbers, ELAM-1 expression, and lining layer hyperplasia in psoriatic arthritis as compared with rheumatoid arthritis. Arthritis Rheum. 1993;36:893–900.
30. Haringman JJ, Gerlag DM, Zwinderman AH, Smeets TJM, Kraan MC, Baeten D, et al. Synovial tissue macrophages: a sensitive biomarker for response to treatment in patients with rheumatoid arthritis. Ann Rheum Dis. 2005;64: 834–8.
31. Berntzen HB, Munthe E, Fagerhol MK. The major leukocyte protein L1 as an indicator of inflammatory joint disease. Scand J Rheumatol. 1988;76:251–6.
32. Brun JG, Jonsson R, Haga HJ. Measurement of plasma calprotectin as an indicator of arthritis and disease activity in patients with inflammatory rheumatic diseases. J Rheumatol. 1994;21:733–8.
33. Brun JG, Haga HJ, Bøe E, Kallay I, Lekven C, Berntzen HB, et al. Calprotectin in patients with rheumatoid arthritis: relation to clinical and laboratory variables of disease activity. J Rheumatol. 1992;19:859–62.
34. Holzinger D, Frosch M, Kastrup A, Prince FHM, Otten MH, Van Suijlekom-Smit LW, et al. The Toll-like receptor 4 agonist MRP8/14 protein complex is a sensitive indicator for disease activity and predicts relapses in systemic-onset juvenile idiopathic arthritis. Ann Rheum Dis. 2012;71:974–80.
35. Pepper RJ, Hamour S, Chavele K, Todd SK, Rasmussen N, Flint SM, et al. Leukocyte and serum S100A8/S100A9 expression reflects disease activity in ANCA-associated vasculitis and glomerulonephritis. Kidney Int. 2013;83: 1150–8.
36. Balzola F, Cullen G, Hoentjen F, Ho GT, Russell R. Fecal calprotectin more accurately reflects endoscopic activity of ulcerative colitis than the Lichtiger index, C-reactive protein, platelets, hemoglobin, and blood leukocytes. Inflamm Bowel Dis Monit. 2013;13:159–60.
37. Rothmund F, Gerss J, Ruperto N, Däbritz J, Wittkowski H, Frosch M, et al. Validation of relapse risk biomarkers for routine use in patients with juvenile idiopathic arthritis. Arthritis Care Res. 2014;66:949–55.
38. Schulze zur Wiesch A, Foell D, Frosch M, Vogl T, Sorg C, Roth J. Myeloid related proteins MRP8/MRP14 may predict disease flares in juvenile

idiopathic arthritis. Clin Exp Rheumatol. 2016;22:368–73.
39. Pepper RJ, Draibe JB, Caplin B, Fervenza FC, Hoffman GS, Kallenberg CGM, et al. The association of serum calprotectin (S100A8/S100A9) levels with disease relapses in PR3-ANCA-associated vasculitis. Arthritis Rheumatol. 2016; [Epub ahead of print].
40. De Vos M, Louis EJ, Jahnsen J, Vandervoort JGP, Noman M, Dewit O, et al. Consecutive fecal calprotectin measurements to predict relapse in patients with ulcerative colitis receiving infliximab maintenance therapy. Inflamm Bowel Dis. 2013;19:2111–7.
41. Ternant D, Ducourau E, Perdriger A, Corondan A, Le Goff B, Devauchelle-Pensec V, et al. Relationship between inflammation and infliximab pharmacokinetics in rheumatoid arthritis. Br J Clin Pharmacol. 2014;78:118–28.
42. Jamnitski A, Krieckaert CL, Nurmohamed MT, Hart MH, Dijkmans BA, Aarden L, et al. Patients non-responding to etanercept obtain lower etanercept concentrations compared with responding patients. Ann Rheum Dis. 2012; 71:88–91.
43. El Miedany Y, El Gaafary M, Youssef S, Ahmed I, Nasr A. Tailored approach to early psoriatic arthritis patients: clinical and ultrasonographic predictors for structural joint damage. Clin Rheumatol. 2015;34:307–13.
44. Schipper LG, Fransen J, den Broeder A, Van Riel PLCM. Time to achieve remission determines time to be in remission. Arthritis Res Ther. 2010;12:R97.
45. Bartlett SJ, Hewlett S, Bingham CO, Woodworth TG, Alten R, Pohl C, et al. Identifying core domains to assess flare in rheumatoid arthritis: an OMERACT international patient and provider combined Delphi consensus. Ann Rheum Dis. 2012;71:1855–60.
46. Heida A, Dijkstra A, Groen H, Muller Kobold A, Verkade H, van Rheenen P. Comparing the efficacy of a web-assisted calprotectin-based treatment algorithm (IBD-live) with usual practices in teenagers with inflammatory bowel disease: study protocol for a randomized controlled trial. Trials. 2015; 16:271.
47. Afif W, Loftus EV Jr, Faubion WA, Kane SV, Bruining DH, Hanson KA, et al. Clinical utility of measuring infliximab and human anti-chimeric antibody concentrations in patients with inflammatory bowel disease. Am J Gastroenterol. 2010;105:1133–9.
48. Nair SC, Welsing PMJ, Choi IYK, Roth J, Holzinger D, Bijlsma JWJ, et al. A personalized approach to biological therapy using prediction of clinical response based on MRP8/14 serum complex levels in rheumatoid arthritis patients. PLoS One. 2016;11:1–12.
49. Garcês S, Antunes M, Benito-Garcia E, da Silva JC, Aarden L, Demengeot J. A preliminary algorithm introducing immunogenicity assessment in the management of patients with RA receiving tumour necrosis factor inhibitor therapies. Ann Rheum Dis. 2014;73:1138–43.
50. Fransen J, Antoni C, Mease PJ, Uter W, Kavanaugh A, Kalden JR, et al. Performance of response criteria for assessing peripheral arthritis in patients with psoriatic arthritis: analysis of data from randomised controlled trials of two tumour necrosis factor inhibitors. Ann Rheum Dis. 2006;65:1373–8.
51. Hammer H, Kvien T, Terslev L. Ultrasound of the hand is sufficient to detect subclinical inflammation in rheumatoid arthritis remission: a post hoc longitudinal study. Arthritis Res Ther. 2017;19:221.

8

Secukinumab provides rapid and sustained pain relief in psoriatic arthritis over 2 years

Iain B. McInnes[1*], Philip J. Mease[2], Georg Schett[3], Bruce Kirkham[4], Vibeke Strand[5], Nicole Williams[6], Todd Fox[7], Luminita Pricop[8], Steffen M. Jugl[7], Kunal K. Gandhi[8], on behalf of the FUTURE 2 Study Group

Abstract

Background: Pain is one of the most important domains affecting health-related quality of life (HRQoL) in patients with psoriatic arthritis (PsA). Secukinumab has demonstrated rapid and sustained improvements in signs and symptoms, including HRQoL, among patients with active PsA. This analysis evaluates the effect of secukinumab on patient-reported pain in PsA through 104 weeks of treatment.

Methods: Pain was assessed through week 104 using clinically relevant measures, including change from baseline in a pain visual analog scale (VAS) and Short Form-36 (SF-36) bodily domain scores; proportion of patients reporting improvements equal to or better than minimum clinically meaningful differences in the pain VAS and SF-36 bodily pain domain scores; and proportion of patients with no, moderate, or extreme pain/discomfort measured by the EuroQoL 5-Dimension 3-Level Questionnaire (EQ-5D-3 L) pain item scores. Correlations of pain measures were analyzed using Pearson's correlation coefficient. Pre-specified analyses of TNF-naïve patients and patients who stopped TNF-inhibitors (TNFis) due to inadequate responses or safety/tolerability (TNF-IR patients) were performed using "as-observed data."

Results: Mean improvements from baseline in pain VAS scores were greater with secukinumab versus placebo by week 3 (− 16.9; $P < 0.0001$ with secukinumab 300 mg and − 12.6; $P < 0.05$ with secukinumab 150 mg) and sustained through week 104. SF-36 bodily pain domain scores were significantly greater with 300 mg secukinumab and secukinumab 150 mg versus placebo by week 4 (16.2 and 16.3, respectively; $P < 0.0001$ for both), and these changes were maintained through week 104. With both secukinumab 300 mg and secukinumab 150 mg, improvements equal to or better than the minimum clinically meaningful differences in pain VAS and SF-36 bodily pain were significant versus placebo at week 3 and week 4, respectively. At week 4, 15%, 9%, and 5% of patients receiving secukinumab 300 mg, secukinumab 150 mg, and placebo, respectively, reported "no pain/discomfort" measured by EQ-5D-3 L; these proportions increased to week 104 with both secukinumab doses. Similarly, improvements in pain measures were significant in both TNF-naïve and TNF-IR patients.

Conclusion: Secukinumab provided rapid and sustained pain relief in PsA over 2 years of treatment. Improvements in pain were reported regardless of prior exposure to TNFis.

Keywords: Pain relief, Psoriatic arthritis, Secukinumab

* Correspondence: iain.McInnes@glasgow.ac.uk
Previously presented in part at: Annual European Congress of Rheumatology; 14–17 June 2017; Madrid, Spain
[1]Institute of Infection, Immunity & Inflammation, College of Medical, Veterinary and Life Sciences, University of Glasgow, 120 University Place, Glasgow G12 8TA, UK
Full list of author information is available at the end of the article

Background

Psoriatic arthritis (PsA) is a chronic progressive, clinically heterogeneous inflammatory arthritis that can manifest as peripheral arthritis, axial disease, enthesitis, dactylitis, and psoriasis of the skin/nails [1, 2]. The disease burden of PsA, taking into account patient-reported outcomes and disease activity measures, is similar to the burden of rheumatoid arthritis and axial spondyloarthritis [3]. A recent analysis from the population-based Multinational Assessment of Psoriasis and Psoriatic Arthritis (MAPP) found that 88% of patients questioned had ongoing joint pain or soreness, and 60% reported > 4 affected joints [4]. The most common locations for joint pain were the knee (41%) followed by finger (26%), hip (19%), ankle (19%), back (18%), and wrist (16%) [4].

The combination of ongoing pain, fatigue, physical impairment, and anxiety likely influence the impact of PsA and reduce health-related quality of life (HRQoL) [5]. Specifically, patients with PsA have impaired HRQoL characterized by poor physical functioning and engagement in daily activities, and pain [6]. In a European League Against Rheumatism (EULAR) initiative to develop and validate the Psoriatic Arthritis Impact of Disease questionnaire (PsAID), patients with PsA identified pain as the most important health domain affecting HRQoL [7]. Additionally, arthritis or joint pain causes a significant economic impact that results in US$6773 greater costs compared to individuals without either [8]. Pain poses an important clinical challenge in the treatment of PsA. In a population-based survey, rheumatologists and dermatologists considered joint pain or swelling to be the critical factor contributing to the severity of PsA [9]. Treatment criteria, scoring indices, and clinical trial domains further reflect the importance of pain in PsA. The Group for Research and Assessment of Psoriasis and Psoriatic Arthritis (GRAPPA) includes pain as an important factor to examine when treating patients with PsA [10]. A patient pain visual analog scale (VAS) score ≤ 15 is one of seven critical criteria for determining minimal disease activity in PsA [11]. Finally, at the Outcome Measures in Rheumatology (OMERACT) 2016 conference, pain was endorsed as part of a core set of domains recommended for study in randomized controlled trials (RCTs) and longitudinal observational studies (LOS) in PsA [12].

Secukinumab, a fully human monoclonal antibody (mAb) that selectively neutralizes interleukin (IL)-17A, has been shown to have significant efficacy in the treatment of moderate-to-severe psoriasis and active PsA, demonstrating rapid onset of action and sustained responses with a consistent safety profile [13, 14]. Since 2015 in the European Union and 2016 in the USA, secukinumab 300 mg and 150 mg have been approved for the treatment of active PsA. In the phase-3 FUTURE 2 study, secukinumab was effective in treating patients not previously exposed (TNF-naïve patients) to TNF-α inhibitors (TNFis) and patients who stopped using up to three previous TNFis due to inadequate responses or for safety/tolerability reasons (TNF-IR patients) [15]. Over 2 years, secukinumab was shown to exhibit rapid and sustained improvements in the signs and symptoms of active PsA, to inhibit radiographic progression, and to improve HRQoL [16, 17]. This post-hoc analysis of FUTURE 2 examines the effect of secukinumab on patient-reported pain in PsA over 104 weeks.

Methods

Details of FUTURE 2 (NCT01752634), an ongoing, multicenter RCT, have been reported previously [15] and will be briefly summarized here.

Patients

FUTURE 2 was conducted at 76 centers throughout Asia, Australia, Europe, and North America, in accordance with the principles of the Declaration of Helsinki, and all centers received approval from independent ethics committees or institutional review boards. Patients included in this trial were aged ≥ 18 years, met the Classification criteria for Psoriatic Arthritis (CASPAR), had ≥ 3 tender and ≥ 3 swollen joints despite treatment with non-steroidal anti-inflammatory drugs (NSAIDs), disease-modifying anti-rheumatic drugs (DMARDs), or TNFis. Patients who had not responded adequately to up to three treatments with TNFis were eligible for inclusion.

A TNFi wash-out period ≥ 4 weeks prior to randomization was mandatory. Patients on concomitant oral corticosteroids who received a stable dose for ≥ 2 weeks prior to randomization (≤ 10 mg/day) and patients who were on methotrexate and received a stable dose for ≥ 4 weeks prior to randomization (≤ 25 mg/week) were allowed throughout the trial. Patients were excluded from the study for previous use of biologic agents other than TNFis; active inflammatory diseases other than PsA; active infection within 2 weeks prior to randomization or a history of chronic, ongoing, or recurrent infections; pregnancy; or malignancy within the past 5 years, with the exception of basal cell carcinoma or actinic keratosis, in-situ cervical cancer, or non-invasive malignant colon polyps.

Study design and assessments

Patients were randomized 1:1:1:1 to receive subcutaneous secukinumab 300 mg, secukinumab 150 mg, secukinumab 75 mg, or placebo at baseline, weeks 1, 2, and 3, and then every 4 weeks from week 4. At week 16, patients were classified as responders (≥ 20% improvement from baseline in tender and swollen joint counts) or non-responders. Placebo-treated patients were randomly assigned again in a 1:1 ratio to receive subcutaneous secukinumab 300 mg or 150 mg every 4 weeks from week 16 (non-responders) or week 24 (responders). This study was blinded from baseline to week 52 and then open label until week 104.

Pain was assessed through week 104 by the mean change from baseline in the pain VAS and Short Form-36 (SF-36) bodily pain domain scores; proportion of patients reporting improvements equal to or better than the minimum clinically meaningful difference (MCID) in the pain VAS score (mean change from baseline ≥ 20%) [18]; proportion of patients reporting improvements equal to or better than the MCID (5-point improvement from baseline) in SF-36 bodily pain domain score [19]; proportion of patients reporting EuroQoL 5-Dimension 3-Level Questionnaire (EQ-5D-3 L) pain item scores of no, moderate, or extreme pain/discomfort; and correlation coefficients for changes from baseline between pain scores.

Statistical methods

Mean changes from baseline in the pain VAS and SF-36 bodily pain domain scores were analyzed using a mixed-effect model for repeated measures (MMRM) through week 24 with treatment regimen, analysis visit, and randomization stratum (TNF-naive or TNF-IR) as factors, weight and baseline score as continuous covariates, and treatment by analysis visit and baseline score by analysis visit as interaction terms, and an unstructured covariance structure. Mean changes from baseline were reported as observed starting from week 28. Frequencies of patient EQ-5D-3 L pain/discomfort domain response were reported using observed data up to week 104. Correlation with pain measures was analyzed using Pearson's correlation coefficient and P values were calculated using the chi-square likelihood ratio test. The proportion of patients with VAS improvement ≥ 20% were reported using as-observed data and P values were calculated using Fisher's exact test. The proportion of patients with improvement ≥ 5 in the SF-36 bodily pain domain score were reported using as-observed data and P values were calculated using Fisher's exact test. Pre-specified subgroup analyses (TNF-naïve and TNF-IR) were performed using MMRM through week 24 and data were reported as observed starting from week 28. Only the results for patients receiving the approved doses – secukinumab 300 mg and secukinumab 150 mg – are reported in this article. Due to the re-randomization of patients in the placebo group at week 16, statistical comparisons of secukinumab versus placebo are presented up to week 16. Analyses were exploratory in nature and conducted without adjustment for multiple comparisons.

Results

Study population

Overall, 397 patients with active PsA were randomized for this trial. Demographics and baseline disease characteristics have been previously reported for patients in this study and are presented in Additional file 1: Table S1. In the overall patient population, mean pain VAS scores were in the range of 55.4–58.9 and mean SF-36 bodily pain scores were in the range of 33.7–37.6. Further, 99% of patients reported moderate-to-extreme pain or discomfort at baseline measured by the EQ-5D-3 L pain/discomfort item. Of 298 patients, 193 (65%) were TNFi naïve at baseline.

Efficacy

Treatment with secukinumab was associated with rapid and sustained relief of pain in patients with PsA. Significant improvements in mean changes from baseline in pain VAS scores were reported beginning at week 3 compared with placebo (– 5.8) with secukinumab 300 mg (–16.9; $P < 0.0001$) and secukinumab 150 mg (–12.6; $P < 0.05$). Improvements in mean changes from baseline in pain VAS scores continued to week 16 and were sustained to week 104 with both doses of secukinumab (Fig. 1a). Additionally, most patients treated with secukinumab reported responses equal to or better than the MCID in the pain VAS response. At week 3, a significantly greater number of patients receiving secukinumab 300 mg had ≥ 20% improvement in pain VAS response compared with placebo (60.6% vs 36.6%; $P < 0.01$). For both doses of secukinumab, the proportion of patients with improvements equal to or better than the MCID in pain VAS scores continued to increase to week 16 and similar levels of attainment were reported at week 104 (Fig. 1b).

A similar trend for reductions in patient-reported pain with secukinumab was reported for SF-36 bodily pain domain scores. At week 4, mean changes from baseline in SF-36 bodily pain scores were significantly greater with both secukinumab 300 mg (16.2) and secukinumab 150 mg (16.3) compared with placebo (5.9; $P < 0.0001$ for both). Continued improvement in SF-36 bodily pain domain scores were reported up to week 12 with both secukinumab doses, and initial improvements were sustained to week 104 for both secukinumab doses (Fig. 2a). Most patients treated with secukinumab also reported equal to or better than the MCID in the SF-36 bodily pain domain score. At week 4, a significantly greater number of patients receiving secukinumab 300 mg (72.3%) and secukinumab 150 mg (73.7%) had improvements ≥ 5 points in SF-36 bodily pain domain score compared with placebo (46.9%; $P < 0.001$ for both). For both doses of secukinumab, the proportion of patients with improvements equal to or better than the MCID in SF-36 bodily pain domain scores were maintained to week 104 (Fig. 2b). The MCID for SF-36 bodily pain domain scores was attained in both anti-TNF-naive and anti-TNF-IR patients receiving secukinumab.

At baseline, only 1% of patients reported no pain or discomfort in the EQ-5D-3 L pain/discomfort item. Following 4 weeks of secukinumab treatment, no pain or

a

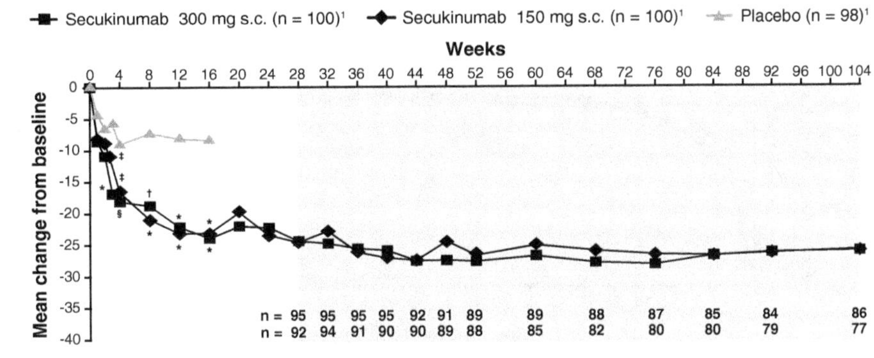

Data values by week for mean change from baseline in pain VAS score

Week	1	2	3	4	8	12	16	20	24	28	32	36	40	44	48	52	60	68	76	84	92	104
SEC 300	-8.5	-10.9	-16.9	-18.1	-18.8	-22.1	-23.9	-22.0	-22.3	-24.4	-24.8	-25.6	-25.9	-27.6	-27.5	-27.7	-26.8	-27.9	-28.2	-26.8	-26.3	-26.1
SEC 150	-8.2	-8.7	-12.6	-16.6	-20.9	-23.2	-23.1	-19.8	-23.5	-24.6	-22.8	-26.2	-27.1	-27.5	-24.5	-26.7	-25.1	-26.0	-26.6	-26.8	-26.4	-25.9
PBO	-4.3	-6.6	-5.8	-9.0	-7.2	-8.1	-8.4	-14.0	-15.9													

b

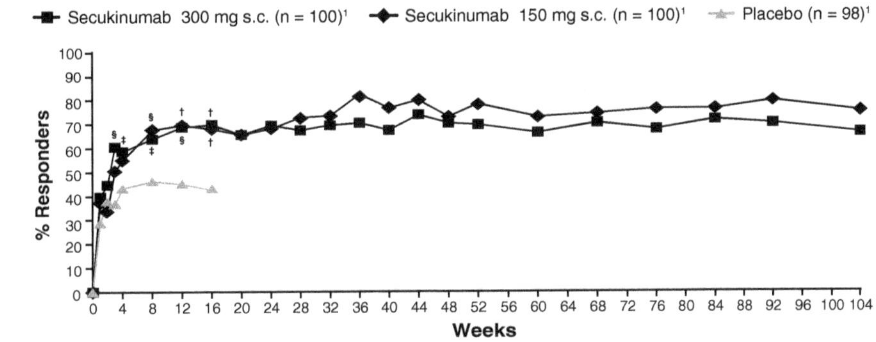

Data values by week for proportion of patients with ≥ 20% improvement in pain VAS response

Week	1	2	3	4	8	12	16	20	24	28	32	36	40	44	48	52	60	68	76	84	92	104
SEC 300	39.8	44.7	60.6	58.8	63.9	68.8	69.8	65.6	69.5	67.4	69.5	70.5	67.4	73.9	70.3	69.7	66.3	70.5	67.8	71.8	70.2	66.3
SEC 150	37.2	33.7	50.5	55.0	67.7	69.7	68.0	65.6	68.1	72.8	73.4	82.4	76.7	80.0	73.0	78.4	72.9	74.4	76.3	76.3	79.7	75.3
PBO	28.7	37.5	36.6	43.3	46.3	45.1	42.5															

Fig. 1 Proportion of patients with ≥ 20% improvement in pain visual analog scale (VAS) score through week 104 (**a**) and proportion of patients with ≥ 20% improvement in pain VAS response (**b**)
Data are presented as LS mean change using MMRM from weeks 1-24, and observed data are presented from weeks 28-104 (shaded area); *P* values are calculated from a MMRM analysis (**a**). Observed data are presented; P values are calculated from Fisher's exact test (**b**)
[1]Number of patients originally randomized to each treatment group. **P* < 0.0001; †*P* < 0.001; ‡*P* < 0.05 §*P* < 0.01 versus placebo
LS, least squares; MMRM, mixed-effect model for repeated measures; PBO, placebo; s.c., subcutaneous; SEC, secukinumab

discomfort was reported by 14.7% of patients receiving secukinumab 300 mg, 9.1% of patients receiving secukinumab 150 mg, and 5.2% of patients receiving placebo (Fig. 3). With secukinumab treatment, the proportion of patients reporting no pain or discomfort continued to increase over time, especially with secukinumab 300 mg and after 2 years of treatment with secukinumab 300 mg almost 30% of patients experienced no pain or discomfort by EQ-5D-3 L.

At weeks 16, 24, 52, and 104, improvements from baseline in mean pain VAS scores were significantly correlated with improvements from baseline in mean SF-36 bodily pain scores (correlation coefficients of – 0.56 to – 0.62; $P < 0.01$ for all) and EQ-5D pain/discomfort domain scores (correlation coefficients of 0.36 to 0.47; $P < 0.01$ for all). Similarly, improvements from baseline in mean SF-36 bodily pain scores were significantly correlated with improvements in EQ-5D pain/discomfort domain scores at weeks 16, 24, 52, and 104 (correlation coefficients of – 0.45 to – 0.52; $P < 0.01$ for all).

Response by prior TNF inadequate response

TNF-naive and TNF-IR patients both demonstrated significant improvements in mean changes from baseline in pain VAS scores and SF-36 bodily pain scores. TNF-naïve patients receiving secukinumab 300 mg reported significant improvements in mean change from baseline in pain VAS score compared with placebo beginning at week 3 (– 19.7 vs – 8.5; $P < 0.01$). With both doses of secukinumab, improvements continued to week 104 (Table 1). Although a similar trend was observed in TNF-IR patients, the magnitude of improvements was

a

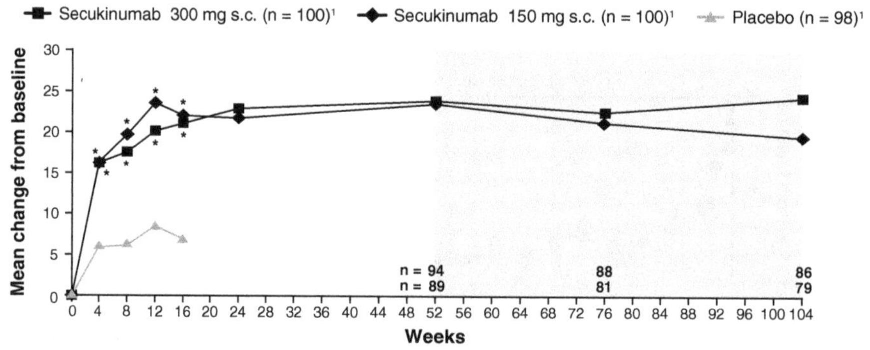

Data values by week for mean change from baseline in SF-36 bodily pain domain score

Week	4	8	12	16	24	52	76	104
SEC 300	16.2	17.6	20.1	21.1	22.9	23.9	22.5	24.3
SEC 150	16.3	19.7	23.6	22.1	21.7	23.5	21.2	19.5
PBO	5.9	6.1	8.5	6.9				

b

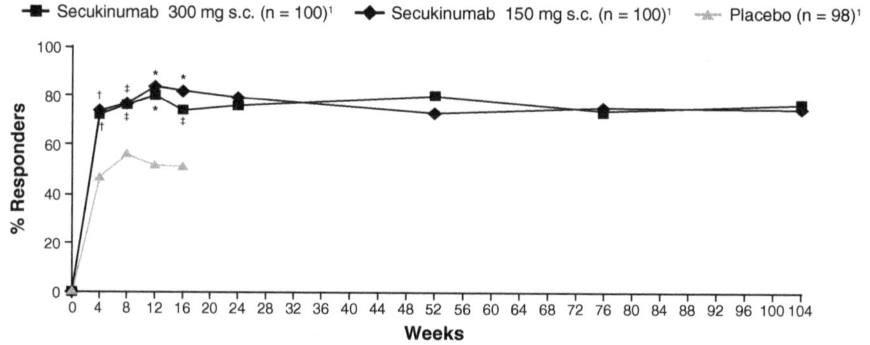

Data values by week for proportion of patients with improvement ≥ 5 in SF-36 bodily pain domain score

Week	4	8	12	16	24	52	76	104
SEC 300	72.3	76.3	80.2	74.0	76.0	79.8	73.9	76.7
SEC 150	73.7	76.8	83.8	82.0	79.2	73.0	75.3	74.7
PBO	46.9	55.8	51.6	51.1				

Fig. 2 Change from baseline in the Short Form-36 (SF-36) bodily pain score through week 104 (**a**) and proportion of patients with improvement ≥ 5 in the SF-36 bodily pain domain score (**b**)
Data are presented as LS mean change using MMRM from weeks 1-24, and observed data are presented from weeks 52-104 (shaded area); *P* values are calculated from a MMRM analysis (**a**). Observed data are presented; *P* values are calculated from Fisher's exact test (**b**)
[1]Number of patients originally randomized to each treatment group. **P* < 0.0001; †*P* < 0.001; ‡*P* < 0.05 versus placebo. LS, least squares; MMRM, mixed-effect model for repeated measures; PBO, placebo; s.c., subcutaneous; SEC, secukinumab

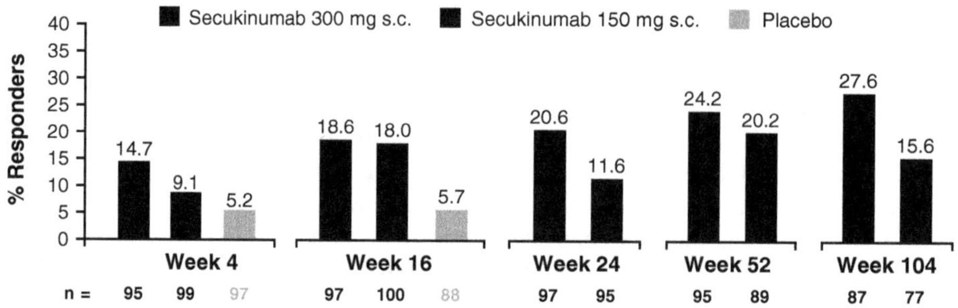

Fig. 3 Proportion of patients with no pain or discomfort in the EuroQoL 5-Dimension (EQ-5D-3 L) domain through week 104
Observed data are presented. Data are presented only for evaluable patients at each time point
s.c., subcutaneous

Table 1 Effect of secukinumab on pain by prior TNF exposure through week 104

	Week 3	Week 4	Week 8	Week 16	Week 24	Week 52	Week 104
TNF-naïve							
Pain VAS, mean change from baseline[a]							
Secukinumab 300 mg	−19.7*	−20.7**	− 20.7*	−27.8****	− 24.0	−30.3	−29.6
Secukinumab 150 mg	−12.8	−15.2	−21.8*	− 25.1***	−26.3	−28.1	−28.3
Placebo	−8.5	−11.3	−10.1	−11.3	–	–	–
SF-36 bodily pain, mean change from baseline[b]							
Secukinumab 300 mg	–	18.4****	18.2*	23.8****	23.9	24.4	24.2
Secukinumab 150 mg	–	18.9****	20.0***	25.4****	25.7	25.8	22.2
Placebo	–	5.6	7.3	8.6	–	–	–
EQ-5D-3 L, no pain or discomfort[c]							
Secukinumab 300 mg	–	–	–	21.5%	24.6%	28.6%	32.8%
Secukinumab 150 mg	–	–	–	22.2%	14.8%	20.3%	17.0%
Placebo	–	–	–	6.9%	–	–	–
TNF-IR							
Pain VAS, mean change from baseline[d]							
Secukinumab 300 mg	−13.1**	−14.9	−16.8**	−18.2**	−20.7	−22.5	−19.3
Secukinumab 150 mg	−14.8*	−21.3*	−21.2*	−21.1*	− 20.0	−23.9	− 20.4
Placebo	−2.1	−5.9	−3.4	−4.4	–	–	–
SF-36 bodily pain, mean change from baseline[e]							
Secukinumab 300 mg	–	15.1	18.7*	18.3*	23.6	23.0	24.5
Secukinumab 150 mg	–	13.6	21.0***	17.9*	16.0	19.0	14.0
Placebo	–	7.8	5.7	5.2	–	–	–
EQ-5D-3 L, no pain or discomfort[f]							
Secukinumab 300 mg	–	–	–	12.5%	12.5%	15.6%	17.2%
Secukinumab 150 mg	–	–	–	10.8%	5.9%	20.0%	12.5%
Placebo	–	–	–	3.3%	–	–	–

Least squares mean change using a mixed-effect model for repeated measures (MMRM) from weeks 1 to 24, and observed data from weeks 52 to 104, for pain visual analog scale (VAS) and Short Form-36 (SF-36) bodily pain scores. Observed data are presented for the EuroQoL 5-Dimension 3-Level Questionnaire (EQ-5D-3 L). At week 16, patients initially randomized to placebo who were non-responders switched to secukinumab treatment. Results are not shown for patients who continued on placebo after week 16. Data are presented only for evaluable patients at each time point. TNF-naïve patients originally randomized to secukinumab 300 mg = 67, to secukinumab 150 mg = 63, and to placebo = 63; patients with inadequate response to TNF (TNF-IR) originally randomized to secukinumab 300 mg = 33, to secukinumab 150 mg = 37, and to placebo = 35. *P* values were calculated from a MMRM analysis

[a]Number of evaluable patients, week 52: 59 for secukinumab 300 mg and 150 mg; week 104: 57 for secukinumab 300 mg and 53 for secukinumab 150 mg

[b]Number of evaluable patients, week 52: 62 for secukinumab 300 mg and 59 for secukinumab 150 mg; week 104: 57 for secukinumab 300 mg and 53 for secukinumab 150 mg

[c]Number of evaluable patients, week 52: 63 for secukinumab 300 mg and 59 for secukinumab 150 mg; week 104: 58 for secukinumab 300 mg and 53 for secukinumab 150 mg

[d]Number of evaluable patients, week 52: 30 for secukinumab 300 mg and 29 for secukinumab 150 mg; week 104: 29 for secukinumab 300 mg and 24 for secukinumab 150 mg

[e]Number of evaluable patients, week 52: 32 for secukinumab 300 mg and 30 for secukinumab 150 mg; week 104: 29 for secukinumab 300 mg and 26 for secukinumab 150 mg

[f]Number of evaluable patients, week 52: 32 for secukinumab 300 mg and 30 for secukinumab 150 mg; week 104: 29 for secukinumab 300 mg and 24 for secukinumab 150 mg

$^{*}P < 0.01$; $^{**}P < 0.05$; $^{***}P < 0.001$; $^{****}P < 0.0001$, versus placebo. TNF, tumor necrosis factor

generally lower. In TNF-IR patients, significant mean improvements from baseline in pain VAS scores were reported at week 3 with secukinumab 300 mg (− 13.1; $P < 0.05$ vs placebo) and secukinumab 150 mg (− 14.8; $P < 0.01$ vs placebo). Due to the smaller number of TNF-IR patients there was more volatility in responses over time. Nonetheless, improvements were maintained over time.

Significant mean improvements from baseline in SF-36 bodily pain scores were also reported by both TNF-naive and TNF-IR patients receiving secukinumab (Table 1). At week 4, mean changes from baseline in SF-36 bodily pain scores in TNF-naïve patients improved by 18.4 with secukinumab 300 mg, by 18.9 with secukinumab 150 mg compared with 5.6 for placebo ($P < 0.0001$ for both versus placebo). Over time, the degrees of improvement in SF-36 bodily pain scores were similar with both doses of secukinumab in TNF-naïve patients. In TNF-IR patients, there were significant mean improvements from baseline in SF-36 bodily pain scores at week 8 with both secukinumab 300 mg (18.7; $P < 0.01$) and 150 mg (21.0; $P < 0.001$) compared to 5.7 with placebo. Mean changes from baseline in SF-36 bodily pain scores were similar over time between TNF-naive and TNF-IR patients with secukinumab 300 mg.

Both TNF-naive and TNF-IR patients also reported improvements in the EQ-5D-3 L pain item scores. At week 16, 22% of TNF-naive patients receiving either dose of secukinumab reported no pain or discomfort compared with 6.9% of patients receiving placebo (Table 1). The proportion of TNF-naive patients receiving secukinumab 300 mg that reported no pain or discomfort continued to increase to week 104 when 32.8% TNF-naive patients had no pain or discomfort. A similar trend was observed in TNF-IR patients but fewer of these patients reported no pain or discomfort compared with TNF-naïve patients. There was a small numerical increase in the number of TNF-IR patients reporting no pain or discomfort at week 104.

Discussion

Pain is one of the most important domains affecting HRQoL in patients with PsA [7], and patients with PsA report role limitations caused by both emotional problems and bodily pain [5, 20]. Pain has also been linked to fatigue in other inflammatory arthritides [21]. Additionally, joint pain has a quantifiable burden to society as demonstrated by work limitations in patients with PsA [22]. Taken together, these findings exemplify the importance of managing pain when treating patients with PsA.

In this post-hoc analysis of the phase-3, FUTURE 2 study, secukinumab 300 mg and secukinumab 150 mg both provided rapid and sustained pain relief to patients with PsA over 2 years' treatment. Improvements in pain with secukinumab were consistent across three different patient-reported measures (pain VAS, SF-36 bodily pain, and EQ-5D-3 L pain/discomfort) and were observed regardless of prior exposure to TNFis. Improvements in pain reported in this trial are consistent with findings of improved pain and HRQoL in other secukinumab trials. In FUTURE 1, improvement was observed in both mean pain VAS and SF-36 bodily pain domain scores [19]. Further, secukinumab 150 mg demonstrated sustained improvement in HRQoL with an SF-36 physical component summary score of 4.89 at week 104 [17]. In FUTURE 2, improved physical function was reported at week 24 with a change from baseline in the Health Assessment Questionnaire Disability Index (HAQ-DI) of − 0.56 with secukinumab 300 mg ($P = 0.004$ vs placebo) and − 0.48 with secukinumab 150 mg ($P = 0.0555$ vs placebo) [15].

In this trial, improvements in pain with secukinumab treatment were sufficient to meet or exceed established definitions for MCID in pain for PsA and were observed irrespective of previous exposure to TNFis. Due to the level of improvement in pain with secukinumab treatment, it is interesting to consider whether pain alleviation is due to overall improvement in inflammation or through a direct role of IL-17 inhibition. Plasma levels of IL-17A are elevated in patients with fibromyalgia and in mice, IL-17 contributes to neuroinflammatory responses and pain hypersensitivity following neuropathic injury [23, 24]. These findings suggest that additional investigation is warranted on the role of IL-17 in other conditions associated with pain such as PsA.

There was significant correlation between the improvement from baseline in mean pain VAS scores and mean SF-36 bodily pain scores and EQ-5D pain/discomfort domain scores and significant correlation between improvement from baseline in mean SF-36 bodily pain scores and EQ-5D pain/discomfort scores. Together these correlations indicate that secukinumab consistently improves pain regardless of the specific measurement used for assessment.

Secukinumab 300 mg and secukinumab 150 mg also improved pain in both TNF-naive and TNF-IR patients measured by the pain VAS, SF-36 bodily pain scores, and EQ-5D-3 L pain/discomfort domain. Not surprisingly, TNF-naïve patients reported numerically greater changes from baseline in all three pain outcomes than those reported by TNF-IR patients.

Limitations of this study include that it was a post-hoc analysis, the lack of an active comparator, and lack of placebo control after week 24.

Conclusions

Secukinumab has previously demonstrated efficacy in treatment of the signs and symptoms of PsA, inhibition of radiographic progression in patients with PsA, and a favorable safety profile [15–17]. In this study, secukinumab provided rapid pain relief for patients with PsA as assessed by multiple clinically relevant patient-reported pain measures. Pain relief began as early as week 3 and improvements were sustained through 104 weeks. Further, improvements in pain were reported by patients regardless of prior exposure to TNFis.

Abbreviations

DMARD: Disease-modifying anti-rheumatic drug; EQ-5D-3 L: EuroQoL 5-Dimension 3-Level Questionnaire; EULAR: European League Against Rheumatism; GRAPPA: Group for Research and Assessment of Psoriasis and Psoriatic Arthritis; HRQoL: Health-related quality of life; IL: Interleukin; LOS: Longitudinal observational studies; MAPP: Multinational Assessment of Psoriasis and Psoriatic Arthritis; MCID: Minimum clinically meaningful difference; MMRM: Mixed-effect model for repeated measures; NSAID: Non-steroidal anti-inflammatory drug; OMERACT: Outcome Measures in Rheumatology; PsA: Psoriatic arthritis; PsAID: Psoriatic Arthritis Impact of Disease; RCT: Randomized controlled trial; SF-36: Short Form-36; TNF: Tumor necrosis factor; TNFi: Tumor necrosis factor-α inhibitor; TNF-IR: TNF inadequate response; VAS: Visual analog scale

Acknowledgements

The authors thank the patients and investigators who participated in the study.

Funding

Technical assistance with editing and styling of the manuscript for submission was provided by Oxford PharmaGenesis Inc. and was funded by Novartis Pharmaceuticals Corporation, East Hanover, NJ, USA. The FUTURE 2 study was funded by Novartis Pharma AG, Basel, Switzerland.

Authors' contributions

The authors were fully responsible for all content and editorial decisions and received no financial support or other form of compensation related to the development of this manuscript. The opinions expressed in the manuscript are those of the authors and Novartis Pharmaceuticals had no influence on the contents. All authors read and approved the final manuscript.

Competing interests

IB McInnes received research grants, consultation fees, or speaker honoraria from AbbVie, Amgen, BMS, Celgene, Janssen, Lilly, Novartis, Pfizer, and UCB. PJ Mease received research grants, consultation fees, or speaker honoraria from AbbVie, Amgen, BMS, Celgene, Crescendo Bioscience, Genentech, Janssen, Eli Lilly, Merck, Novartis, Pfizer, and UCB. G Schett received speaker fees from Abbvie, BMS, Celgene, Chugai, Eli Lilly, Janssen, Novartis, Roche, and UCB. B Kirkham received research support from AbbVie, Novartis, Roche; served as a consultant and speaker for Abbott, BMS, Chugai, MSD, Novartis, Pfizer, Roche, UCB; and participated in speakers bureaus for Abbott, BMS, Chugai, MSD, Novartis, Pfizer, Roche, UCB. V Strand is a founding member of the executive of Outcome Measures in Rheumatoid Arthritis Clinical Trials (OMERACT), an organization that develops outcome measures in rheumatology and receives arms-length funding from 36 companies; a member of the American College of Rheumatology's Clinical Trials Task Force and Chair of the American College of Rheumatology/OMERACT Imaging Subcommittee. Dr. Strand also has served as a consultant and member of advisory boards for AbbVie, Alder, Amgen Corporation, AstraZeneca, Bristol-Myers Squibb, Boehringer Ingelheim, Celltrion, Genentech/Roche, GlaxoSmithKline, Janssen, Eli Lily, Novartis, Pfizer, Regeneron, Sandoz, Sanofi, and UCB. N Williams is a consultant for Novartis through employment at RTI Health Solutions and is an employee of RTI Health Solutions. T Fox, L Pricop, SM Jugl, and KK Gandhi are employees of Novartis and own Novartis stock.

Author details

[1]Institute of Infection, Immunity & Inflammation, College of Medical, Veterinary and Life Sciences, University of Glasgow, 120 University Place, Glasgow G12 8TA, UK. [2]Swedish Medical Center and University of Washington, Seattle, WA, USA. [3]Friedrich-Alexander University of Erlangen-Nuremberg and Universitatsklinikum Erlangen, Erlangen, Germany. [4]Guy's & St Thomas' NHS Foundation Trust, London, UK. [5]Stanford University School of Medicine, Palo Alto, CA, USA. [6]RTI Health Solutions, Durham, NC, USA. [7]Novartis Pharma AG, Basel, Switzerland. [8]Novartis Pharmaceuticals Corporation, East Hanover, NJ, USA.

References

1. Gladman DD. Psoriatic arthritis. Dermatol Ther. 2009;22:40–55.
2. Ritchlin CT, Colbert RA, Gladman DD. Psoriatic arthritis. N Engl J Med. 2017; 376:957–70.
3. Michelsen B, Fiane R, Diamantopoulos AP, Soldal DM, Hansen IJ, Sokka T, et al. A comparison of disease burden in rheumatoid arthritis, psoriatic arthritis and axial spondyloarthritis. PLoS One. 2015;10:e0123582.
4. Kavanaugh A, Helliwell P, Ritchlin CT. Psoriatic arthritis and burden of disease: patient perspectives from the population-based Multinational Assessment of Psoriasis and Psoriatic Arthritis (MAPP) Survey. Rheumatol Ther. 2016;3:91–102.
5. Lee S, Mendelsohn A, Sarnes E. The burden of psoriatic arthritis: a literature review from a global health systems perspective. P T. 2010;35:680–9.
6. Gratacós J, Daudén E, Gómez-Reino J, Moreno JC, Casado MA, Rodriguez-Valverde V. Health-related quality of life in psoriatic arthritis patients in Spain. Reumatol Clin. 2014;10:25–31.
7. Gossec L, de Wit M, Kiltz U, Braun J, Kalyoncu U, Scrivo R, et al. A patient-derived and patient-reported outcome measure for assessing psoriatic arthritis: elaboration and preliminary validation of the Psoriatic Arthritis Impact of Disease (PsAID) questionnaire, a 13-country EULAR initiative. Ann Rheum Dis. 2014;73:1012–9.
8. Williams EM, Walker RJ, Faith T, Egede LE. The impact of arthritis and joint pain on individual healthcare expenditures: findings from the Medical Expenditure Panel Survey (MEPS), 2011. Arthritis Res Ther. 2017;19:38.
9. Lebwohl MG, Kavanaugh A, Armstrong AW, Van Voorhees AS. US perspectives in the management of psoriasis and psoriatic arthritis: patient and physician results from the population-based Multinational Assessment of Psoriasis and Psoriatic Arthritis (MAPP) Survey. Am J Clin Dermatol. 2016; 17:87–97.
10. Coates LC, Kavanaugh A, Mease PJ, Soriano ER, Laura Acosta-Felquer M, Armstrong AW, et al. Group for Research and Assessment of Psoriasis and Psoriatic Arthritis 2015 treatment recommendations for psoriatic arthritis. Arthritis Rheumatol. 2016;68:1060–71.
11. Coates LC, Fransen J, Helliwell PS. Defining minimal disease activity in psoriatic arthritis: a proposed objective target for treatment. Ann Rheum Dis. 2010;69:48–53.
12. Orbai AM, de Wit M, Mease PJ, Callis Duffin K, Elmamoun M, Tillett W, et al. Updating the Psoriatic Arthritis (PsA) Core Domain Set: a report from the PsA Workshop at OMERACT 2016. J Rheumatol. 2017;44:1522–8.
13. Langley RG, Elewski BE, Lebwohl M, Reich K, Griffiths CE, Papp K, et al. Secukinumab in plaque psoriasis—results of two phase 3 trials. N Engl J Med. 2014;371:326–38.
14. Mease PJ, McInnes IB, Kirkham B, Kavanaugh A, Rahman P, van der Heijde D, et al. Secukinumab inhibition of interleukin-17A in patients with psoriatic arthritis. N Engl J Med. 2015;373:1329–39.
15. McInnes IB, Mease PJ, Kirkham B, Kavanaugh A, Ritchlin CT, Rahman P, et al. Secukinumab, a human anti-interleukin-17A monoclonal antibody, in patients with psoriatic arthritis (FUTURE 2): a randomised, double-blind, placebo-controlled, phase 3 trial. Lancet. 2015;386:1137–46.
16. McInnes IB, Mease PJ, Ritchlin CT, Rahman P, Gottlieb AB, Kirkham B, et al. Secukinumab sustains improvement in signs and symptoms of psoriatic arthritis: 2 year results from the phase 3 FUTURE 2 study. Rheumatology (Oxford). 2017;56:1993–2003.
17. Kavanaugh A, Mease PJ, Reimold AM, Tahir H, Rech J, Hall S, et al. Secukinumab for long-term treatment of psoriatic arthritis: a two-year followup from a phase III, randomized, double-blind placebo-controlled study. Arthritis Care Res (Hoboken). 2017;69:347–55.
18. Busse JW, Bartlett SJ, Dougados M, Johnston BC, Guyatt GH, Kirwan JR, et al. Optimal strategies for reporting pain in clinical trials and systematic reviews: recommendations from an OMERACT 12 workshop. J Rheumatol. 2015;42:1962–70.

19. Strand V, Mease P, Gossec L, Elkayam O, van den Bosch F, Zuazo J, et al. Secukinumab improves patient-reported outcomes in subjects with active psoriatic arthritis: results from a randomised phase III trial (FUTURE 1). Ann Rheum Dis. 2017;76:203–7.
20. Husted JA, Gladman DD, Farewell VT, Cook RJ. Health-related quality of life of patients with psoriatic arthritis: a comparison with patients with rheumatoid arthritis. Arthritis Rheum. 2001;45:151–8.
21. Pollard LC, Choy EH, Gonzalez J, Khoshaba B, Scott DL. Fatigue in rheumatoid arthritis reflects pain, not disease activity. Rheumatology (Oxford). 2006;45:885–9.
22. Tillett W, de-Vries C, NJ MH. Work disability in psoriatic arthritis: a systematic review. Rheumatology (Oxford). 2012;51:275–83.
23. Kim CF, Moalem-Taylor G. Interleukin-17 contributes to neuroinflammation and neuropathic pain following peripheral nerve injury in mice. J Pain. 2011; 12:370–83.
24. Pernambuco AP, Schetino LP, Alvim CC, Murad CM, Viana RS, Carvalho LS, et al. Increased levels of IL-17A in patients with fibromyalgia. Clin Exp Rheumatol. 2013;31:S60–3.

9

Inflammatory back pain in psoriatic arthritis is significantly more responsive to corticosteroids compared to back pain in ankylosing spondylitis

Muhammad Haroon[1*], Muddassar Ahmad[1], Muhammad Nouman Baig[2], Olivia Mason[3], John Rice[2] and Oliver FitzGerald[4]

Abstract

Background: The efficacy of corticosteroids in patients with psoriatic arthritis (PsA) and inflammatory back pain has not been studied to date. In this controlled trial, we aimed to investigate the comparative performance of corticosteroids in patients with active axial-PsA (AxPsA) versus those with active ankylosing spondylitis (AS).

Methods: Patients with AxPsA and AS (naïve to biologic therapies), who not only had clinically active disease, but also had bone marrow oedema on magnetic resonance imaging of the sacroiliac joints, were recruited. Clinically active disease was defined as inflammatory back pain (fulfilling Assessment of Spondyloarthritis International Society (ASAS) expert criteria), with spinal pain score (numerical rating scale 0–10) ≥4 and Bath AS Disease Activity Index (BASDAI) score ≥4 despite taking nonsteroidal anti-inflammatory drugs. Moreover, we recruited a control group of patients with non-inflammatory lower back pain. All patients received a single, intra-muscular dose of depot corticosteroid injection (triamcinolone acetonide 80 mg) at baseline. The intra-muscular corticosteroid option was used to overcome any drug compliance issues. Clinical outcome assessments were made at the following time points: baseline, week 2, and week 4. The primary efficacy end point was mean change in Ankylosing Spondylitis Disease Activity Score (ASDAS) at week 2. Key secondary outcomes were mean change in the BASDAI, Bath Ankylosing Spondylitis Functional Index (BASFI) and Ankylosing Spondylitis Quality of Life (ASQoL) at weeks 2 and 4.

Results: In total, 40 patients were recruited (15 with AxPsA, 15 with AS, and 10 controls). At week 2 following corticosteroid treatment, patients with AxPsA had significantly greater improvement in the mean ASDAS compared to patients with AS (1.43 ± 0.39 vs. 1.03 ± 0.30, $p = 0.004$), and also when compared to controls ($p < 0.001$). At week-4, similar significant trend of ASDAS improvement was seen among AxPsA patients compared to AS patients (1.09 ± 0.32 vs. 0.77 ± 0.27, $p = 0.007$) and controls ($p < 0.001$). Similarly, the mean BASDAI, visual analogue scale spinal pain score, ASQoL and BASFI improved significantly among patients with AxPsA compared to patients with AS and controls at week 2 ($p < 0.05$), with this trend also largely maintained at week 4.

Conclusions: Axial inflammation in patients with PsA responds significantly better to corticosteroids than in patients with AS. This furthers the argument and adds to the growing evidence that AxPsA and AS are distinct entities.

Keywords: Corticosteroids, Psoriatic arthritis, Axial psoriatic arthritis, Ankylosing spondylitis, Inflammatory back pain

* Correspondence: mharoon301@hotmail.com
[1]Division of Rheumatology, Department of Medicine, University Hospital Kerry, Tralee, Ireland
Full list of author information is available at the end of the article

Background

Psoriatic arthritis (PsA) is a progressive, immune-mediated musculoskeletal disease with involvement of synovial, entheseal and axial structures. There are varied reports of its prevalence among patients with psoriasis (PsO), and it is becoming clear that PsA is much more common than previously thought. We have shown that 29% of patients with PsO attending dermatology clinics had undiagnosed PsA [1]. PsA was formerly considered a milder form of arthritis but an inception cohort study has shown that 47% of the patients with PsA who presented within 5 months of onset of symptoms had ≥1 erosion by the second year of follow up, despite the fact that the majority had been treated with disease-modifying anti-rheumatic drugs (DMARDs) [2]. More recently, we have also shown that even a 6-month delay from symptom onset to the first visit with a rheumatologist can lead to the development of peripheral joint erosions and worse long-term physical function [3].

It is common that patients with PsA with peripheral arthritis have concomitant inflammatory axial disease, but isolated inflammatory axial disease occurs in fewer than 5% of patients [4]. The reported prevalence of axial disease in patients with PsA is quite variable, and has been reported to be as high as up to 78% [5]. At present there are no approved therapies for treatment of axial involvement in PsA. Most of the treatment response data about axial involvement in SpA come from ankylosing spondylitis (AS) studies, while data about the response of axial involvement in PsA to various treatment strategies are limited [6]. It remains to be seen whether the availability of new therapeutic agents (such as IL-17 inhibitors and IL-23 inhibitors) will have any beneficial effect in patients with axial PsA (AxPsA). The efficacy of corticosteroids in patients with PsA and inflammatory back pain (IBP) has not been studied to date.

AS is a chronic inflammatory disorder of unknown aetiology that principally involves the axial joints and adjacent structures leading to progressive bony fusion of the spine. Nonsteroidal anti-inflammatory drugs (NSAIDs) and biologic drugs such as TNF inhibitors (TNFi) are the principle treatments. Although very little is known about the use of corticosteroids in AS, a recent double-blind, randomised, placebo-controlled trial has shown that 50 mg of prednisolone was only partially effective in patients with active AS, while a dose of 20 mg was not effective [7].

A number of studies have suggested that there are clinical, radiologic, and genetic differences between axial disease in PsA (AxPsA) and AS, suggesting that these are distinct entities [8–10]. Similarly, the studies examining typical AS-associated genetic risks in AxPsA have largely been negative, further supporting the theory that spinal involvement in PsA is genetically different from that seen in AS [11]. However, no study to date has directly compared the therapeutic response in these two diseases. There is only one study that looked at the response of TNFi in active AS (fulfilling modified 1984 New York Criteria for AS) with and without concomitant psoriasis (but no formal diagnosis of PsA) [12]. In this controlled trial, we aimed to investigate the comparative performance of corticosteroids in patients with active axial-PsA versus those with active AS.

Method

All patients attending rheumatology clinics at University Hospital Kerry, who had a confirmed diagnosis of PsA as per the internationally agreed Criteria of the Classification of Psoriatic Arthritis (CASPAR) [13], and AS as per the 1984 Modified New York criteria [14], were suitable for inclusion. Among them, patients with active AxPsA and active AS were recruited in this open-label controlled trial. Active disease was defined as IBP (fulfilling Assessment of Spondyloarthritis International Society (ASAS) expert criteria) [15], with a spinal pain score (numerical rating scale 0–10) ≥4 and Bath Ankylosing Spondylitis Disease Activity Index (BASDAI) score ≥4 despite taking NSAIDS. Furthermore, only those patients with AxPsA and AS with magnetic resonance imaging (MRI)-proven sacroiliac (SI) joint bone marrow oedema [16] (MRI of the sacroiliac joints performed within the 6 months prior to recruitment) were considered for inclusion. Hence, all recruited patients with AxPsA and AS had not only clinically active disease, but also had bone marrow oedema on MRI of the SI joints. Radiographs and MRI scans were reviewed by a consultant radiologist. We further scored inflammation by MRI in the SI joints using the Spondyloarthritis Research Consortium of Canada Magnetic Resonance Imaging Index [17].

All recruited patients were naive to biological therapies such as anti-TNF alpha agents. Moreover, we recruited a control group of patients with non-inflammatory lower back pain attending orthopaedic clinics. Patients in this control group suffered from discogenic lower back pain, and were matched by age, gender and severity of back pain with patients with AxPsA and AS. Patients excluded were those under the age of 18 years and patients with learning difficulties, peripheral joint active polyarthritis, or concomitant fibromyalgia. Patients with monoarthritis or oligoarthritis were included in the study. All patients received a single, intra-muscular dose of depot corticosteroid injection (triamcinolone acetonide 80 mg) at baseline. The intra-muscular corticosteroid option was used to overcome any drug compliance issues. Clinical outcome assessments were made at following time points: baseline, week 2, and week 4. Assessments included the following: spinal pain score (numerical rating scale 0–10), BASDAI, Bath AS Functional Index (BASFI), Ankylosing Spondylitis Quality of Life (ASQoL), Ankylosing Spondylitis Disease

Activity Score (ASDAS), patient global assessment (numeric rating scales 0–10), number of swollen joints (66/68-joint score) and number of tender entheseal sites (Leeds Enthesitis Index). Laboratory outcome assessments included measurement of C-reactive protein (CRP). The primary efficacy end point was the mean change in ASDAS at week 2. Key secondary outcomes were mean change in BASDAI, BASFI, and ASQoL at week 2 and week 4.

ASDAS is a validated composite index that combines patient-oriented measures with a laboratory measure of inflammation (CRP level or erythrocyte sedimentation rate (ESR)) [18], and is used to monitor the actual level of disease activity and to measure response to treatment. As per the recommendations of the Assessment of Spondyloarthritis International Society (ASAS), ASDAS values of 2.1 and 3.5 were selected as cutoff values to define high and very high disease activity, respectively, and ASDAS <1.3 was used as a cutoff to define inactive disease [18]. Similarly, the cutoffs for improvement scores were a change ≥1.1 units for "clinically important improvement" and a change ≥2.0 units for "major improvement" [19].

The study was approved by the local Medical Research Ethics committee (Clinical Research Ethics Committee of the Cork Teaching Hospitals, University College Cork, Ireland; reference number ECM 4, 19/1/16). Written informed consent was obtained from all participants. There were no missing data, as patients were assessed in a dedicated research clinic where all aforementioned clinical, laboratory, and radiographic details were collected.

The required sample size was estimated using the software G*Power 3.1.9.2. With β of 0.8, α of 0.05 and effect size f of 0.25, the total sample size calculated was 30, which reflects actual power of 84%. Statistical analysis was performed using the SPSS software, version 21. Significance was defined as $p < 0.05$ (two-tailed). Baseline descriptive statistics were computed with continuous variables summarised by their means and SD; categorical variables were summarised by proportions. The chi square (X2) statistic was used to investigate the distributions of categorical variables, and continuous variables were analysed using Student's t test.

Results

In total, 40 patients were recruited (15 with AxPsA, 15 with AS, and 10 controls). Table 1 provides the baseline demographic characteristics of these patients, showing that these groups were well-matched by age, gender, and severity of back pain. Sixty percent of the patients with AxPsA were using disease-modifying anti-rheumatic drugs (DMARDs) for their peripheral joint disease. Amongst the AxPsA patients, the mean swollen joint count, tender joint count and Leeds Enthesitis Index was 1.8, 2.7, and 0.2, respectively. The Spondyloarthritis Research Consortium of Canada (SPARCC) score in the AS and AxPsA groups was 24.60 ± 4.68 and 21.86 ± 2.53, respectively.

Table 1 Baseline demographic characteristics and clinical parameters among three patient groups – the axial psoriatic arthritis, ankylosing spondylitis, and control groups

Parameter	Axial psoriatic arthritis	Ankylosing spondylitis	Control
Number of patients	15	15	10
Age in years (mean ± SD)	38.6 ± 7.93	33.9 ± 8.28	40.0 ± 11.6
Duration of back pain - years (mean ± SD)	4.5 ± 1.3	5.4 ± 1.4	5.6 ± 1.7
Gender (female %)	60	46.7	60
CRP (mg/L)	9.00 ± 4.74	7.27 ± 3.61	4.00 ± 1.56
VAS (mean ± SD)	6.60 ± 1.12	6.47 ± 1.13	6.60 ± 1.51
ASQOL (mean ± SD)	11.8 ± 4.19	11.9 ± 3.74	10.0 ± 1.49
BASFI (mean ± SD)	6.40 ± 1.52	6.06 ± 1.49	4.14 ± 1.53
BASDAI (mean ± SD)	5.95 ± 1.24	5.86 ± 1.32	5.18 ± 1.07
ASDAS (mean ± SD)	3.81 ± 0.61	3.75 ± 0.55	2.82 ± 0.67

There were no significant differences ($p > 0.05$) in the parameters listed in Table 1 between patients with axial psoriatic arthritis (AxPsA) and patients with ankylosing spondylitis (AS). Similarly, there were no significant differences ($p > 0.05$) in age, gender, visual analogue scale (VAS) spinal pain score, Ankylosing Spondylitis Quality of Life (ASQoL) or Bath Ankylosing Spondylitis Disease Activity Index (BASDAI) in patients with AxPsA or AS compared with controls

CRP C-reactive protein, *BASFI* Bath Ankylosing Spondylitis Functional Index, *ASDAS* Ankylosing Spondylitis Disease Activity Score

At week 2 following corticosteroid treatment, patients with AxPsA had significantly greater improvement in the mean ASDAS compared to patients with AS (1.43 ± 0.39 vs. 1.03 ± 0.30, $p = 0.004$), and the same was the case when compared to controls ($p < 0.001$, Table 2, Fig. 1). At week 4, patients with AxPsA also had significantly greater improvement in the mean ASDAS compared to both patients with AS (1.09 ± 0.32 vs. 0.77 ± 0.27, $p = 0.007$) and controls ($p < 0.001$). Similarly, the mean BASDAI, VAS spinal pain score, ASQoL and BASFI improved significantly among patients with AxPsA compared to patients with AS and controls at week 2, with this trend also largely maintained at week 4 (Table 2, Figs. 1 and 2). Figure 1 shows the mean changes in ASDAS and BASDAI, and Fig. 2 shows the mean changes in VAS spinal pain score, BASFI, ASQOL, and CRP at baseline, week 2 and week 4 among patients with AxPsA and AS and controls.

Additionally, we compared the mean ASDAS in patients with AS and controls, and found that at week 2 of corticosteroid challenge there was marginal improvement in ASDAS (1.02 ± 0.30 vs. 0.81 ± 0.25, $p = 0.077$), but at week 4 there were no significant mean improvement in ASDAS (0.76 ± 0.27 vs.0.74 ± 0.22, $p = 0.79$). However, there was significantly greater improvement in BASDAI among patients with AS compared to controls at week 2 (1.12 ± 0.33 vs. 0.84 ± 0.24, $p = 0.02$), but at

Table 2 Primary and secondary outcome measure responses at week 2 and week 4 of corticosteroid treatment

Parameter	Axial psoriatic arthritis	Ankylosing spondylitis	Control	*P* value, AxPsA vs. AS
Mean difference from baseline to week 2				
ASDAS	1.43 ± 0.39	1.03 ± 0.30	0.81 ± 0.26	0.004
VAS	2.46 ± 0.91	1.66 ± 1.1	1.0 ± 0.94	0.003
ASQoL	3.80 ± 1.82	2.4 ± 1.72	0.7 ± 0.67	<0.001
BASFI	2.38 ± 0.68	0.95 ± 0.91	0.44 ± 0.41	<0.001
BASDAI	1.93 ± 0.56	1.13 ± 0.33	0.84 ± 0.24	<0.001
Mean difference from baseline to week 4				
ASDAS	1.09 ± 0.32	0.77 ± 0.27	0.73 ± 0.24	0.007
VAS	2.00 ± 0.92	1.33 ± 0.72	1.30 ± 0.82	0.054
ASQoL	3.53 ± 1.35	2.26 ± 1.53	0.70 ± 0.67	<0.001
BASFI	1.76 ± 0.82	0.78 ± 0.63	0.48 ± 0.24	<0.001
BASDAI	1.57 ± 0.49	0.85 ± 0.45	0.62 ± 0.23	<0.001

Data are presented as (mean ± SD)
AxPsA axial psoriatic arthritis, AS ankylosing spondylits, *VAS* visual analogue scale, *ASQoL* Ankylosing Spondylitis Quality of Life, *BASDAI* Bath Ankylosing Spondylitis Disease Activity Index, *BASFI* Bath Ankylosing Spondylitis Functional Index, *ASDAS* Ankylosing Spondylitis Disease Activity Score

week 4 there was no significant improvement in mean BASDAI (0.85 ± 0.45 vs. 0.62 ± 0.23, $p = 0.15$).

Discussion

Inflammatory spinal disease is one of three inflammatory musculoskeletal manifestations that frequently occur in PsA. There are very limited data about the axial involvement in PsA, especially as regards treatment, with treatment guidelines based largely on data from AS trials. To our knowledge, this is the first study to specifically investigate axial disease in PsA. Since at least 50% of patients with PsA develop inflammatory axial disease and it has been shown that limitation of spinal mobility and spinal radiologic changes increase over time, it is important to examine the commonly available therapeutic options [20, 21]. This is especially important as there remains a question as to whether the inflammatory axial disease in PsA may be similar or different to that described in Axial SpA.

The results of our study are important in a number of ways. First, we have carefully compared the efficacy of corticosteroids among patients with AxPsA and AS with IBP and a control group of patients with non-inflammatory lower back pain. This study shows very clearly that patients with AxPsA respond significantly better to corticosteroids than both patients with AS and controls. This observation was quite consistent across the different clinical parameters such as ASDAS, spinal pain score (measured by VAS), BASFI, ASQoL, and BASDAI, and was recorded at both week 2 and week 4. Some attenuation of clinical responses at week 4 compared to week 2 is not surprising and is consistent with gradual wearing-off of the corticosteroid effect over time. Clearly, in our study ASDAS improved significantly in patients with AxPsA both at week 2 and week 4. Furthermore, if we examine the ASDAS improvement criteria, only patients with AxPsA achieved "clinically important improvement" status at week 2. At week 4, there was mild attenuation of the response with the mean change in ASDAS of 1.09 (mean change of 1.1 is required for clinical important improvement) [19].

Second, the significant improvement in IBP in patients with AxPsA compared to those with AS suggests that IBP may have a different pathogenesis in AxPsA and that different therapies might be considered. This is the first study to date comparing the therapeutic response in these two diseases. It is worth noting that the patients with AxPsA in our study responded significantly better to corticosteroids, although they had a relatively lesser burden of bone marrow oedema than the patients with AS: however, patients with AxPsA had other comparable features of back pain. One plausible explanation is that there was more inflammatory involvement in the spine than in the SI joints in these patients with AxPsA, as it has been shown that spinal changes may develop in the absence of SI involvement [22, 23]. Moreover, among patients with AxSpA, spinal inflammation has been observed on MRI in up to half of those without MRI

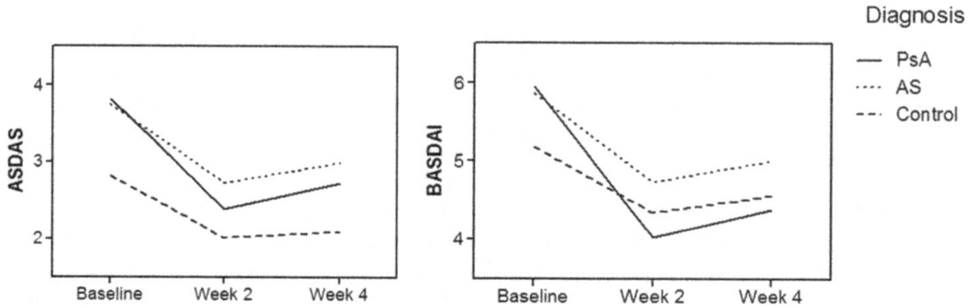

Fig. 1 Changes in mean ankylosing Spondylitis Disease Activity Score (ASDAS) and Bath Ankylosing Spondylitis Disease Activity Index (BASDAI) over time by diagnosis. PsA, psoriatic arthritis; AS, ankylosing spondylitis

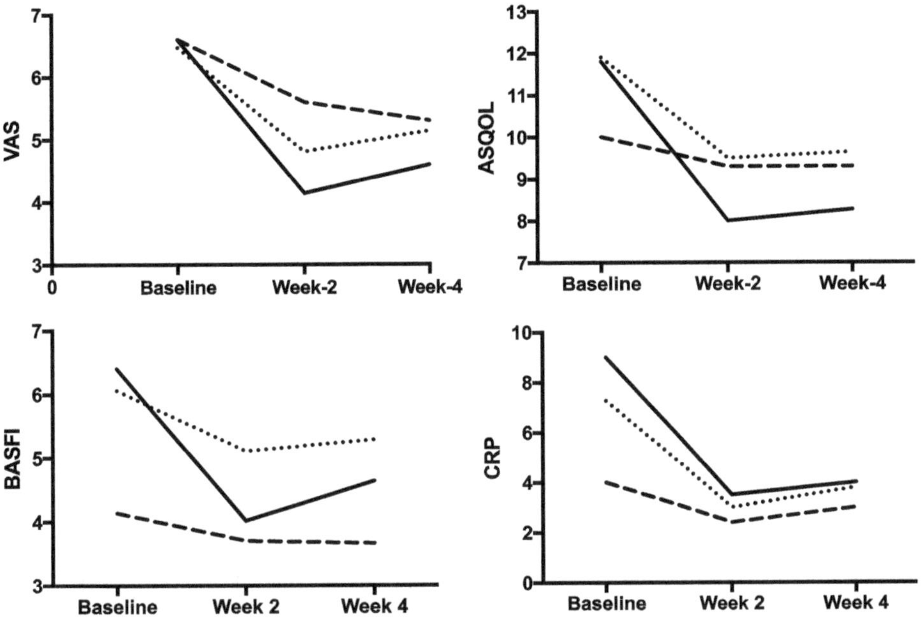

Fig. 2 Changes in mean visual analogue scale (VAS) spinal pain score, Ankylosing Spondylitis Quality of Life (ASQOL), Bath Ankylosing Spondylitis Functional Index (BASFI), and C-reactive protein (CRP) over time by diagnosis. The diagnostic categories are represented similar to Fig. 1

evidence of SI joint inflammation [24, 25]. Unfortunately, we do not have MRI of spine on our patients to further investigate this concept. Another plausible explanation lies in the hypothesis that in PsA there are different primary sites of inflammation, such as synovial-predominant, or enthesis-predominant [26], and this can potentially differentiate patients with AxPsA from those with AS. One can speculate that the IBP in AxPsA is predominantly synovial-based. Interestingly, it has been shown that synovial-based phenotypes in PsA such as joint deformities and joint fusion are associated with *HLA-B*08*, and similarly, sacroiliitis in PsA is most commonly associated with *HLA-B*08* [27]. This is supported by previous studies showing that axial disease in PsA is significantly associated with severe peripheral joint disease [28, 29]. Since PsA is a heterogeneous disease, probably the axial involvement in most of AxPsA patients is predominantly synovial-based and associated with *HLA-B*08*, and in others, entheseal-based and associated with *HLA-B*27* [27]. Given the marked improvement in IBP in AxPsA with corticosteroids, we would propose that standard synthetic (s)DMARDs should be formally tested in active AxPsA, as responses may also be different to those seen in AS where they have not shown benefit.

The strengths of our study include the following: (1) the inclusion of a control group with non-inflammatory lower back pain, and (2) the use of a more robust approach in defining active AxPsA for inclusion of patients in this study - the combination of both active IBP along with the presence of MRI-proven SI joint bone marrow oedema. The rationale to use this approach was the possible disconnect between symptoms of IBP and the imaging diagnosis of sacroiliitis. For example, in a previous study of patients with psoriasis and spondylitic lesions on radiographs, IBP was reported in only 19% [30]. Furthermore, about one third of patients with PsA have asymptomatic sacroiliitis on imaging [31, 32]. We acknowledge that the small number of patients in this study is certainly a limitation of this pilot study; however, given the convincing differential response of IBP to corticosteroid treatment, the study provides useful information worthy of testing in larger and more long-term prospective studies. Genotyping data were not collected, and given such a small sample size this information might not be very helpful. Furthermore, this is an observational, non-randomised study that did not include a placebo-control group. Therefore, the results should be considered as hypothesis-generating rather than proof of efficacy of this treatment. One can argue that patients with AxPsA in our study might have more peripheral arthritis, which usually responds well to corticosteroid therapy, and this potentially could have influenced the axial symptoms along with an impact on measures of axial disease, in particular BASDAI. Measures of joint and entheseal involvement were low in our AxPsA patients with a mean swollen joint count of 1.8, tender joint count of 2.7 and Leeds Enthesitis Index of 0.2. Furthermore, we have analysed the individual questions within the BASDAI questionnaire in our patients, and note that for the questions relating to peripheral arthralgia/swelling and enthesis (question 3 and 4) the average baseline scores were only 2 and 3, suggesting that these peripheral features had little impact on BASDAI scores.

Conclusions

We conclude that axial inflammation in PsA potentially responds significantly better to corticosteroids than in patients with AS. This furthers the argument and adds to the growing evidence that AxPsA and AS are distinct entities. Future studies should further investigate the use of corticosteroids and of sDMARD usage among patients with active IBP in PsA.

Abbreviations

AS: Ankylosing spondylitis; ASAS: Assessment of Spondyloarthritis International Society; ASDAS: Ankylosing Spondylitis Disease Activity Score; ASQoL: Ankylosing Spondylitis Quality of Life; AxPsA: Axial psoriatic arthritis; BASDAI: Bath Ankylosing Spondylitis Disease Activity Index; BASFI: Bath Ankylosing Spondylitis Functional Index; CASPAR: Criteria of the Classification of Psoriatic Arthritis; DMARDs: Disease-modifying anti-rheumatic drugs; IBP: Inflammatory back pain; MRI: Magnetic resonance imaging; NSAIDs: Nonsteroidal anti-inflammatory drugs; PsA: Psoriatic arthritis; PsO: Psoriasis; TNFI: Tumor necrosis factor inhibitors; sDMARDs: synthetic disease-modifying anti-rheumatic drugs; SI: Sacroiliac; VAS: Visual analogue scale

Acknowledgements

Not applicable.

Funding

None.

Authors' contributions

MH, MA, and NB carried out the work, collection and interpretation of data and manuscript drafting. OM contributed to data interpretation and manuscript drafting and editing. MH, JR, and OF conceived the study and its design and were involved in coordination, data interpretation, and manuscript drafting and editing. All authors read and approved the final manuscript.

Consent for publication

Not applicable.

Competing interests

MH has received educational grant supports from Abbvie and Pfizer; OF has received honoraria and grant support and has been a member of advisory boards for Pfizer, Abbvie, MSD, Roche, UCB, and Janssen and Cellgene; MA, NB, OM, and JR have no conflicts of interest.

Author details

[1]Division of Rheumatology, Department of Medicine, University Hospital Kerry, Tralee, Ireland. [2]Department of Orthopaedics, University Hospital Kerry, Tralee, Ireland. [3]CSTAR (Centre for Support and Training in Analysis and Research), University College Dublin, Dublin, Ireland. [4]Department of Rheumatology, St Vincent's University Hospital, Dublin, Ireland.

References

1. Haroon M, Kirby B, FitzGerald O. High prevalence of psoriatic arthritis in patients with severe psoriasis with suboptimal performance of screening questionnaires. Ann Rheum Dis. 2013;72(5):736–40.
2. Kane D, Stafford L, Bresnihan B, FitzGerald O. A prospective, clinical and radiological study of early psoriatic arthritis: an early synovitis clinic experience. Rheumatology (Oxford). 2003;42(12):1460–8.
3. Haroon M, Gallagher P, FitzGerald O. Diagnostic delay of more than 6 months contributes to poor radiographic and functional outcome in psoriatic arthritis. Ann Rheum Dis. 2015;74(6):1045–50.
4. Gladman DD. Axial disease in psoriatic arthritis. Curr Rheumatol Rep. 2007; 9(6):455–60.
5. Battistone MJ, Manaster BJ, Reda DJ, Clegg DO. The prevalence of sacroilitis in psoriatic arthritis: new perspectives from a large, multicenter cohort. A Department of Veterans Affairs Cooperative Study. Skelet Radiol. 1999;28(4): 196–201.
6. Lubrano E, Perrotta FM, Manara M, D'Angelo S, Addimanda O, Ramonda R, Punzi L, Olivieri I, Salvarani C, Marchesoni A. The sex influence on response to tumor necrosis factor-α inhibitors and remission in axial spondyloarthritis. J Rheumatol. 2018;45(2):195–201.
7. Haibel H, Fendler C, Listing J, Callhoff J, Braun J, Sieper J. Efficacy of oral prednisolone in active ankylosing spondylitis: results of a double-blind, randomised, placebo-controlled short-term trial. Ann Rheum Dis. 2014;73(1): 243–6.
8. McEwen C, DiTata D, Lingg C, Porini A, Good A, Rankin T. Ankylosing spondylitis and spondylitis accompanying ulcerative colitis, regional enteritis, psoriasis and Reiter's disease. A comparative study. Arthritis Rheum. 1971;14(3):291–318.
9. Gladman DD, Brubacher B, Buskila D, Langevitz P, Farewell VT. Differences in the expression of spondyloarthropathy: a comparison between ankylosing spondylitis and psoriatic arthritis. Clin Invest Med. 1993;16(1):1–7.
10. Helliwell PS, Hickling P, Wright V. Do the radiological changes of classic ankylosing spondylitis differ from the changes found in the spondylitis associated with inflammatory bowel disease, psoriasis, and reactive arthritis? Ann Rheum Dis. 1998;57(3):135–40.
11. Jadon D, Tillett W, Wallis D, Cavill C, Bowes J, Waldron N, et al. Exploring ankylosing spondylitis-associated ERAP1, IL23R and IL12B gene polymorphisms in subphenotypes of psoriatic arthritis. Rheumatology (Oxford). 2013;52(2):261–6.
12. Braun J, Rudwaleit M, Kary S, Kron M, Wong RL, Kupper H. Clinical manifestations and responsiveness to adalimumab are similar in patients with ankylosing spondylitis with and without concomitant psoriasis. Rheumatology (Oxford). 2010;49(8):1578–89.
13. Taylor W, Gladman D, Helliwell P, et al. Classification criteria for psoriatic arthritis: development of new criteria from a large international study. Arthritis Rheum. 2006;54(8):2665–73.
14. van der Linden S, Valkenburg HA, Cats A. Evaluation of diagnostic criteria for ankylosing spondylitis. A proposal for modification of the New York criteria. Arthritis Rheum. 1984;27(4):361–8.
15. Sieper J, van der Heijde D, Landewé R, Brandt J, Burgos-Vagas R, Collantes-Estevez E, et al. New criteria for inflammatory back pain in patients with chronic back pain: a real patient exercise by experts from the Assessment of SpondyloArthritis international Society (ASAS). Ann Rheum Dis. 2009;68(6):784–8.
16. Lambert RG, Bakker PA, van der Heijde D, Weber U, Rudwaleit M, Hermann KG, et al. Defining active sacroiliitis on MRI for classification of axial spondyloarthritis: update by the ASAS MRI working group. Ann Rheum Dis. 2016;75(11):1958–63.
17. Maksymowych WP, Inman RD, Salonen D, Dhillon SS, Williams M, Stone M, et al. Spondyloarthritis research Consortium of Canada magnetic resonance imaging index for assessment of sacroiliac joint inflammation in ankylosing spondylitis. Arthritis Rheum. 2005;53(5):703–9.
18. van der Heijde D, Lie E, Kvien TK, Sieper J, Van den Bosch F, Listing J, et al. ASDAS, a highly discriminatory ASAS-endorsed disease activity score in patients with ankylosing spondylitis. Ann Rheum Dis. 2009;68(12):1811–8.
19. Machado P, Landewé R, Lie E, Kvien TK, Braun J, Baker D, et al. Ankylosing Spondylitis Disease Activity Score (ASDAS): defining cut-off values for disease activity states and improvement scores. Ann Rheum Dis. 2011;70(1):47–53.
20. Baraliakos X, Coates LC, Braun J. The involvement of the spine in psoriatic arthritis. Clin Exp Rheumatol. 2015;33(5 Suppl 93):S31–5.

21. Chandran V, Barrett J, Schentag CT, Farewell VT, Gladman DD. Axial psoriatic arthritis: Update on a longterm prospective study. J Rheumatol. 2009;36(12): 2744–50.
22. Khan M, Schentag C, Gladman DD. Clinical and radiological changes during psoriatic arthritis disease progression. J Rheumatol. 2003;30(5):1022–6.
23. Taylor WJ, Marchesoni A, Arreghini M, Sokoll K, Helliwell PS. A comparison of the performance characteristics of classification criteria for the diagnosis of psoriatic arthritis. Semin Arthritis Rheum. 2004;34(3):575–84.
24. van der Heijde D, Sieper J, Maksymowych WP, Brown MA, Lambert RG, Rathmann SS, et al. Spinal inflammation in the absence of sacroiliac joint inflammation on magnetic resonance imaging in patients with active nonradiographic axial spondyloarthritis. Arthritis Rheumatol. 2014;66(3):667–73.
25. Jadon DR, Sengupta R, Nightingale A, Lindsay M, Korendowych E, Robinson G, et al. Axial Disease in Psoriatic Arthritis study: defining the clinical and radiographic phenotype of psoriatic spondyloarthritis. Ann Rheum Dis. 2016; 76(4):701–7.
26. FitzGerald O, Haroon M, Giles JT, Winchester R. Concepts of pathogenesis in psoriatic arthritis: genotype determines clinical phenotype. Arthritis Res Ther. 2015;17(1):115.
27. Haroon M, Winchester R, Giles JT, Heffernan E, FitzGerald O. Certain class I HLA alleles and haplotypes implicated in susceptibility play a role in determining specific features of the psoriatic arthritis phenotype. Ann Rheum Dis. 2016;75(1):155–62.
28. Chandran V, Tolusso DC, Cook RJ, Gladman DD. Risk factors for axial inflammatory arthritis in patients with psoriatic arthritis. J Rheumatol. 2010; 37(4):809–15.
29. Haroon M, Winchester R, Giles JT, Heffernan E, FitzGerald O. Clinical and genetic associations of radiographic sacroiliitis and its different patterns in psoriatic arthritis. Clin Exp Rheumatol. 2017;35(2):270–6.
30. Queiro R, Alperi M, Lopez A, Sarasque-Ta C, JI R, Ballina J. Clinical expression, but not disease outcome, may vary according to age at disease onset in psoriatic spondylitis. Joint Bone Spine. 2008;75(5):544–7.
31. Gladman DD. Natural history of psoriatic arthritis. Baillieres Clin Rheumatol. 1994;8(2):379–94.
32. Queiro R, Belzunegui J, González C, De DJSC, Torre JC, et al. Clinically asymptomatic axial disease in psoriatic spondyloarthropathy. A retrospective study. Clin Rheumatol. 2002;21(1):10–3.

Efficacy and safety of secukinumab administration by autoinjector in patients with psoriatic arthritis: results from a randomized, placebo-controlled trial (FUTURE 3)

Peter Nash[1*], Philip J. Mease[2], Iain B. McInnes[3], Proton Rahman[4], Christopher T. Ritchlin[5], Ricardo Blanco[6], Eva Dokoupilova[7], Mats Andersson[8], Radhika Kajekar[9], Shephard Mpofu[8], Luminita Pricop[9] and on behalf of the FUTURE 3 study group

Abstract

Background: The study aimed to assess 52-week efficacy and safety of secukinumab self-administration by autoinjector in patients with active psoriatic arthritis (PsA) in the FUTURE 3 study (ClinicalTrials.gov NCT01989468).

Methods: Patients (≥ 18 years of age; $N = 414$) with active PsA were randomized 1:1:1 to subcutaneous (s.c.) secukinumab 300 mg, 150 mg, or placebo at baseline, weeks 1, 2, 3, and 4, and every 4 weeks thereafter. Per clinical response, placebo-treated patients were re-randomized to s.c. secukinumab 300 or 150 mg at week 16 (nonresponders) or week 24 (responders) and stratified at randomization by prior anti-tumor necrosis factor (TNF) therapy (anti-TNF-naïve, 68. 1%; intolerant/inadequate response (anti-TNF-IR), 31.9%). The primary endpoint was the proportion of patients achieving at least 20% improvement in American College of Rheumatology response criteria (ACR20) at week 24. Autoinjector usability was evaluated by Self-Injection Assessment Questionnaire (SIAQ).

Results: Overall, 92.1% (300 mg), 91.3% (150 mg), and 93.4% (placebo) of patients completed 24 weeks, and 84.9% (300 mg) and 79.7% (150 mg) completed 52 weeks. In the overall population (combined anti-TNF-naïve and anti-TNF-IR), ACR20 response rate at week 24 was significantly higher in secukinumab groups (300 mg, 48.2% ($p < 0.0001$); 150 mg, 42% ($p < 0.0001$); placebo, 16.1%) and was sustained through 52 weeks. SIAQ results showed that more than 93% of patients were satisfied/very satisfied with autoinjector usage. Secukinumab was well tolerated with no new or unexpected safety signals reported.

Conclusions: Secukinumab provided sustained improvements in signs and symptoms in active PsA patients through 52 weeks. High acceptability of autoinjector was observed. The safety profile was consistent with that reported previously.

Keywords: Psoriatic arthritis, Secukinumab, Autoinjector, Interleukin-17a, FUTURE 3 study

* Correspondence: drpnash@tpg.com.au
[1]Department of Medicine, University of Queensland, Brisbane, Australia
Full list of author information is available at the end of the article

Background

Psoriatic arthritis (PsA) is an immune-mediated chronic inflammatory disease that affects peripheral and axial joints, entheses, and skin and is associated with impaired physical function and poor quality of life [1–3].

Nonsteroidal anti-inflammatory drugs (NSAIDs) and nonbiologic disease-modifying anti-rheumatic drugs (DMARDs) are used as first-line therapy for PsA; however, these often only partially control disease symptoms [4].

Introduction of tumor necrosis factor (TNF)-blocking therapy improved the treatment of patients with PsA [5–7]. However, relapse or loss of response to anti-TNF therapy and adverse events (AEs) are common, highlighting an unmet clinical need for improved disease control [8, 9].

The interleukin-17A (IL-17A) pathway is proposed to play a key role in the pathogenesis of PsA [10].

Secukinumab, a fully human monoclonal antibody that selectively neutralizes IL-17A, has shown significant efficacy in the treatment of moderate to severe psoriasis and PsA, with a rapid onset of action, sustained responses, and a favorable safety profile [6, 11–14].

Placebo-controlled, double-blind, phase III trials with secukinumab (FUTURE 1 and FUTURE 2) have reported significant improvements in key clinical domains of PsA sustained through week 104 in FUTURE 2 and week 156 in FUTURE 1 [6, 15–19].

Here we report the primary efficacy and safety results over a 52-week period from the FUTURE 3 study (ClinicalTrials.gov NCT01989468), which involves subcutaneous (s.c.) self-administration of secukinumab via autoinjector in patients with active PsA.

Methods

Patients

Patients included were ≥ 18 years of age, meeting the ClASsification criteria for Psoriatic ARthritis (CASPAR) and having active disease, defined as at least three tender joints out of 78 and at least three swollen joints out of 76, despite previous treatment with NSAIDs, DMARDS, or anti-TNF agents. Patients treated with up to three anti-TNF agents could enroll if they had an inadequate response for at least 3 months or had stopped anti-TNF therapy due to safety/tolerability reasons (anti-TNF-IR), and had an appropriate washout period before randomization.

Concomitant use of oral corticosteroids (≤ 10 mg/day prednisone or equivalent) and methotrexate (MTX; ≤ 25 mg/week) was allowed if the dose was stable for at least 2 weeks and 4 weeks before randomization, respectively.

The exclusion criteria were: previous use of any biological agent other than anti-TNF agents or the use of > 3 anti-TNF agents; active inflammatory diseases other than PsA; active infection in the 2 weeks before randomization, or a history of ongoing, chronic, or recurrent infections, or evidence of tuberculosis infection; history of malignant disease within the past 5 years (excluding basal cell carcinoma or actinic keratosis, in-situ cervical cancer, or noninvasive malignant colon polyps); and pregnancy.

Study design

FUTURE 3 is an ongoing, multicenter, randomized, double-blind, double-dummy, placebo-controlled, parallel-group, 3-year study assessing the use of s.c. secukinumab self-administration with an autoinjector in patients with active PsA.

The study is being conducted at 74 centers across Australia, Bulgaria, Canada, Czech Republic, Germany, Italy, the Netherlands, Russia, Spain, Switzerland, the United Kingdom, and the USA. Following a 10-week screening period, eligible patients were randomized (1:1:1) by means of an interactive response technology (IRT) to one of two secukinumab dose groups (secukinumab 300 mg or 150 mg) or placebo.

Patients in the secukinumab groups received s.c. secukinumab at a dose of 300 mg (2 × 1.0 ml autoinjector) or 150 mg (1.0 ml autoinjector + 1.0 ml placebo autoinjector) at baseline, weeks 1, 2, 3, and 4, and every 4 weeks thereafter. Patients in the placebo group (2 × 1.0 ml placebo autoinjector) were treated according to the same administration schedule as the active drug.

Patients were stratified at randomization based on previous anti-TNF therapy use as anti-TNF-naïve or anti-TNF-IR; at least 60% of patients in each treatment arm (secukinumab 300 mg, secukinumab 150 mg, and placebo) were anti-TNF-naïve.

At week 16, patients were classified either as responders (≥ 20% improvement from baseline in both tender joint count (TJC) and swollen joint count (SJC)) or nonresponders. Placebo patients were re-randomized to receive secukinumab 300 or 150 mg s.c. every 4 weeks at week 16 (nonresponders) or week 24 (responders; Additional file 1: Figure S1).

The study was conducted in accordance with the principles of the Declaration of Helsinki. All centers received approval from independent ethics committees (IECs) or institutional review boards (IRBs). The names of IECs or IRBs that approved the study and the associated approval numbers where applicable are presented in Additional file 1: Table S1. Patients provided written informed consent before starting the study-related procedures.

Outcomes

The primary efficacy endpoint was the proportion of patients achieving an American College of Rheumatology response criterion 20 (ACR20) response at week 24. Secondary endpoints assessed as part of a predefined hierarchical hypothesis-testing strategy at week 24 included: proportion of patients with an ACR50 response; change from baseline in 28-joint Disease Activity Score based on C-reactive protein (DAS28-CRP); proportion of patients achieving Psoriasis Area Severity Index (PASI) 75 response in patients with psoriasis affecting ≥ 3% of body surface area; change from baseline in score of the Short Form-36 Physical Component Summary (SF-36 PCS); PASI 90 response; change from baseline in Health Assessment Questionnaire—Disability Index (HAQ-DI) score; and resolution of dactylitis and enthesitis.

Exploratory endpoints were: Functional Assessment of Chronic Illness Therapy—Fatigue (FACIT-Fatigue); change from baseline in patient's assessment of PsA pain (visual analog scale (VAS)); assessments of all primary and secondary endpoints up to week 52; and subgroup analyses according to previous anti-TNF use (ACR20/50 and DAS28-CRP assessments) and concomitant MTX use (ACR20/50 assessments).

Autoinjector usability was assessed based on investigator/site staff rating scores of successful, hazard-free self-injection and patient rating of autoinjector acceptability. The Self-Injection Assessment Questionnaire (SIAQ) was used to evaluate patients' perceptions before and after self-injection [20]. The SIAQ PRE module was completed by patients before the first self-injection during the baseline visit and assessed three domains (feelings about injections (FL), self-confidence (CO), and satisfaction with self-injection (SA)). The POST module included four domains (FL, CO, pain and skin reactions, and SA) at baseline and weeks 1 and 2.

Safety assessments included evaluation of all AEs and serious AEs (SAEs), together with electrocardiograms, physical examination, vital signs and laboratory assessments, and assessment of anti-secukinumab antibody development (immunogenicity).

Statistical analysis

A sample size of 135 patients per group was estimated to provide about 98% power to detect a treatment difference for the primary endpoint of ACR20 response at week 24 assuming a placebo response of 21% and a secukinumab response of 47% based on Fisher's exact test. Evaluations of efficacy were performed on the full analysis set (FAS), which comprised all randomized patients to whom treatment had been assigned. Closed testing procedures were used to maintain a family-wise error rate of 5% across the secukinumab groups and endpoints (details presented in Additional file 1).

Primary and other binary endpoints were evaluated by means of logistic regression, with treatment and anti-TNF response status as factors and weight as a covariate. Baseline PASI score was a covariate in PASI 75 and PASI 90 analyses. Missing values, including those due to discontinuation of study treatment, were imputed as failures to achieve the given response (nonresponses). Also, patients who did not achieve response based on joint count at week 16 were imputed as nonresponders at week 20 and week 24 (rescue penalty).

Between-group differences in continuous variables were evaluated with the use of a mixed-model repeated-measures (MMRM) approach, with missing data assumed to be missing at random, with treatment, assessment visit, and anti-TNF response status as factors. Weight and baseline values of endpoints were included in the model as continuous covariates, and treatment by analysis visit and baseline score by analysis visit as interaction terms. PASI 75/90 scores were also analyzed using a modified rescue penalty (Additional file 1). Subgroup analyses were carried out on the basis of previous anti-TNF therapy or concomitant MTX treatment.

SIAQ domain scores ranging from 0 to 10 were calculated to assess self-injection experience, with higher scores indicating a better experience for a patient. The percentage of patients who successfully completed self-injection per the instructions for use (IFU) was reported for the overall population at week 1 and SIAQ domain scores were provided by visit.

Safety endpoints were evaluated in the safety set, which included all patients who received at least one dose of the study drug; these endpoints were summarized descriptively. Safety results are presented for the placebo-controlled period and the entire safety-reporting period, which included all safety data up to the cutoff date of the last patient's week 52 visit.

Results

Patients

Overall, 414 patients with active PsA were enrolled in FUTURE 3. At baseline, demographic and disease characteristics were generally balanced across the treatment groups (Table 1). The mean time since the first diagnosis of PsA ranged from 6.6 to 8.3 years. Approximately two-thirds of the patients were anti-TNF-naïve (68.1%) and one-third (31.9%) were anti-TNF-IR, with patients in both subgroups evenly distributed across treatment groups; 53.8% of anti-TNF-IR patients were exposed to ≥ 2 anti-TNF agents. About half (47.6%) of the patients were using MTX at baseline (50.4%, secukinumab 300 mg; 42.8%, secukinumab 150 mg; 49.6%, placebo; Table 1). Of the 414 patients, 128/139 patients (92.1%, secukinumab 300 mg), 126/138 patients (91.3%, secukinumab 150 mg), and 128/137 patients (93.4%, placebo) completed 24 weeks and 337/414 patients (81.4%) completed 52 weeks (Fig. 1). The most common reasons for

Table 1 Demographic and baseline characteristics of patients

Characteristic	Secukinumab 300 mg (*N* = 139)	Secukinumab 150 mg (*N* = 138)	Placebo (*N* = 137)
Age (years), mean (SD)	49.3 (12.9)	50.1 (11.7)	50.1 (12.6)
Male, *n* (%)	67 (48.2)	61 (44.2)	59 (43.1)
Race, *n* (%)			
White	130 (93.5)	129 (93.5)	133 (97.1)
American Indian or Alaska Native	0	2 (1.4)	0
Asian	3 (2.2)	2 (1.4)	4 (2.9)
Other	6 (4.3)	5 (3.6)	0
Weight (kg), mean (SD)	87.1 (19.4)	87.1 (20.0)	82.6 (18.5)
Number of previous anti-TNF treatments for PsA, *n* (%)			
0	95 (68.3)	94 (68.1)	93 (67.9)
1	19 (13.7)	22 (15.9)	20 (14.6)
≥ 2	25 (18.0)	22 (15.9)	24 (17.5)
Time since diagnosis of PsA (years), mean (SD)	8.3 (9.2)	7.7 (8.5)	6.6 (6.9)
MTX use at randomization, *n* (%)	70 (50.4)	59 (42.8)	68 (49.6)
Systemic glucocorticoid use at randomization, *n* (%)	23 (16.5)	24 (17.4)	32 (23.4)
Anti-TNF-naïve, *n* (%)	95 (68.3)	94 (68.1)	93 (67.9)
Patients with specific disease characteristics, *n* (%)			
Psoriasis ≥ 3% of BSA	62 (44.6)	68 (49.3)	59 (43.1)
Presence of dactylitis	46 (33.1)	36 (26.1)	36 (26.3)
Presence of enthesitis	88 (63.3)	95 (68.8)	98 (71.5)
Disease and quality-of-life scores, mean (SD)			
TJC (78 joints)	19.7 (14.8)	23.3 (18.1)	21.9 (16.2)
SJC (76 joints)	8.9 (6.4)	11.2 (9.2)	10.3 (8.6)
DAS28-CRP	4.5 (1.0)	4.6 (1.1)	4.7 (1.1)
PASI[a]	10.1 (8.6)	8.8 (6.4)	10.4 (9.0)
Physician's global assessment (VAS)	51.8 (19.7)	55.2 (16.7)	54.8 (18.1)
HAQ-DI	1.1 (0.7)	1.2 (0.6)	1.2 (0.6)
PsA pain (VAS)	54.8 (23.8)	54.4 (21.4)	53.3 (23.8)
Patient's global assessment (VAS)	59.9 (20.8)	59.8 (22.1)	60.6 (20.9)
SF-36 PCS	39.2 (8.4)	37.9 (7.6)	37.4 (8.5)

BSA body surface area, *DAS28-CRP* 28-joint Disease Activity Score using C-reactive protein, *HAQ-DI* Health Assessment Questionnaire—Disability Index, *MTX* methotrexate, N number of randomized patients, *PASI* Psoriasis Area and Severity Index, *PsA* psoriatic arthritis, *SD* standard deviation, *SF-36 PCS* Short Form-36 Physical Component Summary, *SJC* swollen joint count, *TJC* tender joint count, *TNF* tumor necrosis factor, *VAS* visual analog scale

[a]Assessed in patients with psoriasis on at least 3% of their BSA

discontinuation by 52 weeks were lack of efficacy (5.0%, secukinumab 300 mg; 7.2%, secukinumab 150 mg) and AEs (5.8%, secukinumab 300 mg; 4.3%, secukinumab 150 mg). The most common reason for discontinuation in the initial placebo nonresponder group was lack of efficacy (4.5%, patients re-randomized to secukinumab 300 mg; 11.6%, patients re-randomized to secukinumab 150 mg).

Efficacy

The primary endpoint was met, demonstrating efficacy of secukinumab (150 mg and 300 mg) versus placebo in the ACR20 response at week 24. ACR20 response rates using the conservative estimate of efficacy with missing values imputed as nonresponse were significantly higher in the secukinumab 300 mg (48.2%; $p < 0.0001$) and 150 mg (42.0%; $p < 0.0001$) groups versus placebo (16.1%; Fig. 2). Similarly, ACR50 response rates at week 24 were also significantly higher in the secukinumab 300 mg (34.5%; $p < 0.0001$) and 150 mg (18.8%; $p < 0.05$) groups versus placebo (8.8%; Fig. 3).

ACR20/50 response rates were higher with secukinumab than with placebo in both the anti-TNF-naïve and anti-TNF-IR patients, with response generally being

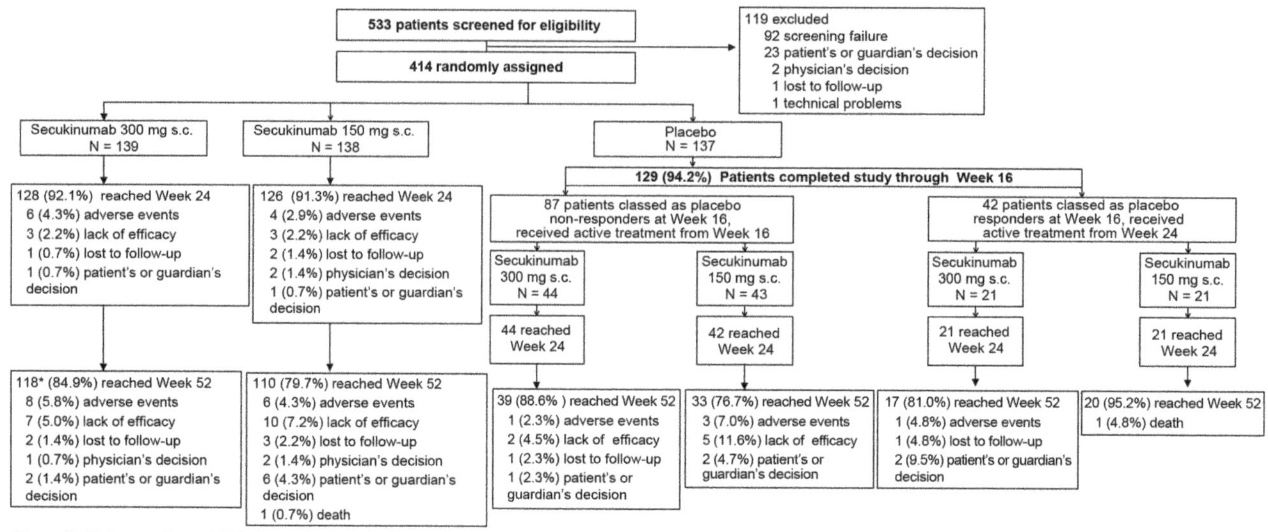

*One patient in the secukinumab 300mg group is categorized as ongoing s.c., subcutaneous

Fig. 1 Patient disposition up to week 52

higher in the anti-TNF-naïve population (Figs. 2 (ACR20) and 3 (ACR50)). At week 24, in anti-TNF-naïve patients the ACR20/50 response rates were 51.6%/41.1% (secukinumab 300 mg), 45.7%/24.5% (secukinumab 150 mg), and 19.4%/11.8% (placebo). In the anti-TNF-IR patients, the ACR20/50 response rates were 40.9%/20.5% in secukinumab 300 mg and 34.1%/6.8% in secukinumab 150 mg versus 9.1%/2.3% in the placebo group (Figs. 2 and 3).

ACR20/50 responses were sustained at week 52 in the overall population (58.3%/33.1% in secukinumab 300 mg group and 47.1%/27.5% in secukinumab 150 mg group). Response rates were also maintained in patients stratified by anti-TNF status through 52 weeks of treatment (Figs. 2 and 3).

Secondary endpoints were assessed in a hierarchical order. At week 24, statistical significance versus placebo was achieved for all secondary endpoints in the secukinumab 300 mg group. In the secukinumab 150 mg group, statistical significance was achieved for DAS28-CRP and PASI 75 scores. Clinical responses at week 24 across secondary endpoints with secukinumab 300 mg and 150 mg were sustained through 52 weeks of treatment (Table 2).

Analysis of PASI 75/90 scores at week 24 using the modified rescue penalty (Additional file 1) resulted in 61.3%/41.9% and 55.9%/39.7% responses with secukinumab 300 and 150 mg, respectively, versus 11.9%/8.5% for placebo ($p < 0.001$).

In anti-TNF-naïve patients, mean change from baseline in the DAS28-CRP score at week 24 was −1.64 ± 0.10 ($p < 0.0001$) and −1.33 ± 0.10 ($p < 0.01$) in the secukinumab 300 and 150 mg groups, respectively, as compared with −0.78 ± 0.14 in the placebo group. In anti-TNF-IR patients, mean change from baseline in DAS28-CRP score was −1.43 ± 0.20 ($p < 0.01$) and −1.06 ± 0.19 ($p > 0.05$) in the secukinumab 300 and 150 mg groups, respectively, as compared with −0.49 ± 0.26 in the placebo group. The mean change from baseline in DAS28-CRP score observed with secukinumab at week 24 was sustained through week 52 regardless of anti-TNF status (anti-TNF-naïve, −1.68 ± 0.10 (secukinumab 300 mg) and −1.44 ± 0.11 (secukinumab 150 mg); anti-TNF-IR, −1.56 ± 0.21 (secukinumab 300 mg) and −1.47 ± 0.21 (secukinumab 150 mg)).

At week 24, ACR20/50 response rates were higher with secukinumab than with placebo in patients with and without concomitant MTX use, and the responses were maintained through 52 weeks of treatment (Additional file 1).

At week 24, mean change from baseline in patient's assessment of PsA pain (VAS) was higher in both the secukinumab 300 and 150 mg groups versus placebo and mean change from baseline in FACIT-Fatigue was higher only in the secukinumab 300 mg group. The changes observed at week 24 in both exploratory endpoints were sustained through 52 weeks of treatment (Table 2).

Observed data at weeks 24 and 52 for the primary, secondary, and exploratory endpoints are presented in Additional file 1: Table S2.

Autoinjector usability and satisfaction assessment

More than 99% of patients in the overall population successfully self-administrated the study drug at week 1. The most common hazard was needle stick in a

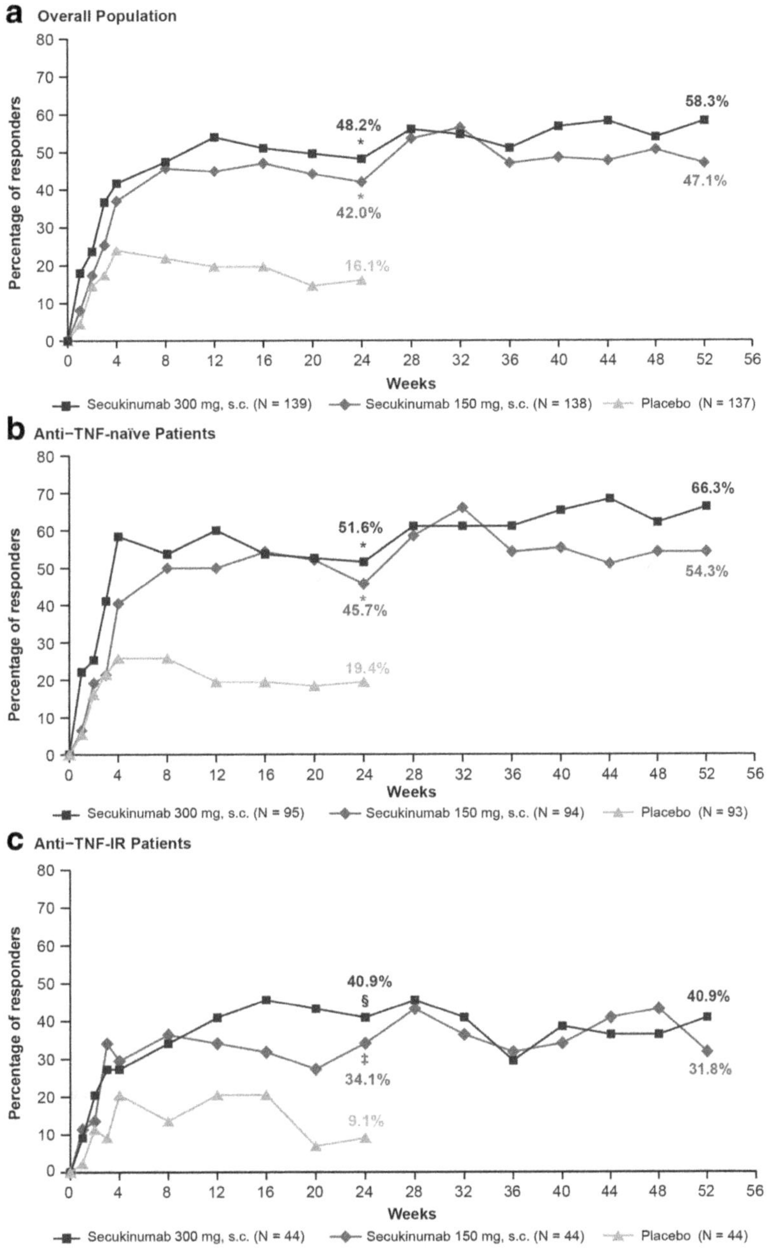

Fig. 2 ACR20 response rates through week 52 in the overall population (**a**) and by anti-TNF status (**b, c**). $^{*}p < 0.0001$, $^{§}p < 0.01$, $^{‡}p < 0.05$ versus placebo. p values adjusted for multiplicity of testing for overall population at week 24. Missing values imputed as nonresponse (nonresponder imputation) through week 52. ACR20 20% improvement in American College of Rheumatology response criteria, IR inadequate response, s.c. subcutaneous, TNF tumor necrosis factor

noncritical area, observed in nine patients overall at randomization and week 1. The scores of FL, CO, and SA were high pre self-injection (FL = 8.22, CO = 6.52, and SA = 6.80) and remained high at week 2 (FL = 8.81, CO = 7.84, and SA = 8.39) in all patients. Patient-reported scores of the three domains by visit and treatment are shown in Additional file 1: Table S3. More than 90% of total patients reported no pain and reaction during or after the injection, and ≥ 88% of patients were either satisfied or very satisfied with the use of the autoinjector devise and found the usage of an autoinjector easy or very easy, with no external help required, as assessed by SIAQ at week 2.

Safety

The incidence of AEs during the placebo-controlled period was similar across the study groups, with a slightly higher number of SAEs reported in the placebo

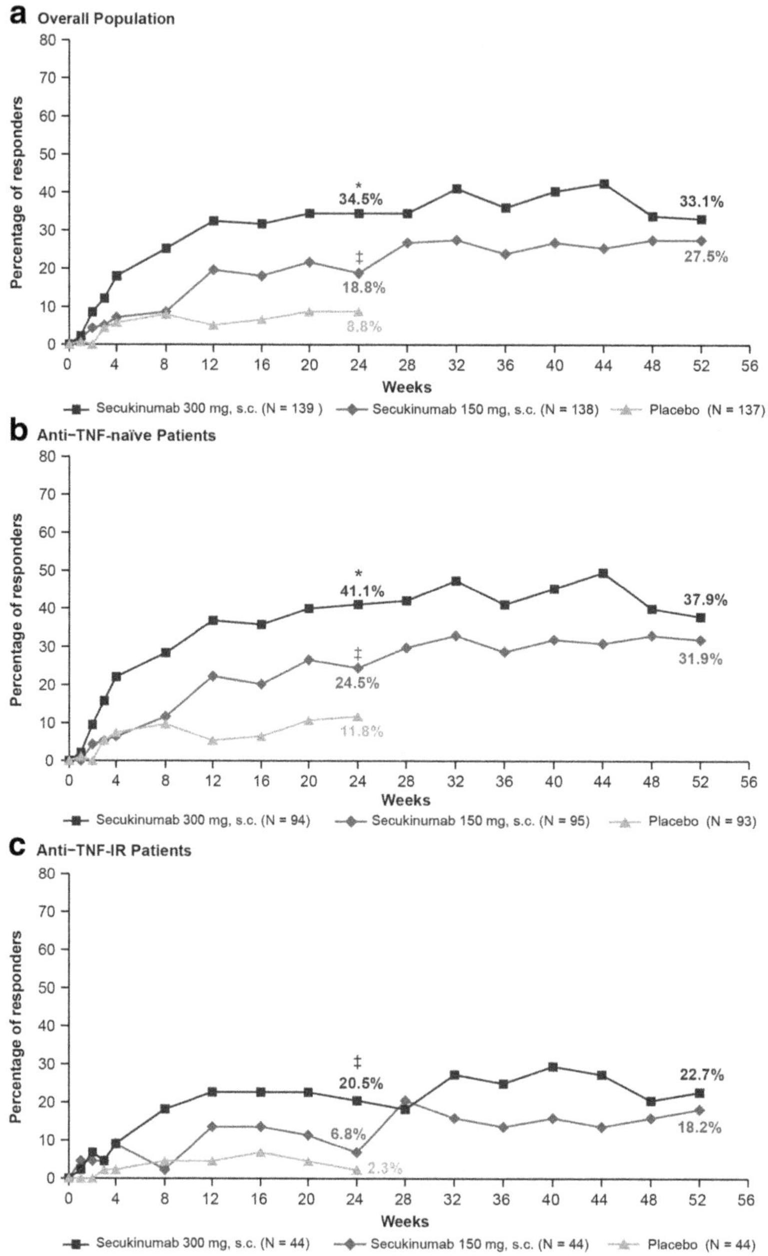

Fig. 3 ACR50 response rates through week 52 in the overall population (**a**) and by anti-TNF status (**b, c**). *$p < 0.0001$, ‡$p < 0.05$ versus placebo. p values adjusted for multiplicity of testing for overall population at week 24. Missing values imputed as nonresponse (nonresponder imputation) through week 52. ACR50 50% improvement in American College of Rheumatology response criteria, IR inadequate response, s.c. subcutaneous, TNF tumor necrosis factor

group (Table 3). Treatment-emergent AEs were reported in 54.7%, 58.0%, and 56.2% of patients receiving secukinumab 300 mg, secukinumab 150 mg, and placebo, respectively. There were no deaths reported during the placebo-controlled 16-week period. Over the entire treatment period (mean ± SD exposure, secukinumab 398.1 ± 112.1 days and placebo 130.7 ± 29.8 days), exposure-adjusted incidence rates (EAIRs) of AEs among patients receiving secukinumab 300 and 150 mg were 194.9 and 192.5 per 100 patient-years, respectively; the corresponding values for SAEs were 8.8 and 10.2 per 100 patient-years, respectively (Table 3). The most frequent SAEs included infections and infestations and musculoskeletal and connective tissue disorders with an EAIR of 1.8 and 2.1, respectively. Details of SAEs through the entire safety period are presented in Additional file 1: Table S4. Two deaths were reported in the secukinumab 150 mg group during the entire 52-week analysis period: one pancreatic carcinoma and one small cell lung cancer (additional details

Table 2 Efficacy of secukinumab at weeks 24 and 52 in the overall population[a]

Endpoint	Week	Secukinumab 300 mg (*N* = 139)	Secukinumab 150 mg (*N* = 138)	Placebo (*N* = 137)
ACR20 response, *n/N* (%)	24	67/139 (48.2)*	58/138 (42.0)*	22/137 (16.1)
	52	81/139 (58.3)	65/138 (47.1)	–
ACR50 response, *n/N* (%)	24	48/139 (34.5)*	26/138 (18.8)‡	12/137 (8.8)
	52	46/139 (33.1)	38/138 (27.5)	–
DAS28-CRP, mean change from baseline ± SE	24	−1.56 ± 0.09*	−1.24 ± 0.1‡	−0.64 ± 0.13
	52	−1.61 ± 0.09	−1.41 ± 0.10	–
PASI 75 response, *n/N* (%)[b]	24	29/62 (46.8)*	34/68 (50.0)‡	6/59 (10.2)
	52	46/62 (74.2)	41/68 (60.3)	–
SF-36 PCS, mean change from baseline ± SE	24	6.46 ± 0.59§	3.42 ± 0.60	2.94 ± 0.83
	52	6.43 ± 0.66	4.49 ± 0.68	–
PASI 90 response, *n/N* (%)[b]	24	21/62 (33.9)§	25/68 (36.8)	4/59 (6.8)
	52	34/62 (54.8)	28/68 (41.2)	–
HAQ-DI score, mean change from baseline ± SE	24	− 0.38 ± 0.04§	− 0.27 ± 0.04	−0.17 ± 0.06
	52	−0.43 ± 0.05	−0.30 ± 0.05	–
Patients with resolution of dactylitis, *n/N* (%)[c]	24	22/46 (47.8)§	14/36 (38.9)	5/36 (13.9)
	52	28/46 (60.9)	19/36 (52.8)	–
Patients with resolution of enthesitis, *n/N* (%)[c]	24	35/88 (39.8)§	35/95 (36.8)	15/98 (15.3)
	52	47/88 (53.4)	44/95 (46.3)	–
Patient's assessment of PsA pain (VAS), mean change from baseline ± SE	24	−18.23 ± 1.97*	−12.46 ± 2.0‡	−3.75 ± 2.81
	52	−20.3 ± 2.1	−11.8 ± 2.2	–
FACIT-Fatigue, mean change from baseline ± SE	24	6.40 ± 0.78†	2.73 ± 0.80	2.07 ± 1.05
	52	6.72 ± 0.9	3.25 ± 0.9	–

Data presented as nonresponder imputation and rescue penalty (binary variables) and mixed-model repeated measures and rescue penalty (continuous variables)
ACR20/50 20%/50% improvement in American College of Rheumatology response criteria; *BSA* body surface area, *DAS28-CRP* 28-joint Disease Activity Score using C-reactive protein, *FACIT-Fatigue* Functional Assessment of Chronic Illness Therapy—Fatigue, *HAQ-DI* Health Assessment Questionnaire—Disability Index, N number of patients, *PASI* Psoriasis Area Severity Index, *PsA* psoriatic arthritis, *SE* standard error, *SF-36 PCS* Short Form-36 Physical Component Summary, *VAS* visual analog scale

*$p < 0.0001$, †$p < 0.001$, §$p < 0.01$, ‡$p < 0.05$ versus placebo. *p* values adjusted for multiplicity of testing for overall population data (except for pain and FACIT-Fatigue)

[a]Prespecified primary and secondary endpoints were analyzed according to a statistical hierarchy except for pain and FACIT-Fatigue. Endpoints are shown in the order of testing

[b]PASI 75 and PASI 90 denote improvements of 75% and 90%, respectively, in the score on the Psoriasis Area Severity Index. Assessed in patients with psoriasis on at least 3% of their BSA

[c]Resolution of dactylitis and enthesitis among those patients with these symptoms at baseline: dactylitis, *N* = 46 (300 mg), 36 (150 mg), and 36 (placebo); enthesitis, *N* = 88 (300 mg), 95 (150 mg),and 98 (placebo)

regarding these patients are available in Additional file 1). Myocardial infarction was reported in one patient with a history of smoking and hyperlipidemia and who was a long-time NSAID user. Suicidal ideation was reported in two patients (one patient each in secukinumab 150 and 300 mg groups); both patients had a prior history of psychiatric disorders and were on related medications. *Candida* infections were reported for 14 patients in the secukinumab dose groups that included eight oral candidiasis (three patients in 300 mg group and five patients in 150 mg group) and four vulvovaginal candidiasis (two patients each in secukinumab 300 mg and secukinumab 150 mg groups). These *candida* infections were diagnosed as nonserious, mild, or moderate in severity by the investigators and did not lead to study withdrawal.

Malignant or unspecified tumors (excluding basal cell and squamous cell carcinomas) were reported in three patients each in the secukinumab 300 mg and 150 mg groups. One patient in the 300 mg group reported inflammatory bowel disease (moderate). Neutropenia was reported in three patients: one patient in the 300 mg group and two patients in the 150 mg group. This included Grade 3 leukopenia (one patient each in the 300 and 150 mg groups) and Grade 3 neutropenia (one patient in 150 mg group). Injection-site reactions were reported by six patients in the secukinumab 300 mg and seven patients in the secukinumab 150 mg group. Treatment-emergent anti-secukinumab antibodies (positive during study but negative at baseline) were detected in four patients, while neutralizing antibodies were not detected in any patients.

Table 3 Safety profile during the placebo-controlled period and the entire safety-reporting period

Variable	Through week 16 (placebo-controlled period)			Entire safety-data period		
	Secukinumab 300 mg (*N* = 139)	Secukinumab 150 mg (*N* = 138)	Placebo (*N* = 137)	Any secukinumab 300 mg (*N* = 204)	Any secukinumab 150 mg (*N* = 202)	Any secukinumab (*N* = 406)
Exposure to study treatment (days), mean ± SD				403.8 ± 108.3	392.3 ± 115.8	398.1 ± 112.1
Any AE	76 (54.7)	80 (58.0)	77 (56.2)	164 (194.9)	156 (192.5)	320 (193.7)
Any serious AE	3 (2.2)	5 (3.6)	9 (6.6)	19 (8.8)	21 (10.2)	40 (9.5)
Discontinued due to AEs[a]	3 (2.2)	5 (3.6)	5 (3.6)	9 (4.4)	13 (6.4)	22 (5.4)
Death[b]	0	0	0	0	2 (1.0)	2 (0.5)
Common AEs[c]						
Nasopharyngitis	13 (9.4)	11 (8.0)	13 (9.5)	47 (25.0)	30 (15.5)	77 (20.2)
Upper respiratory tract infection	7 (5.0)	6 (4.3)	5 (3.6)	23 (10.9)	19 (9.3)	42 (10.1)
Diarrhea	4 (2.9)	7 (5.1)	2 (1.5)	16 (7.5)	15 (7.2)	31 (7.4)
Back pain	5 (3.6)	4 (2.9)	1 (0.7)	16 (7.5)	12 (5.7)	28 (6.6)
Headache	6 (4.3)	9 (6.5)	6 (4.4)	11 (5.1)	15 (7.3)	26 (6.1)
Arthralgia	4 (2.9)	1 (0.7)	1 (0.7)	12 (5.5)	13 (6.3)	25 (5.9)
Bronchitis	3 (2.2)	2 (1.4)	5 (3.6)	15 (6.9)	9 (4.3)	24 (5.6)
Fatigue	5 (3.6)	4 (2.9)	2 (1.5)	7 (3.2)	15 (7.3)	22 (5.2)
Urinary tract infection	6 (4.3)	3 (2.2)	2 (1.5)	13 (6.0)	9 (4.2)	22 (5.1)
AEs of special interest						
Myocardial infarction	0	0	0	0	1 (0.5)	1 (0.2)
Neutropenia	0	0	0	1 (0.4)	2 (0.9)	3 (0.7)
Candida infection	0	2 (1.4)	2 (1.5)	6 (2.7)	8 (3.8)	14 (3.2)
IBD	0	0	1 (0.7)	1 (0.4)	0	1 (0.2)

Data are number (%) or number (incidence per 100 patient-years). In the analysis of the entire study period, the secukinumab groups include any patients who received the stated dose of secukinumab, including those who were randomly assigned to the placebo group at baseline and who underwent a second randomization to active treatment at week 16/24

AE adverse event, *IBD* inflammatory bowel disease, N number of patients, *SD* standard deviation

[a]Exposure-adjusted incidence rates were not calculated for discontinuations because of AEs and death

[b]Two deaths reported in the secukinumab 150 mg group: one due to pancreatic carcinoma and one due to small cell lung cancer on day 173 and day 227, respectively

[c]The most common AEs are reported as the preferred terms from the *Medical Dictionary for Regulatory Activities* and occurred at an incidence of at least 5 per 100 patient-years in the pooled secukinumab group during the entire treatment period

Discussion

In this phase III trial, self-administration of secukinumab using an autoinjector in patients with PsA improved the signs and symptoms, skin measures, and physical function through 52 weeks of treatment. The ACR20/50 response rates with both secukinumab doses (300 and 150 mg) at week 24 were significantly higher than with placebo and were sustained through week 52. At week 24, significant outcomes with secukinumab 300 and 150 mg versus placebo were also observed in other clinically relevant domains of PsA, which were sustained through week 52. Patients were imputed as nonresponders based on joint count for all of the binary variables. These nonresponders included patients who were responding to variables with no/low correlation to joint assessment (e.g., PASI 75/90) at week 16. To overcome this, PASI 75/90 responses were also analyzed using a modified, variable-specific rescue penalty. The modified rescue penalty showed notably higher response rates for PASI 75 and PASI 90 compared to the original method in both secukinumab groups, with a minimal increase in the placebo group.

Results of this study are in agreement with the findings of earlier studies, which also showed significant improvements in the signs and symptoms of PsA with secukinumab 300 and 150 mg [6, 16, 18, 21]. Responses with secukinumab 150 mg observed in the present study, however, were lower than the responses observed in previous studies, with no obvious explanation other than interstudy variation.

In the subgroup analysis by previous anti-TNF use, clinical responses were observed with secukinumab in both anti-TNF-naïve and anti-TNF-IR populations, with responses generally greater in the anti-TNF-naïve subgroup. Substantial evidence suggests that treatment with anti-TNF agents reduces disease activity in patients with

PsA [5–7]. However, some patients do not tolerate or respond well to these agents, and these refractory patients are commonly managed by switching from one anti-TNF to another. Glintborg et al. [22] reported that switching of anti-TNF agents in PsA patients was associated with decreasing ACR20 response rates from 47% with first-line anti-TNF therapy to 22% and 18% among patients switching to a second or third biologic, respectively. In this study, more than 50% of the patients in the anti-TNF-IR subgroup had received two or three anti-TNF agents and the ACR20 response rates at week 24 were 40.9% (secukinumab 300 mg) and 34.1% (secukinumab 150 mg). Higher responses observed with secukinumab 300 mg compared with 150 mg in patients previously exposed to anti-TNF agents are consistent with previous studies [6, 15, 16, 18] and provide additional supporting evidence that secukinumab 300 mg is an appropriate treatment option for this group of patients. Improvements with secukinumab through 52 weeks were similar in both concomitant MTX and without MTX subgroups.

This study showed the utility of the autoinjector device. More than 88% of patients were satisfied using the autoinjector and reported little or no pain at all. Moreover, the majority of the patients found usage of an autoinjector easy or very easy, with no external help required. These observations are in agreement with those recently reported for the secukinumab autoinjector in the psoriasis JUNCTURE trial [23].

The safety profile of secukinumab in this study was based on 398.1 patient-years of exposure to any secukinumab dose and showed no new or unexpected safety signals, and was consistent with earlier reports of secukinumab in PsA [16] and psoriasis [13]. The overall incidence of AEs up to week 16 was comparable between secukinumab dose groups and placebo. No dose dependence was observed for secukinumab. The majority of the AEs reported during the entire treatment period were nonserious and mild to moderate. All serious AEs in any secukinumab group for the entire treatment period were single events with no specific trends or clusters. The rate of discontinuations because of AEs with secukinumab was low, with two deaths reported during the study. *Candida* infections were reported more frequently with secukinumab (3.4%) than with placebo (1.5%); all were manageable with no treatment discontinuations. Since IL-17 plays a role in mucocutaneous defense against bacterial and fungal infections [24], continuous observation for *candida* infections is needed for these patients. Immunogenicity with secukinumab was low and was not associated with a loss of efficacy or with immunogenicity-related AEs.

This study has some limitations. This trial was not designed to identify a difference between doses. The long-term efficacy and safety of secukinumab compared to placebo could not be determined as patients on placebo had to be given rescue medication after a short period due to ethical consideration and study design, which was consistent with clinical trials of other biologic agents.

Conclusions

In summary, self-administration of subcutaneous secukinumab provided sustained improvements at 52 weeks across multiple clinical domains in patients with active PsA. Patients reported high levels of satisfaction with the autoinjector and considered it easy to use and not painful. The safety profile of secukinumab showed no new or unexpected safety signals during this time.

Abbreviations

ACR: American College of Rheumatology; AE: Adverse event; CASPAR: ClASsification criteria for Psoriatic ARthritis; CO: Self-confidence; DAS-28 CRP: 28-joint Disease Activity Score based on C-reactive protein; DMARD: Disease-modifying anti-rheumatic drug; FACIT: Functional Assessment of Chronic Illness Therapy; FAS: Full analysis set; FL: Feelings about injections; HAQ-DI: Health Assessment Questionnaire—Disability Index; IEC: Independent ethics committee; IFU: Instructions for use; IL: Interleukin; IRB: Institutional review board; IRT: Interactive response technology; MMRM: Mixed-model repeated-measures; MTX: Methotrexate; NSAID: Nonsteroidal anti-inflammatory drug; PASI: Psoriasis Area Severity Index; PsA: Psoriatic arthritis; s.c.: Subcutaneous; SA: Satisfaction with self-injection; SF-36 PCS: Short Form-36 Physical Component Summary; SIAQ: Self-Injection Assessment Questionnaire; SJC: Swollen joint count; TJC: Tender joint count; TNF: Tumor necrosis factor; TNF-IR: Tumor necrosis factor inhibitor inadequate responder; VAS: Visual analog scale

Acknowledgements

The authors thank the patients who participated in this study, the study investigators, and John Gallagher, medical consultant for Novartis Pharma AG, Basel, Switzerland. Manuscript writing support was provided by Santoshkumar Tota, Novartis Healthcare Pvt. Ltd, Hyderabad, India.

Funding

Novartis Pharma AG (Basel, Switzerland).

Authors' contributions

All authors had access to the data, contributed to its interpretation, and collaborated in the development of the manuscript. The initial draft of the manuscript was written by a medical writer employed by the study sponsor. All authors critically reviewed and provided feedback on subsequent versions. All authors made the decision to submit the manuscript for publication and vouch for the accuracy and completeness of the data and fidelity of this report to the study protocol. All authors read and approved the final manuscript.

Competing interests

PN has received research grants for clinical trials and honoraria for lectures and advice from Novartis, AbbVie, Roche, Pfizer, BMS, Janssen, and Celgene. PJM has received grant/research support from AbbVie, Amgen, BMS, Celgene, Crescendo Bioscience, Genentech, Janssen, Lilly, Merck, Novartis, Pfizer, and UCB; been a consultant for AbbVie, Amgen, BMS, Celgene, Crescendo Bioscience, Genentech, Janssen, Lilly, Merck, Novartis, Pfizer, and UCB; and on the speakers' bureau for AbbVie, Amgen, BMS, Celgene, Crescendo Bioscience, Genentech, Janssen, Lilly, Merck, Novartis, Pfizer, and UCB. IBM has received research grants, consultation fees, or speaker honoraria from AbbVie, Amgen, BMS, Celgene, Janssen, Lilly, Novartis, Pfizer, and UCB. PR has received consulting fees from Abbott, AbbVie, Amgen, BMS, Celgene, Janssen, Novartis, Pfizer and Roche; and been a consultant for pharmaceutical companies dealing with biologic agents in rheumatology. CTR has received research grants, consultation fees, or speaker honoraria from Amgen, UCB, AbbVie, Novartis, and Janssen. RB has received research grants from AbbVie, MSD, and Roche; consulting fees from AbbVie, Pfizer, Roche, Bristol-Myers, Janssen, and MSD; and was on the speakers' bureau for AbbVie, Pfizer, Roche, Bristol-Myers, Janssen, and MSD. ED has no competing interests. MA, RK, SM, and LP are employees of Novartis. RK, SM, and LP own Novartis stock.

Author details

[1]Department of Medicine, University of Queensland, Brisbane, Australia. [2]Swedish Medical Centre and University of Washington, Seattle, WA, USA. [3]University of Glasgow, Glasgow, UK. [4]Memorial University of Newfoundland, St. John's, NL, Canada. [5]Allergy/Immunology and Rheumatology Division, University of Rochester, Rochester, NY, USA. [6]Hospital Universitario Marqués de Valdecilla, IDIVAL, Santander, Spain. [7]Medical Plus, s.r.o., Uherské Hradiště, and University of Veterinary and Pharmaceutical Sciences, Faculty of Pharmacy, Brno, Czech Republic. [8]Novartis Pharma AG, Basel, Switzerland. [9]Novartis Pharmaceuticals Corporation, East Hanover, NJ, USA.

References

1. Gladman DD, Farewell VT, Pellett F, Schentag C, Rahman P. HLA is a candidate region for psoriatic arthritis. evidence for excessive HLA sharing in sibling pairs. Hum Immunol. 2003;64:887–9.
2. Rosen CF, Mussani F, Chandran V, Eder L, Thavaneswaran A, Gladman DD. Patients with psoriatic arthritis have worse quality of life than those with psoriasis alone. Rheumatology. 2012;51:571–6.
3. Raychaudhuri SK, Saxena A, Raychaudhuri SP. Role of IL-17 in the pathogenesis of psoriatic arthritis and axial spondyloarthritis. Clin Rheumatol. 2015;34:1019–23.
4. Gossec L, Smolen JS, Ramiro S, de Wit M, Cutolo M, Dougados M, et al. European League Against Rheumatism (EULAR) recommendations for the management of psoriatic arthritis with pharmacological therapies: 2015 update. Ann Rheum Dis. 2016;75:499–510.
5. Carneiro S, Azevedo VF, Bonfiglioli R, Ranza R, Goncalves CR, Keiserman M, et al. Recommendations for the management and treatment of psoriatic arthritis. Rev Bras Reumatol. 2013;53:227–41.
6. Mease PJ. Biologic therapy for psoriatic arthritis. Rheum Dis Clin N Am. 2015;41:723–38.
7. Saad AA, Ashcroft DM, Watson KD, Symmons DP, Noyce PR, Hyrich KL, et al. Efficacy and safety of anti-TNF therapies in psoriatic arthritis: an observational study from the British Society for Rheumatology Biologics Register. Rheumatology (Oxford). 2010;49:697–705.
8. Fagerli KM, Lie E, van der Heijde D, Heiberg MS, Kalstad S, Rodevand E, et al. Switching between TNF inhibitors in psoriatic arthritis: data from the NOR-DMARD study. Ann Rheum Dis. 2013;72:1840–4.
9. Golmia RP, Martins AH, Scheinberg M. When anti-TNF fails, anti-IL12-23 is an alternate option in psoriasis and psoriatic arthritis. Rev Bras Reumatol. 2014; 54:247–9.
10. Raychaudhuri SP, Raychaudhuri SK, Genovese MC. IL-17 receptor and its functional significance in psoriatic arthritis. Mol Cell Biochem. 2012;359:419–29.
11. Blauvelt A, Reich K, Tsai TF, Tyring S, Vanaclocha F, Kingo K, et al. Secukinumab is superior to ustekinumab in clearing skin of subjects with moderate-to-severe plaque psoriasis up to 1 year: results from the CLEAR study. J Am Acad Dermatol. 2017;76:60–9. e9
12. Hueber W, Patel DD, Dryja T, Wright AM, Koroleva I, Bruin G, et al. Effects of AIN457, a fully human antibody to interleukin-17A, on psoriasis, rheumatoid arthritis, and uveitis. Sci Transl Med. 2010;2:52ra72.
13. Langley RG, Elewski BE, Lebwohl M, Reich K, Griffiths CE, Papp K, et al. Secukinumab in plaque psoriasis—results of two phase 3 trials. N Engl J Med. 2014;371:326–38.
14. Thaci D, Blauvelt A, Reich K, Tsai TF, Vanaclocha F, Kingo K, et al. Secukinumab is superior to ustekinumab in clearing skin of subjects with moderate to severe plaque psoriasis: CLEAR, a randomized controlled trial. J Am Acad Dermatol. 2015;73:400–9.
15. Kavanaugh A, McInnes IB, Mease PJ, Hall S, Chinoy H, Kivitz AJ, et al. Efficacy of subcutaneous secukinumab in patients with active psoriatic arthritis stratified by prior tumor necrosis factor inhibitor use: results from the randomized placebo-controlled FUTURE 2 Study. J Rheumatol. 2016;43: 1713–7.
16. McInnes IB, Mease PJ, Kirkham B, Kavanaugh A, Ritchlin CT, Rahman P, et al. Secukinumab, a human anti-interleukin-17A monoclonal antibody, in patients with psoriatic arthritis (FUTURE 2): a randomized, double-blind, placebo-controlled, phase 3 trial. Lancet. 2015;386:1137–46.
17. Mease P, McInnes IB. Secukinumab: a new treatment option for psoriatic arthritis. Rheumatol Ther. 2016;3:5–29.
18. McInnes IB, Mease PJ, Ritchlin CT, Rahman P, Gottlieb AB, Kirkham B, Kajekar R, Delicha EM, Pricop L, Mpofu S. Secukinumab sustains improvement in signs and symptoms of psoriatic arthritis: 2 year results from the phase 3 FUTURE 2 study. Rheumatology (Oxford). 2017;56:1993–2003.
19. Mease PJ, Kavanaugh A, Reimold A, Tahir H, Rech J, Hall S, et al. Secukinumab provides sustained improvements in the signs and symptoms of active psoriatic arthritis through 3 years: efficacy and safety results from a phase 3 trial. Arthritis Rheumatol. 2016;68(10). http://acrabstracts.org/abstract/secukinumab-provides-sustained-improvements-in-the-signs-andsymptoms-of-active-psoriatic-arthritis-through-3-years-efficacy-and-safety-results-from-a-phase-3-trial/.
20. Keininger D, Coteur G. Assessment of self-injection experience in patients with rheumatoid arthritis: psychometric validation of the Self-Injection Assessment Questionnaire (SIAQ). Health Qual Life Outcomes. 2011;9:2.
21. Kavanaugh A, Mease PJ, Reimold AM, Tahir H, Rech J, Hall S, et al. Secukinumab for long-term treatment of psoriatic arthritis: 2-year follow-up from a phase 3, randomized, double-blind, placebo-controlled study. Arthritis Care Res (Hoboken). 2017;69:347–55.
22. Glintborg B, Ostergaard M, Krogh NS, Andersen MD, Tarp U, Loft AG, et al. Clinical response, drug survival, and predictors thereof among 548 patients with psoriatic arthritis who switched tumor necrosis factor alpha inhibitor therapy: results from the Danish Nationwide DANBIO Registry. Arthritis Rheum. 2013;65:1213–23.
23. Lacour JP, Paul C, Jazayeri S, Papanastasiou P, Xu C, Nyirady J, et al. Secukinumab administration by autoinjector maintains reduction of plaque psoriasis severity over 52 weeks: results of the randomized controlled JUNCTURE trial. J Eur Acad Dermatol Venereol. 2017;31:847–56.
24. Gaffen SL, Hernandez-Santos N, Peterson AC. IL-17 signaling in host defense against Candida albicans. Immunol Res. 2011;50:181–7.

11

The association between sonographic enthesitis and radiographic damage in psoriatic arthritis

Ari Polachek[1], Richard Cook[2], Vinod Chandran[3,4,5], Dafna D. Gladman[6] and Lihi Eder[7*]

Abstract

Background: To examine the association between sonographic enthesitis and the severity of radiographic features of damage in the peripheral and axial joints in psoriatic arthritis (PsA).

Methods: A cross-sectional analysis was conducted in patients with PsA. The MAdrid Sonography Enthesitis Index (MASEI) scoring system was used to quantify the extent of sonographic entheseal abnormalities. Radiographic damage in the peripheral joints and spine was assessed by the modified Steinbrocker score (mSS), Modified New York Criteria for sacroiliitis, and the modified Stoke Ankylosing Spondylitis Spine Score (mSASSS). The association between MASEI and the extent of radiographic damage was assessed using negative binomial and logistic regression. The results were expressed in terms of the regression coefficient estimates and their exponentiated values (e^{β}) or odds ratios (OR), and 95% confidence intervals (CI).

Results: Two hundred and twenty three patients were analyzed; 58% were males, with mean ± SD age of 55.9 ± 12. 9 years and PsA duration of 16.7 ± 12.4 years. Regression analyses yielded an association between higher MASEI scores (10 units increase) and peripheral joint damage including mSS (e^{β} = 1.42, 95% CI: 1.15, 1.72), joint ankylosis (OR = 1.93, 95% CI: 1.37, 2.72), arthritis mutilans (OR = 1.77, 95% CI: 1.23, 2.54), and periostitis (OR = 1.41, 95% CI: 1.08, 1.84). Similarly, an association was found between higher MASEI scores and axial damage as measured by mSASSS (e^{β} = 2.18, 95% CI: 1.16, 4.09) and sacroiliitis (OR = 1.33, 95% CI: 1.03, 1.72).

Conclusions: The severity of sonographic enthesitis is a potential marker of radiographic peripheral and axial joint damage in PsA.

Keywords: Spondyloarthritis, Pathogenesis, Ultrasound, Steinbrocker, Sacroiliitis, Spondylitis

Background

Psoriatic arthritis (PsA) is an inflammatory musculoskeletal disease affecting up to a third of psoriasis patients [1, 2]. PsA can affect different locations including the synovial joint, bone, fat pad, bursa, adjacent tendons, and entheses [3]. Enthesitis is a unique feature of the spondyloarthritis (SpA) disease group in general, and of PsA in particular [4, 5]. Clinical enthesitis is a common finding occurring in a third of PsA patients [6, 7].

There are a few imaging modalities that can assist in enthesitis assessment apart from physical examination. Conventional radiography, which usually shows erosions at the enthesis and enthesophytes [8], is limited by its ability to detect mainly chronic irreversible bone damage rather than active inflammation. Another modality is magnetic resonance imaging (MRI) that can demonstrate both active lesions, as entheseal thickness, soft tissue edema, and adjacent bone marrow edema, as well as chronic lesions including erosions and enthesophytes [9]. However, in a recent study that evaluated whole-body MRI, enthesitis was found in only 18% of the patients with PsA and the ability to read images from some locations was technically limited [10]. Musculoskeletal ultrasound (US) assessment is inexpensive, readily available, relatively easy to perform and can evaluate a number of entheseal locations in a short period of time [11]. Several studies

* Correspondence: lihi.eder@wchospital.ca
[7]Department of Medicine, University of Toronto, Women's College Research Institute, Women's College Hospital, Room 6326, 76 Grenville Street, Toronto, ON M5S 1B2, Canada
Full list of author information is available at the end of the article

found higher sensitivity and specificity of US assessment of the entheses compared with clinical examination [12–15]. Therefore, US has emerged as the preferred modality to assess enthesitis.

The primacy of enthesitis in the pathogenesis of SpA and PsA is a matter of debate. According to the synovio-entheseal model, suggested by McGonagle et al. enthesitis is the initial site of musculoskeletal inflammation in SpA [16]. A few animal model studies support this hypothesis by reporting a link between mechanical stress, enthesitis, and the development of arthritis that is similar to PsA [17–19]. In addition, in a small study that followed 30 psoriasis patients for 3.5 years, the presence of sonographic features of thickness of the quadriceps tendon predicted the development of PsA [20]. However, overall there is limited information about the association between enthesitis and disease outcomes in patients with PsA. We hypothesized that since enthesitis play a role in the pathogenesis of PsA it may serve as a marker of more severe disease outcomes in PsA, alternatively, enthesitis may play a direct role in the development of joint damage in PsA.

Hence, the main objective of the present study was to examine the association between sonographic enthesitis and the severity of radiographic features of damage in the peripheral and axial joints in patients with PsA.

Methods

Setting and study population

A cross-sectional study of patients enrolled in the Toronto PsA cohort was conducted. The cohort consists of patients with PsA who are referred to the University of Toronto PsA clinic for the management of their PsA. The patients are enrolled in an ongoing prospective cohort study aimed at assessing prognostic factors in PsA. Each patient is assessed at 6–12-month intervals according to a standard protocol. For the present study, randomly available consecutive patients were recruited for a single ultrasound assessment. The recruitment was completed during two separated time periods: June 2011 to October 2012 (this group of patients participated in our previous study about enthesitis in PsA [21]) and January 2014 to December 2015. Patients were recruited independently of their clinical and radiographic information. All patients satisfied the Classification for Psoriatic Arthritis (CASPAR) criteria [22].

Information collected includes demographics, lifestyle habits including smoking, co-morbid conditions, medications, height, weight, counts of tender swollen and damaged joints, dactylitis, clinical enthesitis assessment according to the SPondyloArthritis Research Consortium Canada (SPARCC) index [22], psoriasis area and severity index (PASI) and the presence of psoriatic nail involvement. The study was approved by the University Health Network Research Ethics Board. All patients signed an informed consent form.

Ultrasound assessment of enthesitis

A single rheumatologist (LE), who has 7 years of experience in musculoskeletal US and assessment of sonographic enthesitis, performed all US scanning using a MyLab 70 XVG scanner (Esaote, Florence, Italy) equipped with a 6–18 MHz linear transducer (Esaote). Power Doppler settings were standardized with a Doppler frequency of 8.3–10 MHz (depending on body habitus), pulse repetition frequency of 750 Hz, and a wall filter of 2. The following entheseal sites that are part of the MAdrid Sonographic Enthesitis Index (MASEI) scoring system were scanned bilaterally: quadriceps tendon insertion to the patella, patellar tendon insertion to the patella, and tibial tuberosity, Achilles tendon and plantar fascia insertions into the calcaneus, and triceps tendon insertion to the olecranon process. Each tendon was scanned in both longitudinal and transverse planes, and the scan images were stored as short video files for later reading. Each examination took about 20 minutes. The patients were placed in a supine position to assess the patellar and quadriceps entheses. The knee was placed in 30° flexion to assess grayscale abnormalities and in full extension to assess vascularization. Then the patients were placed in a prone position with the feet over the end of the examination table for assessment of the Achilles tendon and plantar fascia entheses. The triceps tendon enthesis was assessed with the elbow flexed to 90° [23].

The MASEI was used to generate a global score (range, 0–136) that reflects the severity of entheseal abnormalities in each patient [24]. The enthesopathy US grayscale features of this index include: thickening and structural changes of the tendon insertion, calcific deposits at the tendon insertion, bony changes including erosions and enthesophyte formation as defined by de Miguel et al. [24]. The thickness of the enthesis was measured at the insertion of the deeper tendon margin into the bone in a longitudinal axis. Bursitis was defined as a well circumscribed, localized anechoic or hypoechoic area at the site of an anatomical bursa, which was compressible by the transducer. Vascularization was assessed by the power Doppler within 2 mm of the cortical bone insertion. The sonographic elementary lesions described above are illustrated in Fig. 1. The total MASEI score was further categorized into: (1) bone score, including calcific deposits, erosions and enthesophytes and (2) soft tissue score, including thickening and structural changes of the tendon insertion, bursitis and vascularization. The categorization of sonographic enthesitis scores to chronic/bone score and inflammatory/soft tissue score have been previously used by others [25]. Reading of the US scans was performed independently from the clinical

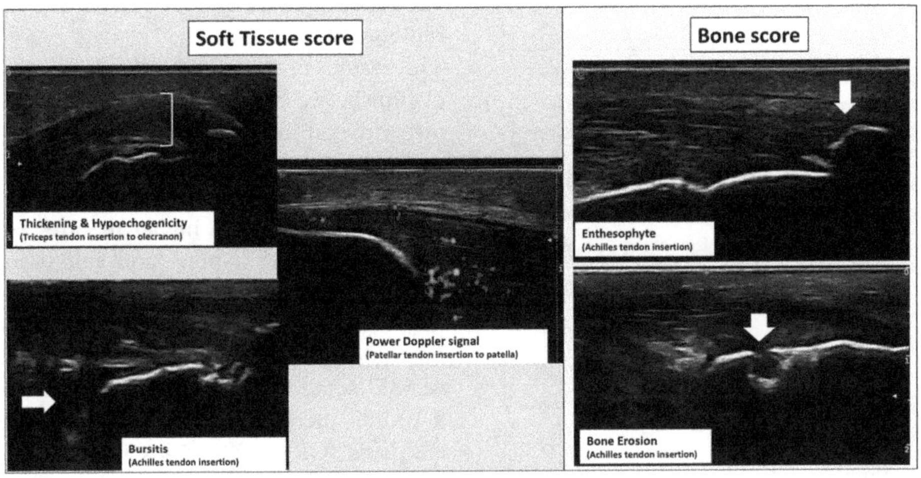

Fig. 1 Elementary lesions of enthesitis included in the Madrid Sonography Enthesitis Index (MASEI)

and radiographic data by a single reader (LE). The intra-observer intra-class correlation coefficient for MASEI was 0.8 [23].

Radiographic joint damage assessment

According to the Toronto PsA clinic protocol, conventional radiography assessment that includes hands, feet, spine, and sacroiliac joints is conducted every 2 years. The reading is performed by at least two rheumatology experts in PsA who were blinded to the US results (DDG, VC).

Peripheral joint damage in 42 joints of the hands and feet was assessed by the modified Steinbrocker score (mSS) [8]. According to this method each joint is scored on a scale ranging from 0 to 4: 0 for normal; 1 for juxta-articular osteopenia or soft tissue swelling; 2 for erosion; 3 for erosion and joint space narrowing, and 4 for total joint destruction. The total mSS is the sum of all scores that are equal or greater than 2 (range 0–168). A score of 1 is not counted towards the total mSS; therefore only definite erosive damage is considered. This method is used to follow radiographic damage in our cohort as it has proved to be valid, reliable, sensitive to change, and feasible to perform in a clinic setting [8]. Additional radiographic features of peripheral joint damage recorded included joint ankylosis, arthritis mutilans that was defined as bone resorption affecting more than 50% of the joint and periostitis that was defined as juxta-articular new bone formation. Axial joint damage was assessed by the modified New York criteria for sacroiliitis [26] and the modified Stoke Ankylosing Spondylitis Spine Score (mSASSS) for spinal damage (score range 0–72) [27].

Statistical analysis

The analysis was restricted to patients with complete data. Continuous data were described by the mean ± SD and categorical variables were expressed as frequencies and percentages. The association between MASEI score (by 10 units increase, the primary predictor) and the various radiographic features of joint damage (outcomes) was assessed through the use of negative binomial regression models [28] with count responses (mSS and mSASSS) and logistic regression for binary data (ankylosis, mutilans, sacroiliitis, and periostitis).

The initial regression model included only MASEI score as a single co-variate. Multiple regression analyses were then performed in which each regression model xadjusted for age, sex, body mass index (BMI), PsA duration, smoking (past, current, never), and current use of disease-modifying antirheumatic drugs (DMARDs) and biologic medications. A sensitivity analysis was performed with "ever use" instead of "current use" of DMARDs and biologics as model covariates. For negative binomial regression models the effect of MASEI score was expressed through its regression coefficient (β) along with its exponential value (e^{β}) and their 95% confidence intervals (CI); the exponentiated value e^{β} is interpreted as the multiplicative effect of 10 units change of MASEI score on the mean response while the other covariates remain unchanged. Odds ratios (OR) were used to express the effect of 10 units increase in the MASEI score in logistic regression models. The effect of a covariate was considered statistically significant if the P value was less than 0.05. The statistical analyses were performed using SAS version 9.4 (SAS Institute, Inc., Cary, NC, USA)

Results

Baseline characteristics

Two hundred and twenty-three patients were included in the analysis (nine patients were excluded due to missing data). Their mean age was 56 ± 12.9 years (57.9% males) with a mean PsA duration of 16.9 ± 12.4 years (Table 1). Their mean tender and swollen joint counts were 2.5 ± 5.3

Table 1 Characteristics of the study population at the time of the assessment ($N = 223$)

Variable	Value
Demographics:	
Age (years), mean ± SD	56 ± 12.9
Male gender, n (%)	129 (57.9)
PsA duration (years), mean ± SD	16.9 ± 12.4
Psoriasis skin disease duration (years), mean ± SD	28.1 ± 14.5
BMI, mean ± SD	29.8 ± 6.1
Smoking	
Current, n (%)	29 (13)
Past, n (%)	70 (31.4)
Clinical activity measures:	
Tender joints count, mean ± SD	2.5 ± 5.3
Swollen joint count, mean ± SD	1.1 ± 3.3
Clinical enthesitis, n (%)	31 (13.9)
Dactylitis, n (%)	9 (4)
PASI, mean ± SD	2.6 ± 5.8
Nail lesions, n (%)	59 (26.4)
HLA-B*27	34 (15.5)
Radiographic evaluation:	
modified Steinbrocker score	
mean ± SD	18.7 ± 33.6
median (25th, 75th percentile)	4 (0, 20)
Arthritis mutilans, n (%)	20 (9)
Joint ankylosis, n (%)	26 (11.7)
Periostitis, n (%)	49 (22.2)
mSASSS,	
mean ± SD	1.7 ± 7.2
median (25th, 75th percentile)	0 (0, 0)
Sacroiliitis, n (%),	82 (37.1)
Sonographic evaluation:	
MASEI, mean ± SD	15.7 ± 12.6
Treatment:	
DMARDs – current use, n (%)	102 (45.7)
DMARDs – ever use, n (%)	181 (81.2)
Biologics – current use, n (%)	119 (53.4)
Biologics – ever use, n (%)	130 (58.3)

PsA psoriatic arthritis, *BMI* body mass index, BOD*PASI* psoriasis area and severity index, *HLA-B*27* human leukocyte antigen B*27, *mSASSS* modified Stoke Ankylosing Spondylitis Spine Score, *MASEI* MAdrid Sonography Enthesitis Index, *DMARDs* disease-modifying antirheumatic drugs

and 1.1 ± 3.3, respectively. Clinical enthesitis was found in 13.9% of the patients.

The mean MASEI score was 15.6 ± 12.6 and the mean mSS was 18.7 ± 33.6. With respect to axial radiographic damage, the mean mSASSS was 1.7 ± 7.2 and 37.1% of the patients had sacroiliitis.

The association between MASEI and peripheral radiographic damage

The results of the statistical analyses assessing the association between MASEI score and the various measures of peripheral joint damage are shown in Table 2. Multiple regression analysis yielded an association between MASEI score and mSS so that a 10-unit increase in MASEI was associated with a 42% higher mSS ($e^{\beta} = 1.42$, 95% CI 1.15, 1.72). Both MASEI bone and soft tissue subscores were independently associated with mSS. In addition, an association was found between a MASEI score and additional outcomes of peripheral joint damage (Table 3). A higher MASEI score was also associated with ankylosis such that a 10-unit increase in MASEI almost doubled the odds of ankylosis (OR = 1.93, 95% CI 1.37, 2.72). Similarly, both MASEI bone and soft tissue subscores were associated with this outcome. Finally, an association was found between MASEI score (10 units increase) and arthritis mutilans (OR 1.77, 95% CI 1.23, 2.54) and periostitis (OR 1.41, 95% CI 1.08, 1.84). When the components of the MASEI score were examined separately, only MASEI bone score was associated with these outcomes.

The association between MASEI and axial radiographic damage

The results of the regression models assessing the association between MASEI score and the various measures of axial joint damage are shown in Table 3 and 4. Multiple regression analyses yielded an association between a higher MASEI score (10 units increase) and mSASSS (e^{β} 2.18, 95% CI 1.16, 4.09). Both the MASEI bone and soft tissue subscores were associated with higher mSASSS scores. In addition, an association was found between a higher MASEI score (10 units increase) and the presence of sacroiliitis (OR 1.33, 95% CI 1.03, 1.72). MASEI bone subscore was associated with sacroiliitis, but the MASEI soft tissue subscore was not.

Sensitivity analysis

In a sensitivity analysis, the model covariates "current use of DMARDs" and "current use of biologics" were replaced by "ever use of DMARDs" and "ever use of biologics". No significant changes in the results were observed (data not shown).

Discussion

It was Ball in 1971 who primarily set the foundations for the significance of enthesitis in SpA, by suggesting that the enthesis is centrally affected in ankylosing spondylitis (AS) patients, while the synovial joint is the main target of the inflammatory involvement in rheumatoid arthritis (RA) patients [29]. A few decades later, McGonagle and colleagues contributed significantly to the understanding of enthesitis as a key feature in SpA [16, 30]. Over

Table 2 The association between MASEI and modified Steinbroker score - negative binomial regression

Variable*	Univariate regression			Multiple regression**		
	estimate (SE)	exp$^{(Estimate)}$ (95% CI)	*P* value	estimate (SE)	exp$^{(Estimate)}$ (95% CI)	*P* value
MASEI – total	0.48 (0.11)	1.61 (1.30, 1.99)	<0.001	0.35 (0.10)	1.42 (1.15, 1.73)	<0.001
MASEI – bone score	0.86 (0.19)	2.36 (1.63, 3.38)	<0.001	0.64 (0.18)	1.89 (1.33, 2.69)	<0.001
MASEI – soft tissue score	0.63 (0.20)	1.88 (1.26, 2.77)	0.002	0.37 (0.18)	1.44 (1.03, 2.05)	0.03

MASEI MAdrid Sonography Enthesitis Index
*10 units increase in MASEI
**Each model was adjusted for age, sex, PsA duration, BMI, smoking, current use of DMARDs and biologics

the years, this idea was recognized by different organizations as the Assessment of Spondyloarthritis International Group (ASAS) that included it in their classification criteria for both axial and peripheral SpA and by the Group for Research and Assessment of Psoriasis and Psoriatic Arthritis (GRAPPA) who included it in the stem requirements of the CASPAR criteria [21, 31, 32].

The current study provides novel data regarding the association between enthesitis and features of severity in patients with PsA. The study found that a higher MASEI score, which reflects more severe enthesitis, is associated with severity of peripheral radiographic joint damage as measured by mSS. Furthermore, the severity of enthesitis was associated with proliferative and erosive features of joint damage including joint ankylosis, arthritis mutilans and periostitis. Additionally, a higher enthesitis score was associated with features of axial radiographic damage, including syndesmophytes and sacroiliitis.

According to the synovio-entheseal complex model, enthesitis is the primary lesion that triggers the related inflammation in the adjacent synovial joint [16]. This hypothesis is supported by a study that compared early SpA to early RA patients and demonstrated that knee synovitis was associated with entheseal abnormalities only in the SpA group [33]. Additional studies from the same group found associations between enthesitis and various features of SpA as dactylitis, tenosynovitis, arthritis mutilans, distal interphalangeal joint involvement, and psoriatic nail disease [34]. Supporting the importance of enthesitis in peripheral musculoskeletal inflammation in PsA, other studies that compared PsA and RA patients found that sonographic entheseal abnormalities in the fingers were identified only in the PsA group [4, 5]. Finally, a recent study in transgenic TNFα mice demonstrated that the initial signs of inflammation were found at the entheses and subsequently new bone formation appeared at entheseal sites and correlated with

Table 3 The association between MASEI score and features of radiographic damage – Logistic regression analysis

Variable*	Univariate regression		Multiple regression**	
	OR (95% CI)	*P* value	OR (95% CI)	*P* value
Joint ankylosis				
MASEI total	2.05 (1.52 2.75)	<0.001	1.93 (1.37, 2.72)	<0.001
MASEI – bone score	3.49 (2.09, 5.85)	<0.001	3.24 (1.75, 6.01)	<0.001
MASEI – soft tissue score	2.59 (1.55, 4.31)	<0.001	2.96 (1.36, 4.22)	0.003
Arthritis mutilans				
MASEI total	1.96 (1.43, 2.69)	<0.001	1.77 (1.23, 2.54)	0.002
MASEI – bone score	3.94 (2.24, 6.93)	<0.001	3.77 (1.84, 7.70)	<0.001
MASEI – soft tissue score	2.00 (1.15, 3.50)	0.014	1.71 (0.90, 3.26)	0.102
Periostitis				
MASEI total	1.48 (1.17, 1.88)	0.001	1.41 (1.08, 1.84)	0.013
MASEI – bone score	2.05 (1.35, 3.11)	<0.001	1.88 (1.17, 3.02)	0.009
MASEI – soft tissue score	1.65 (1.07, 2.53)	0.022	1.52 (0.96, 2.41)	0.07
Sacroiliitis				
MASEI total	1.36 (1.10, 1.70)	0.005	1.33 (1.03, 1.72)	0.027
MASEI – bone score	2.12 (1.42, 3.16)	<0.001	2.24 (1.40, 3.61)	<0.001
MASEI – soft tissue score	1.23 (0.84, 1.83)	0.285	1.10 (0.71, 1.70)	0.664

MASEI MAdrid Sonography Enthesitis Index
*10 units increase in MASEI
**Each model was adjusted for age, sex, PsA duration, BMI, smoking, current use of DMARDs and biologics

Table 4 The association between MASEI and mSASSS – negative binomial regression

Variable*	Univariate model			Multivariable model**		
	estimate (SE)	exp$^{(Estimate)}$ (95% CI)	*P* value	estimate (SE)	exp$^{(Estimate)}$ (95% CI)	*P* value
MASEI – total	0.65 (0.25)	1.92 (1.17, 3.09)	0.009	0.78 (0.32)	2.18 (1.16, 4.09)	0.02
MASEI – bone score	1.23 (0.42)	3.42 (1.52, 7.69)	0.003	1.51 (0.51)	4.52 (1.68, 12.18)	0.003
MASEI – soft tissue score	1.04 (0.50)	2.89 (1.06, 7.61)	0.04	0.70 (0.69)	2.01 (0.52, 7.77)	0.31

MASEI MAdrid Sonography Enthesitis Index
*10 units increase in MASEI
**Each model was adjusted for age, sex, PsA duration, BMI, smoking, current use of DMARDs and Biologics

the degree of inflammation [19]. In accordance with these findings, our study found an association between the extent of enthesitis and peripheral joint damage.

However, there are studies that could not confirm the specific link between enthesitis and SpA [35, 36]. Paramarta et al. found the same prevalence of entheseal involvement in SpA and RA patients [35]. Ibrahim et al. found similar sonographic entheseal scores in patients with PsA and RA [36]. However, the significantly older age of the RA group in their study may have accounted for the higher entheseal score in this group leading to the similarity in scores. Overall, the discrepancies between the different studies can be attributed to the lack of standardization manifesting with diversity in several aspects including the type of the patients, the sample size, disease manifestations, enthesitis sites scanned, sonographic indices, and imaging equipment.

Unfortunately, there are only a few longitudinal studies that may address the controversy regarding the primacy of enthesitis in the pathogenesis of SpA [20, 37]. Tinazzi et al. found that thickness of the quadriceps tendon predicated the development of clinical PsA in a small cohort of psoriasis patients [20]. El-Miedany et al. evaluated 126 psoriasis patients by clinical, radiological and sonographic measures over a period of 1 year [37]. However, this study did not differentiate between the two pathologies as it found that both sonographic enthesitis and synovitis at baseline were predictors of joint damage in new-onset PsA patients. Finally, a recent study in 41 psoriasis patients found that arthralgia and baseline MRI synovitis in the hand joints predicted the development of clinical PsA after 1 year of follow-up [38]. The detection of periarticular inflammation in only 4% of the patients raises a question regarding the reliability of this tool for enthesitis evaluation.

Enthesitis is a widespread condition that can involve the peripheral as well as the axial skeleton. The location of inflammation in spondylitis is at the entheses, where the ligaments attach to the vertebrae [39]. Several studies showed an association between clinical enthesitis [measured by the Maastricht Ankylosing Spondylitis Enthesis Score (MASES)] and both higher disease activity [measured by the Bath Ankylosing Spondylitis Disease Activity Index (BASDAI)] and worse functional status [40, 41]. In addition, Muche et al. reported that enthesitis in the sacroiliac region, as detected by MRI, was more common in advanced sacroiliitis [42]. Our study found an association between sonographic enthesitis and axial damage, including both spondylitis and sacroiliitis. In contrast to our study, Alcalde et al. did not find a correlation between sonographic enthesitis and radiographic sacroiliitis [43]. However, their study is not entirely comparable to ours for several reasons: first, the study population included AS and not PsA patients, second, the sample size was much smaller including only 44 patients and lastly, the sonographic enthesitis index included less entheseal sites and did not include Power Doppler vascularization assessment.

The agreement between sonographic and clinical assessment of enthesitis is an area of interest in rheumatology due to the limited specificity and sensitivity of the latter method [15]. A few studies that compared these two modalities found low to moderate agreement [43, 44]. Recently, van der Ven et al. reported that adding US evaluation in psoriasis patients who had entheseal tenderness on clinical examination reduced the rate of enthesitis by 64% [45]. In this regard, it should be mentioned that the MASEI score includes entheseal lesions that represent irreversible damage from prior active enthesitis, such as enthesophytes and erosions, in addition to active lesions such as vascularization. Thus, the sonographic score may be high in patients who sustained entheseal damage from prior enthesitis who may be in remission at the time of assessment.

This study has several limitations. First, the association between sonographic enthesitis in sites located adjacent to large joints and radiographic damage of small joints in the hands and feet is indirect and may not suggest a causal link. Identifying enthesitis in the small joints is a difficult task, which may explain why there is no such enthesitis index. In addition, radiographic damage in large joints is less common and hence there is no standardized damage index for these sites. Thus, although the study cannot support a direct causal link between enthesitis and the development of peripheral or axial joint damage, the strong association observed between the extent of enthesitis and a number of features of joint damage in the peripheral and axial joints suggest that enthesitis may be a marker of more severe PsA phenotypes.

An additional limitation of the study includes its cross-sectional nature that does not allow making causal inferences. Furthermore, we assessed the associations between enthesitis at a single time point and radiographic damage that has accumulated over time. However, MASEI score includes a bone damage subcategory which reflects irreversible entheseal bone damage (e.g., enthesophytes and erosions) that has accumulated over time. Furthermore, all regression analyses showed that these chronic bone lesions were more strongly associated with radiographic joint damage than the soft tissue lesions. Lastly, treatments may have modified the relationship as we controlled for treatment only at the time of assessment, although it is expected that effective treatment for enthesitis, such as biologics, would have weakened the association. However, our sensitivity analyses that included the use of biologics and DMARDs at any point during the disease did not significantly modify the results.

This study has several strengths. To our knowledge, this is the largest study thus far that explored the association between sonographic enthesitis and radiographic joint damage in PsA. The use of sonographic enthesitis as a primary predictor improved the accuracy of assessing this important feature over physical examination [15]. In addition, the PsA cohort in this study is well phenotyped, which enables to control for multiple confounders.

Conclusions

The results of the study suggest that the severity of sonographic enthesitis is a potential marker of radiographic peripheral and axial joint damage in PsA. The association was found with both erosive and proliferative bone lesions. These findings raise the question of whether enthesitis has a role in the pathogenesis of articular damage in PsA. Further longitudinal studies in early PsA patients are required in order to establish the precise cause and effect relationships between enthesitis, synovitis, and joint damage.

Abbreviations

AS: Ankylosing spondylitis; ASAS: Assessment of Spondyloarthritis International Group; BMI: Body mass index; CASPAR: Classification for psoriatic arthritis; CI: Confidence interval; DMARDs: Disease-modifying antirheumatic drugs; GRAPPA: Group for Research and Assessment of Psoriasis and Psoriatic Arthritis; MASEI: MAdrid Sonography Enthesitis Index; MRI: Magnetic resonance imaging; mSASSS: modified Stoke Ankylosing Spondylitis Spine Score; mSS: modified Steinbrocker score; OR: Odds ratios; PASI: Psoriasis area and severity index; PsA: Psoriatic arthritis; RA: Rheumatoid arthritis; SpA: Spondyloarthritis; SPARCC: SPondyloArthritis Research Consortium Canada; US: Ultrasound

Acknowledgements

Not applicable.

Funding

No funding was received for this study.

Disclosures

The University of Toronto Psoriatic Arthritis Program is supported by a grant from the Krembil Foundation. Ari Polachek was supported by an educational grant from Janssen Canada. Lihi Eder is supported by a New Investigator Salary Grant from the Arthritis Society and the Canadian Association of Psoriasis Patients. The authors declare that they do not have any potential conflicts of interests

Authors' contributions

AP contributed to study conception and design, analysis and interpretation of the data and preparation of the manuscript. RC contributed to analysis and interpretation of the data and preparation of the manuscript. VC contributed to study conception and design, analysis and interpretation of the data and preparation of the manuscript. DDG contributed to study conception and design, analysis and interpretation of the data and preparation of the manuscript. LE contributed to study conception and design, analysis and interpretation of the data and preparation of the manuscript. All authors read and approved the final manuscript.

Consent for publication

Not applicable.

Competing interests

The authors declare that they have no competing interests.

Author details

[1]Centre for Prognostic Studies in the Rheumatic Diseases, Toronto Western Hospital, University of Toronto, 1-412, 399 Bathurst Street, Toronto, ON M5T 2S8, Canada. [2]Department of Statistics and Actuarial Science, University of Waterloo, Waterloo, ON, Canada. [3]Department of Medicine and Laboratory Medicine, Institute of Medical Science, University of Toronto, Toronto, ON, Canada. [4]Department of Pathobiology, Institute of Medical Science, University of Toronto, Toronto, ON, Canada. [5]Centre for Prognosis Studies in the Rheumatic Diseases, Krembil Research Institute, Toronto Western Hospital, Toronto, ON, Canada. [6]Center for Prognostic Studies in the Rheumatic Diseases, Toronto Western Hospital, University of Toronto, Toronto, ON, Canada. [7]Department of Medicine, University of Toronto, Women's College Research Institute, Women's College Hospital, Room 6326, 76 Grenville Street, Toronto, ON M5S 1B2, Canada.

References

1. Haroon M, Kirby B, FitzGerald O. High prevalence of psoriatic arthritis in patients with severe psoriasis with suboptimal performance of screening questionnaires. Ann Rheum Dis. 2013;72:736–40.
2. Ogdie A, Langan S, Love T, Haynes K, Shin D, Seminara N, et al. Prevalence and treatment patterns of psoriatic arthritis in the UK. Rheumatology (Oxford). 2013;52:568–75.
3. Gladman DD, Chandran V. Observational cohort studies: lessons learnt from the University of Toronto Psoriatic Arthritis Program. Rheumatol (Oxford). 2011;50:25–31.
4. Fournié B, Margarit-Coll N, Champetier de Ribes TL, Zabraniecki L, Jouan A, Vincent V, et al. Extrasynovial ultrasound abnormalities in the psoriatic finger. Prospective comparative power-doppler study versus rheumatoid arthritis. Joint Bone Spine. 2006;73:527–31.
5. Zabotti A, Salvin S, Quartuccio L, De Vita S. Differentiation between early rheumatoid and early psoriatic arthritis by the ultrasonographic study of the synovio-entheseal complex of the small joints of the hands. Clin Exp Rheumatol. 2016;34:459–65.

6. Polachek A, Li S, Chandran V, Gladman D. Clinical enthesitis in a prospective longitudinal psoriatic arthritis cohort: incidence, prevalence, characteristics and outcome. Arthritis Care Res (Hoboken). 2016. Epub ahead of print.
7. Ranza R, Carneiro S, Qureshi AA, Martins G, Rodrigues JJ, Romiti R, et al. Prevalence of psoriatic arthritis in a large cohort of Brazilian patients with psoriasis. J Rheumatol. 2015;42:829–34.
8. Rahman P, Gladman DD, Cook RJ, Zhou Y, Young G, Salonen D. Radiological assessment in psoriatic arthritis. Br J Rheumatol. 1998;37:760–5.
9. Eshed I, Bollow M, Mcgonagle DG, Tan AL, Althoff CE, Asbach P. MRI of enthesitis of the appendicular skeleton in spondyloarthritis. Ann Rheum Dis. 2007;66:1553–9.
10. Poggenborg RP, Eshed I, Østergaard M, Sørensen IJ, Møller JM, Madsen OR. Enthesitis in patients with psoriatic arthritis, axial spondyloarthritis and healthy subjects assessed by 'head-to-toe' whole-body MRI and clinical examination. Ann Rheum Dis. 2015;74:823–9.
11. Gandjbakhch F, Terslev L, Joshua F, Wakefield RJ, Naredo E, D'Agostino MA. Ultrasound in the evaluation of enthesitis: status and perspectives. Arthritis Res Ther. 2011;13:R188.
12. Wiell C, Szkudlarek M, Hasselquist M, Møller JM, Vestergaard A, Nørregaard J. Ultrasonography, magnetic resonance imaging, radiography, and clinical assessment of inflammatory and destructive changes in fingers and toes of patients with psoriatic arthritis. Arthritis Res Ther. 2008;10:402.
13. Husic R, Gretler J, Felber A, Graninger WB, Duftner C, Hermann J. Disparity between ultrasound and clinical findings in psoriatic arthritis. Ann Rheum Dis. 2014;78:1529–36.
14. Balint PV, Kane D, Wilson H, McInnes IB, Sturrock RD. Ultrasonography of entheseal insertions in the lower limb in spondyloarthropathy. Ann Rheum Dis. 2002;10:905–10.
15. Zabotti A, Bandinelli F, Batticciotto A, Scirè CA, Iagnocco A, Sakellariou G. Musculoskeletal ultrasonography for psoriatic arthritis and psoriasis patients: a systematic literature review. Rheumatol (Oxford). 2017. Epub ahead of print.
16. McGonagle D, Lories RJU, Tan AL, Benjamin M. The concept of a "Synovio-Entheseal complex" and its implications for understanding joint inflammation and damge in psoriatic arthritis and beyond. Arthritis Rheum. 2007;56:2482–92.
17. Lories RJ, Derese I, Luyten FP. Modulation of bone morphogenetic protein signaling inhibits the onset and progression of ankylosing enthesitis. J Clin Invest. 2005;115:1571–9.
18. Braem K, Carter S, Lories RJ. Spontaneous arthritis and ankylosis in male DBA/1 mice: further evidence for a role of behavioral factors in "stress-induced arthritis". Biol Proced Online. 2012;14:10.
19. Jacques P, Lambrecht S, Verheugen E, Pauwels E, Kollias G, Armaka M, et al. Proof of concept: enthesitis and new bone formation in spondyloarthritis are driven by mechanical strain and stromal cells. Ann Rheum Dis. 2014;73:437–45.
20. Tinazzi I, McGonagle D, Biasi D, Confente S, Caimmi C, Girolomoni G, et al. Preliminary evidence that subclinical enthesopathy may predict psoriatic arthritis in patients with psoriasis. J Rheumatol. 2011;38:2691–2.
21. Eder L, Jayakar J, Thavaneswaran A, Haddad A, Chandran V, Salonen D, et al. Is the MAdrid Sonographic Enthesitis Index useful for differentiating psoriatic arthritis from psoriasis alone and healthy controls? J Rheumatol. 2014;41:466–72.
22. Taylor W, Gladman D, Helliwel P, Marchesoni A, Mease P, Mielants H. Classification criteria for psoriatic arthritis: development of new criteria from a large international study. Arthritis Rheum. 2006;54:2665–73.
23. Maksymowych WP, Mallon C, Morrow S, Shojania K, Olszynki WP, Wong RL, et al. Development and validation of the spondyloarthritis research consortium of Canada (SPARCC) enthesitis index. Ann Rheum Dis. 2009;68:948–63.
24. de Miguel E, Cobo T, Munoz-Fernandez S, Naredo E, Uson J, Acebes JC, et al. Validity of enthesis ultrasound assessment in spondyloarthropathy. Ann Rheum Dis. 2009;68:169–74.
25. Aydin SZ, Ash ZR, Tinazzi I, Castillo-Gallego C, Kwok C, Wilson C, et al. The link between enthesitis and arthritis in psoriatic arthritis: a switch to a vascular phenotype at insertions may play a role in arthritis development. Ann Rheum Dis. 2013;72:992–5.
26. van der Linden S, Valkenburg HA, Cats A. Evaluation of diagnostic criteria for ankylosing spondylitis. A proposal for modifi cation of the New York criteria. Arthritis Rheum. 1984;27:361–8.
27. Spoorenberg A, de Vlam K, van der Linden S, Dougados M, Mielants H, van de Tempel H, et al. Radiological scoring methods in ankylosing spondylitis. Reliability and change over 1 and 2 years. J Rheumatol. 2004;31:125–32.
28. Hilbe JM. Negative binomial regression, vol. 77. secondth ed. New York: Cambridge University Press; 2012. p. 611–2.
29. Ball J. Enthesopathy of rheumatoid arthritis and ankylosing spondylitis. Ann Rheum Dis. 1971;30:213–23.
30. McGonagle D, Gibbon W, Emery P. Classification of inflammatory arthritis by enthesitis. Lancet. 1998;352:1137–40.
31. Rudwaleit M, van der Heijde D, Landewé R, Listing J, Akkoc N, Brandt J, et al. The development of Assessment of SpondyloArthritis international Society classification criteria for axial spondyloarthritis (part II): validation and final selection. Ann Rheum Dis. 2009;68:777–83.
32. Rudwaleit M, van der Heijde D, Landewé R, Akkoc N, Brandt J, Chou CT, et al. The Assessment of SpondyloArthritis International Society classification criteria for peripheral spondyloarthritis and for spondyloarthritis in general. Ann Rheum Dis. 2011;70:25–31.
33. McGonagle D, Gibbon W, O'Connor P, Green M, Pease C, Emery P. Characteristic MRI entheseal changes of knee synovitis in spondyloarthropathy. Arthritis Rheum. 1998;41:694–700.
34. McGonagle D, Tan AL. The enthesis in psoriatic arthritis. Clin Exp Rheumatol. 2015;33(5 Suppl 93):S36–9.
35. Paramarta JE, van der Leij C, Gofita I, Yeremenko N, van de Sande MG, de Hair MJ, et al. Peripheral joint inflammation in early onset spondyloarthritis is not specifically related to enthesitis. Ann Rheum Dis. 2014;73:735–40.
36. Ibrahim G, Groves C, Chandramohan M, Beltran A, Valle R, Reyes B, et al. Clinical and ultrasound examination of the Leeds Enthesitis Index in psoriatic arthritis and rheumatoid arthritis. ISRN Rheumatol. 2011;2011: 731917.
37. El Miedany Y, El Gaafary M, Youssef S, Ahmed I, Nasr A. Tailored approach to early psoriatic arthritis patients: clinical and ultrasonographic predictors for structural joint damage. Clin Rheumatol. 2015;34:307–13.
38. Faustini F, Simon D, Oliveira I, Kleyer A, Haschka J, Englbrecht M, et al. Subclinical joint inflammation in patients with psoriasis without concomitant psoriatic arthritis: a cross-sectional and longitudinal analysis. Ann Rheum Dis. 2016;75(12):2068–74.
39. Hermann KG, Baraliakos X, van der Heijde DM, Jurik AG, Landewé R, Marzo-Ortega H, et al. Descriptions of spinal MRI lesions and definition of a positive MRI of the spine in axial spondyloarthritis: a consensual approach by the ASAS/OMERACT MRI study group. Ann Rheum Dis. 2012;71:1278–88.
40. Spadaro A, Iagnocco A, Perrotta FM, Modesti M, Scarno A, Valesini G. Clinical and ultrasonography assessment of peripheral enthesitis in ankylosing spondylitis. Rheumatol (Oxford). 2011;50:2080–6.
41. Rezvani A, Bodur H, Ataman S, Kaya T, Buğdaycı DS, Demir SE. Correlations among enthesitis, clinical, radiographic and quality of life parameters in patients with ankylosing spondylitis. Mod Rheumatol. 2014;24:651–6.
42. Muche B, Bollow M, François RJ, Sieper J, Hamm B, Braun J. Anatomic structures involved in early- and late-stage sacroiliitis in spondylarthritis: a detailed analysis by contrast-enhanced magnetic resonance imaging. Arthritis Rheum. 2003;48:1374–84.
43. Alcalde M, Acebes JC, Cruz M, González-Hombrado L, Herrero-Beaumont G, Sánchez-Pernaute O. A sonographic enthesitic index of lower limbs is a valuable tool in the assessment of ankylosing spondylitis. Ann Rheum Dis. 2007;66:1015–9.
44. Hamdi W, Chelli-Bouaziz M, Ahmed MS, Ghannouchi MM, Kaffel D, Ladeb MF, et al. Correlations among clinical, radiographic, and sonographic scores for enthesitis in ankylosing spondylitis. Joint Bone Spine. 2011;78:270–4.
45. van der Ven M, Karreman MC, Weel AE, Tchetverikov I, Vis M, Nijsten TE, Hazes JM, et al. Adding ultrasound to clinical examination reduced frequency of enthesitis in primary care psoriasis patients with musculoskeletal complaints. Clin Exp Rheumatol. 2016;34:1020–25.

12

Residual disease activity and treatment adjustments in psoriatic arthritis in current clinical practice

Leonieke J. J. van Mens[1*], Marleen G. H. van de Sande[1], Inka A. Fluri[1], Sadaf Atiqi[1], Arno W. R. van Kuijk[2†] and Dominique L. P. Baeten[1†]

Abstract

Background: With expanding therapeutic possibilities for treatment of psoriatic arthritis (PsA) it will be increasingly important to determine residual disease and define when to adjust treatment. The rationale behind treatment decisions in current daily clinical practice and the relationship with residual disease activity has not been investigated. The aim of this study was to assess current clinical practice on defining residual disease and subsequent treatment decisions made in PsA patients.

Methods: This cross-sectional study scored disease activity and treatment decisions prospectively in 142 consecutive PsA patients visiting the outpatient clinic for routine follow up. Disease activity parameters were scored by patient and the treating rheumatologist; the rheumatologist additionally registered his opinion on the presence of remaining disease activity despite current treatment (further mentioned as remaining disease) and subsequent treatment decisions.

Results: Two thirds (90/142) of patients had remaining disease activity according to the treating rheumatologist. Almost half (46%) of these patients had moderate to high disease activity according to the clinical Disease Activity Index for Psoriatic Arthritis (cDAPSA). Residual disease activity was determined by joint disease and pain rather than by active psoriasis. Demographic and clinical features were similar between groups with or without residual disease. Among patients with remaining disease activity, 74% were treated with either a conventional synthetic disease-modifying anti-rheumatic drug (csDMARD) only or a first TNF-inhibiting biological agent, suggesting opportunities for treatment modification. However, treatment adjustment was initiated in only 21 (23%) of the 90 patients with residual disease. When comparing patients with remaining disease activity with and without treatment adjustment, we found no differences in objective disease activity measures, such as joint counts and patient scores. These data suggest that treatment is not adjusted in a large majority of patients with residual disease activity, although options for treatment changes are available.

Conclusions: Remaining disease activity is present in almost two thirds of patients with PsA when scored by the treating rheumatologist, but triggers treatment adjustment in only a minority. Further research to understand why disease activity does not lead to treatment adjustment is required to enable implementation of treatment strategies in clinical practice.

Keywords: Psoriatic arthritis, Clinical practice, Treatment decisions, Residual disease activity, Treatment strategies

* Correspondence: l.j.vanmens@amc.uva.nl
†Equal contributors
[1]Department of Clinical Immunology & Rheumatology, Amsterdam Rheumatology and immunology Center, Academic Medical Center/University of Amsterdam, Meibergdreef 9, 1105 AZ Amsterdam, The Netherlands
Full list of author information is available at the end of the article

Background

Treatment options for psoriatic arthritis (PsA) increased significantly in the last decade with leflunomide and tumor necrosis factor (TNF) inhibitors (TNFi) becoming part of our standard therapeutic arsenal [1]. Several other new treatments became available in recent years, including ustekinumab, apremilast, and secukinumab [2–5]. Additionally, the first trial comparing target-steered treatment vs standard care in PsA, the Tight Control of Psoriatic Arthritis (TICOPA) trial, demonstrated that not only the availability of treatments but also the strategy on how to use these treatments determines the clinical outcome. The treat-to-target arm of the study shows significantly better outcomes in peripheral arthritis, skin, and patient reported outcomes in comparison with the standard-care arm, with more patients reaching a minimal disease activity state in the treat-to-target arm [6]. Therefore, the combination of additional treatment options and better treatment strategies holds great promise to improve the outcome in PsA in daily clinical practice.

Intriguingly, the few available publications on real-life clinical PsA practice indicate that not many patients are in a minimal disease state despite treatment [7]. Potential reasons for residual disease activity in this group of patients could be categorized as follows: (1) patients not responding to all available treatments - for this category, new treatment options obviously open up new perspectives; (2) patients in whom comorbidities, side effects, and/or incompliance result in the inability or unwillingness to use available medication - in this case, new treatments may not have an additional value; and (3) patients in whom the currently available treatments are not optimally used - this category could benefit from stricter definition and implementation of treatment strategies.

To quantify the presence of remaining disease activity in PsA in daily clinical practice and understand the underlying reasons, we set up a cross-sectional cohort documenting disease activity and treatment use in consecutive patients with PsA and analyzed the treatment decisions that were made by the treating rheumatologist. Importantly, the available treatment options in clinical practice during the inclusion period of this study were limited to conventional disease modifying anti-rheumatic drugs (csDMARDs), such as methotrexate and leflunomide, and TNFi. Ustekinumab became available for use in clinical practice just before this study and was therefore not a common drug to prescribe at the time.

Methods

This observational cross-sectional study was conducted at the rheumatology outpatient clinics of two centers in Amsterdam (AMC and Reade) between October 2014 and September 2015. Sixteen participating rheumatologists recruited consecutive patients with PsA visiting their outpatient clinic, including a total of 152 patients. The inclusion criteria were (1) clinical diagnosis of psoriatic arthritis, (2) age 18 years or older, (3) disease duration of at least 6 months, (4) fulfillment of the Classification Criteria for Psoriatic Arthritis (CASPAR) [8], and (5) current or previous treatment with synthetic and/or biological DMARD therapy. Patients currently participating in a clinical trial were excluded from the study. This observational study did not require ethical approval and/or patient informed consent as the Medical Research Involving Human subjects Act (WMO) does not apply to these types of studies in the Netherlands, as confirmed by the Ethics Committee of the Academic Medical Center/University of Amsterdam. The study was conducted in accordance with the Declaration of Helsinki (2008) and International Conference on Harmonization (ICH)/Good Clinical Practice (GCP) standards.

Data collection

Data on demographics, disease characteristics, current treatment, treatment history, and medical history were extracted from the patient files by the study physician (LvM). To reflect decision-making in real-life clinical practice, the disease activity scores and the statements on the presence of remaining disease and the decisions on treatment adjustment were made by the treating rheumatologist during a routine clinical visit. At the time of the visit the treating rheumatologist performed a physical examination, collected outcome measures, and answered questions on remaining disease activity and treatment modifications. Physical assessments included scoring of swelling and tenderness of the joints (swollen joint count (SJC)66/tender joint count (TJC)68), an enthesitis count, recording the number of enthesial sites with enthesitis according to the rheumatologist, and a dactylitis count. Disease activity measures were the Physician global Assessment on disease activity (VAS-PhysGlobal) and a Physician Assessment of psoriatic skin activity (VASPhysSkin) on a visual analog scale (VAS) of 0–10 cm and the Bath Ankylosing Spondylitis Activity Disease Index (BASDAI). The following questions were answered by the rheumatologist. Do you think there is remaining disease activity in this patient, despite current treatment regimen? (further mentioned in this manuscript as "remaining disease"). Will you start additional therapy or change current therapy for the remaining disease activity? If yes, what will you start or change? If no, what is the reason not to treat this remaining disease activity?

Patients completed the Patient Global Assessment of Disease Activity (VASPtGlobal) on a VAS of 0–10 cm and the Patient Assessment Of Pain (VASPtPain) on a VAS of 0–10 cm. To grade the severity of the disease activity in a composite index, we used the clinical Disease Activity in PsA score (cDAPSA) calculated as SJC66 + TJC68 + VASptglobal + VASptPain and divided by categories: remission, cDAPSA ≤4; low disease activity, cDAPSA >4 and ≤13; moderate disease activity, cDAPSA >13 and ≤27; and high disease activity, cDAPSA >27 [9, 10].

Data analysis

Data are presented as mean and standard deviation (SD) or as median and interquartile range (IQR) where applicable. Statistical comparisons between remaining disease groups and treatment yes/no groups were performed using the t test or, alternatively, the Mann-Whitney U test when data were not normally distributed. Statistical tests were two-sided and P values <0.05 were considered statistically significant. Analysis was performed in SPSS (V22.0).

Results

A total of 152 patients were included, and data scored by the rheumatologist and patient scores were available for 142 patients. The remaining 10 were excluded from analysis as either the physician or the patient data were missing. Disease characteristics and demographics are shown in Table 1.

We first analyzed the disease activity present in patients with or without residual disease according to their treating rheumatologist. Fifty-two patients were considered by the treating rheumatologist not to have remaining disease activity (Table 1). These patients indeed had low disease activity in all measured objective disease domains: there were only three patients with a swollen joint count >0, three patients with a tender joint count >0, and no patients at all with dactylitis or enthesitis. The median skin severity score was 1 on the 10-point scale. This was confirmed by patient-reported severity and pain scores (median VASpatient global and VASpt pain score of 1 out of 10). Accordingly, all patients were in remission (36/52) or low disease activity (15/52) (there was insufficient data on one patient to calculate the cDAPSA) as defined by the cDAPSA composite score.

Of the 142 patients, 90 (63%) were considered in the opinion of the treating rheumatologist to have remaining disease activity (Table 1). This was supported by disease activity across all measured domains, with 31% of patients having at least one swollen joint (including 16% with three or more swollen joints), 60% having one or more tender joints, 18% having enthesitis, 9% having dactylitis, and 30% who had a VASphys skin score >2. This was reflected by higher scores in patient-reported severity of pain and in the global health score (median score of 5/10). The cDAPSA composite score indicated that 46% of these patients had moderate to high disease activity. Overall, these data indicate that almost two thirds of the patients had some kind of objective residual disease activity, with almost half of those having even moderate to high disease activity. The remaining disease activity was mainly determined by joint disease and pain rather than by skin psoriasis, partly driven by an overall low burden of skin psoriasis in this cohort.

In order to better define which patients had remaining disease activity, we compared demographic and clinical features between those with and without residual disease activity. There were no differences in gender, disease duration, comorbidity, current treatment duration, or number of previously used csDMARDS. Residual disease activity was more frequently reported in patients treated with a csDMARD only (66%) or a second TNFi (69%) in comparison with patients on their first TNFi (44%) (P = 0.019). As 74% of the patients with residual disease activity were currently treated with either a csDMARD only or a first TNFi, this suggests that treatment modification could be an option.

We asked the rheumatologist whether the presence of remaining disease activity would lead to a treatment adjustment. Of the 90 patients with remaining disease activity, treatment was modified in only 21 (23%). These treatment adjustments included start of analgesic treatment (n = 6), local or intramuscular corticosteroid therapy (n = 5), switch of csDMARD to another csDMARD (n = 4), referral to other specialists (hand surgeon, orthopedic surgery) (n = 2), start of a second and a third TNFi in a patient already using TNFi treatment (n = 2), addition of a csDMARD to current TNFi therapy (n = 1), and start of a TNFi in a patient only using csDMARDs (n = 1).

In order to understand why treatment adjustment was only initiated in 23% of the patients with remaining disease activity, we compared those with and without treatment adjustment for clinical and demographic features (Table 2). With the exception of VAS physician (median 3 (IQR 2–5) vs 2 (2–3), P = 0.007), none of the disease activity measures were different between the two groups, not even objective measures such as the SJC. Also demographic features such as gender, disease duration, and treatment durations were similar (Table 2). However, treatment was less frequently changed in patients already treated with a second TNFi (in 3/24 (13%) of patients) in comparison with the csDMARD only or first TNFi groups (15/51 (28%) and 4/14 (29%), respectively).

We additionally investigated the reasons not to adjust treatment. In 39/69 (57%) patients, the rheumatologist judged the complaints as "minor". This group included 8 patients with a SJC ≥1, 19 with a TJC ≥1, and 6 with an enthesitis. cDAPSA scores categorized these patients as having moderate disease activity (n = 12), low disease activity (n = 19), and remission (n = 5) (with 4 patients

Table 1 Clinical characteristics and disease activity of patients with and without residual disease activity

	Total group (*n* = 142)	Residual disease activity according to rheumatologist (*n* = 90)	No residual disease activity according to rheumatologist (*n* = 52)	Residual disease vs no residual disease *P* value
Age mean (SD)	53.0 (12.6)	53.6 (6.3)	51.9 (13.6)	0.000
Male/female *n/n*	92/60	53/37	33/19	0.865
Disease duration diagnosis mean (SD)	10.3 (7.9)	11.0 (9.2)	10.1 (6.8)	0.494
on treatment > 6 months, %	93	86	94	0.618
Current only DMARD user *n* (%)	110 (49)	52 (58)	23 (44)	0.032
Current first TNF user *n* (%)	32 (22)	14 (16)	18 (35)	
Current > 1 TNF user *n* (%)	35 (24)	24 (27)	11 (21)	
Swollen joints	0 (0–0)	0 (0–1)	0 (0–0)	0.000
SJC of 0, *n* (%)	111 (77)	63 (70)	49 (94)	
SJC of 1, *n* (%)	10 (7)	8 (9)	2 (4)	
SJC of 2, *n* (%)	5 (3)	5 (6)	0 (0)	
SJC of ≥ 3, *n* (%)	15 (10)	14 (16)	1 (2)	
Tender joints	1 (0–2)	1 (0–3)	0 (0–0)	0.000
TJC of 0, *n* (%)	82 (57)	36 (40)	46 (88)	
TJC of 1, *n* (%)	21 (13)	16 (18)	5 (10)	
TJC of 2, *n* (%)	12 (13)	12 (13)	0 (-)	
TJC of 3, *n* (%)	25 (17)	24 (27)	1 (2)	
Number of dactylitic digits	0 (0–0)	0 (0–0)	0 (0–0)	0.017
Dactylitis count of 1, *n* (%)	8 (6)	8 (9)	0 (-)	
Number of enthesitis points	0 (0–0)	0 (0–0)	0 (0–0)	0.001
Enthesitis count of 1, *n* (%)	14 (10)	14 (16)	0 (-)	
Enthesitis count of 2–4, *n* (%)	2 (1)	2 (2)	0 (-)	
VAS physician skin severity	1 (0–2)	1 (1–2.5)	1 (0–1)	0.000
VAS physician overall disease activity	1 (1–3)	2 (1–4)	1 (0–1)	0.000
VAS patient global disease activity	2 (1–6)	5 (2–7)	1 (0–2)	0.000
VAS pt pain	2 (1–6)	5 (2–7)	1 (0–2)	0.000
BASDAI	2,65 (1–4.8)	4.1 (2.5–5.9)	0.9 (0.4–1.8)	0.000
cDAPSA remission, *n* (%)	45 (32)	9 (10)	36 (69)	0.000
cDAPSA low disease activity, *n* (%)	49 (35)	34 (38)	15 (29)	
cDAPSA moderate disease activity, *n* (%)	35 (25)	35 (39)	0 (-)	
cDAPSA high disease activity, *n* (%)	6 (4)	6 (7)	0 (-)	
cDAPSA missing, *n* (%)	7 (5)	6 (7)	1 (2)	

Values are median (IQR) unless stated otherwise. Significance of the comparisons was determined by independent sample *t* test for continuous variables and the Mann-Whitney *U* test for non-normally distributed variables. The comparisons within cDAPSA groups were determined by the Kruskall-Wallis test
csDMARD conventional synthetic disease-modifying anti-rheumatic drugs, *BASDAI* Bath Ankylosing Spondylitis Disease Activity Index, *TNFi* tumor necrosis factor inhibitor, *SJC* swollen joint count, *TJC* tender joint count, *VAS* visual analog scale, *cDAPSA* clinical Disease Activity in PsA score

having incomplete data to calculate the cDAPSA score). In the remaining 30 patients the following reasons were reported: patients' preference not to adjust medication (10/69 (14%)); absence of additional treatment options (5/69 (7%)) (these patients were all currently treated with a second or third TNFi); lack of compliance and/or adverse events(5/69 (7%)); and other reasons (20/69 (29%)) (more than one reason could be reported per patient). Other reasons included: disease activity reflects symptoms of comorbidity instead of the PsA (non-inflammatory joint problems/disease including osteoarthritis of the knee/hand, trigger finger, meniscal tear, and recent fracture) ($n = 4$); awaiting therapeutic effect of recent change ($n = 3$); side effects resulted in a disruption of treatment; recently restarted therapy ($n = 3$); no therapeutic options left for this patient ($n = 2$); first awaiting results of magnetic resonance imaging (MRI) ($n = 1$); task of the dermatologist ($n = 2$); comorbidity prohibits

Table 2 Disease activity in patients with residual disease activity resulting or not resulting in additional treatment

	Total group ($n = 90$)	Additional treatment ($n = 21$)	No additional treatment ($n = 69$)	Additional treatment vs No additional treatment P value
Age, mean (SD)	53.6 (12.2)	52.6 (10.8)	53.9 (12.7)	0.270
Male/female, *n/n*	53/37	15/6	38/31	0.167
Disease duration diagnosis mean, (SD)	11.0 (9.2)	10.8 (8.6)	11.2 (9.4)	0.837
On treatment > 6 months, %	92	90	93	0.057
Swollen joints	0 (-0–1)	0 (0–1.5)	0 (0–1)	0.359
SJC of 0, *n* (%)	63 (70)	13 (62)	50 (72)	
SJC of 1, *n* (%)	8 (9)	3 (14)	5 (7)	
SJC of 2, *n* (%)	5 (6)	2 (10)	3 (4)	
SJC of ≥3, *n* (%)	14 (16)	3 (14)	11 (16)	
Tender joints	1 (0–3)	1 (0–2)	1 (0–3)	0.923
TJC of 0, *n* (%)	36 (40)	7 (33)	29 (42)	
TJC of 1, *n* (%)	16 (18)	8 (38)	8 (12)	
TJC of 2, *n* (%)	12 (13)	2 (10)	10 (15)	
TJC of ≥3, *n (%)*	25 (27)	4 (20)	21 (30)	
Number of dactylitic digits	0 (0–0)	0 (0–0)	0 (0–0)	0.310
Dactylitic digits ≥1, *n* (%)	8 (9)	3 (14)	5 (8)	
Number of enthesitis points	0 (0–0)	0 (0–0)	0 (0–0)	0.384
Enthesitis points ≥1, *n* (%)	16 (18)	5 (24)	11 (16)	
VAS physician skin severity	1 (1–3)	2 (1–3.5)	1 (1–2)	0.478
VAS physician overall disease activity	2 (1–4)	3 (2–5)	2 (1–3)	0.007
VAS patient global disease activity	5 (2–7)	6 (3–7)	5 (2–7)	0.157
VAS pt pain	5 (2–7)	6 (3–7)	4 (2–7)	0.225
BASDAI	4.1 (2.5–5.9)	4.2 (2.7–5.8)	3.7 (2.5–5.9)	0.907
cDAPSA remission, *n* (%)	9 (10)	1 (5)	8 (12)	0.594
cDAPSA low disease activity, *n* (%)	34 (38)	7 (33)	27 (39)	
cDAPSA moderate disease activity, *n* (%)	35 (39)	11 (52)	23 (33)	
cDAPSA high disease activity, *n* (%)	6 (7)	2 (10)	4 (6)	
cDAPSA missing, *n* (%)	6 (7)	0	6 (9)	

Numbers are median (IQR) unless stated otherwise. Significance of the comparisons is determined by independent sample *t* test for continues variables and the Mann-Whitney *U* test for non-normally distributed variables. The comparisons within the cDAPSA groups were determined by the Kruskall-Wallis test
SJC swollen joint count, *TJC* tender joint count, *VAS* visual analog scale, *BASDAI* Bath Ankylosing Spondylitis Disease Activity Index, *cDAPSA* clinical Disease Activity in PsA score

treatment intensification ($n = 2$; one patient was recently diagnosed with breast cancer and one patient had undergone surgery complicated by insufficient wound healing); side effects limit use of optimal dosage for treatment ($n = 1$); patient is incompliant to therapy ($n = 1$). Overall, judgment by the rheumatologist and/or patient rather than objective hurdles to intensify treatment (absence of additional treatment options, lack of compliance, intolerance) drove the decision not to modify treatment despite the presence of residual disease activity.

Discussion

This prospective, cross-sectional study in 142 patients with PsA in daily clinical practice showed that despite being on stable treatment and follow up, almost two third of the patients were considered by the treating rheumatologist to have residual disease activity. Almost half (46%) of these patients had moderate to high disease activity according to the cDAPSA. Residual disease activity was determined by joint disease and pain rather than by active psoriasis. Our findings are perfectly aligned with recently published data from Michelsen et al., showing that only a few patients with PsA fulfilled remission criteria and only 25% fulfilled minimal disease activity (MDA) in daily clinical practice [7]. Whereas these data suggest that a majority of patients may benefit from treatment modification and/or intensification, certainly in an era with emerging novel treatment options, treatment was adjusted in only 21 patients with PsA (23%) with residual disease activity in our cohort. While the cDAPSA showed moderate to high disease activity in almost half of these patients, the rheumatologists reported in a majority of patients that (a) the residual disease was not substantial enough to justify treatment adjustment or (b) that the patient did not wish to adjust treatment. When comparing patients with remaining disease activity with and without treatment adjustment, we found no differences in objective disease activity measures, such as joint counts and patient scores. And albeit remaining disease was more prevalently found in patients treated with either csDMARDs alone or a second TNFi treatment, these groups were not more likely to receive a treatment adjustment. These data suggest that treatment is not adjusted in a large majority of patients with residual disease activity, although options for treatment changes are still available.

The only published treat-to-target study in PsA (TICOPA) reported that despite the clear protocol stating that treatment be adjusted when MDA was not fulfilled, in 37% no treatment adjustment followed [6]. Reported reasons for non-escalation (and not following the TICOPA study protocol) were (1) recent start of current therapy, (2) comorbidity, (3) no therapeutic options left, and (4) unable to tolerate the escalated dose. In our cohort, only a few patients had started or adjusted treatment recently or had severe comorbidity resulting in contraindications for TNFi or csDMARDs. As in TICOPA, the absence of therapeutic options was a decisive factor in a fraction of patients, as we observed more patients with residual disease activity in the group treated with a second TNFi, keeping in mind the new treatments such as ustekinumab only recently came to market and apremilast and secukinumab were not available at the time of our study. Intriguingly, however, residual disease activity was more frequently reported not only in patients treated with a second TNFi (69%), or first TNFi (44%), but also in patients on a csDMARD only (66%). In the latter group, the addition of a TNFi was at that time a very obvious, well-validated and recommended therapeutic alternative, which was not used despite ongoing disease activity [5, 11]. Important to note, in the Netherlands csDMARDS, TNFi, and the newer treatments are approved treatments. They are available and reimbursed to all patients with active PsA when prescribed by a rheumatologist, therefore payer issues can be excluded as an argument for not adjusting treatment.

Collectively, these data suggest that absence of treatment modification/intensification was not due to the absence of therapeutic options in a vast majority of patients. Alternative reasons for not adjusting treatment in patients with PsA with residual disease activity despite additional therapeutic options could include (1) lack of structural disease activity assessment in clinical practice, (2) limited availability of evidence that aggressive treatments result in improved short-term and long-term clinical outcomes, and (3) poor implementation of guidelines and treatment strategies in clinical practice.

As to lack of structural disease activity assessment in clinical practice, Coates et al. reported that PsA-specific measurements are not often used in routine clinical practice and that a target for treatment is defined in less than half of the visits [12]. Measuring activity in all domains and consensus on the definition of residual disease activity are warranted here as guidelines recommend "to achieve the lowest possible level of disease activity in all domains of disease". Although the present study required a systematic evaluation of the different domains of PsA (arthritis, pain, enthesitis, dactylitis, skin) the rheumatologist was not asked to integrate these data in a comprehensive disease activity measure. Relying exclusively on the activity of the joints and/or more global questions, could potentially explain why the rheumatologists considered the complaints as minor in 57% of the patients with PsA with residual disease activity. It would be interesting to study if the use of a comprehensive measure such as MDA or a treat-to-target strategy based on MDA or DAPSA/cDAPSA would change the rheumatologist's opinion on disease activity in the same patients.

A second factor to consider is the familiarity of the rheumatologist with the evidence that profound disease suppression is associated with better short-term and long-term outcomes in PsA. MDA is a well-validated measure [13]. Post-hoc analyses show that a sustained MDA state upon treatment results in better clinical and radiological outcomes [14, 15]. The TICOPA trial confirmed the benefit of the treat-to-target approach in a randomized clinical trial with better clinical and patient-reported outcomes in the treat-to-target arm compared with standard clinical care [6]. Importantly, the data from TICOPA became available after the inclusion of patients in the present study was completed. It would be interesting to assess if the availability of these new data would change the opinion of the rheumatologist.

The third and final factor is to what extent guidelines and treatment strategies are really implemented in daily clinical practice. The implementation of guidelines in rheumatology clinical practice has been shown to be a challenge. Studies in rheumatoid arthritis indicate that there is a discrepancy between the reported acceptance of guidelines and the application of these in clinical practice [16, 17]. The IRIS study even showed that despite participation in 2 years of educational training, rheumatologists seem to be reluctant to apply recommendations in real-life clinical practice [18]. These factors could play a role in PsA as well, and attention to the implementation of concepts and guidelines may even be the most important factor to consider when developing treatment strategies for PsA.

As this was a real-life, non-interventional study, the limitations to our study include (a) we did not have any influence on the treatment strategy applied by the rheumatologists; however, csDMARDS (oral and subcutaneous) and TNFi are available and reimbursed to all patients with active PsA when prescribed by a rheumatologist; (b) we incorporated measurements feasible for use in our current clinical practice and therefore did not include a measurement of nail disease or physical functioning, and did not collect laboratory or radiological data; (c) not including multiple additional measurements resulted in an inability to calculate more comprehensive measures of PsA disease activity such as the Psoriatic Arthritis Disease Activity Score (PASDAS) or MDA, capturing more domains of the disease. Nevertheless, the DAPSA and cDAPSA are measurements suggested for use in the treat-to-target setting of PsA [10]; and (d) we did not have sufficient power to study different subsets of patients.

Conclusions

Within the limits of this cross-sectional evaluation, we conclude that residual disease activity was present in almost two thirds of patients with PsA in a daily clinical practice cohort but triggered treatment adjustment in only a quarter of those patients. Subjective opinions of the rheumatologist and/or the patient rather than comorbidities or a lack of treatment options drove the decision not to adjust treatment despite residual disease activity. With the increasing availability of novel drugs to treat PsA and the ongoing efforts on a consensus for treatment target, better understanding as to why residual disease activity does not lead to treatment adjustment in clinical practice is a third important pillar in developing and implementing treatment strategies to improve outcome in PsA.

Acknowledgements
We would like to thank all patients for their participation and the clinicians in AMC and Reade for their help in the recruitment of patients and the assessments done during their outpatient clinics.

Funding
This work was supported by an unrestricted grant from UCB.

Authors' contributions
Study conception and design: LvM, AvK, and DB. Acquisition of the data: LvM, IF and SA. Analysis or interpretation of the data: LvM, AvK, and DB. All authors were involved in drafting the article or revising it critically for important intellectual content and all authors approved the final version to be published.

Consent for publication
Not applicable.

Competing interests
LvM, IF, and SA: none declared. MvdS has received speakers/consultancy fees from Takeda, Tillotts, and Benecke MSD. DB has received research grants and speakers/consultancy fees from Pfizer, MSD, AbbVie, UCB, Novartis, Janssen, and Boehringer Ingelheim, and speakers/consultancy fees from Eli Lilly, Roche, BMS, and Glenmark, and is currently an employee of UCB. AvK has received speakers/consultancy fees from Celgene, Janssen-Cilag, Novartis, MSD, and Roche.

Author details
[1]Department of Clinical Immunology & Rheumatology, Amsterdam Rheumatology and immunology Center, Academic Medical Center/University of Amsterdam, Meibergdreef 9, 1105 AZ Amsterdam, The Netherlands.
[2]Rheumatology, Amsterdam Rheumatology and immunology Center | Reade, Amsterdam, The Netherlands.

References

1. Ramiro S, Smolen JS, Landewé R, van der Heijde D, Dougados M, Emery P, et al. Pharmacological treatment of psoriatic arthritis: a systematic literature review for the 2015 update of the EULAR recommendations for the management of psoriatic arthritis. Ann Rheum Dis. 2015. doi: 10.1136/annrheumdis-2015-208466.
2. Kavanaugh A, Puig L, Gottlieb AB, Ritchlin C, You Y, Li S, et al. Efficacy and safety of ustekinumab in psoriatic arthritis patients with peripheral arthritis and physician-reported spondylitis: post-hoc analyses from two phase III, multicentre, double-blind, placebo-controlled studies (PSUMMIT-1/PSUMMIT-2). Ann Rheum Dis. 2016;1. doi: 10.1136/annrheumdis-2015-209068.
3. Kavanaugh A, Mease PJ, Gomez-Reino JJ, Adebajo AO, Wollenhaupt J, Gladman DD, et al. Treatment of psoriatic arthritis in a phase 3 randomised, placebo-controlled trial with apremilast, an oral phosphodiesterase 4 inhibitor. Ann Rheum Dis. 2014;73:1020–6. doi: 10.1136/annrheumdis-2013-205056.
4. Mease PJ, McInnes IB, Kirkham B, Kavanaugh A, Rahman P, van der Heijde D, et al. Secukinumab Inhibition of interleukin-17A in patients with psoriatic arthritis. N Engl J Med. 2015;373:1329–39. doi: 10.1056/NEJMoa1412679.
5. Gossec L, Smolen JS, Ramiro S, de Wit M, Cutolo M, Dougados M, et al. European League Against Rheumatism (EULAR) recommendations for the management of psoriatic arthritis with pharmacological therapies: 2015 update. Ann Rheum Dis. 2015. 10.1136/annrheumdis-2015-208337.
6. Coates LC, Moverley AR, McParland L, Brown S, Navarro-Coy N, O'Dwyer JL, et al. Effect of tight control of inflammation in early psoriatic arthritis (TICOPA): a UK multicentre, open-label, randomised controlled trial. Lancet. 2015;386:2489–98. doi: http://www.thelancet.com/pdfs/journals/lancet/PIIS0140-6736(15)00347-5.pdf.
7. Michelsen B, Diamantopoulos AP, Høiberg HK, Soldal DM, Kavanaugh A, Haugeberg G. Need for improvement in current treatment of psoriatic arthritis: study of an outpatient clinic population. J Rheumatol. 2017. doi: 10.3899/jrheum.160973.
8. Taylor W, Gladman D, Helliwell P, Marchesoni A, Mease P, Mielants H. Classification criteria for psoriatic arthritis: development of new criteria from a large international study. Arthritis Rheum. 2006;54:2665–73.
9. Schoels MM, Aletaha D, Alasti F, Smolen JS. Disease activity in psoriatic arthritis (PsA): defining remission and treatment success using the DAPSA score. Ann Rheum Dis. 2015. doi: 10.1136/annrheumdis-2015-207507.
10. Smolen JS, Schöls M, Braun J, Dougados M, FitzGerald O, Gladman DD, et al. Treating axial spondyloarthritis and peripheral spondyloarthritis, especially psoriatic arthritis, to target: 2017 update of recommendations by an international task force. Ann Rheum Dis. 2017. doi: 10.1136/annrheumdis-2017-211734.

11. Coates LC, Kavanaugh A, Mease PJ, Soriano ER, Laura Acosta Felquer M, Armstrong AW, et al. Group for research and assessment of psoriasis and psoriatic arthritis: treatment recommendations for psoriatic arthritis 2015. Arthritis Rheumatol (Hoboken, NJ). 2016;67. doi: 10.1002/art.39573.
12. Coates LC, Helliwell PS. Treating to target in psoriatic arthritis: how to implement in clinical practice. Ann Rheum Dis. 2015;27. doi: 10.1136/annrheumdis-2015-208617.
13. Coates LC, Fransen J, Helliwell PS. Defining minimal disease activity in psoriatic arthritis: a proposed objective target for treatment. Ann Rheum Dis. 2010;69:48–53.
14. Kavanaugh A, van der Heijde D, Beutler A, Gladman D, Mease P, Krueger GG, et al. Radiographic progression of patients with psoriatic arthritis who achieve minimal disease activity in response to golimumab therapy: results through 5 years of a randomized, placebo-controlled study. Arthritis Care Res (Hoboken). 2016;68:267–74.
15. Van Der Heijde D, Landewé R, Baraliakos X, Houben H, Van Tubergen A, Williamson P, et al. Radiographic findings following two years of infliximab therapy in patients with ankylosing spondylitis. Arthritis Rheum. 2008;58: 3063–70.
16. Krüger K, Karberg K. "Treat-To-Target" aus der Sicht der niedergelassenen Rheumatologie. Z Rheumatol. 2011;70:664–9. German.
17. Littlejohn G, Roberts L, Arnold M, Bird P, Burnet S, de Jager J, et al. A multicenter, observational study shows high proportion of Australian rheumatoid arthritis patients have inadequate disease control. Int J Rheum Dis. 2013;16: 532–8.
18. Gvozdenović E, Allaart CF, van der Heijde D, Ferraccioli G, Smolen JS, Huizinga TWJ, et al. When rheumatologists report that they agree with a guideline, does this mean that they practise the guideline in clinical practice? Results of the International Recommendation Implementation Study (IRIS). RMD Open. 2016;2:e000221.

13

The epidemiology of psoriatic arthritis in Israel

Lihi Eder[1,2*], Arnon Dov Cohen[3,4], Ilan Feldhamer[3], Sari Greenberg-Dotan[3], Erez Batat[3] and Devy Zisman[5,6]

Abstract

Background: There is limited information on the epidemiology of psoriatic arthritis (PsA) in general and in Middle Eastern populations in particular. The aims of this study were to estimate the prevalence and incidence rates of PsA and their temporal trends in the general population in Israel.

Methods: In this study, a cohort of adult patients with PsA was derived from the database of Clalit Health Services (CHS), Israel's largest health fund, with over 4.4 million members. The crude and age- and sex-standardized prevalence and incidence rates of PsA from 2006 to 2015 in the general population were calculated. The variation in PsA prevalence was assessed in relation to several demographic factors.

Results: Among the 2,931,199 individuals aged 18 years and older registered in the CHS database in 2015, 4490 patients had a diagnosis of PsA (322 incident cases), resulting in overall crude prevalence and incidence rates of 0. 153% (95% CI 0.149%, 0.158%) and 10.9 (95% CI 9.8, 12.3) per 100,000 population, respectively. The reported prevalence of PsA in Israel has doubled between 2006 and 2015 (from 0.073% to 0.153%). In contrast, the global incidence rate remained stable, with a gradual increase in incidence among individuals aged 51 to 70 years. PsA is associated with Jewish ethnicity, high socioeconomic status, and higher body mass index.

Conclusions: The prevalence and incidence of PsA in Israel are within the range of previous estimates from Southern European populations. An increase in the reported prevalence of PsA was observed over the past decade in the general population in Israel.

Keywords: Psoriasis, Psoriatic arthritis, Spondyloarthritis, Epidemiology, Middle East

Background

Psoriasis is a chronic inflammatory skin condition affecting 2–3% of the general population in Europe and North America [1, 2]. Psoriatic arthritis (PsA) is a chronic, potentially destructive inflammatory arthritis affecting people with psoriasis. There is limited data about the population-based epidemiology of PsA. Researchers have estimated that the prevalence of PsA in the general population ranges from 0.05% to 0.67%, whereas the incidence rates range from 6.1 to 41.3 [3–7] per 100,000 population. The majority of these studies were conducted in Europe and North America among people of European origin. Researchers in recent studies in East Asia reported significantly lower prevalence and incidence rates of PsA among Asian individuals [8–10]. There is very little data about the epidemiology of PsA in Middle Eastern populations from various ethnic groups [11, 12]. Assessing the epidemiology of PsA in such populations could contribute to the understanding of the worldwide burden of the disease. Furthermore, because PsA susceptibility is strongly affected by environmental and genetic factors, studying the epidemiology of the disease in ethnically diverse populations from different geographic regions could potentially contribute to the understanding of underlying mechanisms of the disease. The aims of this study were to estimate the prevalence of PsA and its variation among different age, sex, and ethnic subgroups in the general population in Israel and to assess the temporal trends in the population-based prevalence and incidence of PsA in Israel over the past decade.

* Correspondence: lihi.eder@wchospital.ca
[1]Women's College Research Institute, Women's College Hospital, Suite 6326, 76 Grenville St, Toronto, Ontario M5S 1B2, Canada
[2]Department of Medicine, University of Toronto, Toronto, ON, Canada
Full list of author information is available at the end of the article

Methods

Patients and setting

The study was conducted using data from 2002 to 2015 stored in the Clalit Health Services (CHS) database. CHS is one of the four not-for-profit health maintenance organizations that provide hospital- and community-based medical services, including medical treatments, diagnostic tests, and hospitalizations, for the Israeli population. All Israeli residents are required by law to choose to be covered by one of the health maintenance organizations, of which CHS is the largest, providing medical services to approximately 4.4 million enrollees (52% of Israel's population). The population served by CHS is broadly representative of the Israeli population in terms of demographics, geographic distribution, and ethnic diversity. The CHS database includes detailed demographics and clinical data, including sociodemographic information derived from Israel's Central Bureau of Statistics and the National Insurance Institute (Social Security). The database has real-time input from pharmaceutical, medical, and administrative operating systems. The data are compiled into a centralized data warehouse from electronic medical records from primary care and specialist clinics, hospitals, pharmacies, and laboratories. CHS also coordinates a chronic disease registry, and all affiliated primary care physicians provide clinical information on all subjects aged > 20 years with any of 110 chronic diseases based on International Classification of Diseases, Ninth Revision (ICD-9), codes. The CHS database has been used in numerous epidemiological studies, including in the field of psoriatic disease [13, 14].

The study population included all subjects aged 18 years and older and enrolled in CHS at any point between 2006 and 2015. Patients were followed from the time of enrollment in CHS until death, their leaving CHS, or the end of the study in December 2015. The primary analysis of the global and subgroup prevalence of PsA was conducted using the entire CHS population of 2015. The temporal trends in the prevalence and incidence rates of PsA from 2006 to 2015 were assessed. For this analysis, the study populations included all CHS members aged 18 years and older for each assessed year. All data in this study were anonymous to the investigators. The study was approved by the research ethics board of Carmel Medical Center.

Case definition of PsA and psoriasis

In a pilot study, an algorithm for identification of patients with PsA in the CHS database was validated [15]. Two rheumatologists reviewed the medical records of a random sample of 205 patients who received their initial diagnostic code of PsA (ICD-9 code 696.0) in 2014. Based on the medical chart review, a decision was made regarding the disease status: (1) definite/probable/possible PsA, (2) not PsA, or (3) insufficient/no data to verify diagnosis. Several candidate algorithms were tested to determine the one providing the highest positive predictive value. The selected algorithm comprised one of the following conditions: (1) PsA diagnosis assigned at least once by a rheumatologist; (2) permanent diagnosis code assigned by a primary care physician combined with use of synthetic or biologic disease-modifying antirheumatic drugs; or (3) PsA code listed in a hospitalization discharge summary. This algorithm had positive predictive value, sensitivity, and specificity of 90.5%, 88.7%, and 88.1%, respectively.

The methodology for identification of patients with psoriasis in the CHS database has been described previously [16–18]. Briefly, patients were defined as having psoriasis when there was at least one documented diagnosis of psoriasis in the medical records assigned by a CHS dermatologist or when psoriasis was listed in the diagnoses of hospital discharge letters.

Additional information

The following variables were extracted from the database: age, sex, socioeconomic status (SES), ethnicity (Jewish or Arab), area of residence (urban vs. rural), and body mass index (BMI). SES was classified as low, middle, or high according to the neighborhood socioeconomic scores established by the Israel Central Bureau of Statistics as a proxy for SES, represented by a Z-score comparing the Israeli neighborhood mean SES with the neighborhood of a subject [19].

Statistical analysis

The crude and age- and sex-standardized annual prevalence and incidence rates (with corresponding 95% CIs) were calculated for PsA by dividing the number of patients with PsA (aged 18 and over) by the total number of CHS enrollees (aged 18 and over) in the relevant year over the period 2006–2015. The CHS information is available from 2002; however, a 4-year "run-in" period was used to distinguish between incident and prevalent PsA cases. Thus, the prevalence and incidence rates are reported from 2006 onward. Disease onset is defined as the date of the first qualifying health services contact for which a diagnosis of PsA is provided. Patients with such first contacts were considered incident cases of PsA. Prevalent cases were carried forward from the first date they received the diagnosis of PsA until they died, left CHS, or the study ended (December 2015). Annual sex- and age-specific prevalence and incidence rates were calculated for 10-year age groups and expressed as proportions (95% CIs) using the 2006 Israeli population for direct age and sex standardization [20].

In addition, the crude prevalence of PsA (in 2015) was reported separately for each of the following subgroups: sex (males vs. females), ethnicity (Jewish vs. Arab), SES (high, moderate, low), area of residence (urban vs. rural), and BMI category (underweight, normal, overweight, obese). Information about model covariates was obtained for the year of 2015 from the CHS database. The first BMI recorded in the database in 2015 was used. SES was recorded at the end of the calendar year for all patients. Univariable and multivariable logistic regression analyses were conducted to assess the association between the above-detailed variables and PsA compared with the general population. Only patients with complete data were included in the analysis (27.9% of the subjects had missing BMI). A sensitivity analysis was conducted by removing BMI from the regression model. The results were expressed as ORs with 95% CIs.

Results

Among the 2,931,199 individuals aged 18 years and older registered in the CHS database in 2015, 4490 patients had a diagnosis of PsA; of those, 322 patients had a new diagnosis of PsA, resulting in an overall crude prevalence rate of 0.153% (95% CI 0.149%, 0.158%) and incidence rate of 10.9 (95% CI 9.8, 12.3) per 100,000 population (Table 1). Additionally, 110,201 patients had a diagnosis of psoriasis, resulting in an overall crude prevalence of 3.759% (95% CI 3.738%, 3.781%). The prevalence of PsA among patients with psoriasis (in 2015) was 4.07%.

The prevalence of PsA was slightly higher in females (0.159%; 54% of patients) than in males (0.147%; 46% of patients). The prevalence of PsA peaked in the seventh decade of life, at 0.327%. The age at diagnosis of PsA was higher than reported in previous cohorts from Europe and North America, because over half the patients were diagnosed after the age of 50 years (Fig. 1).

Most patients with PsA had a recorded diagnosis of psoriasis (3869 patients [86.2%]). In the majority (2371 [61.3%]), the diagnosis of PsA was recorded following the diagnosis of psoriasis. In 1061 patients (27.4%), the diagnoses of PsA and psoriasis were recorded in the same year, and in the remaining 11.3% of patients, the diagnosis of PsA preceded the diagnosis of psoriasis.

Temporal trend in the prevalence and incidence of PsA from 2006 to 2015

The crude prevalence of PsA doubled during the study period, from 0.073% in 2006 to 0.153% in 2015 (Table 2). A similar increase was observed in the age- and sex-standardized PsA prevalence: from 0.067% in 2006 to 0.137% in 2015 (204% increase). The crude and the age- and sex-standardized incidence rates remained stable from 2006 to 2015 with (approximately 11 per 100,000 population). The prevalence and incidence rates increased in similar degrees in both sexes over time (data not shown). The temporal trends in sex-standardized prevalence and incidence of PsA by age groups are shown in Fig. 2. A more pronounced increase in the prevalence of PsA was observed in the older age groups (61–70 and > 70 years). A gradual upward trend in the incidence rate was observed among middle-aged individuals (51–60, 61–70 years).

Factors associated with PsA

The prevalence of PsA was associated with several demographic and lifestyle factors, as shown in Table 3. The sex distribution of PsA was overall balanced. An association was found between the level of SES and PsA. PsA was most frequent in people with a higher SES (high SES prevalence 0.201%, adjusted OR high vs. low SES 1.29; 95% CI 1.19, 1.42), followed by middle SES (moderate SES prevalence 0.167%, OR middle vs. low SES 1.11; 95% CI 1.03, 1.20) and lowest in the low SES (prevalence 0.116%). Additionally, the distribution of PsA varied by ethnicity, with higher prevalence in individuals of Jewish ethnicity compared with Arabs (adjusted OR 1.64, 95% CI 1.47, 1.82). Last, in accordance with previous literature [21], PsA was more frequent in overweight (prevalence 0.201%; OR 1.41; 95% CI 1.30, 1.54) and obese individuals (prevalence 0.266%; OR 1.80;

Table 1 Prevalence and incidence of psoriatic arthritis in Israel by age and sex in 2015

Age group (years)	Males			Females			All				
	PsA (*n*)	Total (N)	Prevalence (%)	PsA (*n*)	Total (N)	Prevalence (%)	PsA (*n*)	New PsA (N)	Total (N)	Prevalence (%)	Incidence[a]
18–30	73	370,656	0.019	129	389,179	0.033	202	34	759,835	0.027	4.5
31–40	275	306,169	0.089	286	303,310	0.094	561	50	609,479	0.092	8.2
41–50	348	208,302	0.167	359	210,432	0.171	707	62	418,734	0.169	14.8
51–60	482	188,410	0.255	548	209,250	0.262	1,030	79	397,660	0.259	19.9
61–70	569	178,702	0.318	674	201,982	0.333	1,243	60	380,684	0.326	15.8
71–80	225	94,914	0.237	278	121,381	0.229	503	27	216,295	0.232	12.5
>80	93	56,517	0.164	151	91,995	0.164	244	10	148,512	0.164	6.7
All	2065	1,403,670	0.147	2425	1,527,529	0.159	4490	322	2,931,119	0.153	10.9

PsA Psoriatic arthritis
[a]Per 100,000 population

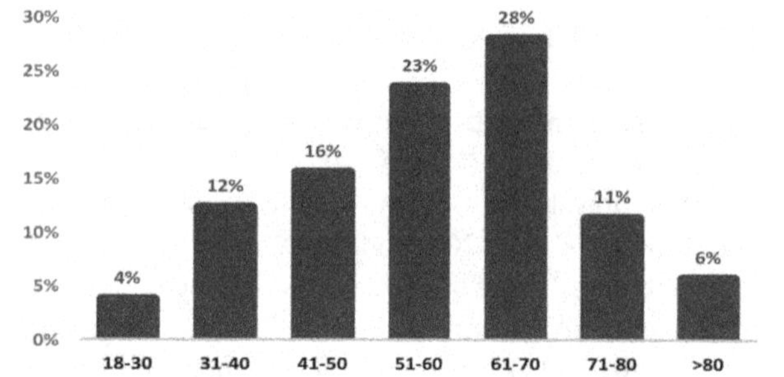

Fig. 1 The distribution of age at diagnosis of psoriatic arthritis among all patients

95% CI 1.65, 1.97) than in people with normal weight (prevalence 0.104%). A sensitivity analysis that removed BMI from the regression model showed essentially the same results (data not shown).

Discussion

In this population-based study, the temporal trends in the prevalence and incidence of PsA in Israel over the past decade were described. The following major findings are presented:

1. In 2015, the prevalence of PsA in the adult population in Israel was 0.153%, and the incidence rate was 10.9 per 100,000 population.
2. The reported prevalence of PsA in Israel has doubled over the past decade. In contrast, the global incidence rate remained relatively stable, except for a gradual increase in the rate among individuals aged 51 to 70 years.
3. PsA was more frequent in people from the following groups: Jewish ethnicity, higher SES, and higher BMI.

The population-based epidemiology of PsA has been investigated mostly in European populations. Limited information exists about the epidemiology of PsA in other ethnic groups and geographic regions, in particular in Middle Eastern populations. Researchers in a few small clinic-based studies assessed epidemiologic features of PsA in Iranian and Turkish patients [11, 12]. To the best our knowledge, this is the first large-scale population-based study that provides information about the prevalence of PsA in a Middle Eastern population including two ethnically diverse subpopulations. Our estimates of the prevalence of PsA in Israel (0.153%) fall well within the prevalence range reported in other population-based studies in Southern European countries, including Greece (0.06–0.17%) [22, 23] and Turkey (0.05%) [11], but tended to be lower than estimates in the United States (0.25%) [24] and Northern European countries such as Sweden (0.25%) [25], Norway (0.19–0.67%) [6, 26], the United Kingdom (0.19%) [3], and Iceland (0.16%) [27]. Moreover, the prevalence of PsA was significantly higher than the reported prevalence in East Asian populations, which is less than 0.10% [9, 10]. Fewer studies assessed the incidence of PsA. Overall, our estimated incidence rate of 10.9 cases per 100,000 population fell within previous estimates in other European populations, which ranged from 6.1 to 41.3 per 100,000 population [4, 6, 7]. The variation in prevalence rates may be attributed to genetic and environmental factors but also to variations in study designs and case definitions. In general, surveys that were based on self-reported diagnosis of PsA found higher prevalence rates than studies that relied on medical records and health administrative data.

The prevalence of PsA among patients with psoriasis in our study was 4.07%, which is lower than the estimated prevalence in other population-based studies (ranging from

Table 2 Crude and age- and sex-standardized prevalence and incidence of psoriatic arthritis in Israel by year (2006–2015)

Year	Prevalence of PsA				Incidence of PsA		
	Total population (*N*)	PsA (*n*)	Crude prevalence (%)	Standardized prevalence (%) (95% CI)[a]	New PsA (*n*)	Crude incidence#	Standardized incidence[a] (95% CI)[b]
2006	2,620,136	1910	0.073	0.067 (0.065, 0.070)	277	10.6	10.4 (9.5, 11.4)
2007	2,648,067	2132	0.081	0.075 (0.072, 0.077)	251	9.8	9.3 (8.4, 10.3)
2008	2,676,404	2425	0.091	0.084 (0.081, 0.086)	308	11.5	11.4 (10.4, 12.4)
2009	2,705,397	2663	0.098	0.091 (0.088, 0.093)	278	10.3	10.1 (9.2, 11.1)
2010	2,734,705	2938	0.107	0.099 (0.096, 0.102)	303	11.1	11.1 (10.1, 12.1)
2011	2,777,279	3237	0.117	0.107 (0.104, 0.110)	330	11.9	11.7 (10.8, 11.8)
2012	2,816,452	3531	0.125	0.114 (0.111, 0.117)	382	12.5	12.3 (11.3, 13.3)
2013	2,861,934	3866	0.135	0.122 (0.119, 0.125)	354	13.4	13.1 (12.0, 14.1)
2014	2,905,530	4223	0.145	0.131 (0.128, 0.134)	404	13.9	13.5 (12.5, 14.6)
2015	2,931,199	4490	0.153	0.137 (0.134, 0.141)	322	11.0	10.6 (9.7, 11.6)

PsA Psoriatic arthritis
[a]Age- and sex-standardized to Israel population in 2006
[b]Crude and standardized rates are per 100,000 population

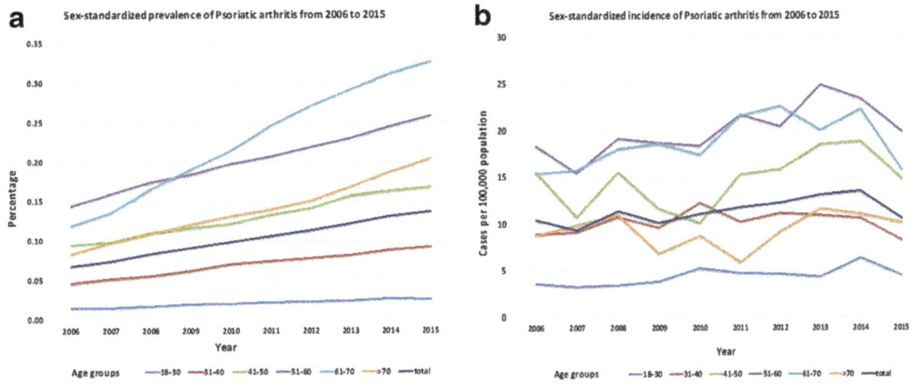

Fig. 2 Sex-standardized prevalence (**a**) and incidence (**b**) of psoriatic arthritis in Israel by age group from 2006 to 2015

4.6% to 11%) [3, 24, 28]. Possible explanations may include the low prevalence of the HLA-B27 antigen in the Israeli population [29], the older peak age of diagnosis of PsA observed in our cohort (range 60 to 70 years) [3, 26, 27], or possibly other genetic and environmental factors that are unique to our population.

We have demonstrated that the crude and age-adjusted prevalence of PsA doubled during the study period. These findings are in line with recent studies from Europe and Asia in which researchers reported an increase in the prevalence and incidence of psoriasis and PsA over time [7, 9, 30, 31]. The observed increase in prevalence may be partially attributed to an increase in the incidence rate among individuals aged 51 to 70 years, which is the peak age of diagnosis of PsA in Israel. Increased awareness of PsA among physicians over the past decade, possibly promoted by the publication of the Classification Criteria for Psoriatic Arthritis (CASPAR) criteria in 2006, educational activities among specialists, the introduction of effective biologic medications for PsA, and the increased use of sensitive diagnostic modalities (e.g., ultrasound) likely contributed to the observed time period effect. Additionally, with the increasing awareness of the disease, it is possible that rheumatologists are more likely to classify a disease as "PsA" rather than "spondyloarthritis," which may explain some of the increase in occurrence over the past decade. Other potential causes, such as increased occurrence of known risk factors for PsA (e.g., obesity) at the population level or changes in the population demographics (e.g., immigration of high-risk groups), are less likely to contribute to the observed increase over such a short time period.

Table 3 Prevalence of psoriatic arthritis by demographic characteristics (in 2015) and their association with psoriatic arthritis by logistic regression analysis

	Prevalence (%)	Univariable model		Multivariable model[a]	
		OR	95% CI	OR	95% CI
Sex					
Female	0.159	1.08	1.02, 1.15	1.03	0.96, 1.10
Male	0.147	1.00		1.00	
Socioeconomic status					
High	0.204	1.76	1.63, 1.90	1.29	1.19, 1.42
Middle	0.167	1.44	1.35, 1.55	1.11	1.03, 1.20
Low	0.116	1.00		1.00	
Ethnicity					
Jewish	0.175	2.13	1.95, 2.33	1.64	1.47, 1.82
Arab	0.082	1.00		1.00	
Residential area					
Urban	0.151	0.82	0.73, 0.92	1.02	0.89, 1.15
Rural	0.184	1.00		1.00	
BMI, kg/m^2					
> 30	0.266	2.57	2.37, 2.80	1.80	1.65, 1.97
25–30	0.200	1.94	1.78, 2.10	1.41	1.30, 1.54
18.5–25	0.106	1.00		1.00	
< 18.5	0.068	0.63	0.47, 0.86	0.98	0.72, 1.33

BMI Body mass index
[a]The model was also adjusted for age group
CI Confidence Interval, *OR* Odds Ratio

Several demographic factors were associated with the occurrence of PsA. As in other studies, PsA was almost equally distributed between women and men (female/male ratio 1.08) [3]. Other factors that influenced the occurrence of PsA were ethnicity, SES, and BMI. The prevalence of PsA was almost twofold higher in the Jewish population than among Arab individuals. This difference in disease occurrence may be related to variations in genetic structure, environmental exposures, or issues related to healthcare use [21]. With regard to impact of genetic heterogeneity within the Jewish population on the occurrence of PsA, information about family origin is unavailable in the CHS database.

This study has several limitations that should be taken into consideration. First, we could not capture patients with PsA who did not seek medical attention or those who were undiagnosed as having PsA. Nonetheless, we estimated the proportion of the population that places a burden on the healthcare system. Second, the case definition is based on diagnostic coding from electronic medical records that are based on physician diagnoses. This may have led to misclassification of cases. This risk, however, was minimized by selection of an algorithm with high accuracy that used data based largely on a diagnosis by relevant specialists. The primary strength of the study is the use of a large representative sample of over half the Israeli population. Consequently, the results of the study could be generalized to the broader population beyond those patients included in our study.

Conclusions

In summary, the epidemiology of PsA is much less studied than in many other rheumatic diseases. High-quality real-world data about the epidemiology of PsA is of clear importance for understanding the burden of the disease on society. Our study, which included over 4000 patients with PsA, is one of the largest population-based studies to date and is the first to include an evaluation of the prevalence of PsA in Middle Eastern individuals. The prevalence of PsA in the adult Israeli population in 2015 was 0.153%. The reported prevalence of PsA has doubled over the past decade, highlighting the rising medical needs and economic burden of this patient population. Further studies are needed to continue monitoring this trend and understand its underlying causes.

Abbreviations

BMI: Body mass index; CHS: Clalit Health Services; PsA: Psoriatic arthritis; SES: Socioeconomic status

Acknowledgements

Not applicable.

Funding

No funding was received for this study. LE is supported by a New Investigator Salary Award from the Arthritis Society and the Canadian Association of Psoriasis Patients.

Authors' contributions

LE, ADC, IF, SGD, EB, and DZ conceived of and designed the study. LE, ADC, IF, and DZ analyzed and interpreted the data. LE, ADC, IF, SGD, EB, and DZ prepared the manuscript. All authors read and approved the final manuscript.

Consent for publication

Not applicable.

Competing interests

The authors declare that they have no competing interests.

Author details

[1]Women's College Research Institute, Women's College Hospital, Suite 6326, 76 Grenville St, Toronto, Ontario M5S 1B2, Canada. [2]Department of Medicine, University of Toronto, Toronto, ON, Canada. [3]Chief Physician's Office, Central Headquarters, Clalit Health Services, Tel Aviv, Israel. [4]Siaal Research Center for Family Medicine and Primary Care, Faculty of Health Sciences, Ben-Gurion University of the Negev, Be'er-Sheva, Israel. [5]Department of Rheumatology, Carmel Medical Center, Haifa, Israel. [6]The Ruth and Bruce Rappaport Faculty of Medicine, Technion—Israel Institute of Technology, Haifa, Israel.

References

1. Gelfand JM, Weinstein R, Porter SB, Neimann AL, Berlin JA, Margolis DJ. Prevalence and treatment of psoriasis in the United Kingdom: a population-based study. Arch Dermatol. 2005;141:1537–41.
2. Langley RG, Krueger GG, Griffiths CE. Psoriasis: epidemiology, clinical features, and quality of life. Ann Rheum Dis. 2005;64 Suppl 2:ii18–25.
3. Ogdie A, Langan S, Love T, Haynes K, Shin D, Seminara N, et al. Prevalence and treatment patterns of psoriatic arthritis in the UK. Rheumatology (Oxford). 2013;52:568–75.
4. Alamanos Y, Voulgari P, Drosos A. Incidence and prevalence of psoriatic arthritis: a systematic review. J Rheumatol. 2008;35:1354–8.
5. Stolwijk C, van Onna M, Boonen A, van Tubergen A. Global prevalence of spondyloarthritis: a systematic review and meta-regression analysis. Arthritis Care Res (Hoboken). 2016;68:1320–31.
6. Hoff M, Gulati AM, Romundstad PR, Kavanaugh A, Haugeberg G. Prevalence and incidence rates of psoriatic arthritis in central Norway: data from the Nord-Trondelag health study (HUNT). Ann Rheum Dis. 2015;74:60–4.
7. Egeberg A, Kristensen LE, Thyssen JP, Gislason GH, Gottlieb AB, Coates LC, et al. Incidence and prevalence of psoriatic arthritis in Denmark: a nationwide register linkage study. Ann Rheum Dis. 2017;76(9):1591–7.
8. Oh EH, Ro YS, Kim JE. Epidemiology and cardiovascular comorbidities in patients with psoriasis: a Korean nationwide population-based cohort study. J Dermatol. 2017;44(6):621–9.
9. Wang TS, Hsieh CF, Tsai TF. Epidemiology of psoriatic disease and current treatment patterns from 2003 to 2013: a nationwide, population-based observational study in Taiwan. J Dermatol Sci. 2016;84:340–5.
10. Li R, Sun J, Ren LM, Wang HY, Liu WH, Zhang XW, et al. Epidemiology of eight common rheumatic diseases in China: a large-scale cross-sectional survey in Beijing. Rheumatology (Oxford). 2012;51:721–9.
11. Cakir N, Pamuk ON, Dervis E, Imeryuz N, Uslu H, Benian O, et al. The prevalences of some rheumatic diseases in western Turkey: Havsa study. Rheumatol Int. 2012;32:895–908.
12. Jamshidi F, Bouzari N, Seirafi H, Farnaghi F, Firooz A. The prevalence of psoriatic arthritis in psoriatic patients in Tehran. Iran Arch Iran Med. 2008;11:162–5.
13. Shapiro J, Cohen AD, Weitzman D, Tal R, David M. Psoriasis and cardiovascular risk factors: a case-control study on inpatients comparing psoriasis to dermatitis. J Am Acad Dermatol. 2012;66:252–8.
14. Zisman D, Bitterman H, Shalom G, Feldhamer I, Comanesther D, Batat E, et al. Psoriatic arthritis treatment and the risk of herpes zoster. Ann Rheum Dis. 2016;75:131–5.
15. Eder L, Cohen AD, Feldhamer I, Greenberg-Dotan S, Batat E, Zisman D. Validity of diagnostic codes and point prevalence of psoriatic arthritis in Israel – a population-based study [abstract 1697]. Arthritis Rheumatol. 2016; 68(Suppl 10).
16. Cohen AD, Sherf M, Vidavsky L, Vardy DA, Shapiro J, Meyerovitch J. Association between psoriasis and the metabolic syndrome: a cross-sectional study. Dermatology. 2008;216:152–5.
17. Cohen AD, Dreiher J, Shapiro Y, Vidavsky L, Vardy DA, Davidovici B, et al. Psoriasis and diabetes: a population-based cross-sectional study. J Eur Acad Dermatol Venereol. 2008;22:585–9.
18. Dreiher J, Weitzman D, Shapiro J, Davidovici B, Cohen AD. Psoriasis and chronic obstructive pulmonary disease: a case-control study. Br J Dermatol. 2008;159:956–60.
19. Filc D, Davidovich N, Novack L, Balicer RD. Is socioeconomic status associated with utilization of health care services in a single-payer universal health care system? Int J Equity Health. 2014;13:115.
20. Statistical Abstract of Israel 2006. Israeli Central Bureau of Statistics. http://www.cbs.gov.il/reader/shnaton/shnatonh_new.htm?CYear=2006&Vol=57&CSubject=2. Accessed 22 Jan 2017.

21. Love TJ, Zhu Y, Zhang Y, Wall-Burns L, Ogdie A, Gelfand JM, et al. Obesity and the risk of psoriatic arthritis: a population-based study. Ann Rheum Dis. 2012;71:1273–7.
22. Trontzas P, Andrianakos A, Miyakis S, Pantelidou K, Vafiadou E, Garantziotou V, et al. Seronegative spondyloarthropathies in Greece: a population-based study of prevalence, clinical pattern, and management. The ESORDIG study Clin Rheumatol. 2005;24:583–9.
23. Alamanos Y, Papadopoulos NG, Voulgari PV, Siozos C, Psychos DN, Tympanidou M, et al. Epidemiology of psoriatic arthritis in northwest Greece, 1982-2001. J Rheumatol. 2003;30:2641–4.
24. Gelfand JM, Gladman DD, Mease PJ, Smith N, Margolis DJ, Nijsten T, et al. Epidemiology of psoriatic arthritis in the population of the United States. J Am Acad Dermatol. 2005;53:573.
25. Haglund E, Bremander AB, Petersson IF, Strombeck B, Bergman S, Jacobsson LT, et al. Prevalence of spondyloarthritis and its subtypes in southern Sweden. Ann Rheum Dis. 2011;70:943–8.
26. Madland TM, Apalset EM, Johannessen AE, Rossebo B, Brun JG. Prevalence, disease manifestations, and treatment of psoriatic arthritis in Western Norway. J Rheumatol. 2005;32:1918–22.
27. Love TJ, Gudbjornsson B, Gudjonsson JE, Valdimarsson H. Psoriatic arthritis in Reykjavik, Iceland: prevalence, demographics, and disease course. J Rheumatol. 2007;34:2082–8.
28. Karreman MC, Weel AE, van der Ven M, Vis M, Tchetverikov I, Nijsten TE, et al. Prevalence of psoriatic arthritis in primary care patients with psoriasis. Arthritis Rheumatol. 2016;68:924–31.
29. Elkayam O, Segal R, Caspi D. Human leukocyte antigen distribution in Israeli patients with psoriatic arthritis. Rheumatol Int. 2004;24:93–7.
30. Danielsen K, Olsen AO, Wilsgaard T, Furberg AS. Is the prevalence of psoriasis increasing? A 30-year follow-up of a population-based cohort. Br J Dermatol. 2013;168:1303–10.
31. Icen M, Crowson CS, McEvoy MT, Dann FJ, Gabriel SE, Maradit KH. Trends in incidence of adult-onset psoriasis over three decades: a population-based study. J Am Acad Dermatol. 2009;60:394–401.

14

Abatacept reduces synovial regulatory T-cell expression in patients with psoriatic arthritis

Agnes Szentpetery[1], Eric Heffernan[2], Martina Gogarty[3], Lisa Mellerick[4], Janet McCormack[5], Muhammad Haroon[1], Musaab Elmamoun[1], Phil Gallagher[1], Genevieve Kelly[6], Aurelie Fabre[4,5], Brian Kirby[6] and Oliver FitzGerald[1*]

Abstract

Background: The aim was to study changes in immunohistochemical expression markers of synovial and skin inflammation, clinical outcomes and magnetic resonance imaging (MRI) scores with abatacept treatment in patients with psoriatic arthritis (PsA).

Methods: Biological-treatment-naïve PsA patients with active disease including synovitis of a knee were enrolled in this single-centre, crossover study. Patients were randomised to receive intravenous abatacept 3 mg/kg of body weight or placebo infusion on day 1, 15 and 29; thereafter abatacept 10 mg/kg of body weight was administered every 28 days for 5 months. Clinical data were collected at each visit. Synovial biopsy of the involved knee was obtained at baseline and 2 and 6 months. MRI of the same knee and skin biopsy was performed prior to arthroscopy.

Results: Fifteen patients were recruited. Significant improvements in the joint-related measures were observed; 90% were European League Against Rheumatism criteria responders and 30% achieved psoriasis area severity index (PASI)50 at 6 months. Reduction in synovitis ($P = 0.016$) and vascularity ($P = 0.039$) macroscopic scores consistent with decrease in total MRI score ($P = 0.016$) were noticed. Abatacept decreased the immunohistological expression of FOXP3+ cells ($P = 0.027$), specifically the expression of CD4+FOXP3+ regulatory T cells (Tregs) ($P = 0.008$) in the synovium over 6 months. There was no significant clinical or immunohistological change in any of the skin measures.

Conclusion: This is the first study assessing synovial and psoriatic skin immunpathological changes following abatacept treatment in PsA. Reduction in Treg expression in the synovium but not in the psoriatic lesion suggests abnormal Treg function in PsA with differential suppressive capacity in the synovium compared to the lesional skin. The results of this study demonstrate that abatacept 10 mg/kg of body weight might be an effective treatment option for joint disease in patients with PsA.

Keywords: Abatacept, Psoriatic arthritis, Synovium, Skin, Regulatory T-cell, FOXP3

* Correspondence: oliver.fitzgerald@ucd.ie
[1]Department of Rheumatology, St. Vincent's University Hospital, Dublin, Ireland
Full list of author information is available at the end of the article

Background

Psoriatic arthritis (PsA) is a chronic immune-mediated inflammatory disease that affects peripheral joints, entheses and axial sites along with skin and nails. In addition to the characteristic extra-articular features, such as uveitis and inflammatory bowel disease, PsA is also associated with comorbidities [1, 2].

Interplay between the adaptive and innate immune system, activation of T cells and subsequent production of inflammatory cytokines such as TNF, interferon (IFN)-γ, IL-17 and IL-22 have a dominant pathogenic role in psoriatic plaques [3, 4]. In PsA, CD8+ T cells may represent key players that recognise antigens presented by human leukocyte antigen (HLA) class 1 molecules [5]. CD8+ T cells are found in greater numbers in synovial fluid and in entheseal sites while CD4+ T cells are more abundant in synovial tissue [5–7].

Regulatory T cells (Tregs) are a subset of CD4+ CD25high T lymphocytes that require forkhead box transcription factor (FOXP3) for their suppressive function [4, 8, 9]. Tregs derived from the thymus mediate suppression through a contact-dependent mechanism including cytotoxic T-lymphocyte antigen 4 (CTLA-4) [10]. Increased Treg expression compared to normal skin has been reported in psoriatic lesions, irrespective of the disease severity. Previous studies indicated an abnormal phenotype and impaired function of synovial Tregs in rheumatoid arthritis (RA) and increased FOXP3 expression in synovial CD4+ T cells in rheumatoid factor (RF)-negative RA and PsA compared to seropositive RA [10–12]. Tregs isolated from peripheral blood and psoriatic skin have dysfunctional activity in suppressing effector T-cell responses in psoriasis [13–16].

Due to the heterogeneity of PsA, identifying appropriate treatment for each individual can be challenging. Patients with peripheral arthritis that does not respond to disease-modifying antirheumatic drugs (DMARDs) are recommended for treatment with apremilast or biologic agents (TNFi, IL-12/23i and IL17i), IL-12/23i and IL17i) are recommended [17]. Since not all patients respond to these agents and many patients' initial responses wane over time due to immunogenicity, poor tolerability and/or adverse events, it has been important to develop new therapies that target other key cytokines and immunologic pathways [18]. Targeting T cells, the main mediators of the pathogenic processes in PsA, can potentially have a significant role in the future immunotherapy of the disease.

Abatacept is a soluble, fully human fusion protein consisting of the extracellular domain of CLTA-4 linked to human IgG1 [19]. Abatacept selectively binds to CD80/86 on antigen-presenting cells blocking the costimulatory interaction with CD28 on T-cells, and thereby inhibits optimal T-cell activation and decreases production of inflammatory cytokines such as TNFα, INFγ, IL-2 and IL-6 [20–22]. Abatacept is approved in RA and juvenile idiopathic arthritis [23, 24]. One phase 2 randomised controlled trial of abatacept in PsA showed significant American College of Rheumatologists (ACR)20 responses, but only modest improvement in skin measures compared to placebo (PBO) [25]. More recently, a randomised, placebo-controlled, phase 3 trial of abatacept in PsA reported benefits of abatacept in ACR20 responses, regardless of TNFi exposure, with modest benefit on psoriasis lesions [26].

A few studies have evaluated synovial changes after different therapies in PsA [27], but the effect of abatacept on synovial and skin tissue has not been previously studied. Therefore, our aim was to study changes in immunohistochemical markers of synovial and skin inflammation, including FOXP3 expression, after introducing abatacept treatment in PsA. Secondary objectives were to (1) assess clinical outcomes and magnetic resonance imaging (MRI) changes over time, (2) evaluate the impact of a short period of abatacept 3 mg/kg of body weight treatment compared to PBO and (3) investigate if cell markers of synovial inflammation correlate with disease activity measures and MRI synovitis scores.

Methods

Patients

PsA patients fulfilling the classification criteria for psoriatic arthritis (CASPAR) [28] with active disease of ≥3 months duration (tender joint count ≥3 and swollen joint count ≥3), aged 18 to 80 years were recruited. Patients had to have clinical synovitis of the knee and have agreed to undergo synovial biopsies. Presence of a psoriatic skin lesion was not requisite. Participants must not have been exposed to a previous biologic DMARD. Methotrexate (MTX) was the only concomitant synthetic DMARD (sDMARD) permitted in the study. Patients who were on a stable dose of MTX (7.5–25 mg/week) for >3 months prior to randomisation remained on this stable dose for the duration of the study. A decrease in the MTX dosage was allowed in cases of toxicity. The use of a stable dose of prednisolone <10 mg/day or its equivalent, and of a nonsteroidal anti-inflammatory drug (NSAID) was permitted during the study. Decrease in NSAIDs was permitted but only if due to toxicity.

Key exclusion criteria were concurrent autoimmune diseases or skin conditions other than plaque psoriasis, arthritis mutilans, pregnancy, breast feeding, evidence of latent or active tuberculosis, evidence of chronic or clinically significant infection or malignancy.

Informed, written consent was obtained from all study participants according to the Declaration of Helsinki. The study was approved by St. Vincent's Healthcare Group Ethics and Medical Research Committee.

Study design and treatment

This study was a single-centre, placebo-controlled, crossover study of 15 patients with PsA. Patients were randomised to receive abatacept 3 mg/kg of body weight (approved dosing for RA) or PBO infusions on day 1, 15 and 29; thereafter abatacept 10 mg/kg of body weight was administered every 28 days for 5 months (on day 57, 85, 113, 141 and 169). Treatments were administered as a 30-minute intravenous infusion; dosing was calculated based on body weight at screening (500 mg, 750 mg and 1000 mg for patients weighing <60 kg, 60–100 kg and >100 kg, respectively).

Clinical and laboratory assessments

Demographic data collected included age, sex, psoriasis and psoriatic arthritis disease duration, menopausal status, previous use of sDMARDs, current use of MTX, oral corticosteroids and calcium and vitamin D supplements. Clinical assessments were performed at each visit. Clinical variables included disease activity score in 28 joints (DAS28) with four variables (DAS28-erythrocyte sedimentation rate (ESR) and DAS28-C-reactive protein (CRP)), tender joint count (TJC) 28 and 68, swollen joint count (SJC) 28 and 66, number of digits with dactylitis, enthesitis score based on the Leeds enthesitis index (LEI), number of affected nails on the hands (0–10) and psoriasis area severity index (PASI) [29, 30]. Patients' self-reported parameters such as duration of early morning stiffness (EMS), visual analogue scale for global health (GVAS), pain and fatigue scores, health assessment questionnaire (HAQ), dermatology life quality index (DLQI) and PsA-specific quality of life score (PsAQol) were recorded [30, 31]. Laboratory assessments included a recording of the following parameters: RF positivity, antibodies against cyclic citrullinated peptides (aCCP), ESR and CRP.

Efficacy and safety assessments

Joint and skin-related response to abatacept or PBO was assessed using the European League Against Rheumatism (EULAR) response criteria and a 50% improvement in the PASI score (PASI50) [32]. Safety evaluations were obtained at each visit including routine laboratory tests and monitoring of adverse events (AEs) for severity of the event (mild, moderate, severe or very severe), the investigator's opinion of its relationship to abatacept/PBO treatment (not related, unlikely or possibly related) and information on outcomes.

Synovial and skin biopsies

Arthroscopy of the same involved knee joint was performed using a Wolf (Illinois, USA) 2.7-mm needle arthroscope under local anaesthesia at three time points (day 1, 57 and 169). Macroscopic synovitis and vascularity were scored on a visual analogue scale (VAS) (0–100 mm). Synovial membrane biopsies were obtained from at least six sites within the joint (suprapatellar pouch, medial and lateral gutters, infrapatellar and tibiofemoral regions and cartilage pannus junction near the patellar rim) using 1.5-mm grasping forceps [33, 34].

Under local anaesthesia, patients underwent a 6-mm-punch skin biopsy at three time points (day -28, 54 and 166). Biopsies were taken from the centre of a target psoriasis lesion from the same plaque [15].

Immunohistochemical analysis

Synovial and skin biopsies were embedded in Tissue-Tek optimal cutting temperature (OCT) compound (Sakura, Zoeterwoude, The Netherlands) and stored at -80 °C. Cryostat sections (7 μm) were mounted on slides coated with 3-aminopropyltriethoxysilane (Sigma-Aldrich St. Louis, MO, USA), air-dried overnight, wrapped in foil and stored at -80 °C. A routine three-stage immunoperoxidase labelling technique was used [35]. Tissue sections were thawed and acetone-fixed for 10 minutes. Immunostaining was performed on the Dako Autostainer 48 Link. Sections were processed using the Dako Envision FLEX Mouse Linker kit according to the manufacturer's instructions. DAB was used as the chromogen and slides were counterstained with hematoxylin. The synovial and skin sections were incubated with mouse monoclonal antibodies against T-cell-specific markers CD3 (1:25), CD4 (1:20), CD8 (1:50), CD31 (Dako Ready to use Antibody, Clone numbers: CD3 – F7.2.38, CD4 – 4B12, CD8 – C8/144B, CD31 – JC70A) (Dako, Glostrup, Denmark), and FOXP3 (1:500) (Abcam, Cambridge, UK, Clone: 236A/E7). Sections were also incubated with an appropriate isotype-matched mouse monoclonal antibody (IgG1). Negative control slides omitting the secondary antibodies were also stained.

CD3, CD4 and CD8 expression in the biopsies were scored using a well-established semi-quantitative scoring method on a 5-point scale ranging from 0 to 4 (0 = no staining, 1 ≤ 25%, 2 = 25–50%, 3 = 50–75%, 4 ≥ 75% staining). For evaluation of CD4+ cells, only cells with lymphocyte morphology were included as CD4 can be expressed by macrophages [36, 37]. CD31-expressing microvessels were assessed under × 400 magnification by counting the number of vessels staining per five high power fields (HPF) on two levels when available (=10 HPF/slides). The result for one biopsy was extrapolated from two HPFs, due to the size of the tissue sample. Intranuclear staining for FOXP3 expression was assessed in a semi-quantitative manner as a percentage over 300 cells. (More specifically, 300 lymphocytes were counted at objective × 40 in "hot spots", both in lymphoid aggregates and lymphoid infiltrates, and the number of FOXP3+ cells was divided by 3 to obtain a percentage;

the result was then the average rounded up or down to the nearest whole number.)

Immunofluorescence staining of synovial tissue

To examine synovial tissue co-localization of CD4 with FOXP3, dual immunofluorescence staining was performed on cryostat synovial sections. Cryostat sections were defrosted at room temperature for 20 minutes and fixed in acetone for 10 minutes. Slides were washed in PBS for 5 minutes. Non-specific binding was blocked using 1% casein in PBS for 20 minutes. Slides were co-incubated with rabbit monoclonal antibody against CD4 (1:500, Abcam, Clone: EPR6855) and mouse monoclonal anti-FOXP3 antibody (1:500, Abcam, Clone: 236A/E7). IgG control antibodies were used as negative controls. Following overnight incubation in a humidified chamber at 4 °C, immunofluorescence sections were co-incubated with Alexa 488 goat anti-mouse superclonal™ secondary antibody (1:200, Invitrogen) and Cy™3-conjugated goat anti-rabbit secondary antibody (1:500, Jackson ImmunoResearch) for 60 minutes. Sections were mounted with Antifade (Molecular Probes) and assessed by immunofluorescence microscopy (Olympus BX51). The number of CD4+FOXP3+ Tregs at baseline and 6 months was scored manually by two independent readers on cryostat sections by identifying cells that had clear signals for co-expression of CD4 and FOXP3 on merged images.

Magnetic resonance imaging

MRI scan of the same involved knee was performed in each patient 3 days prior to arthroscopy at baseline, 2 and 6 months using a 1.5 T Signa Excite HD MRI scanner (GE Healthcare, UK) and a dedicated eight-channel array HD knee surface coil, with patients lying supine. The examinations performed included intravenous contrast (Gadolinium diethylenetriamine penta-acetic acid) enhanced, T1-weighted, fat-suppressed pulse sequences in coronal, sagittal and axial planes. The following scanning parameters were used: coronal, repetition time (TR) 640 ms; echo time (TE) 16; slice thickness 4/1 mm; field of view (FOV) 18; NEX 2; matrix 512 × 256; sagittal, TR 500; TE 16; slice thickness 4/1 mm; FOV 22; NEX 2; matrix 256 × 192 axial, TR 440; TE 11; slice thickness 3/1.5 mm; FOV 16; NEX 3; matrix 224 × 192.

Images were scored using the psoriatic arthritis MRI synovitis score (PsAMRIS) semi-quantitative method by one consultant radiologist with a special interest in musculoskeletal radiology, who was blind to patient identity and scan chronology. Each knee was divided into four anatomical regions ((medial (MED) and lateral (LAT) parapatellar recesses, intercondylar notch (ICN) and suprapatellar pouch (SPP)) and a synovitis score ranging from 0 to 3 was assigned to each region (0 = normal synovium, 1 = diffuse, even thickening, 2 = nodular thickening, 3 = gross, nodular thickening) based on the overall impression of the severity of synovial abnormality in the three orthogonal scanning planes. A total MRI synovitis score (MRIS) from the four regional scores ranging from 0 to 12 was calculated and used for analysis [38, 39].

Statistical analysis

Statistical analysis was performed using SPSS for Windows version 20.0 (Armonk, NY, USA). Baseline characteristics were described using mean (SD), median (IQR) for continuous variables and percentage for counts. The Wilcoxon test and the paired sample t test were used to compare responses to abatacept treatment for clinical measures, synovitis macroscopic scores and immunohistological staining scores at 0 vs 2 months, 2 vs 6 months and 0 vs 6 months. To measure the effect of the first 2 months of abatacept or PBO treatment over time on cell markers of inflammation in the group we used a general linear model (GLM) repeated measure (within-subject factor: 0, 2 and 6-month time points, between-subject factors: abatacept and PBO treatment groups, and treatment duration). Correlation between synovial cell markers, macroscopic scores, clinical parameters and MRI scores were analysed using Pearson correlation. $P < 0.05$ was considered as statistically significant.

Results

Demographic and disease-specific characteristics of the patients

Fifteen patients (8 female and 7 male) with mean age of 45 (±14.6) years were recruited, and 14 subjects were randomised. Seven patients received abatacept 3 mg/kg of body weight and seven patients were given PBO infusions on day 1, 15 and 29. Eleven patients received he abatacept dose of 10 mg/kg of body weight from day 57. In total 10 patients completed the study (Fig. 1). Out of 14 randomised subjects, 2 patients dropped out due to commitment issues (1 patient in the 3 mg/kg of body weight treatment arm and 1 in the PBO arm) and 2 patients were withdrawn because of an acute disease flare (1 patient in the 10 mg/kg of body weight treatment arm on day 71 and 1 in the PBO arm on day 40). Demographic and disease-specific characteristics of the group are summarised in Table 1. All patients were of Caucasian race. Mean disease duration was 18 years for psoriasis and 10 years for PsA. Four patients were on a stable dose of MTX at the time of recruitment (one patient in the 3 mg/kg of body weight treatment arm and three in the PBO arm) and stayed on the same dose of MTX, the remainder had not received any prior DMARDs; one patient (PBO arm) was on a stable dose of prednisolone 5 mg/day.

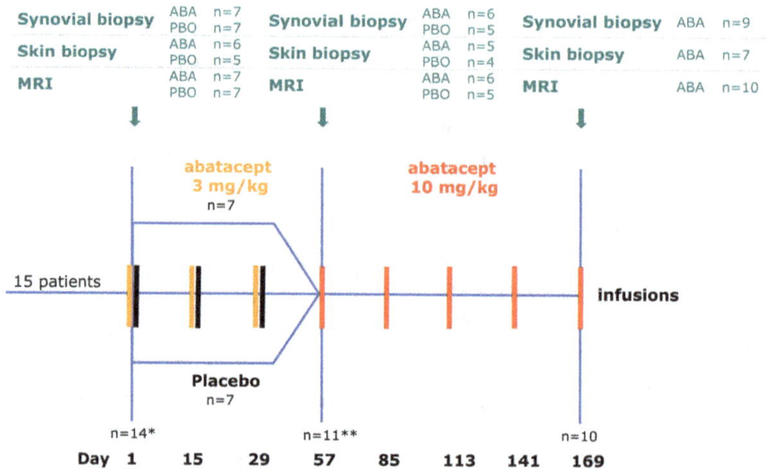

Fig. 1 Study design. Numbers of patients who underwent synovial and skin biopsies, and magnetic resonance imaging (*MRI*) in the abatacept (*ABA*) and placebo (*PBO*) study arms at each time point. *One patient was not randomized (screening visit and first MRI only). **Four patients were withdrawn from the study (two patients due to commitment issues (one in the 3 mg/kg of body weight treatment arm and one in the PBO arm)

Clinical responses of arthritis and psoriasis

All patients had active joint disease at baseline as reflected by both physicians' assessments and patients' reported outcome measures (PROMs), such as morning stiffness, pain, global health, fatigue, HAQ or PsAQoL scores. Mean TJC68, SJC66, DAS28-ESR and DAS28-CRP were 11.5 (±11), 6.9 (±7.4), 4.9 (±1) and 4.7 (±0.9), respectively. Skin-related measures showed mild to moderate psoriasis with mean PASI, DLQI and nail scores 4.5 (±4.6), 4.8 (±7.2) and 5 (±3.8), respectively (Table 1). DAS28-ESR ($P = 0.01$) and DAS28-CRP ($P = 0.042$) improved as early as 2 months. Significant improvements in most of the joint-related measures and PROMs were observed at 6 months compared to 2 months and to baseline (data not shown). There was very little change in skin-related outcomes. Change in PASI and DLQI from 2 to 6 months was -5.4 (±11.7) and -4.2 (±11.1) in the treatment, and -1.15 (±2.6) and 0.17 (±2.2) in the PBO group, respectively.

According to the EULAR response criteria 73% and 90% of patients were EULAR responders after 2 and 6 months of treatment (46% and 80% good responders, 27% and 10% moderate responders, respectively). PASI50 response at 2 and 6 months was seen in only 9% and 30% of the patients.

Improvement of knee synovitis on MRI

MRI scans were available at 0, 2 and 6 months for 15, 11 and 10 patients, respectively. MRI synovitis scores improved in each anatomical region of the knee throughout the study. Mean total MRIS at baseline, 2 and 6 months were 8.1 (±3), 7.3 (±3.8) and 6.2 (±4.3), respectively. There was a significant reduction in total MRIS from 2 to 6 months ($P = 0.047$) and from 0 to 6 months ($P = 0.016$). MRIS at 6 months was associated with change in DAS28-CRP from 2 to 6 months (rho = -0.63, $P = 0.049$).

Macroscopic evaluation of the synovium

Synovial inflammation as assessed by arthroscopy showed significant improvement throughout the study. Mean macroscopic scores at baseline and 2 and 6 months were 73 (±22.1), 41 (±29.7) and 44.4 (±34.3) for synovitis, and 59 (±29.7), 46 (±27.6) and 34 (±29.6) for vascularity, respectively. Significant reduction in synovitis scores was noted from 0 to 2 months and from 0 to 6 months ($P = 0.016$), and in vascularity scores from 0 to 6 months ($P = 0.039$).

Immunohistological analyses of synovial and skin tissues

Synovial and skin biopsies were available at 0, 2 and 6 months for 14, 11 and 9 patients, and for 11, 9 and 7 patients, respectively. Mean scores of immunohistological expression of CD3, CD4, CD8, FOXP3 and CD31 in the synovium and in the skin prior to and following treatment are summarised in Table 2. There was a trend toward reduction in CD8+ T cells, a reduction in CD4 expression ($P = 0.073$) and a significant reduction in FOXP3 expression ($P = 0.027$) in the synovium following treatment at 6 months. Figure 2 shows representative, single-stained images of decrease in CD4+ cells and in FOXP3+ cells prior to and at 6 months after abatacept treatment. FOXP3 expression was observed mostly in lymphoid follicles; some peri-vascular staining was seen and some lining layer staining was occasionally observed.

We did not find significant change in synovial CD3, CD8 or CD31 expression during the study period. A trend toward reduction in CD3+, CD4+ and CD8+ T

Table 1 Patients' demographic and clinical characteristics at baseline

Variable	Value
Demographic parameters	
Age (years)	45 (±14.6)
Female/male, *n* (%)	8 (53)/7 (47)
Age onset of psoriasis (years)	23 (±15)
Psoriasis disease duration (years)	18 (±12)
Age onset of PsA (years)	35 (±15)
PsA disease duration (years)	10 (±9.6)
Previous sDMARDs, *n* (%)	3 (20)
Concomitant sDMARDs (methotrexate), *n* (%)	4 (27)
Currently taken corticosteroids, *n* (%)	1 (7)
Clinical parameters, physician's assessment	
aCCP+, n (%)	0
RF+, *n* (%)	1 (7)
ESR (mm/h)	27 (±11)
CRP (mg/L)	19 (±10.4)
DAS28-ESR	4.9 (±1)
DAS28-CRP	4.7 (±0.9)
TJC 68	11.5 (±11)
SJC 66	6.9 (±7.4)
Dactylitis (0–20)	1.1 (±1.8)
Enthesitis (0–6)	1.6 (±1.6)
Nail (0–10)	5 (±3.8)
PASI (0–72)	4.5 (±4.6)
Clinical parameters, patient-reported	
Stiffness (minutes)	46 (±35.9)
Pain (0–10)	5.9 (±3.1)
GVAS (0 – 100)	56 (±28.6)
Fatigue (0–10)	5.9 (±2.8)
HAQ (0–3)	0.9 (±0.7)
DLQI (0–30)	4.8 (±7.2)
PsAQol (0–20)	8.6 (±5.7)

Results are presented as mean ± SD, median (IQR) or percentage. Dactylitis, the number of affected digits. Enthesitis score is based on the Leeds enthesitis index. Nail, the number of affected nails on the hands. Stiffness is early morning stiffness. Pain scale ranges from 0 = no pain to 10 = pain as bad as it could be. The visual analogue scale for global health (GVAS) ranges from 0 = worst imaginable health state to 100 = best imaginable health state. The fatigue scale ranges from 0 = no fatigue to 10 = fatigue as bad as it could be. The health assessment questionnaire HAQ scale ranges from 0 = no difficulty to 3 = unable to perform activity. *PsA* psoriatic arthritis, *aCCP* antibodies against cyclic citrullinated peptides, *RF* rheumatoid factor, *sDMARD* synthetic disease-modifying antirheumatic drug, *aCCP* antibodies against cyclic citrullinated peptides, *RF* rheumatiod factor, *ESR* erythrocyte sedimentation rate, *CRP* C-reactive protein, *DAS28-ESR/CRP* disease activity score based on a 28-joint assessment of pain or swelling using the ESR/CRP-based formula (www.das-score.nl), *TJC* tender joint count, *SJC* swollen joint count, *PASI* psoriasis area and severity index, *DLQI* dermatology life quality index, PsAQol psoriatic arthritis-specific quality of life score

cells was also seen in the lesional skin in particular in the first 2 months; however, significant change in expression was not observed for any of the cell markers over the 6-month treatment period.

Dual immunofluorescence staining of synovial tissue

Recent studies have proposed that FOXP3 is not only expressed by Tregs, but can be expressed by other types of lymphoid or myeloid cells, and by some non-haematopoietic cells such as epithelial cells [40]. To further specify the phenotype of FOXP3+ cells we performed dual immunofluorescence staining on synovial tissue sections with anti-CD4 and anti-FOXP3 antibodies.

Figure 3a-c shows representative images of immunofluorescent staining in synovial tissue (nuclear staining of FOXP3 (green), CD4+ T lymphocytes (red), and double-stained CD4+FOXP3+ T lymphocytes (green nuclear staining surrounded by red cytoplasmic staining). CD4 co-localized with FOXP3 mostly in lymphoid follicles. Figure 3d demonstrates quantification of double-stained CD4+FOXP3+ cells in synovial tissue at baseline and 6-months post treatment. Significant reduction ($P = 0.008$) in the number of double stained CD4+FOXP3+ T-cells was found in patients (n = 9) following 6 months abatacept treatment compared to baseline.

The impact of a short period of treatment with abatacept 3 mg/kg of body weight or placebo on clinical outcomes and cell markers

Abatacept 3 mg/kg of body weight or PBO was given to 7 patients in each arm on day 1, 15 and 29. Clinical outcomes, PROMs, and cell markers of synovial and skin inflammation were compared between the two treatment arms at 0 and 2 months. Disease activity measures and cell markers or their change over 2 months did not show significant difference between the abatacept and PBO groups (data not shown), with two exceptions: the MRIS was higher at baseline ($P = 0.02$) and FOXP3 expression in the skin was lower at 2 months ($P = 0.028$) in the treatment group compared to the PBO arm. The GLM repeated measure showed that the short PBO treatment did not have a significant effect on the changes in expression of cell markers of synovial and skin inflammation between baseline and 2 and 6 months in the whole group.

Macroscopic evaluation of synovial inflammation correlates with reduction in synovial cell markers

Both synovitis and vascularity scores correlated with FOXP3 expression at 2 months (rho = 0.7, $P = 0.024$ and rho = 0.65, $P = 0.041$, respectively), and improvement in vascularity score correlated with reduction in FOXP3 expression from 2 to 6 months (rho = 0.64, $P = 0.034$).

Table 2 Synovial and skin immunohistological expression of CD3, CD4, CD8, FOXP3 and CD31 prior to and following abatacept treatment

	Baseline		2 Months		6 Months	P value		
						0 vs 2 months		0 vs 6 months
	ABA	PBO	ABA	PBO	ABA	ABA	PBO	ABA
Synovium								
CD3	2.66 (±1.2)	1.8 (±0.8)	2.3 (±1)	2.25 (±1.5)	2.22 (±1.3)	0.679	0.824	0.739
CD4	2.83 (±1.2)	2.4 (±1.5)	2.3 (±0.8)	2.75 (±1.3)	1.78 (±1.1)	0.296	1	0.073
CD8	1.66 (±0.8)	2 (±1)	1.3 (±1)	1.75 (±1)	1.33 (±0.7)	0.576	0.604	0.129
FOXP3	5 (±6)	4.4 (±4.4)	2.8 (±2.2)	4.6 (±4)	1.13 (±2.4)	0.407	0.807	0.027*
CD31	78.3 (±53.9)	85.6 (±50.2)	67.6 (±75.9)	155.5 (±136)	73.22 (±69.9)	0.621	0.482	0.813
Skin								
CD3	2.6 (±0.8)	2.4 (±0.9)	2.25 (±1.5)	2.5 (±2.1)	2.43 (±1.1)	0.718	0.717	0.891
CD4	3.5 (±0.5)	2.8 (±1.1)	2.75 (±0.9)	4 (±0)	3.14 (±0.9)	0.182	1	0.891
CD8	2 (±0.6)	1.75 (±1)	1.5 (±0.6)	2 (±1.4)	1.71 (±0.8)	0.718	0.423	0.577
FOXP3	16 (±9.5)	9.2 (±10.7)	9.5 ±4.5	17.5 ±2.1	13.14 ±8.3	0.743	0.709	0.497
CD31	61.2 (±38)	65.4 (±20.5)	75.5 ±17.1	64.5 ±10.6	54.71 ±17.2	0.788	0.749	0.612

The Wilcoxon test and the paired sample *t* test were used for analysis. Results are presented as mean ± SD
Number of ABA samples at 0, 2 and 6 months: synovial n = 7, n = 6, n = 9; skin n = 6, n = 5, n = 7, respectively. Number of PBO samples at 0 and 2 months: synovial n = 7, n = 5; skin n = 5, n = 4, respectively. Expression of CD3, CD4 and CD8 was scored on a 5-point scale (0–4). CD31 expression was scored by the number of positive vessels/10 high power fields. Forkhead box protein transcription factor 3 (FOXP3) expression was scored as %/300 cells. *ABA* abatacept group, *PBO* placebo group. *Statistically significant

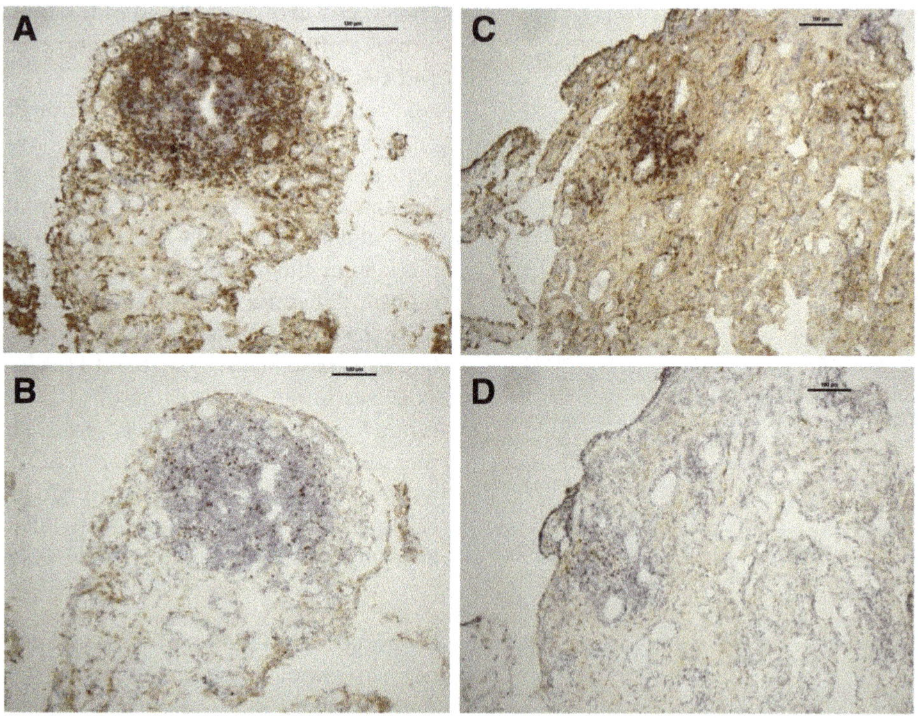

Fig. 2 Immunohistological comparison of the expression of CD4+ and forkhead box protein transcription factor 3-positive (FOXP3+) T cells (magnification × 10) in the synovial tissue prior to and at 6 months after abatacept treatment (patient #6). Baseline images show focal infiltration of CD4+ T cells (**a**) and FOXP3+ T cells (**b**) in a villus. Decrease in CD4 expression and significant reduction in the number of FOXP3+ T cells are shown (**c** and **d**, respectively)

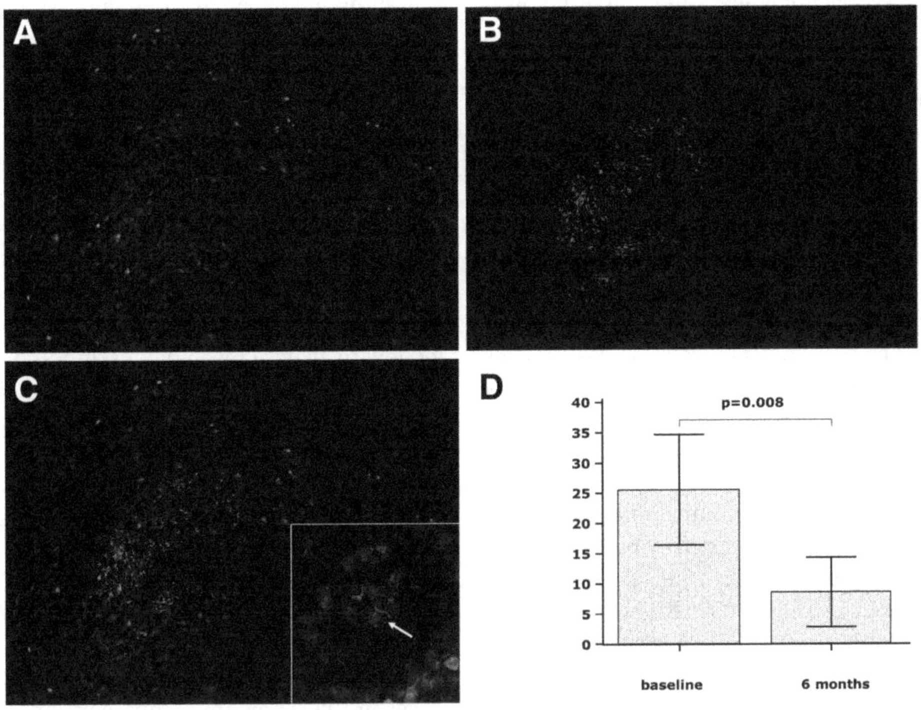

Fig. 3 Representative images of immunofluorescent staining in cryostat synovial sections in a patient. **a** Nuclear staining of forkhead box protein transcription factor 3 (FOXP3) (*green*), **b** CD4+ T lymphocytes (*red*), **c** double-stained CD4+FOXP3+ T lymphocytes (*green* nuclear staining surrounded by *red* cytoplasmic staining), insert shows magnification × 40, *white arrow* points to a double-stained CD4+FOXP3+ T cell. **d** Reduction in the number of double-stained CD4+FOXP3+ T cells from baseline to 6 months. Magnification of photomicrographs × 20

Safety

AEs were reported in a total of 12 patients (86%). Four patients (57%) in the treatment arm receiving abatacept 3 mg/kg of body weight, 6 patients (86%) in the PBO arm, and 8 patients (73%) who received the dose of 10 mg/kg of body weight from day 57 experienced mild or moderate AEs. There were no cases of acute infusion reaction. AEs possibly related to abatacept or PBO as per the investigator's opinion were reported in one (headache, influenza-like symptoms) and two (diarrhea, flare of psoriasis and arthritis) cases, respectively. There were no serious adverse events.

Discussion

This single-centre, placebo-controlled, crossover study demonstrates that abatacept reduced the immunohistological expression of CD4+ T cells and specifically reduced FOXP3+ Treg expression in the synovium over 6 months. Abatacept 10 mg/kg treatment significantly improved clinical measures including MRI synovitis scores and arthritis-related PROMs in PsA with little effect on skin-related outcomes.

Clinical efficacy of abatacept has been reported in patients with active RA, including those with an inadequate response to MTX or TNF inhibitors [41], in early type 1 diabetes mellitus, and more recently, in primary Sjögren's syndrome [21, 42]. Whilst there was no major clinical response to treatment with abatacept 10 mg/kg of body weight in a phase-2 open-label 24-week trial in ankylosing spondylitis [43], Mease et al. reported efficacy of abatacept on joint symptoms in PsA and identified a differential dosage effect of abatacept, with the dose of 10 mg/kg of body weight having more therapeutic effect on arthritis than the 3 mg/kg regimen [25]. In line with this study, we did not notice significant improvement in joint-related outcomes with the dose of 3 mg/kg of body weight, whereas the 10 mg/kg regimen led to significant improvements in most joint-related measures at 6 months. Similarly, MRI synovitis scores improved significantly over time only after administering the dose of 10 mg/kg of body weight. Abatacept has been shown to have some clinical benefit in the treatment of psoriasis [4]. In an open-label phase-1 study of abatacept in psoriasis, 50% or greater improvement of skin involvement was achieved in patients using doses of 25 and 50 mg/kg of body weight, and the same doses correlated best with the reduction of epidermal hyperplasia and the decrease in activated T cells in the skin [44, 45]. We observed very little improvement in the PASI or DLQI over 6 months, but the treatment doses of 3 and 10 mg/kg of body weight may have been too low to be of clinical benefit.

Studies assessing synovial changes after initiating antirheumatic therapy are limited in PsA. From these studies it can be concluded that successful treatment leads to deactivation of endothelium, reduced vascularity and reduction in infiltrating immune cells [27]. Immunpathological changes in the synovium following abatacept treatment in PsA was evaluated in a single case report, and suggested regression of synovial inflammation in a patient refractory to TNF inhibitors [46]. We found significant reduction in macroscopic scores for both synovitis and vascularity after 6 months of abatacept therapy. A trend toward reduction in CD8+ and CD4+ T cells was observed throughout the study, but a statistically significant effect of the treatment was only detected for the reduction in the number of FOXP3+ Tregs in the synovium.

Tregs play a central role in immune tolerance, suppressing not only autoimmune responses but also aberrant or excessive immune responses to non-self-antigens [4] Data on the presence of FOXP3+ Tregs in inflamed synovial tissue are controversial. Enrichment of Tregs in the inflamed joints was reported in a large cohort of patients with chronic inflammatory arthritis, including patients with PsA [47], whilst another study showed only scarce synovial membrane expression of FOXP3+ T cells during relapse in inflammatory arthritis [12]. Deficiencies in Treg function have been also identified in different autoimmune diseases, including RA and psoriasis. Anti-TNF therapy has been shown to induce a potent population of Tregs in patients with RA; however, after cessation of treatment the natural Treg defect persisted [11, 13–15]. It has been suggested that reduced expression and functional abnormalities in Treg-associated CTLA-4 could contribute to abnormal Treg function in RA and may represent a target for therapy [11]. Data for the effects of abatacept on Treg cell function are limited and conflicting. Bonelli et al. showed that abatacept increased the frequency of Treg cells in RA and inhibited their suppressive capacity [48], whilst another study in RA reported enhanced suppressive capacity of Tregs isolated from peripheral blood [49]. Whether the reduction in FOXP3 expression in the synovium we observed after abatacept treatment is protective or pathogenic remains unclear, since our study did not include detailed phenotypic or functional analyses of the Tregs. However, in view of the significant improvement seen in arthritis measures we speculate that the reduction in potentially dysfunctional Tregs may be protective. In line with our observations, a lack of retention of Tregs has been reported after successful anti-inflammatory treatment with intra-articular glucocorticoid injection, suggesting that a specific treatment that modulates local FOXP3+ Treg numbers and function would be of benefit for patients with joint inflammation [12].

A study investigating the role of Tregs in the pathogenesis of psoriasis found increased Treg expression in lesional skin compared to normal skin, in particular in the chronic plaque type of psoriasis, irrespective of disease severity [15]. It has been proposed that the differential dosage effect of abatacept in PsA that was reported in a previous study may be due to the suppression of Tregs at higher doses [19, 25]. In this study, we did not observe a better skin response with low-dose abatacept, possibly due to the small sample size, although the study by Abrams et al. [45] suggests that the abatacept doses used in our study may well have been too low to achieve meaningful skin response.

In contrast to changes seen in the synovial tissue, we did not demonstrate significant immunohistological change in skin involvement in response to abatacept. Different cytokine milieu in the joints compared to the skin may account for this. A recent comparative genomic profiling study of the synovium versus skin lesions in PsA revealed clearly distinct gene expression patterns in the skin compared to the synovium with a stronger IL-17 gene signature in the skin, and more equivalent TNF and IFN-γ gene signatures in both tissues. The authors found fewer Tregs in the synovium compared to the skin; however, the difference was not significant [50].

Conclusions

In conclusion, this is the first study to assess both synovial and psoriatic skin immunopathological changes following abatacept treatment in PsA. The results of the study suggest that treatment with abatacept 10 mg/kg of body weight is associated with significant improvement in the joint-related clinical outcomes but not skin-related outcomes in biologic DMARD-naïve PsA patients and might be an effective treatment option in patients with PsA. We observed different patterns of efficacy of abatacept in the joints and in lesional skin. Reduction in FOXP3+ T-cell expression in the synovium but not in the psoriatic lesion following abatacept treatment may indicate abnormal Treg function in PsA with differential suppressive capacity in the synovium compared to the skin. Comprehensive studies are required on both the distribution and function of Tregs, together with their complex interactions with the local inflammatory milieu present in the psoriatic skin lesion and inflamed synovium in PsA.

Abbreviations

aCCP: Antibodies against cyclic citrullinated peptides; AEs: Adverse events; CASPAR: Classification criteria for psoriatic arthritis; CRP: C-reactive protein; CTLA-4: Cytotoxic T-lymphocyte Antigen 4; DAS28: Disease activity score 28; DLQI: Dermatology life quality index; DMARDs: Disease-modifying antirheumatic drugs; EMS: Early morning stiffness; ESR: Erythrocyte sedimentation rate; EULAR: European League Against Rheumatism; FOXP3: Forkhead box transcription factor; GVAS: Visual analogue scale for global health; HAQ: Health assessment questionnaire; HPF: High-power fields; IgG1: Immunoglobulin G1; IL: Interleukin; INFγ: Interferon gamma; JIA: Juvenile idiopathic arthritis; LEI: Leeds enthesitis index; MRI: Magnetic resonance imaging; MRIS: Total MRI synovitis score; MTX: Methotrexate;

NSAID: Nonsteroidal anti-inflammatory drug; PASI: Psoriasis Area Severity Index; PBO: Placebo; PBS: Phosphate-buffered saline; PDE4i: Phosphodiesterase 4 inhibitor; PROMs: Patients' reported outcome measures; PsA: Psoriatic arthritis; PsAQol: PsA-specific quality of life score; RA: Rheumatoid arthritis; RF: Rheumatoid factor; SJC: Swollen joint count; TJC: Tender joint count; TNFi: Tumour necrosis factor alpha inhibitor Tregs, Regulatory T cells

Acknowledgements

The authors thank all the patients who participated in the study. We are grateful to Prof. Douglas Veale, Dr Carl Orr, Dr Len Harty and Dr Emese Balogh for obtaining the synovial biopsies and to Dr Anne Marie Tobin and Dr Karoline Adamzik for performing skin biopsies. We would also like to thank Ms Katalin Hodosi for reviewing the statistical analyses. The authors gratefully acknowledge Ms Anne Marie Baker, Ms Martina Cooney and Dr Monika Biniecka their valuable contribution to the study.

Funding

Bristol Myers Squibb provided the study drug and an unrestricted research grant.

Authors' contributions

OF was the principal investigator who obtained the research grant, and was responsible for the study design and overseeing the study. AS was responsible for study recruitment and data collection, performed the statistical analysis and drafted the manuscript. EH carried out MRI scoring and contributed to data interpretation. MG carried out immunohistochemical analysis. LM assisted with immunohistochemical analysis and data acquisition. JMc carried out immunohistochemical analysis and contributed to data interpretation. MH was responsible for study recruitment and data collection. ME contributed to data collection and interpretation. PG participated in designing the study and its coordination. GK was responsible for obtaining skin biopsies and contributed to data interpretation. AF was responsible for overseeing immunohistochemical analysis and carried out immunohistochemical scoring. BK was the co-principal investigator of the study and participated in its design and coordination. All authors read and approved the final manuscript.

Authors' information

Not applicable.

Competing interests

OF was supported by research grants from Pfizer, AbbVie, BMS and UCB. AS, EH, MG, LM, JMcC, MH, ME, PG, GK, AF and BK declare that they have no competing interests.

Consent for publication

Not applicable.

Author details

[1]Department of Rheumatology, St. Vincent's University Hospital, Dublin, Ireland. [2]Department of Radiology, St. Vincent's University Hospital, Dublin, Ireland. [3]School of Biochemistry and Immunology, TCD, Dublin, Ireland. [4]Department of Histopathology, St. Vincent's University Hospital, Dublin, Ireland. [5]Research Pathology, Immunohistochemistry Core Facility, UCD Conway Institute, UCD School of Medicine, Dublin, Ireland. [6]Department of Dermatology, St. Vincent's University Hospital, Dublin, Ireland.

References

1. Fitzgerald O, Winchester R. Psoriatic arthritis: from pathogenesis to therapy. Arthritis Res Ther. 2009;11:214.
2. Haroon M, FitzGerald O. Psoriatic arthritis: complexities, comorbidities and implications for the clinic. Expert Rev Clin Immunol. 2016;12:406–16.
3. Diani M, Altomare G, Reali E. T cell responses in psoriasis and psoriatic arthritis. Autoimmun Rev. 2015;14:286–92.
4. Cai Y, Fleming C, Yan J. New insights of T cells in the pathogenesis of psoriasis. Cell Mol Immunol. 2012;9:302–9.
5. FitzGerald O, Haroon M, Giles JT, Winchester R. Concepts of pathogenesis in psoriatic arthritis: genotype determines clinical phenotype. Arthritis Res Ther. 2015;17:115.
6. Veale DJ. New therapies and new goals for psoriatic arthritis. Arthritis Rheum. 2011;63:874–6.
7. Mortezavi M, Thiele R, Ritchlin C. The joint in psoriatic arthritis. Clin Exp Rheumatol. 2015;33:S20–5.
8. Hoeppli RE, Wu D, Cook L, Levings MK. The environment of regulatory T cell biology: cytokines, metabolites, and the microbiome. Front Immunol. 2015;6:61.
9. Appel H, Wu P, Scheer R, Kedor C, Sawitzki B, Thiel A, et al. Synovial and peripheral blood CD4 + FoxP3+ T cells in spondyloarthritis. J Rheumatol. 2011;38:2445–51.
10. Ryder LR, Bartels EM, Woetmann A, Madsen HO, Odum N, Bliddal H, et al. FoxP3 mRNA splice forms in synovial CD4+ T cells in rheumatoid arthritis and psoriatic arthritis. APMIS. 2012;120:387–96.
11. Flores-Borja F, Jury EC, Mauri C, Ehrenstein MR. Defects in CTLA-4 are associated with abnormal regulatory T cell function in rheumatoid arthritis. Proc Natl Acad Sci U S A. 2008;105:19396–401.
12. Raghavan S, Cao D, Widhe M, Roth K, Herrath J, Engstrom M, et al. FOXP3 expression in blood, synovial fluid and synovial tissue during inflammatory arthritis and intra-articular corticosteroid treatment. Ann Rheum Dis. 2009; 68:1908–15.
13. Sugiyama H, Gyulai R, Toichi E, Garaczi E, Shimada S, Stevens SR, et al. Dysfunctional blood and target tissue CD4+ CD25high regulatory T cells in psoriasis: mechanism underlying unrestrained pathogenic effector T cell proliferation. J Immunol. 2005;174:164–73.
14. Soler DC, McCormick TS. The dark side of regulatory T cells in psoriasis. J Invest Dermatol. 2011;131:1785–6.
15. Yun WJ, Lee DW, Chang SE, Yoon GS, Huh JR, Won CH, et al. Role of CD4CD25FOXP3 regulatory T cells in psoriasis. Ann Dermatol. 2010;22:397–403.
16. Buckner JH. Mechanisms of impaired regulation by CD4(+)CD25(+)FOXP3(+) regulatory T cells in human autoimmune diseases. Nat Rev Immunol. 2010; 10:849–59.
17. Coates LC, Kavanaugh A, Mease PJ, Soriano ER, Laura Acosta Felquer M, Armstrong AW, et al. Group for research and assessment of psoriasis and psoriatic arthritis: treatment recommendations for psoriatic arthritis 2015. Arthritis Rheumatol. 2016;68:1060–71.
18. Mease P. A short history of biological therapy for psoriatic arthritis. Clin Exp Rheumatol. 2015;33:S104–8.
19. Iannone F, Lapadula G. The inhibitor of costimulation of T cells: Abatacept. J Rheumatol. 2012;39:100–2.
20. Moreland L, Bate G, Kirkpatrick P. Abatacept. Nat Rev Drug Discov. 2006;5: 185–6.
21. Orban T, Bundy B, Becker DJ, DiMeglio LA, Gitelman SE, Goland R, et al. Co-stimulation modulation with abatacept in patients with recent-onset type 1 diabetes: a randomised, double-blind, placebo-controlled trial. Lancet. 2011; 378:412–9.
22. Weisman MH, Durez P, Hallegua D, Aranda R, Becker JC, Nuamah I, et al. Reduction of inflammatory biomarker response by abatacept in treatment of rheumatoid arthritis. J Rheumatol. 2006;33:2162–6.
23. Ruderman EM, Pope RM. The evolving clinical profile of abatacept (CTLA4-Ig): a novel co-stimulatory modulator for the treatment of rheumatoid arthritis. Arthritis Res Ther. 2005;7 Suppl 2:S21–5.
24. Genovese MC, Becker JC, Schiff M, Luggen M, Sherrer Y, Kremer J, et al. Abatacept for rheumatoid arthritis refractory to tumor necrosis factor alpha inhibition. N Engl J Med. 2005;353:1114–23.
25. Mease P, Genovese MC, Gladstein G, Kivitz AJ, Ritchlin C, Tak PP, et al. Abatacept in the treatment of patients with psoriatic arthritis: results of a six-month, multicenter, randomized, double-blind, placebo-controlled, phase II trial. Arthritis Rheum. 2011;63:939–48.
26. Mease PJ, Gottlieb AB, van der Heijde D, FitzGerald O, Johnsen A, Nys M, et al. Efficacy and safety of abatacept, a T-cell modulator, in a randomised, double-blind, placebo-controlled, phase III study in psoriatic arthritis. Ann Rheum Dis. 2017:1–9. doi:10.1136/annrheumdis-2016-210724.
27. van Kuijk AW, Tak PP. Synovitis in psoriatic arthritis: immunohistochemistry, comparisons with rheumatoid arthritis, and effects of therapy. Curr Rheumatol Rep. 2011;13:353–9.
28. Taylor W, Gladman D, Helliwell P, Marchesoni A, Mease P, Mielants H, et al. Classification criteria for psoriatic arthritis: development of new criteria from a large international study. Arthritis Rheum. 2006;54:2665–73.

29. Healy PJ, Helliwell PS. Measuring clinical enthesitis in psoriatic arthritis: assessment of existing measures and development of an instrument specific to psoriatic arthritis. Arthritis Rheum. 2008;59:686–91.
30. Coates LC, Mumtaz A, Helliwell PS, Mease PJ, Callis-Duffin K, Krueger GG, et al. Development of a disease severity and responder index for psoriatic arthritis (PsA)–report of the OMERACT 10 PsA special interest group. J Rheumatol. 2011;38:1496–501.
31. Finlay AY, Khan GK. Dermatology Life Quality Index (DLQI)–a simple practical measure for routine clinical use. Clin Exp Dermatol. 1994;19:210–6.
32. Fransen J, van Riel PL. The Disease Activity Score and the EULAR response criteria. Rheum Dis Clin North Am. 2009;35:745–57.
33. van de Sande MG, Gerlag DM, Lodde BM, van Baarsen LG, Alivernini S, Codullo V, et al. Evaluating antirheumatic treatments using synovial biopsy: a recommendation for standardisation to be used in clinical trials. Ann Rheum Dis. 2011;70:423–7.
34. Veale DJ. The role of arthroscopy in early arthritis. Clin Exp Rheumatol. 1999; 17(1):37–8.
35. Gogarty M, Fitzgerald O. Immunohistochemistry of the inflamed synovium. Methods Mol Med. 2007;135:47–63.
36. van Kuijk AW, Reinders-Blankert P, Smeets TJ, Dijkmans BA, Tak PP. Detailed analysis of the cell infiltrate and the expression of mediators of synovial inflammation and joint destruction in the synovium of patients with psoriatic arthritis: implications for treatment. Ann Rheum Dis. 2006;65:1551–7.
37. Tak PP, Smeets TJ, Daha MR, Kluin PM, Meijers KA, Brand R, et al. Analysis of the synovial cell infiltrate in early rheumatoid synovial tissue in relation to local disease activity. Arthritis Rheum. 1997;40:217–25.
38. Rhodes LA, Grainger AJ, Keenan AM, Thomas C, Emery P, Conaghan PG. The validation of simple scoring methods for evaluating compartment-specific synovitis detected by MRI in knee osteoarthritis. Rheumatology (Oxford). 2005;44:1569–73.
39. Glinatsi D, Bird P, Gandjbakhch F, Mease PJ, Boyesen P, Peterfy CG, et al. Validation of the OMERACT Psoriatic Arthritis Magnetic Resonance Imaging Score (PsAMRIS) for the hand and foot in a randomized placebo-controlled trial. J Rheumatol. 2015;42:2473–9.
40. Devaud C, Darcy PK, Kershaw MH. Foxp3 expression in T regulatory cells and other cell lineages. Cancer Immunol Immunother. 2014;63:869–76.
41. Massarotti EM. Clinical and patient-reported outcomes in clinical trials of abatacept in the treatment of rheumatoid arthritis. Clin Ther. 2008;30:429–42.
42. Meiners PM, Vissink A, Kroese FG, Spijkervet FK, Smitt-Kamminga NS, Abdulahad WH, et al. Abatacept treatment reduces disease activity in early primary Sjogren's syndrome (open-label proof of concept ASAP study). Ann Rheum Dis. 2014;73:1393–6.
43. Song IH, Heldmann F, Rudwaleit M, Haibel H, Weiss A, Braun J, et al. Treatment of active ankylosing spondylitis with abatacept: an open-label, 24-week pilot study. Ann Rheum Dis. 2011;70:1108–10.
44. Abrams JR, Lebwohl MG, Guzzo CA, Jegasothy BV, Goldfarb MT, Goffe BS, et al. CTLA4Ig-mediated blockade of T-cell costimulation in patients with psoriasis vulgaris. J Clin Invest. 1999;103:1243–52.
45. Abrams JR, Kelley SL, Hayes E, Kikuchi T, Brown MJ, Kang S, et al. Blockade of T lymphocyte costimulation with cytotoxic T lymphocyte-associated antigen 4-immunoglobulin (CTLA4Ig) reverses the cellular pathology of psoriatic plaques, including the activation of keratinocytes, dendritic cells, and endothelial cells. J Exp Med. 2000;192:681–94.
46. Canete JD, Celis R, Hernandez V, Pablos JL, Sanmarti R. Synovial immunopathological changes associated with successful abatacept therapy in a case of severe refractory psoriatic arthritis. Ann Rheum Dis. 2010;69: 935–6.
47. Cao D, van Vollenhoven R, Klareskog L, Trollmo C, Malmstrom V. CD25brightCD4 + regulatory T cells are enriched in inflamed joints of patients with chronic rheumatic disease. Arthritis Res Ther. 2004;6:R335–46.
48. Bonelli M, Goschl L, Bluml S, Karonitsch T, Hirahara K, Ferner E, et al. Abatacept (CTLA-4Ig) treatment reduces T cell apoptosis and regulatory T cell suppression in patients with rheumatoid arthritis. Rheumatology (Oxford). 2016;55:710–20.
49. Alvarez-Quiroga C, Abud-Mendoza C, Doniz-Padilla L, Juarez-Reyes A, Monsivais-Urenda A, Baranda L, et al. CTLA-4-Ig therapy diminishes the frequency but enhances the function of Treg cells in patients with rheumatoid arthritis. J Clin Immunol. 2011;31:588–95.
50. Belasco J, Louie JS, Gulati N, Wei N, Nograles K, Fuentes-Duculan J, et al. Comparative genomic profiling of synovium versus skin lesions in psoriatic arthritis. Arthritis Rheumatol. 2015;67:934–44.

15

Minimal disease activity and impact of disease in psoriatic arthritis

Rubén Queiro[1*], Juan D. Cañete[2], Carlos Montilla[3], Miguel Abad[4], María Montoro[5], Susana Gómez[5], Ana Cábez[5] and on behalf of the MAAPS study group

Abstract

Background: Patients with psoriatic arthritis (PsA) experience functional impairment and reduced quality of life, and thus patient global assessment in PsA is explained mainly by the physical, but also by the psychological, aspect of the disease. To assess the prevalence of minimal disease activity (MDA) in Spanish patients with PsA, we examined their characteristics and the association between MDA and the impact of the disease as assessed by the PsA Impact of Disease (PsAID) questionnaire.

Methods: A cross-sectional multicenter study was carried out in patients who fulfilled the Classification for Psoriatic Arthritis (CASPAR) criteria with at least 1 year of disease duration, and who were treated with biological or conventional synthetic (cs) disease-modifying anti-rheumatic drugs (DMARDs) according to routine clinical practice in Spain. Patients were considered in MDA if they met at least 5/7 of the MDA criteria. The association between MDA and the recently developed PsAID questionnaire was also recorded.

Results: Of 227 patients included, 133 (58.6%) were in the MDA state (52% with antitumor necrosis factor (anti-TNF) α monotherapy, 24% with csDMARD monotherapy, and 24% with anti-TNFα in combination with csDMARD). Using multivariate logistic regression analysis, male gender (odds ratio (OR) 2.74, $p = 0.001$), a sedentary lifestyle (OR 3.13, $p = 0.002$), familial history of PsA (OR 0.38, $p = 0.036$), C-reactive protein (CRP) level (OR 0.92, $p = 0.010$), and use of corticoids (OR 0.33, $p = 0.007$) were considered features related to MDA. MDA patients had a significantly lower impact of the disease according to PsAID (mean total score (SD): MDA 3.3 (3.1) vs. non-MDA 7.1 (5.2); $p < 0.001$).

Conclusions: Nearly 60% of Spanish PsA patients achieve MDA in routine clinical practice. MDA remains one of the most useful therapeutic targets for PsA since patients who reached this state also had a significantly lower impact of disease according to PsAID.

Keywords: Minimal disease activity, Psoriatic arthritis, PsAID, Therapeutic objective

Background

Psoriatic arthritis (PsA) is a chronic inflammatory musculoskeletal disease that is usually seronegative for rheumatoid factor, associated with psoriasis, and with a prevalence of 0.02–0.42% in the general population and 13.8–30% among patients with psoriasis [1, 2]. PsA is a heterogeneous condition with articular and extra-articular manifestations including a combination of peripheral arthritis, axial disease, enthesitis, dactylitis, and skin and nail disease.

The target of therapy for PsA is to reach a state of remission or, at least, minimal disease activity (MDA). For patients with PsA, the heterogeneity among disease manifestations as well as the need to validate outcome measures makes the definition of remission challenging [3]. Clinical remission requires achieving disease quiescence in all disease domains [3]. In 2010, Coates et al. [4] developed a composite outcome measure as a target of treatment for patients with PsA that encompasses most of the disease domains. These criteria for MDA

* Correspondence: rubenque7@yahoo.es
[1]Department of Rheumatology, HU, Central de Asturias, Av. Roma, s/n, 33011 Oviedo, Asturias, Spain
Full list of author information is available at the end of the article

were validated using interventional trial data [5]. Recent studies have found that MDA could be a reliable target for antitumor necrosis factor alpha (anti-TNF) therapy [6–8].

PsA has a high impact on the lives of patients [9, 10]. Patients with PsA experience significant disability and reduced quality of life, resulting from emotional distress and functional impairment associated with psoriatic skin lesions, as well as arthritis-related joint pain [9, 10]. A prominent benefit of treatment with anti-TNF in PsA patients has been an improvement in patient-reported outcomes (PROs), including health-related quality of life [11]. Recently Gossec et al. have developed and validated the PsA Impact of Disease (PsAID) questionnaire which can be used to calculate a score reflecting the impact of PsA on the lives of patients [12].

Measures that assess outcomes in rheumatic diseases should not only capture the major domains of the disease, but also capture the vision of the patient for improvement in their overall health. The aim of this study was to determine the MDA rate in patients with PsA, to describe their characteristics, and to evaluate the association between MDA and the impact of the disease as assessed by the PsAID questionnaire in routine clinical practice.

Methods

This was an observational, cross-sectional, multicenter study carried out at twenty-five rheumatology outpatient clinics over the whole of Spain. The study included outpatients of both genders over 18 years of age diagnosed with PsA according to the Classification for Psoriatic Arthritis (CASPAR) criteria [13] with at least 1 year of disease duration, with hand and foot radiological tests carried out during the 6 months prior to the study visit, and receiving treatment with biological and conventional synthetic (cs) disease-modifying anti-rheumatic drugs (DMARDs).

All patients provided their informed written consent. In accordance with Spanish recommendations, the study was approved by the Clinical Research Ethics Committee of La Fe Hospital and was conducted in accordance with the principles contained in the Declaration of Helsinki for studies in humans. Data were collected between May 2014 and February 2015 at a single visit.

Patient data collection included demographics and clinical characteristics (age, sex, body mass index, educational level and employment status, toxic habits, and comorbidities), detailed PsA clinical history (evolution time of PsA, time from onset of skin and articular symptoms, pattern of PsA at onset (peripheral, axial, mixed), enthesitis, dactylitis, involvement of distal interphalangeal joint, familial history (psoriasis, PsA, ankylosing spondylitis, others), C-reactive protein (CRP) levels, erythrocyte sedimentation rate (ESR), positive human leukocyte antigen-B27 (HLA-B27)), and record of current use of medications (nonsteroidal anti-inflammatory drugs (NSAIDs), infiltrations, biological and csDMARDs, and corticoids). Radiological findings (erosions in hands and feet, joint space narrowing on hands or feet, sacroilitis, syndesmophytes) from radiological tests carried out during the 6 months prior to the study visit were also recorded. The Psoriasis Area Severity index (PASI) [14] was assessed. In addition, patients completed self-reported questionnaires including the Health Assessment Questionnaire (HAQ) [15], the Bath Ankylosing Spondylitis Disease Activity Index (BASDAI) [16], and the PsAID [12].

Patients were considered in MDA when they met ≥5 of the following criteria: tender joint count ≤1, swollen joint count ≤1, PASI score ≤1 or body surface area ≤3%, patient pain visual analog scale (VAS) score ≤15, patient global disease activity VAS score ≤20, HAQ score ≤0.5, and tender entheseal points ≤1.

The PsAID questionnaire [12] reflects the impact of PsA from the perspective of the patient. It is comprised of 12 physical and psychological domains. Each domain is rated from 0 to 10 with a different weighting. The total score is divided by 20. The final score has a range from 0 (best status) to 10 (worst status) with a cutoff of 4 [12].

Statistical methodology

A descriptive statistical analysis of all the variables was performed, including central tendency and dispersion measures for continuous variables, and absolute and relative frequencies for categorical variables. Patients were analyzed and distributed into two groups according to MDA status. Student's t test, Mann-Whitney U test or Kruskall Wallis H test were used to compare quantitative variables and Pearson's chi-square or Fisher exact tests were used for qualitative variables. Univariate and multivariate models were carried out to identify factors independently associated with MDA. Tests were two-tailed with a significance level of 5%. Data were analyzed using SPSS V19.0 statistical software.

Results

Of the 227 included patients, 133 (58.6%) were in MDA at the study visit. Figure 1 shows the proportion of patients that fulfilled each MDA criterion according to MDA state. The most common active domains were global disease activity VAS score ≤20 and HAQ <0.5, achieved by 58.6% and 77.4% of MDA patients, respectively (Fig. 1).

Demographic and clinical characteristics of the study population with respect to the presence of MDA are shown in Table 1. Most of the patients were men (54.2%) with a mean (SD) age of 53.2 (12.4) years. Overall, 57.7% (MDA 47.9% vs. non-MDA 57.4%; $p = 0.197$) of patients suffered from at least one concomitant

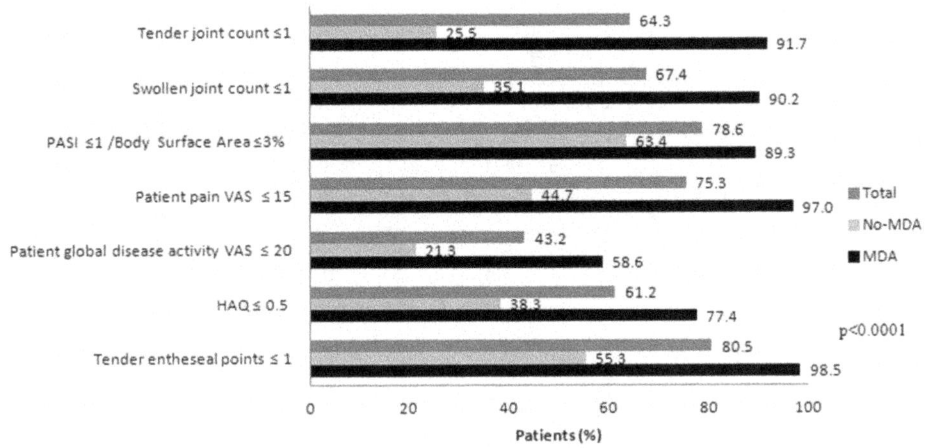

Fig. 1 MDA criteria according to MDA state. *HAQ* Health Assessment Questionnaire, *MDA* minimal disease activity, *PASI* Psoriasis Area and Severity Index, *VAS* Visual analogue scale

disease, the most frequent being dislipemia (MDA 33.1% vs. non-MDA 26.6%; $p = 0.295$), hypertension (MDA 26.3% vs. non-MDA 28.7%; $p = 0.688$), and obesity (MDA 24.1% vs. non-MDA 17.0%; $p = 0.201$; Table 1).

Of the total patients, 54.6% were employed (MDA 60.9% vs. non-MDA 45.7%) and 5.7% had temporary or full disability to work due to PsA (MDA 1.5% vs. non-MDA 11.7%; $p < 0.001$). Regarding PsA condition, 83.3% of the patients were diagnosed with peripheral disease (oligoarticular 51.6%, polyarticular 48.4%). Dactylitis, enthesitis, and distal interphalangeal joints were detected in 49.3%, 35.7%, and 41.0% of patients, respectively.

Overall, 49.3% of the patients had familial history of psoriasis, and 12.3% had a history of PsA, which was significantly more frequent in non-MDA patients than in those who achieved the MDA state (19.1% vs. 7.5%; $p < 0.05$; Table 1). Disease duration was 9.6 (7.7) years and the musculoskeletal symptoms onset occurred nearly 10 years after the skin symptoms appeared (Table 1). At the study visit, MDA patients had fewer hand erosions than non-MDA patients (30.8% vs. 44.7%; $p < 0.05$; Table 1). The mean (SD) CRP level was 3.6 (6.2) mg/L, (MDA 2.8 (3.9) mg/L vs. non-MDA 4.7 (8.2) mg/L; $p < 0.05$), the mean (SD) ESR value was 14.76 (12.4) mm/h, and 23 (17.6%) of 131 patients tested for HLA-B27 were positive.

MDA patients had a significantly lower impact of the disease as measured by PsAID (MDA 3.3 (3.1) vs. non-MDA 7.1 (5.2); $p < 0.001$; Table 1). Eighty-eight (66.7%) of MDA patients vs. 34 (37.4%) of non-MDA patients obtained a PsAID score <4 ($p < 0.0001$). Statistically significant differences were observed between MDA and non-MDA patients for all PsAID domains ($p < 0.001$; Fig. 2). Similarly, patients with MDA presented a significantly lower total score on PASI, BASDAI, and HAQ questionnaires compared with those who had not achieved MDA ($p < 0.001$; Table 1).

Multivariate analysis showed that male gender increased the odds of having achieved MDA (odds ratio (95% confidence interval) 2.75 (1.47–5.12); $p = 0.001$) as well as living a sedentary life (3.13 (1.50–6.53); $p = 0.002$), while having a familial history of PsA (0.39 (0.16–0.94); $p = 0.038$), current elevated CRP level (0.92 (0.86–0.98); $p = 0.010$) or use of corticosteroids (0.33 (0.15–0.74); $p = 0.007$) decreased the odds of having achieved MDA (Table 2).

Treatments at the study visit are shown in Table 3. MDA was achieved by 62.7% of the patients who received anti-TNF alone, by 52.5% receiving anti-TNF plus csDMARDs treatment, and by 62.7% receiving monotherapy with csDMARDS (Table 3). Overall, the most frequent anti-TNFs used were etanercept (37.5%) and adalimumab (31.3%), and among the csDMARDs the most common was methotrexate (76.0%).

Statistically significant differences were not observed between non-MDA and MDA patients regarding use of any kind of treatment with the exception of corticoids (Table 3). The proportion of patients who received corticoids was significantly higher among non-MDA than MDA patients (59% non-MDA vs. 41% MDA; $p < 0.05$; Table 3).

Discussion

Remission or low disease activity is the goal of therapy in PsA. In this study, 58.6% of the patients were in a MDA state. This prevalence is in concordance with that reported in other studies [6–8]. Recent prospective studies, also carried out in the clinical setting, demonstrated that up to 64% of patients treated with anti-TNFα drugs achieved MDA after 12 months [6–8]. A similar rate (60%) was also reported in a PsA cohort of 344 patients receiving biological and non-biological DMARDs [17].

Table 1 Demographic and clinical characteristics of the study population

	Total *n* = 227	MDA *n* = 133	No MDA *n* = 94	*p*
Male, *n* (%)	123 (54.2)	82 (61.7)	41 (43.6)	<0.05
Age, mean (SD), years	53.2 (12.4)	53.5 (13.3)	52.8 (10.9)	NS
Smoker, *n* (%)	41 (18.1)	19 (14.3)	22 (23.4)	NS
Comorbidities, *n* (%)				
Dyslipemia	69 (30.4)	44 (33.1)	25 (26.6)	NS
HBP	62 (27.3)	35 (26.3)	27 (28.7)	NS
Obesity	48 (21.1)	32 (24.1)	16 (17.0)	NS
DM	23 (10.1)	15 (11.3)	8 (8.5)	NS
PsA characteristics				
PsA clinical pattern, *n* (%)				NS
Axial	8 (3.5)	3 (2.3)	5 (5.3)	
Peripheral	189 (83.3)	113 (85.0)	76 (80.9)	
Mixed	30 (13.2)	17 (12.8)	13 (13.8)	
Familial history, *n* (%)				
Psoriasis	112 (49.3)	64 (48.1)	48 (51.1)	NS
PsA	28 (12.3)	10 (7.5)	18 (19.1)	<0.05
Ankylosing spondylitis	2 (0.9)	2 (1.5)	0 (0.0)	NS
PsA duration, mean (SD), years	9.6 (7.7)	9.80 (8.1)	9.38 (7.3)	NS
Skin symptoms duration, mean (SD), years	22.1 (14.7)	20.6 (14.3)	24.2 (15.1)	NS
Articular symptoms duration, mean (SD), years	12.1 (9.3)	11.8 (8.8)	12.7 (9.9)	NS
PsA status at study visit				
Radiologic findings				
Erosions in hands, *n* (%)	83 (36.6)	41 (30.8)	42 (44.7)	<0.05
Joint in hands with erosion, mean (SD)	4.3 (4.2)	4.9 (4.5)	3.7 (3.9)	NS
Erosions in feet, *n* (%)	67 (29.5)	38 (28.6)	29 (30.9)	NS
Joint in feet with erosion, mean (SD)	3.7 (3.4)	3.9 (3.3)	3.5 (3.7)	NS
PsAID, mean (SD)	4.9 (4.5)	3.3 (3.1)	7.1 (5.2))	<0.001
PASI, mean (SD)	1.6 (3.8)	0.9 (1.6)	2.8 (5.7)	<0.05
BASDAI*, mean (SD)	2.8 (2.4)	2.0 (1.8)	3.6 (2.5)	<0.001
HAQ, mean (SD)	0.8 (0.6)	0.3 (0.5)	0.5 (0.6)	<0.001

BASDAI Bath Ankylosing Spondylitis Disease Activity Index, *DM* diabetes mellitus, *HAQ* Health Assessment Questionnaire, *HBP* high blood pressure, *MDA* minimal disease activity, *NS* not significant, *PASI* Psoriasis Area and Severity Index, *PsA* psoriatic arthritis, *PsAID* Psoriatic Arthritis Impact of Disease, *SD* standard deviation.
*Performed only in subjects with axial disease

The less frequently achieved MDA criteria by the MDA population were patient global disease activity VAS score ≤20 and HAQ <0.5; this latter measure focused on physical disability and pain. This finding is in line with previous results [6], and might reflect the patient's perception not only of damage but also of active disease. In fact, meeting MDA criteria does not exclude the presence of a small amount of disease activity [17]. However, MDA is a good therapeutic target in PsA, as patients who reach this state have better functional status and lower impact of disease.

In line with our results, male sex has been identified previously as a predictor not only of MDA [18] but also of response to treatment with anti-TNFα therapy [6–8]. However, we found that a sedentary lifestyle is a factor associated with MDA, which could be in contradiction with previous studies where obesity and metabolic syndrome have been associated with a lower probability of achieving MDA [19–21]. Indeed, the benefit of programs that encourage physical activity has been reported recently [22]. Although unexpected and controversial, according to the hypothesis that mechanical stress is associated with musculoskeletal inflammation, a sedentary lifestyle in PsA could reduce clinical complications associated with strenuous physical activity [23].

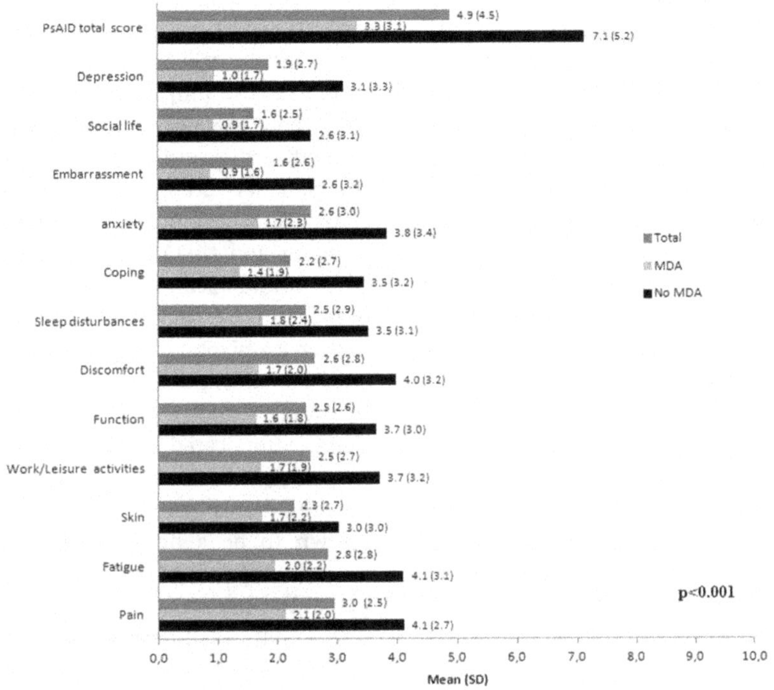

Fig. 2 Psoriatic Arthritis Impact of Disease (*PsAID*) score according to minimal disease activity (*MDA*) state

There has been evidence of genetic predisposition to PsA, although there is no specific gene for the disease [24, 25]. In our study, the presence of a familial history of PsA was related with non-MDA. It may represent an effect of genetics both in the severity and in the capability to respond to drugs, although it is an open thesis that calls for additional research. On the contrary, in our study having a familial history of psoriasis did not present a relationship with MDA. Similarly, a recent study showed that the severity of psoriasis and the proportion of patients with comorbidities were not affected by the presence of a family history of psoriasis [26].

In PsA, the most common inflammatory indicators (ESR and CRP) used for the evaluation of disease activity in rheumatoid arthritis are within normal levels in half of the patients [27]. However, when these two markers are increased, their utility is undeniable [27]. Baseline high CRP and ESR are predictors for MDA [6].

Table 2 Multivariate logistic regression analysis

	p value	Adjusted OR (95% CI)
Sex (men)	0.001	2.746 (1.473–5.119)
Sedentary lifestyle	0.002	3.127 (1.497–6.534)
PsA familial history	0.038	0.387 (0.159–0.938)
C-reactive protein	0.010	0.920 (0.864–0.980)
Corticoids	0.007	0.335 (0.151–0.745)

CI confidence interval, *PsA* psoriatic arthritis, *OR* odds ratio

Table 3 PsA treatment at study visit

	Total	MDA	No MDA	*p*
Treatment pattern, *n* (%)				NS
Anti-TNF monotherapy	110	69 (62.7)	41 (37.3)	
DMARDS and anti-TNF	61	32 (52.5)	29 (47.5)	
DMARDS monotherapy	51	32 (62.7)	19 (37.3)	
Anti-TNF*, *n* (%)	112	64 (57.1)	48 (42.9)	NS
Etanercept	42	26 (61.9)	16 (38.1)	
Adalimumab	35	22 (62.9)	13 (37.1)	
Infliximab	15	6 (40.0)	9 (60.0)	
Golimumab	13	7 (53.8)	6 (46.2)	
Mean (SD) time, months	45.7 (34.7)	50.5 (35.0)	40.2 (33.8)	NS
DMARDS*, *n* (%)	171	101 (59.1)	70 (40.9)	NS
Metotrexate	130	76 (58.5)	54 (41.5)	
Leflunomide	32	17 (53.1)	15 (46.9)	
Mean (SD) time, months	73.7 (70.4)	71.8 (71.8)	76.4 (69.7)	NS
NSAIDs**, *n* (%)	114	62 (54.4)	52 (45.6)	NS
Infiltrations**, *n* (%)	48	27 (56.3)	21 (43.8)	NS
Corticoids**, *n* (%)	39	16 (41.0)	23 (59.0)	<0.05

*Monotherapy or combination therapy
**Combination therapy
anti-TNF anti-tumor necrosis factor, *DMARDS* disease-modifying anti-rheumatic drugs, *NS* not significant, *NSAIDs* nonsteroidal anti-inflammatory drugs

Conversely, in this cross-sectional study, we found that having increased CRP level at the study visit has a very slight relationship to non-MDA status. Being a transversal study, it may only reflect the patients who are in a state of greater activity.

We also identified use of therapy with corticoids as a possible factor related to non-MDA state. This could reflect that physicians were more likely to prescribe corticosteroids in severe/difficult cases. On the other hand, several authors have indicated that systemic therapy with corticoids hinders the control of skin manifestations and should therefore not be used routinely, but only for a limited period of time [28, 29]. Systemic use of corticosteroids improves skin psoriasis, but their withdrawal triggers relapses in the form of a "rebound effect", producing recurrence of the skin manifestations or transformation into the generalized pustular form [28, 29].

Heterogeneity and complexity of PsA are challenging for the clinical measure of the disease, both from the patient's perspective and from the physician's view. Patients with PsA experience functional impairment and reduced quality of life, so patient global assessment in PsA is explained mainly by the physical, but also by the psychological aspect, of the disease [30]. PROs, such as the novel PsAID questionnaire [12], are important instruments to evaluate healthcare interventions and to reflect the impact of PsA on patients' lives. There are few studies that have reported results with this tool [31]. In the present study, we observed that MDA state and lower impact of the disease are associated. Thus, statistically significant differences were observed between MDA and non-MDA patients in all physical and psychological PsAID domains. These findings suggest that PsAID information seems to be in consonance with the MDA state and could be a useful tool for assessing PsA from the patient's point of view.

An adequate therapeutic approach for PsA depends on the type and severity of the skin and joint involvements [32]. Anti-TNF drugs have been shown to significantly inhibit joint damage [33–35]. In the present study, MDA was achieved by a significant proportion of patients (63%) receiving anti-TNF or csDMARD monotherapy. Interestingly, we found a lower, but not meaningful, proportion of patients receiving anti-TNF concomitantly with csDMARDS (52.5%) in the MDA state compared with those treated with anti-TNF alone. This could be due to concomitant therapy being administered to more severe patients who have more difficulty achieving a MDA state.

Moreover, ad hoc analysis results from clinical trials indicated that concomitant use of methotrexate and anti-TNF was not more effective in achieving a response [32, 36]. A recent study showed that methotrexate administered in combination with etanercept in patients with PsA may not provide significantly greater improvement in arthritis or psoriasis symptoms than etanercept monotherapy [36]. Despite the advances in therapy for PsA, there remain many patients who fail to respond and lose efficacy over time [32]. In the present study, 41.4% of the patients did not achieve the MDA state, although statistically significant differences were not observed between non-MDA and MDA patients regarding the use of non-biological DMARDs and biological DMARDs. Some authors suggested that the TNFα pathway might not have a pivotal role in driving the inflammation in such patients, and these patients might benefit from other treatments targeted at different inflammatory pathways that are implicated in the disease activity [7, 32].

Some limitations derived from the cross-sectional nature of this study should be borne in mind. PsA is known to be a heterogeneous disorder, with progression highly variable between individuals. The data presented here are a photograph of a specific moment of the state of illness of patients with a long evolution of the disease. We cannot be sure what proportion of patients achieved MDA state due to the natural history of the disease and what success treatment had on outcome. Thus, it is difficult to know whether the management of these patients was as appropriate as it should have been. Furthermore, we do not know the proportion of patients who reached sustained MDA and how long they remained in this state. A further limitation is related to the study being designed to include patients on conventional or biological DMARDs, representing the majority of PsA cases followed in the Rheumatology Department. PsA patients that only require NSAIDs or corticosteroids are usually followed in general practice and therefore they were not included.

Despite these limitations, this multicenter study shows the treatment response of a representative Spanish population with PsA in a routine clinical setting. In addition, a further strength of this study is the use of the novel PsAID questionnaire, which allowed a precise interpretation of the patient-perceived impact of the disease.

To summarize, in this study we report that a significant proportion of PsA patients achieve a MDA state in normal clinical practice, reflecting a management of PsA in Spain similar to that which has been published in other countries. The PsAID could be an additional useful tool to assess PsA interventions in clinical practice, although further studies are needed to confirm it.

Conclusions

This study supports the use of MDA and PsAID as two of the main assessment tools for PsA in routine clinical practice.

Abbreviations

BASDAI: Bath Ankylosing Spondylitis Disease Activity Index; CASPAR: Classification for Psoriatic Arthritis; CRP: C-reactive protein; csDMARD: Conventional synthetic disease-modifying anti-rheumatic drug; DMARD: Disease-modifying anti-rheumatic drug; ESR: Erythrocyte sedimentation rate; HAQ: Health Assessment Questionnaire; HLA-B27: Human leukocyte antigen-B27; MDA: Minimal disease activity; NSAID: Nonsteroidal anti-inflammatory drug; PASI: Psoriasis Area Severity Index; PRO: Patient-reported outcome; PsA: Psoriatic arthritis; PsAID: Psoriatic Arthritis Impact of Disease; TNF: Tumor necrosis factor; VAS: Visual analog scale

Acknowledgements

MAAPS (Minimal Activity in Psoriatic Arthritis) study group: J.C. Torre Alonso (H. Monte Naranco, Oviedo, Spain); J.A Román-Ivorra (HU. La Fe, Valencia, Spain); J. Sanz (HU. Puerta de Hierro, Madrid, Spain); J. Salvatierra (HU. San Cecilio, Granada, Spain); J. Calvo-Alén (HU. Sierrallana, Torrelavega, Spain); A. Sellas (Vall d´Hebron, Barcelona, Spain); F.J. Rodriguez (Santa Lucia, Cartagena, Spain); A. Bermúdez (Virgen de la Arrixaca, Murcia, Spain); M.Romero (Complejo hospitalario Jaén, Spain); M. Riesco (Rheumatology H. Juan Ramón Jiménez, Huelva, Spain); J.C Cobeta (H. Royo Villanova, Zaragoza, Spain); F.Medina (H. Puerta del Mar, Cádiz, Spain); A. Aragón (H. Getafe, Madrid, Spain); ML. García (HU. Basurto, Bilbao, Spain); A. Urruticoechea (H. Can Misses, Ibiza, Spain); CM. González (HU. Gregorio Marañón, Madrid, Spain); E. Judez (CU. Albacete, Spain); B. González (HU. Nta. Sra de la Candelaria, Tenerife, Spain); P. Fernández (HU. 12 de Octubre, Madrid, Spain); L. Pantoja (H. del Bierzo, Leon, Spain); R. Morlá (H. Sant Pau y Sta. Tecla, Tarragona, Spain). The authors are grateful to Mª Luz Samaniego and Eva Pascual for their valuable contribution in statistical analyses and all the initial steps of the study, respectively. We are also grateful to Esther Tapia for helping us with the medical writing of this manuscript.

Funding

This study was funded by Pfizer, S.L.U.

Authors' contributions

RQ, JDC, CM, MA, MM, SG, and AC participated in the original idea and design of the study, interpreted results of analysis, and actively reviewed and criticized the manuscript for important intellectual content. All authors helped to draft the manuscript, and they read, modified and approved the final version.

Competing interests

JDC has received fees for speaking and/or consulting from AbbVie, Boehringer, Bristol, Celgene, Janssen, MSD/Schering Plough, Novartis and Pfizer. MM, SG, and AC are employees of Pfizer, S.L.U. The remaining authors declare that they have no competing interests.

Consent for publications

Not applicable.

Author details

[1]Department of Rheumatology, HU, Central de Asturias, Av. Roma, s/n, 33011 Oviedo, Asturias, Spain. [2]Department of Rheumatology, HU, Clinic and IDIBAPS, C/Villarroel, 170-08036 Barcelona, Spain. [3]Department of Rheumatology, HU, Parque Natural de las Batuecas 17, Cabrerizos, Salamanca Cp 37193, Spain. [4]Department of Rheumatology HU, Virgen del Puerto, Paraje Valcorchero s/n, 10600 Plasencia, Spain. [5]Medical Department, Pfizer, Avenida de Europa, 20 B, 28108 Alcobendas, Madrid, Spain.

References

1. Chandran V, Raychaudhuri SP. Geoepidemiology and environmental factors of psoriasis and psoriatic arthritis. J Autoimmun. 2010;34(3):J314–21.
2. Ibrahim G, Waxman R, Helliwell PS. The prevalence of psoriatic arthritis in people with psoriasis. Arthritis Rheum. 2009;61(10):1373–8.
3. Kavanaugh A, Fransen J. Defining remission in psoriatic arthritis. Clin Exp Rheumatol. 2006;24(6 Suppl 43):S-7.
4. Coates LC, Fransen J, Helliwell PS. Defining minimal disease activity in psoriatic arthritis: a proposed objective target for treatment. Ann Rheum Dis. 2010;69(1):48–53.
5. Coates LC, Helliwell PS. Validation of minimal disease activity criteria for psoriatic arthritis using interventional trial data. Arthritis Care Res (Hoboken). 2010;62(7):965–9.
6. Perrotta FM, Marchesoni A, Lubrano E. Minimal disease activity and remission in psoriatic arthritis patients treated with anti-TNF-alpha drugs. J Rheumatol. 2016;43(2):350–5.
7. Haddad A, Thavaneswaran A, Ruiz-Arruza I, Pellett F, Chandran V, Cook RJ, et al. Minimal disease activity and anti-tumor necrosis factor therapy in psoriatic arthritis. Arthritis Care Res (Hoboken). 2015;67(6):842–7.
8. Lubrano E, Parsons WJ, Perrotta FM. Assessment of response to treatment, remission, and minimal disease activity in axial psoriatic arthritis treated with tumor necrosis factor inhibitors. J Rheumatol. 2016;43(5):918–23.
9. Strand V, Sharp V, Koenig AS, Park G, Shi Y, Wang B, et al. Comparison of health-related quality of life in rheumatoid arthritis, psoriatic arthritis and psoriasis and effects of etanercept treatment. Ann Rheum Dis. 2012; 71(7):1143–50.
10. Borman P, Toy GG, Babaoglu S, Bodur H, Ciliz D, Alli N. A comparative evaluation of quality of life and life satisfaction in patients with psoriatic and rheumatoid arthritis. Clin Rheumatol. 2007;26(3):330–4.
11. Saad AA, Ashcroft DM, Watson KD, Symmons DP, Noyce PR, Hyrich KL. Improvements in quality of life and functional status in patients with psoriatic arthritis receiving anti-tumor necrosis factor therapies. Arthritis Care Res (Hoboken). 2010;62(3):345–53.
12. Gossec L, de Wit M, Kiltz U, Braun J, Kalyoncu U, Scrivo R, et al. A patient-derived and patient-reported outcome measure for assessing psoriatic arthritis: elaboration and preliminary validation of the Psoriatic Arthritis Impact of Disease (PsAID) questionnaire, a 13-country EULAR initiative. Ann Rheum Dis. 2014;73(6):1012–9.
13. Taylor W, Gladman D, Helliwell P, Marchesoni A, Mease P, Mielants H. Classification criteria for psoriatic arthritis: development of new criteria from a large international study. Arthritis Rheum. 2006;54(8):2665–73.
14. Chandran V, Gottlieb A, Cook RJ, Duffin KC, Garg A, Helliwell P, et al. International multicenter psoriasis and psoriatic arthritis reliability trial for the assessment of skin, joints, nails, and dactylitis. Arthritis Rheum. 2009;61(9):1235–42.
15. Blackmore MG, Gladman DD, Husted J, Long JA, Farewell VT. Measuring health status in psoriatic arthritis: the Health Assessment Questionnaire and its modification. J Rheumatol. 1995;22(5):886–93.
16. Garrett S, Jenkinson T, Kennedy LG, Whitelock H, Gaisford P, Calin A. A new approach to defining disease status in ankylosing spondylitis: the Bath Ankylosing Spondylitis Disease Activity Index. J Rheumatol. 1994;21(12):2286–91.
17. Coates LC, Cook R, Lee KA, Chandran V, Gladman DD. Frequency, predictors, and prognosis of sustained minimal disease activity in an observational psoriatic arthritis cohort. Arthritis Care Res (Hoboken). 2010;62(7):970–6.
18. Theander E, Husmark T, Alenius GM, Larsson PT, Teleman A, Geijer M, et al. Early psoriatic arthritis: short symptom duration, male gender and preserved physical functioning at presentation predict favourable outcome at 5-year follow-up. Results from the Swedish Early Psoriatic Arthritis Register (SwePsA). Ann Rheum Dis. 2014;73(2):407–13.
19. Costa L, Caso F, Ramonda R, Del PA, Cantarini L, Darda MA, et al. Metabolic syndrome and its relationship with the achievement of minimal disease activity state in psoriatic arthritis patients: an observational study. Immunol Res. 2015;61(1-2):147–53.
20. Di Minno MN, Peluso R, Iervolino S, Lupoli R, Russolillo A, Scarpa R, et al. Obesity and the prediction of minimal disease activity: a prospective study in psoriatic arthritis. Arthritis Care Res (Hoboken). 2013;65(1):141–7.
21. Eder L, Thavaneswaran A, Chandran V, Cook RJ, Gladman DD. Obesity is associated with a lower probability of achieving sustained minimal disease activity state among patients with psoriatic arthritis. Ann Rheum Dis. 2015;74(5):813–7.
22. Chimenti MS, Triggianese P, Conigliaro P, Santoro M, Lucchetti R, Perricone R. Self-reported adherence to a home-based exercise program among patients affected by psoriatic arthritis with minimal disease activity. Drug Dev Res. 2014;75 Suppl 1:S57–9.
23. Jacques P, McGonagle D. The role of mechanical stress in the pathogenesis of spondyloarthritis and how to combat it. Best Pract Res Clin Rheumatol. 2014;28(5):703–10.

24. Barnas JL, Ritchlin CT. Etiology and pathogenesis of psoriatic arthritis. Rheum Dis Clin North Am. 2015;41(4):643–63.
25. FitzGerald O, Haroon M, Giles JT, Winchester R. Concepts of pathogenesis in psoriatic arthritis: genotype determines clinical phenotype. Arthritis Res Ther. 2015;17:115.
26. Lopez-Estebaranz JL, Sanchez-Carazo JL, Sulleiro S. Effect of a family history of psoriasis and age on comorbidities and quality of life in patients with moderate to severe psoriasis: results from the ARIZONA study. J Dermatol. 2016;43(4):395–401.
27. Punzi L, Podswiadek M, Oliviero F, Lonigro A, Modesti V, Ramonda R, et al. Laboratory findings in psoriatic arthritis. Reumatismo. 2007;59 Suppl 1:52–5.
28. Griffiths CE. Therapy for psoriatic arthritis: sometimes a conflict for psoriasis. Br J Rheumatol. 1997;36(4):409–10.
29. Menter A, Gottlieb A, Feldman SR, Van Voorhees AS, Leonardi CL, Gordon KB, et al. Guidelines of care for the management of psoriasis and psoriatic arthritis: Section 1. Overview of psoriasis and guidelines of care for the treatment of psoriasis with biologics. J Am Acad Dermatol. 2008;58(5):826–50.
30. Talli S, Etcheto A, Fautrel B, Balanescu A, Braun J, Canete JD, et al. Patient global assessment in psoriatic arthritis—what does it mean? An analysis of 223 patients from the Psoriatic arthritis impact of disease (PsAID) study. Joint Bone Spine. 2016;83(3):335–40.
31. Salaffi F, Di CM, Carotti M, Farah S, Gutierrez M. The Psoriatic Arthritis Impact of Disease 12-item questionnaire: equivalence, reliability, validity, and feasibility of the touch-screen administration versus the paper-and-pencil version. Ther Clin Risk Manag. 2016;12:631–42.
32. Veale DJ. Psoriatic arthritis: recent progress in pathophysiology and drug development. Arthritis Res Ther. 2013;15(6):224.
33. Iervolino S, Di Minno MN, Peluso R, Lofrano M, Russolillo A, Di MG, et al. Predictors of early minimal disease activity in patients with psoriatic arthritis treated with tumor necrosis factor-alpha blockers. J Rheumatol. 2012;39(3):568–73.
34. Mease PJ, Kivitz AJ, Burch FX, Siegel EL, Cohen SB, Ory P, et al. Etanercept treatment of psoriatic arthritis: safety, efficacy, and effect on disease progression. Arthritis Rheum. 2004;50(7):2264–72.
35. Antoni C, Krueger GG, de Vlam K, Birbara C, Beutler A, Guzzo C, et al. Infliximab improves signs and symptoms of psoriatic arthritis: results of the IMPACT 2 trial. Ann Rheum Dis. 2005;64(8):1150–7.
36. Combe B, Behrens F, McHugh N, Brock F, Kerkmann U, Kola B, et al. Comparison of etanercept monotherapy and combination therapy with methotrexate in psoriatic arthritis: results from 2 clinical trials. J Rheumatol. 2016;43(6):1063–7.

16

Mitigation of disease- and treatment-related risks in patients with psoriatic arthritis

Martin Bergman[1*] and Amy Lundholm[2]

Abstract

Psoriatic arthritis is a part of the family of diseases referred to as spondyloarthropathies, a diverse group of chronic inflammatory disorders with common clinical, radiographic, and genetic features. Peripheral arthritis is the most common symptom of psoriatic arthritis and patients also frequently experience involvement of the entheses, spine, skin, and nails. Due to the diverse clinical spectrum of disease severity, tissues affected, and associated comorbidities, the treatment of psoriatic arthritis can be challenging and it is necessary to mitigate risks associated with both the disease and its treatment. These risks include disease-specific, treatment-related, and psychological risks. Disease-specific risks include those associated with disease progression that can limit functional status and be mitigated through early diagnosis and initiation of treatment. Risks also arise from comorbidities that are associated with psoriatic arthritis such as cardiovascular disease, obesity, diabetes mellitus, and gastrointestinal inflammation. Patient outcomes can be affected by the treatment strategy employed and the pharmacologic agents administered. Additionally, it is important for physicians to be aware of risks specific to each therapeutic option. The impact of psoriatic arthritis is not limited to the skin and joints and it is common for patients to experience quality-of-life impairment. Patients are also more likely to have depression, anxiety, and alcoholism. This article reviews the many risks associated with psoriatic arthritis and provides guidance on mitigating these risks.

Keywords: Psoriatic arthritis, Disease-specific risks, Treatment-related risks, Psychological risks, Comorbidities, Quality of life, Risk, Review

Background

Psoriatic arthritis (PsA) is a member of the spondyloarthropathies (SpA) family of diseases, a diverse group of chronic inflammatory rheumatic disorders with common clinical, radiographic, and genetic features [1, 2]. There are a wide variety of clinical and anatomic characteristics that distinguish PsA from other chronic rheumatic diseases such as rheumatoid arthritis (RA) and other forms of SpA [3, 4]. The primary regions affected in patients with PsA are the peripheral joints, entheses (connective tissue between tendon or ligament and bone), and axial sites, often in an asymmetrical pattern, in addition to psoriasis of the skin and nails [4, 5]. In addition to the larger joints, the small joints of the fingers, including the distal interphalangeal (DIP) joints—which are generally spared by RA—and toes are also typically involved in PsA [5]. Further, up to 43% of patients with PsA experience sacroiliitis (inflammation of the sacroiliac [SI] joint) in the spinal column [6]. Dactylitis (swelling of an entire digit) is also common in patients with PsA and is a marker of disease progression [7]. Although PsA is commonly associated with the presence of psoriasis, skin disease and joint inflammation do not always present concurrently [2].

The prevalence of PsA in the United States is 0.25% [8]. However, the prevalence of PsA in patients with psoriasis is substantially higher, with approximately 30% of individuals reported to have both conditions [9]. PsA is reportedly more common in women than in men compared with ankylosing spondylitis [5, 10]. Although it is important to recognize that there may be some degree of selection bias in this regard (due to conventional wisdom and teaching that women are unlikely to develop ankylosing spondylitis).

* Correspondence: mjbergman@prodigy.net
[1]Taylor Hospital, 8 Morton Avenue, Suite 304, Ridley Park, PA 19078, USA
Full list of author information is available at the end of the article

The differentiation of PsA from RA can be aided by certain clinical characteristics. Unlike RA, PsA is not associated with circulating autoantibodies [3, 11]. Patients with PsA are usually seronegative (absence of circulating rheumatoid factor) and a negative test for rheumatoid factor is one component of the ClASsification criteria for Psoriatic Arthritis (CASPAR) [2, 12]. Additionally, PsA and RA typically have distinct patterns of inflammatory joint damage, which can be distinguished through specific clinical and radiological changes. The clinical pathology of PsA typically presents in the distal interphalangeal and axial joints, with an asymmetrical distribution, whereas RA is primarily symmetrically distributed in the metacarpophalangeal and wrist joints [3]. However, PsA may also present as a symmetrical arthropathy or as an oligoarthropathy. The vascular pathology of PsA is distinct from RA and is characterized by a hypervascularized network of elongated, tortuous vessels [3]. Whereas RA primarily results in bone and cartilage resorption, PsA has both bone destruction and formation traits [13]. Both patients with RA and PsA experience erosion that leads to resorption of cortical bone, but additional formation of bony spurs is observed along insertion sites of entheses only in patients with PsA [13].

Like other forms of SpA, susceptibility to PsA is associated with the human leukocyte antigen B27 (HLA-B27) gene [2]. The strength of the association between HLA-B27 and disease susceptibility varies among different SpA subtypes as well as between ethnic groups and the presence of HLA-B27 in combination with other major histocompatibility complex class alleles may influence the pattern of axial or peripheral disease presentation [14].

The clinical spectrum of PsA is extremely diverse in both disease severity and tissues affected, and this disorder often occurs in conjunction with several associated comorbidities [4, 15]. The array of symptoms, coupled with the wide range in severity and disease course, presents difficult challenges for treatment [16]. Mitigation of risks associated with the disease itself, its treatment, and associated comorbidities are all important considerations when managing patients with PsA (Table 1). This review will discuss and highlight the many risks associated with PsA, with the aim to help improve awareness of risks among physicians and to provide guidance in mitigating these risks.

Table 1 PsA risk framework

Disease-related risks (including functional concerns)

- Assessment of symptoms (pain, stiffness, swelling, rash)
  - Physical examination
  - Joint examination
  - PASI
- Functional assessment
  - Imaging (X-rays, MRI)
- Quality of life (social interaction, sexual health, body image)
  - SF-36 subscales
  - EuroQoL-5 dimension
  - PsAQoL
  - Pain Disability Index
  - PsAID
  - Work ability
- Documentation of extra-articular manifestations and/or comorbidities
- Poor balance/risk of falls
  - Fractures

Treatment-related risks

- Contraindications
  - NSAIDs in patients with IBD, CV disease
- Adverse events
  - Liver damage with methotrexate (obese patients particularly at risk)
- Poor compliance/persistence
  - Reduced efficacy of biologics
- Routine laboratory monitoring with biologics
- Immunogenicity with biologics

Psychosocial risks

- Mental health (particularly depression, but also anxiety)
  - SF-36 subscales
  - PsAID
  - DASS-21
- Alcohol abuse
- Self-esteem issues (especially in younger patients)
- Social participation
  - PsAID

CV cardiovascular, *DASS-21* Depression and Anxiety Stress Scale, *IBD* inflammatory bowel disease, *MRI* magnetic resonance imaging, *NSAIDs* nonsteroidal anti-inflammatory drugs, *PASI* Psoriasis Area and Severity Index, *PsAID* Psoriatic Arthritis Impact of Disease, *PsAQoL* Psoriatic Arthritis Quality of Life Questionnaire, *SF-36* Short-form 36

Disease-specific risks

Risks associated with disease progression

Early diagnosis and treatment of PsA is important because the disease not only causes functional impairment over time, but also may increase the risk of mortality in affected patients [15]. Unfortunately, early detection methods for PsA remain limited and the disease is often underdiagnosed due to symptoms going unrecognized [15]. Common initial symptoms include arthritis in the upper and lower limbs (Table 2).

For proper treatment of PsA, it is necessary to consider all aspects of the disease, including clinical pathology and psychological issues [15]. Further, worse outcomes in patients with PsA are associated with a delay in diagnosis, disability, and joint damage, whereas male sex and lower burden of inflammation at presentation were predictors of improved patient outcomes [17–19]. The presence of specific HLA alleles can also identify patients likely to sustain joint damage [19].

Maintaining good functional status is the primary aim of pharmacologic treatment in patients with PsA. Although the recommended approaches to the diagnosis, therapy, and follow-up of patients with PsA have changed numerous times over the past decade, the goal of treatment is remission or, alternatively, low disease activity or minimal disease activity (MDA) if remission is not attainable [20, 21]. Loss of physical functioning directly impairs

Table 2 First signs and symptoms attributable to psoriatic spondyloarthritis [74]

First signs and symptoms, n (%)	Psoriatic spondyloarthritis		
	≤2 years (*n* = 51)	>10 years (*n* = 187)	*P* value
Low back pain	13 (26)	31 (17)	0.15
Sacroiliac syndrome	6 (12)	17 (9)	0.59
Neck pain	1 (2)	14 (7)	0.20
Dactylitis	5 (10)	17 (9)	0.79
Arthritis, lower limbs	29 (57)	131 (70)	0.08
Arthritis, upper limbs	27 (53)	106 (57)	0.63
Enthesitis	5 (10)	15 (8)	0.78

(Adapted from: Rojas-Vargas M et al. First signs and symptoms of spondyloarthritis—data from an inception cohort with a disease course of two years or less (REGISPONSER-Early). Rheumatology (Oxford). 2009;48(4):404–409)
Significance obtained by the chi-square test for contingency tables
Comparison of REGISPONSER-Early (≤2 years) vs REGISPONSER-Late (>10 years)

patient quality of life (QoL) and results in increased direct and indirect costs associated with the disease [22]. For example, decreased functional status can prevent patients from performing daily activities of living, such as washing and dressing [23].

Clinicians should be aware of the relevant extra-articular manifestations of PsA and its associated comorbidities, which result in considerable morbidity and mortality [24]. At least 1 extra-articular immune-mediated inflammatory disease is present in 94.7% of patients with PsA and the most common of these are psoriasis (94%), uveitis (1.3%), and inflammatory bowel disease (0.7%) [25]. The extra-articular manifestations and comorbidities associated with PsA can also significantly impact QoL and must be considered in the management of PsA [23].

Risks associated with comorbidities

Patients with PsA have a higher prevalence and incidence of cardiovascular (CV) disease than the general population [24, 26]. This increased risk is due to both a higher prevalence of traditional risk factors such as hypertension, obesity, diabetes, and hyperlipidemia, and also to nonconventional risk factors, for example, those related to chronic systemic inflammation, including higher levels of C-reactive protein and erythrocyte sedimentation rate [24, 27]. Interestingly, suppression of inflammation in patients with PsA has been linked with improvements in surrogate markers of CV risk, such as increased carotid intima media thickness and endothelial dysfunction [28]. Further, the presence of metabolic syndrome and insulin resistance, which are also more common in patients with PsA, are associated with increased severity of PsA and increased risk of CV disease [29, 30]. These findings suggest that systemic inflammation may play an important role in driving CV risk in patients with PsA.

Obesity is reported in 35% of patients with PsA and has been suggested as a potential risk factor for developing PsA [31, 32]. Obesity may also impact disease activity and response to therapy, possibly through increased production of inflammatory cytokines [33]. For instance, irrespective of the kind of therapy used, obesity is associated a lower probability of achieving MDA and it is speculated that the chronic pro-inflammatory state, the biomechanical effect of heavy weight on the joints, and the altered pain threshold associated with obesity may be factors responsible preventing achievement of MDA [32].

PsA is associated with diabetes mellitus and the rate of diabetes mellitus is significantly higher in patients with PsA than in those with RA (odds ratio 1.56; 95% confidence interval [CI] 1.07–2.28; $P = 0.02$) [34]. Caution should be used if prescribing glucocorticoids because they are associated with an approximately 30% increase in the risk for developing diabetes mellitus in patients with psoriasis or PsA [35]. Some dermatologists consider psoriasis as a contraindication for use of corticosteroids, due to concerns of converting plaque psoriasis into pustular psoriasis. However, corticosteroids are still often used across various practice settings, including dermatology.

A strong relationship has been noted between gastrointestinal (GI) inflammation and joint inflammation in various forms of SpA [36]. However, the prevalence of inflammatory bowel disease in patients with PsA is less clearly defined [24]. Of note, there is a significantly increased risk of Crohn's disease in women with psoriasis (relative risk [RR] 3.86, 95% CI 2.23–6.67) that is further increased in women with both psoriasis and PsA (RR 6.43, 95% CI 2.04–20.32) [37].

Patients with PsA also suffer from sleep disturbances and diminished sleep quality that are associated with generalized pain, anxiety, enthesitis, increased levels of C-reactive protein, and increased erythrocyte sedimentation rate [38]. The prevalence of depression in patients with PsA is 22.2%, compared with 9.6% in patients with psoriasis alone, and the estimated prevalence in the general population (9%) [39]. Similarly, the prevalence of anxiety among patients with PsA is reported as 36.6%, compared with 24.4% in patients with psoriasis alone [39].

Mitigation of disease-specific risks

Mitigation and evaluation of disease-specific risks is dependent upon prompt and accurate diagnosis. Currently, the primary objectives in clinical rheumatology are early diagnosis and initiation of treatment because diagnostic delays are a significant contributor to poor patient outcomes [4, 15]. Even short delays (6 months) from symptom onset to first visit with a rheumatologist have been observed to contribute to development of peripheral joint erosions and worse long-term physical function [40]. To this end, remission in PsA has been attributed to early diagnosis and treatment.

Disease-related risks should be evaluated through good patient history and use of metrics specific to PsA [41]. These include evaluation of physical function and skin involvement, as well as joint examination (tender joint count, swollen joint count, entheseal assessment). Additionally, physicians should be aware of the possibility of PsA when diagnosing and treating patients who suffer from pre-existing psoriasis. Tracking of metrics over time should be undertaken to detect whether medications are ameliorating disease severity. Imaging may be used for diagnosis and following disease progression over time [41]. In recent years, magnetic resonance imaging (MRI) and ultrasonography have been increasingly used for assessment of PsA and have provided additional information on the pathogenesis of PsA [15].

Treatment with drugs is necessary for patients with PsA and recommended treatment guidelines tailored to individual PsA characteristics are shown in Fig. 1 [16]. Although it is important for patients with PsA to remain active, it is typically not possible to manage disease symptoms through physical therapy alone.

Treatment-related risks

Risks associated with treatment strategy

Early recognition and intervention with therapy is key to controlling disease progression in patients with PsA [15]. The tumor necrosis factor (TNF) inhibitors etanercept, infliximab, adalimumab, golimumab, and certolizumab pegol have been shown to improve signs and symptoms of PsA [42–46]. Additionally, apremilast (an oral phosphodiesterase-4 inhibitor), abatacept (a T cell selective costimulation modulator), ustekinumab (an interleukin- [IL-] 12/23 inhibitor), and secukinumab (an IL-17A inhibitor) have also shown varying degrees of efficacy in the treatment of PsA [47–53]. Approved agents are discussed in more detail in the following section.

Treat-to-target is a therapeutic concept derived from RA and other diseases [54, 55], which has been proposed for all forms of SpA [20, 41, 54, 56]. With this approach, a clear target, such as remission or low disease activity, is identified and the goal is to sustain this response over time, with an understanding of the need to treat flares and keep tight control of disease activity [55]. A universal definition of the target (e.g., remission, prevention of flare of disease) is required for the treat-to-target approach and, in SpA, remission and sustained low disease activity have been suggested as possible targets [20, 55]. Although definitions of remission or MDA in SpA have been proposed, none have been widely accepted or endorsed and given the multifaceted nature of SpA, a composite of outcome measures may be most useful [54, 57].

The Tight Control of Psoriatic Arthritis (TICOPA) trial, an open-label, randomized, controlled study, has recently provided evidence on the benefit of treating-to-target in PsA [58]. This study compared treat-to-target versus standard of care in newly diagnosed patients with PsA receiving methotrexate (MTX), a combination of disease-modifying antirheumatic drugs (DMARDs), or TNF inhibitors. Results from TICOPA demonstrated that tight control of disease activity using a step-up dosing regimen to achieve MDA (reviewed and adjusted, if necessary, every 4 weeks) significantly improved joint outcomes compared with standard of care (per the treating physician, reviewed every 12 weeks). After 48 weeks, the odds of achieving an American College of Rheumatology (ACR) 20% criteria for improvement (ACR20 response) nearly doubled (odds ratio 1.91; 95% CI, 1.03–3.55; $P = 0.0392$) without any unexpected serious adverse events (AEs) [58].

Risks associated with pharmacologic treatment

The complexities of PsA pathology suggest the need to identify suitable therapies to address the different combinations of clinical manifestations [21]. Traditional treatments for PsA include nonsteroidal anti-inflammatory drugs (NSAIDs), steroids, and synthetic DMARDs [59]. NSAIDs are effective for relieving musculoskeletal symptoms due to joint inflammation, but have no efficacy on psoriatic skin lesions and are associated with AEs including renal toxicity, gastrointestinal toxicity, and the risk of developing CV events [59]. Traditional DMARD treatment options for PsA include sulfasalazine and MTX [16, 59, 60]. There is debate over the efficacy of MTX and randomized trials have generally been unable to show efficacy [59, 61, 62]. Additionally, MTX is ineffective in treating axial inflammation and there is little evidence to support its use for other symptoms such as enthesitis [59, 62]. However, in the placebo-controlled Methotrexate in Psoriatic Arthritis (MIPA) trial (that showed no benefit with respect to the primary endpoint of PsA response criteria), treatment with MTX resulted in a significant improvement over placebo in both patient and physician global assessments, as well as Psoriasis Area and Severity Index (PASI) scores at 6 months [61, 62]. Nonetheless, the MIPA authors asserted that their findings questioned the classification of MTX as a DMARD in the setting of PsA, with recognition that there are safety concerns associated with MTX therapy [61]. In particular, the use of MTX in obese patients may lead to potential liver damage [63]. Alcohol abuse and the high prevalence of fatty liver in obese patients may contribute to the development of liver damage and the presence of fatty liver can also impede monitoring for liver damage.

Current targeted treatment options approved for PsA include biologics (TNF inhibitors, ustekinumab, and secukinumab) and the small molecule apremilast [3, 59]. These therapies are typically recommended for use after inadequate response to at least one DMARD but early escalation can be considered, especially for patients with poor prognostic factors such as raised inflammatory markers or high active-disease joint counts [16]. For patients who fail a

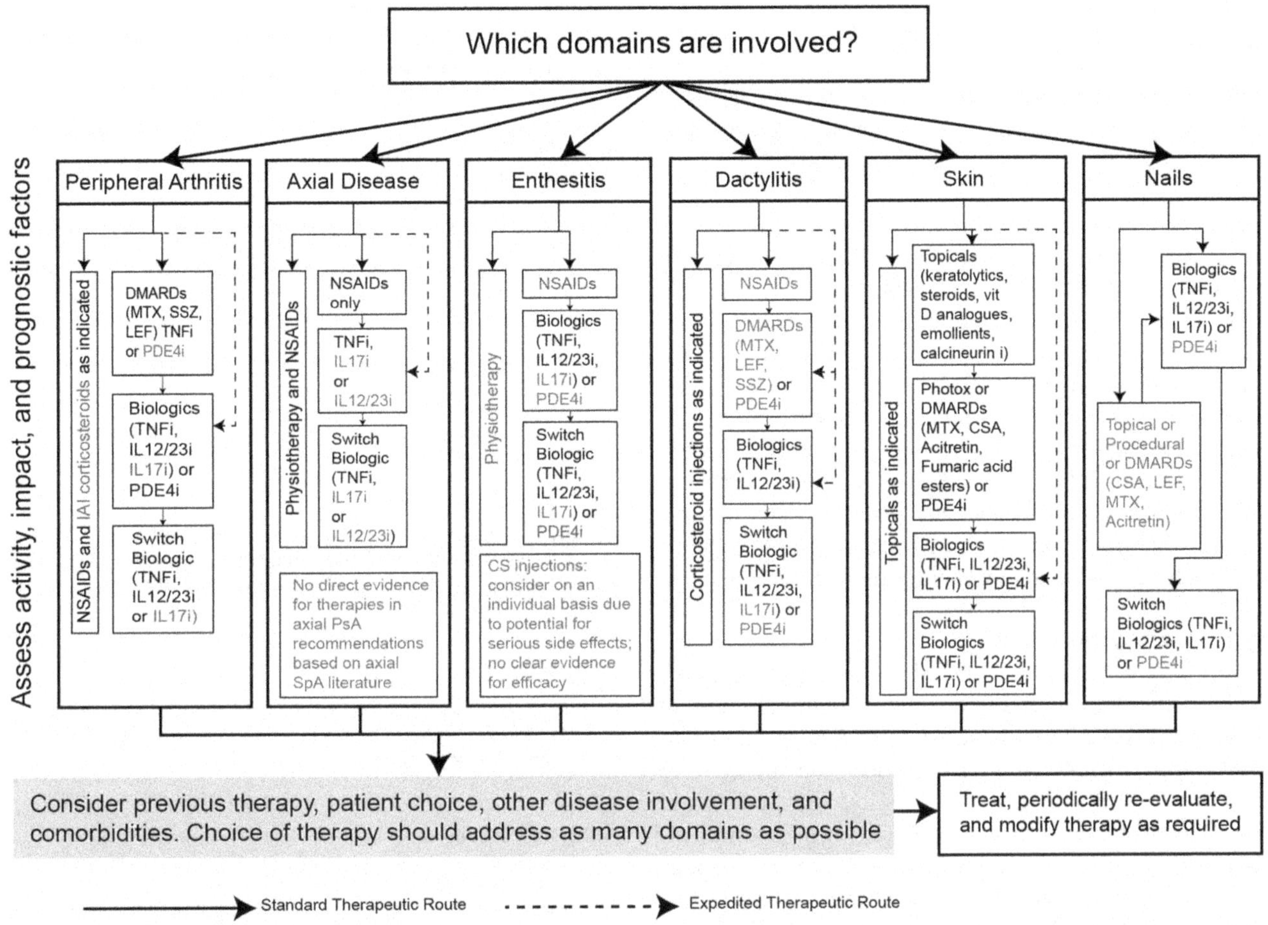

Grey text identifies conditional recommendations for drugs without current regulatory approvals or where recommendations are based on abstract data only. CS = corticosteroids, CSA = cyclosporine, DMARDs = disease modifying anti-rheumatic drugs, IAI = intra-articular injection, IL17i = interleukin 17 inhibitors, IL12/23i = interleukin 12/23 inhibitors, LEF = leflunomide, MTX = methotrexate, NSAIDs = nonsteroidal anti-inflammatory drugs, PDE4i = phosphodiesterase 4 inhibitor (apremilast), SSZ = sulfasalazine, TNFi = tumor necrosis factor inhibitor

Fig. 1 GRAPPA treatment schema for active PsA [16]. Reprinted with permission from: Coates LC et al. Group for Research and Assessment of Psoriasis and Psoriatic Arthritis 2015 treatment recommendations for psoriatic arthritis. Arthritis Rheumatol 2016;68(5):1060–1071

biologic therapy, the GRAPPA guidelines provide a conditional recommendation for switching to a different biologic agent within a drug class or to a drug with a different mode of action [16]. While switching TNF inhibitors can be effective, response rates tend to diminish with successive TNF inhibitor use [64]. There has been investigation of combining TNF inhibitors with a DMARD to prolong biologic persistence but a clear benefit of combination therapy was not observed [65]. There are currently two biologics (secukinumab and ustekinumab) available for treatment of PsA with a different mechanisms of action than TNF inhibition [50, 51, 53]. A concern with all biologic therapies for PsA is an increased risk for infections and patients should be monitored for the development of serious infections that would necessitate discontinuation of treatment until the infection resolves. Reactivation of tuberculosis has been observed with TNF inhibitors and patients must be monitored for active tuberculosis while receiving these agents.

Additionally, response to biologic agents can be limited by immunogenicity and the development of antidrug antibodies [66]. Antidrug antibodies have been observed in 29% of patients receiving adalimumab and 21% of patients receiving infliximab and their presence was significantly correlated with low drug levels and high levels of disease activity [66]. This study also reported that MTX significantly decreased the prevalence of antidrug antibodies, and use of MTX should be considered for patients treated with TNF inhibitors. With secukinumab and ustekinumab, treatment-emergent antidrug antibodies were reported in 0.2% to 0.3% and 9.3%, respectively, of patients from phase 3 trials [49, 52, 53]. In patients receiving ustekinumab and MTX, antidrug antibodies were less common (6.4%) than in those only receiving ustekinumab (12.3%) [52].

Treatment of skin disease associated with PsA can include phototherapy such as ultraviolet B or oral psoralen followed by ultraviolet A (PUVA) [67]. PUVA therapy carries an increased risk of skin cancer compared with other forms of ultraviolet light treatment and patients receiving this treatment should be monitored for skin cancer [67, 68].

Risks associated with poor compliance

Patient compliance to therapy is an underlying concern in the management of PsA. In patients treated with TNF inhibitors, age has been associated with increased compliance and female sex, comorbidity, and poor clinical condition at baseline have been associated with decreased compliance [69]. Poor adherence can reduce therapeutic efficacy and increase medical costs due to the need for more aggressive treatments [69, 70]. In general, there is the potential for reduced compliance if a patient cannot observe their disease directly, although this is less likely in patients with PsA because skin involvement is more common.

Psychosocial risks

The impact of PsA is not limited to the skin and joints and patients often experience substantial impairment in QoL [71]. There is an increased risk of depression and anxiety in patients with PsA, which can complicate treatment [71]. Symptoms of depression and anxiety are associated with low treatment adherence in chronic diseases and can impair the ability of patients to self-manage [72]. Physicians should remain cognizant of depressive behaviors such as alcoholism, nonsocial behavior, drug addiction, and suicide ideation and even though treatment of PsA can improve symptoms of depression and anxiety, it is still important for physicians to identify individuals who would benefit from referral for counseling.

Patients with both PsA and psoriasis experience worse QoL than those with only psoriasis [73]. Additionally, this difference in QoL was not due to differences in other comorbidities between patients with and without joint involvement [73]. Collectively, further efforts should be made by physicians to identify patients with PsA who should be referred for counseling as well as to monitor changes in these psychosocial issues over the course of treatment.

Conclusions

Among patients with PsA, a major emphasis of comprehensive care should be aimed at mitigating risks and improving physical health-related QoL. As outlined above, this may be achieved by early diagnosis, prevention of disease progression, treatment of PsA-associated physical morbidity, mitigation of treatment-related risk, and treatment of associated medical comorbidity. Various agents, including newer biologics, have approved indications for use in the PsA population—providing the clinician and patients with choices of agents based on their specific disease symptoms. Overall, management of patients with PsA is complex and requires the adoption of a more patient-focused multidisciplinary approach.

Abbreviations

ACR: American College of Rheumatology; AEs: Adverse events; CASPAR: ClASsification criteria for Psoriatic Arthritis; CI: Confidence interval; CV: Cardiovascular; DIP: Distal interphalangeal; DMARDs: Disease-modifying antirheumatic drugs; GI: Gastrointestinal; GRAPPA: Group for Research and Assessment of Psoriasis and Psoriatic Arthritis; HLA: Human leukocyte antigen; IBD: Inflammatory bowel disease; IL: Interleukin; MDA: Minimal disease activity; MIPA: Methotrexate in Psoriatic Arthritis; MRI: Magnetic resonance imaging; MTX: Methotrexate; NSAIDs: Nonsteroidal anti-inflammatory drugs; PASI: Psoriatic Area and Severity Index; PsA: Psoriatic arthritis; PUVA: Psoralen followed by ultraviolet A; QoL: Quality of life; RA: Rheumatoid arthritis; RR: Relative risk; SI: Sacroiliac; SpA: Spondyloarthropathies; TICOPA: Tight Control of Psoriatic Arthritis; TNF: Tumor necrosis factor

Acknowledgements

Technical assistance with editing and styling of the manuscript for submission was provided by Oxford PharmaGenesis Inc. and was funded by Novartis Pharmaceuticals Corporation.

Funding

The authors were fully responsible for all content and editorial decisions and received no financial support or other form of compensation related to the development of this manuscript.

Authors' contributions

MB conceived of the concept for this review, participated in its design and coordination, and drafted and reviewed the content of the manuscript. AL conceived of the concept for this review, participated in its design and coordination, and drafted and reviewed the content of the manuscript. Both authors read and approved the final manuscript.

Competing interests

MB is a consultant/speaker for Abbvie, Amgen, Celgene, Genentech, Horizon, Iroko, Janssen, Novartis, and Pfizer, and holds stock in Merck, BMS, Pfizer, and Johnson & Johnson. AL has no competing interests to declare.

Consent for publication

Not applicable.

Author details

[1]Taylor Hospital, 8 Morton Avenue, Suite 304, Ridley Park, PA 19078, USA. [2]Lankenau Medical Center, Wynnewood, PA, USA.

References

1. Collantes E, Zarco P, Muñoz E, Juanola X, Mulero J, Fernández-Sueiro JL, et al. Disease pattern of spondyloarthropathies in Spain: description of the first national registry (REGISPONSER)—extended report. Rheumatology (Oxford). 2007;46:1309–15.
2. Zochling J, Smith EU. Seronegative spondyloarthritis. Best Pract Res Clin Rheumatol. 2010;24:747–56.
3. Veale DJ, Fearon U. What makes psoriatic and rheumatoid arthritis so different? RMD Open. 2015;1:e000025.
4. Haroon M, FitzGerald O. Psoriatic arthritis: complexities, comorbidities and implications for the clinic. Expert Rev Clin Immunol. 2016;12:405–16.
5. Amherd-Hoekstra A, Näher H, Lorenz HM, Enk AH. Psoriatic arthritis: a review. J Dtsch Dermatol Ges. 2010;8:332–9.

6. Gladman DD, Antoni C, Mease P, Clegg DO, Nash P. Psoriatic arthritis: epidemiology, clinical features, course, and outcome. Ann Rheum Dis. 2005;64 Suppl 2:ii14–7.
7. Brockbank JE, Stein M, Schentag CT, Gladman DD. Dactylitis in psoriatic arthritis: a marker for disease severity? Ann Rheum Dis. 2005;64:188–90.
8. Gelfand JM, Gladman DD, Mease PJ, Smith N, Margolis DJ, Nijsten T, et al. Epidemiology of psoriatic arthritis in the population of the United States. J Am Acad Dermatol. 2005;53:573.
9. Mease PJ, Gladman DD, Papp KA, Khraishi MM, Thaci D, Behrens F, et al. Prevalence of rheumatologist-diagnosed psoriatic arthritis in patients with psoriasis in European/North American dermatology clinics. J Am Acad Dermatol. 2013;69:729–35.
10. Haroon NN, Paterson JM, Li P, Haroon N. Increasing proportion of female patients with ankylosing spondylitis: a population-based study of trends in the incidence and prevalence of AS. BMJ Open. 2014;4:e006634.
11. Sanmarti R, Graell E, Perez ML, Ercilla G, Viñas O, Gómez-Puerta JA, et al. Diagnostic and prognostic value of antibodies against chimeric fibrin/filaggrin citrullinated synthetic peptides in rheumatoid arthritis. Arthritis Res Ther. 2009;11:R135.
12. Taylor W, Gladman D, Helliwell P, Marchesoni A, Mease P, Mielants H, et al. Classification criteria for psoriatic arthritis: development of new criteria from a large international study. Arthritis Rheum. 2006;54:2665–73.
13. Schett G, Coates LC, Ash ZR, Finzel S, Conaghan PG. Structural damage in rheumatoid arthritis, psoriatic arthritis, and ankylosing spondylitis: traditional views, novel insights gained from TNF blockade, and concepts for the future. Arthritis Res Ther. 2011;13 Suppl 1:S4.
14. Londono J, Santos AM, Peña P, Calvo E, Espinosa LR, Reveille JD, et al. Analysis of HLA-B15 and HLA-B27 in spondyloarthritis with peripheral and axial clinical patterns. BMJ Open. 2015;5:e009092.
15. Liu JT, Yeh HM, Liu SY, Chen KT. Psoriatic arthritis: epidemiology, diagnosis, and treatment. World J Orthop. 2014;5:537–43.
16. Coates LC, Kavanaugh A, Mease PJ, Soriano ER, Laura Acosta-Felquer M, Armstrong AW, et al. Group for Research and Assessment of Psoriasis and Psoriatic Arthritis 2015 treatment recommendations for psoriatic arthritis. Arthritis Rheumatol. 2016;68:1060–71.
17. Gladman DD, Hing EN, Schentag CT, Cook RJ. Remission in psoriatic arthritis. J Rheumatol. 2001;28:1045–8.
18. Saber TP, Ng CT, Renard G, Lynch BM, Pontifex E, Walsh CA, et al. Remission in psoriatic arthritis: is it possible and how can it be predicted? Arthritis Res Ther. 2010;12:R94.
19. Eder L, Gladman DD. Predictors for clinical outcome in psoriatic arthritis - what have we learned from cohort studies? Expert Rev Clin Immunol. 2014;10:763–70.
20. Smolen JS, Braun J, Dougados M, Emery P, Fitzgerald O, Helliwell P, et al. Treating spondyloarthritis, including ankylosing spondylitis and psoriatic arthritis, to target: recommendations of an international task force. Ann Rheum Dis. 2014;73:6–16.
21. Elyoussfi S, Thomas BJ, Ciurtin C. Tailored treatment options for patients with psoriatic arthritis and psoriasis: review of established and new biologic and small molecule therapies. Rheumatol Int. 2016;36:603–12.
22. Zhu TY, Tam LS, Lee VW, Hwang WW, Li TK, Lee KK, et al. Costs and quality of life of patients with ankylosing spondylitis in Hong Kong. Rheumatology (Oxford). 2008;47:1422–5.
23. Singh JA, Strand V. Spondyloarthritis is associated with poor function and physical health-related quality of life. J Rheumatol. 2009;36:1012–20.
24. Ogdie A, Schwartzman S, Husni ME. Recognizing and managing comorbidities in psoriatic arthritis. Curr Opin Rheumatol. 2015;27:118–26.
25. Zarco P, González CM, Rodríguez de la Serna A, Peiró E, Mateo I, Linares L, et al. Extra-articular disease in patients with spondyloarthritis. Baseline characteristics of the spondyloarthritis cohort of the AQUILES study. Reumatol Clin. 2015;11:83–9.
26. Horreau C, Pouplard C, Brenaut E, Barnetche T, Misery L, Cribier B, et al. Cardiovascular morbidity and mortality in psoriasis and psoriatic arthritis: a systematic literature review. J Eur Acad Dermatol Venereol. 2013;27 Suppl 3:12–29.
27. Zhu TY, Li EK, Tam LS. Cardiovascular risk in patients with psoriatic arthritis. Int J Rheumatol. 2012;2012:714321.
28. Jamnitski A, Symmons D, Peters MJ, Sattar N, McInnes I, Nurmohamed MT. Cardiovascular comorbidities in patients with psoriatic arthritis: a systematic review. Ann Rheum Dis. 2013;72:211–6.
29. Bostoen J, Van Praet L, Brochez L, Mielants H, Lambert J. A cross-sectional study on the prevalence of metabolic syndrome in psoriasis compared to psoriatic arthritis. J Eur Acad Dermatol Venereol. 2014;28:507–11.
30. Haroon M, Gallagher P, Heffernan E, FitzGerald O. High prevalence of metabolic syndrome and of insulin resistance in psoriatic arthritis is associated with the severity of underlying disease. J Rheumatol. 2014;41:1357–65.
31. Soltani-Arabshahi R, Wong B, Feng BJ, Goldgar DE, Duffin KC, Krueger GG. Obesity in early adulthood as a risk factor for psoriatic arthritis. Arch Dermatol. 2010;146:721–6.
32. Eder L, Thavaneswaran A, Chandran V, Cook RJ, Gladman DD. Obesity is associated with a lower probability of achieving sustained minimal disease activity state among patients with psoriatic arthritis. Ann Rheum Dis. 2015;74:813–7.
33. Versini M, Jeandel PY, Rosenthal E, Shoenfeld Y. Obesity in autoimmune diseases: not a passive bystander. Autoimmun Rev. 2014;13:981–1000.
34. Labitigan M, Bahče-Altuntas A, Kremer JM, Reed G, Greenberg JD, Jordan N, et al. Higher rates and clustering of abnormal lipids, obesity, and diabetes mellitus in psoriatic arthritis compared with rheumatoid arthritis. Arthritis Care Res (Hoboken). 2014;66:600–7.
35. Solomon DH, Love TJ, Canning C, Schneeweiss S. Risk of diabetes among patients with rheumatoid arthritis, psoriatic arthritis and psoriasis. Ann Rheum Dis. 2010;69:2114–7.
36. Elewaut D, Matucci-Cerinic M. Treatment of ankylosing spondylitis and extra-articular manifestations in everyday rheumatology practice. Rheumatology (Oxford). 2009;48:1029–35.
37. Li WQ, Han JL, Chan AT, Qureshi AA. Psoriasis, psoriatic arthritis and increased risk of incident Crohn's disease in US women. Ann Rheum Dis. 2013;72:1200–5.
38. Gezer O, Batmaz I, Sariyildiz MA, Sula B, Ucmak D, Bozkurt M, et al. Sleep quality in patients with psoriatic arthritis. Int J Rheum Dis. 2014. doi:10.1111/756-185X.12505. [Epub ahead of print].
39. McDonough E, Ayearst R, Eder L, Chandran V, Rosen CF, Thavaneswaran A, et al. Depression and anxiety in psoriatic disease: prevalence and associated factors. J Rheumatol. 2014;41:887–96.
40. Haroon M, Gallagher P, FitzGerald O. Diagnostic delay of more than 6 months contributes to poor radiographic and functional outcome in psoriatic arthritis. Ann Rheum Dis. 2015;74:1045–50.
41. Rohekar S, Chan J, Tse SM, Haroon N, Chandran V, Bessette L, et al. 2014 Update of the Canadian Rheumatology Association/spondyloarthritis research consortium of Canada treatment recommendations for the management of spondyloarthritis. Part I: principles of the management of spondyloarthritis in Canada. J Rheumatol. 2015;42:654–64.
42. Mease PJ, Kivitz AJ, Burch FX, Siegel EL, Cohen SB, Ory P, et al. Etanercept treatment of psoriatic arthritis: safety, efficacy, and effect on disease progression. Arthritis Rheum. 2004;50:2264–72.
43. Mease PJ, Fleischmann R, Deodhar AA, Wollenhaupt J, Khraishi M, Kielar D, et al. Effect of certolizumab pegol on signs and symptoms in patients with psoriatic arthritis: 24-week results of a phase 3 double-blind randomised placebo-controlled study (RAPID-PsA). Ann Rheum Dis. 2014;73:48–55.
44. Antoni C, Krueger GG, de Vlam K, Birbara C, Beutler A, Guzzo C, et al. Infliximab improves signs and symptoms of psoriatic arthritis: results of the IMPACT 2 trial. Ann Rheum Dis. 2005;64:1150–7.
45. Mease PJ, Gladman DD, Ritchlin CT, Ruderman EM, Steinfeld SD, Choy EH, et al. Adalimumab for the treatment of patients with moderately to severely active psoriatic arthritis: results of a double-blind, randomized, placebo-controlled trial. Arthritis Rheum. 2005;52:3279–89.
46. Kavanaugh A, McInnes I, Mease P, Krueger GG, Gladman D, Gomez-Reino J, et al. Golimumab, a new human tumor necrosis factor α antibody, administered every four weeks as a subcutaneous injection in psoriatic arthritis: twenty-four-week efficacy and safety results of a randomized, placebo-controlled study. Arthritis Rheum. 2009;60:976–86.
47. Kavanaugh A, Mease PJ, Gomez-Reino JJ, Adebajo AO, Wollenhaupt J, Gladman DD, et al. Treatment of psoriatic arthritis in a phase 3 randomised, placebo-controlled trial with apremilast, an oral phosphodiesterase 4 inhibitor. Ann Rheum Dis. 2014;73:1020–6.
48. Mease P, Genovese MC, Gladstein G, Kivitz AJ, Ritchlin C, Tak PP, et al. Abatacept in the treatment of patients with psoriatic arthritis: results of a six-month, multicenter, randomized, double-blind, placebo-controlled, phase II trial. Arthritis Rheum. 2011;63:939–48.
49. Mease PJ, McInnes IB, Kirkham B, Kavanaugh A, Rahman P, van der Heijde D, et al. Secukinumab inhibition of interleukin-17A in patients with psoriatic arthritis. N Engl J Med. 2015;373:1329–39.
50. McInnes IB, Kavanaugh A, Gottlieb AB, Puig L, Rahman P, Ritchlin C, et al. Efficacy and safety of ustekinumab in patients with active psoriatic arthritis: 1 year results of the phase 3, multicentre, double-blind, placebo-controlled PSUMMIT 1 trial. Lancet. 2013;382:780–9.

51. McInnes IB, Sieper J, Braun J, Emery P, van der Heijde D, Isaacs JD, et al. Efficacy and safety of secukinumab, a fully human anti-interleukin-17A monoclonal antibody, in patients with moderate-to-severe psoriatic arthritis: a 24-week, randomised, double-blind, placebo-controlled, phase II proof-of-concept trial. Ann Rheum Dis. 2014;73:349–56.
52. Ritchlin C, Rahman P, Kavanaugh A, McInnes IB, Puig L, Li S, et al. Efficacy and safety of the anti-IL-12/23 p40 monoclonal antibody, ustekinumab, in patients with active psoriatic arthritis despite conventional non-biological and biological anti-tumour necrosis factor therapy: 6-month and 1-year results of the phase 3, multicentre, double-blind, placebo-controlled, randomised PSUMMIT 2 trial. Ann Rheum Dis. 2014;73:990–9.
53. McInnes IB, Mease PJ, Kirkham B, Kavanaugh A, Ritchlin CT, Rahman P, et al. Secukinumab, a human anti-interleukin-17A monoclonal antibody, in patients with psoriatic arthritis (FUTURE 2): a randomised, double-blind, placebo-controlled, phase 3 trial. Lancet. 2015;386:1137–46.
54. Miedany YE. Treat to target in spondyloarthritis: the time has come. Curr Rheumatol Rev. 2014;10:87–93.
55. Wendling D. Treating to target in axial spondyloarthritis: defining the target and the arrow. Expert Rev Clin Immunol. 2015;11:691–3.
56. Schoels MM, Braun J, Dougados M, Emery P, Fitzgerald O, Kavanaugh A, et al. Treating axial and peripheral spondyloarthritis, including psoriatic arthritis, to target: results of a systematic literature search to support an international treat-to-target recommendation in spondyloarthritis. Ann Rheum Dis. 2014;73:238–42.
57. Coates LC, Fransen J, Helliwell PS. Defining minimal disease activity in psoriatic arthritis: a proposed objective target for treatment. Ann Rheum Dis. 2010;69:48–53.
58. Coates LC, Moverley AR, McParland L, Brown S, Navarro-Coy N, O'Dwyer JL, et al. Effect of tight control of inflammation in early psoriatic arthritis (TICOPA): a UK multicentre, open-label, randomised controlled trial. Lancet. 2015;386:2489–98.
59. Kang EJ, Kavanaugh A. Psoriatic arthritis: latest treatments and their place in therapy. Ther Adv Chronic Dis. 2015;6:194–203.
60. Gossec L, Smolen JS, Gaujoux-Viala C, Ash Z, Marzo-Ortega H, van der Heijde D, et al. European League Against Rheumatism recommendations for the management of psoriatic arthritis with pharmacological therapies. Ann Rheum Dis. 2012;71:4–12.
61. Kingsley GH, Kowalczyk A, Taylor H, Ibrahim F, Packham JC, McHugh NJ, et al. A randomized placebo-controlled trial of methotrexate in psoriatic arthritis. Rheumatology (Oxford). 2012;51:1368–77.
62. Mease PJ. Spondyloarthritis: is methotrexate effective in psoriatic arthritis? Nat Rev Rheumatol. 2012;8:251–2.
63. Berends MA, Snoek J, de Jong EM, van de Kerkhof PC, van Oijen MG, van Krieken JH, et al. Liver injury in long-term methotrexate treatment in psoriasis is relatively infrequent. Aliment Pharmacol Ther. 2006;24:805–11.
64. Glintborg B, Østergaard M, Krogh NS, Andersen MD, Tarp U, Loft AG, et al. Clinical response, drug survival, and predictors thereof among 548 patients with psoriatic arthritis who switched tumor necrosis factor α inhibitor therapy: results from the Danish Nationwide DANBIO Registry. Arthritis Rheum. 2013;65:1213–23.
65. Mease PJ, Collier DH, Saunders KC, Li G, Kremer JM, Greenberg JD. Comparative effectiveness of biologic monotherapy versus combination therapy for patients with psoriatic arthritis: results from the Corrona registry. RMD Open. 2015;1:e000181.
66. Zisapel M, Zisman D, Madar-Balakirski N, Arad U, Padova H, Matz H, et al. Prevalence of TNF-α blocker immunogenicity in psoriatic arthritis. J Rheumatol. 2015;42:73–8.
67. Menter A, Korman NJ, Elmets CA, Feldman SR, Gelfand JM, Gordon KB, et al. Guidelines of care for the management of psoriasis and psoriatic arthritis: Section 5. Guidelines of care for the treatment of psoriasis with phototherapy and photochemotherapy. J Am Acad Dermatol. 2010;62:114–35.
68. Archier E, Devaux S, Castela E, Gallini A, Aubin F, Le Maitre M, et al. Carcinogenic risks of psoralen UV-A therapy and narrowband UV-B therapy in chronic plaque psoriasis: a systematic literature review. J Eur Acad Dermatol Venereol. 2012;26 Suppl 3:22–31.
69. López-González R, León L, Loza E, Redondo M, de Yébenes MJG, Carmona L. Adherence to biologic therapies and associated factors in rheumatoid arthritis, spondyloarthritis and psoriatic arthritis: a systematic literature review. Clin Exp Rheumatol. 2015;33:559–69.
70. Blum MA, Koo D, Doshi JA. Measurement and rates of persistence with and adherence to biologics for rheumatoid arthritis: a systematic review. Clin Ther. 2011;33:901–13.
71. Lee S, Mendelsohn A, Sarnes E. The burden of psoriatic arthritis: a literature review from a global health systems perspective. P T. 2010;35:680–9.
72. Betteridge N, Boehncke WH, Bundy C, Gossec L, Gratacós J, Augustin M. Promoting patient-centred care in psoriatic arthritis: a multidisciplinary European perspective on improving the patient experience. J Eur Acad Dermatol Venereol. 2016;30:576–85.
73. Rosen CF, Mussani F, Chandran V, Eder L, Thavaneswaran A, Gladman DD. Patients with psoriatic arthritis have worse quality of life than those with psoriasis alone. Rheumatology (Oxford). 2012;51:571–6.
74. Rojas-Vargas M, Muñoz-Gomariz E, Escudero A, Font P, Zarco P, Almodovar R, et al. First signs and symptoms of spondyloarthritis—data from an inception cohort with a disease course of two years or less (REGISPONSER-Early). Rheumatology (Oxford). 2009;48:404–9.

17

Psoriatic arthritis is associated with bone loss of the metacarpals

Alexander Pfeil[1*], Laura Krojniak[1], Diane M. Renz[2], Lisa Reinhardt[1], Marcus Franz[3], Peter Oelzner[1], Gunter Wolf[1] and Joachim Böttcher[4]

Abstract

Background: BoneXpert (BX) is a newly developed medical device based on digital X-ray radiogrammetry to measure human cortical bone thickness. The aim of this study was to quantify cortical bone loss of the metacarpals in patients with psoriatic arthritis (PsA) and compare these findings with other radiological scoring methods.

Methods: The study includes 104 patients with verified PsA. The BX method was used to measure the Metacarpal Index (MCI) at the metacarpal bones (II–IV). Additionally, the T-score of the MCI (T-score$_{MCI}$) was calculated. Radiographic severity was determined by the Psoriatic Arthritis Ratingen Score (Proliferation Score and Destruction Score) as published by Wassenberg et al. and the Psoriatic Arthritis modified van der Heijde Sharp Score (Joint Space Narrowing Score and Erosion Score).

Results: For the total PsA study cohort, the T-score$_{MCI}$ was significantly reduced by -1.289 ± 1.313 SD. The MCI negatively correlated with the Proliferation Score ($r = -0.732$; $p < 0.001$) and the Destruction Score ($r = -0.771$; $p < 0.001$) of the Psoriatic Arthritis Ratingen Score. Lower coefficients of correlations were observed for the Psoriatic Arthritis modified van der Heijde Sharp Score. In this context, a severity-dependent and PsA-related periarticular demineralisation as measured by the MCI was quantified. The strongest reduction of −30.8 % ($p < 0.01$) was observed for the MCI in the Destruction Score.

Conclusions: The BX MCI score showed periarticular demineralisation and severity-dependent bone loss in patients with PsA. The measurements of the BX technique were able to sensitively differentiate between the different stages of disease manifestation affecting bone integrity and thereby seem to achieve the potential to be a surrogate marker of radiographic progression in PsA.

Keywords: BoneXpert, Digital X-ray radiogrammetry, Bone mineral density, Psoriatic arthritis, Cortical bone loss, Periarticular demineralisation

Background

Psoriatic arthritis (PsA) is an inflammatory disease characterised by progressive joint destruction and related disability based on enthesitis as well as synovitis, often affecting the small joints of the hand [1]. The radiographic damage in PsA presents a wide spectrum of joint destruction which includes periarticular demineralisation and erosions, joint space narrowing, ankyloses of the joints, malalignment and subluxation of the affected joints and new bony formation with periosteal reaction and ankylosis [2, 3] which are the consequence of the chronic inflammation. Plain radiography has been the gold standard for many decades to assess radiographic damage and progression of PsA and the effectiveness of therapy for individual assessment of each patient and also in clinical trials. In the last decades, scoring methods (e.g. Psoriatic Arthritis Ratingen Score and Psoriatic Arthritis modified van der Heijde Sharp Score (SHS Score)) were established to measure the radiographic damage in PsA [3].

Digital X-ray radiogrammetry (DXR) is a computer-based technique for measuring cortical thickness, and functions as a marker for metacarpal cortical bone mineral density with high precision and reproducibility [4, 5]. A

* Correspondence: alexander.pfeil@med.uni-jena.de
[1]Department of Internal Medicine III, Jena University Hospital—Friedrich Schiller University Jena, Erlanger Allee 101, Jena 07747, Germany
Full list of author information is available at the end of the article

common application of DXR is the quantification of inflammatory-associated periarticular metacarpal bone loss in patients with RA [6]. Periarticular bone loss detected by DXR is strongly associated with disease activity in RA [7] and radiographic progression [8]. Additionally, two initial studies investigated periarticular bone loss in PsA [9, 10].

BoneXpert (BX) is a more advanced DXR technique using computer-assisted diagnosis software for the analysis of the metacarpal bones [11–18]. This new version is now available for the measurement of the Metacarpal Index (MCI) and the quantification of periarticular mineralisation in adults. The clinical advantage of the BX technique consists of its integration into a PACS system as well as into a PACS workflow to reveal a direct image analysis and quantification of periarticular bone loss.

The aim of this study was to evaluate the presence of periarticular cortical bone loss of the metacarpals in patients with PsA using BX and to compare these findings with the established radiological scoring methods. If BX is able to measure bone loss more sensitively it may be considered a surrogate marker of disease progression in the clinical setting.

Methods

Study population

A total of 104 PsA patients (57 female, 47 male) fulfilling the CASPAR criteria [19] were included in the study. Radiographs of the hand were performed on all subjects using standardised technical conditions. There was no pre-selection due to severity of PsA or if steroid therapy had been given. All patients were treated either with non-steroidal anti-inflammatory drugs or disease-modifying antirheumatic drugs (details see Table 1).

Measurement of cortical hand bone mass by BX

The BX system (version 2.3.0.4; Visiana, Holte, Denmark) is a computer-assisted diagnostic technique for the radiogeometrical analysis of the metacarpal bones on plain radiographs. All plain radiographs (anterior–posterior projection) of the non-dominant hand were acquired by the same X-ray devices using standardised conditions.

The edge of each metacarpal diaphysis was defined using 32 points which corresponded to the same anatomical locations across all subjects [20, 21]. Two of the points corresponded to the proximal and distal ends of the metacarpal bone, and these markers were used to define the bone axis. The length (L) of the bone was measured along this axis, including the epiphysis. A region of interest (ROI) was positioned at 44 % of L from the proximal end of the bone, and it extended to 25 % of L. The ROIs were located at the metacarpal bones II–IV (see Fig. 1). In this region, the inner and outer edges of the cortical bone partition were determined as follows: the outer cortical edge was the location with the maximal gradient and the inner cortical edge was detected as an intensity maximum [21].

Table 1 Baseline characteristics of the study cohort

	Total study group
Total, *n*	104
Women	57
Men	47
Age (years), mean ± SD	54.7 ± 12.3
Height (cm), mean ± SD	168 ± 9.0
Weight (kg), mean ± SD	79 ± 16.7
Body mass index, mean ± SD	27.6 ± 5.2
Disease duration (years), mean ± SD	9.6 ± 6.7
Tender joint count (0–28 joints), mean ± SD	2.5 ± 2.5
Swollen joint count (0–28 joints), mean ± SD	2.3 ± 2.5
C-reactive protein (mg/l), mean ± SD	9.8 ± 14.2
Erythrocyte sedimentation rate (mm/hour), mean ± SD	16.3 ± 17.1
Corticosteroids, *n* (%)	
Yes (mean dose 5 mg/day)	28 (26.9)
No	76 (73.1)
Non-steroidal anti-inflammatory drug, *n* (%)	49 (47.1)
Synthetic disease-modifying antirheumatic drugs, *n* (%)	42 (40.4)
Biological disease-modifying antirheumatic drugs, *n* (%)	13 (12.5)

SD standard deviation

Based on the ROI for each metacarpal bone, the average width (W) and the average cortical thickness (T) were determined and expressed as the mean for the metacarpal bones II–IV in millimetres [21].

The cortical area (A) was estimated by the defined formula for a cylindrically symmetric bone model [21]:

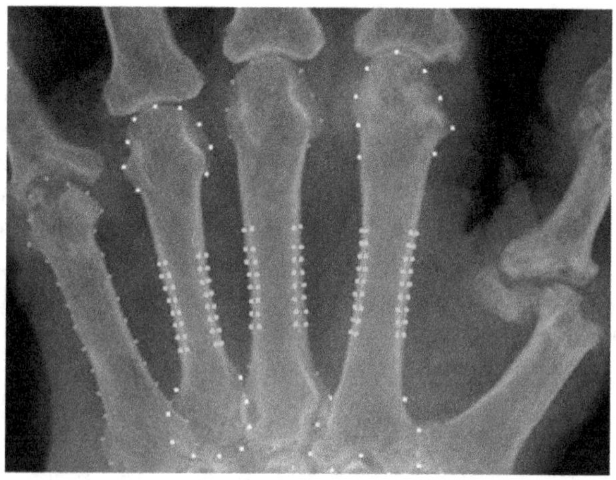

Fig. 1 Screen view of BX analysis with the positioned ROI (*green dots*) for the measurement of cortical thickness at metacarpals II–IV

$$A = \pi \, T \, W \, (1 - T/W).$$

Additionally, the MCI was computed as the T divided by the W which was later refined to [21]:

$$MCI = A / W^2$$

Based on the A as well as the metacarpal bone length (L) and W, the Bone Health Index (BHI) was computed as:

$$BHI = A \, / \, \left(W^{1.333} L^{0.333}\right)$$

Scoring of hand radiographs

Each radiograph of the PsA cohort was scored by two independent radiologists using the same scoring methods. In the cases of ambiguity, a third highly experienced radiologist reviewed the radiographs for a final decision.

Psoriatic Arthritis Ratingen Score

The Destruction Score and the Proliferation Score published by Wassenberg et al. [22] are bicompartment scores used to determine the extent of destructive change (destruction) and the presence of bony growth (proliferation) regarding the joints of the hand and feet in PsA.

The Destruction Score segment indicates the percentage of the joint surface destruction of the articulation with the following scoring: score 0 = normal, score 1 = one or more erosions with destruction of up to 10 %, score 2 = 11–25 %, score 3 = 26–50 %, score 4 = 51–75 % and score 5 = >75 % joint surface destruction.

The Proliferation Score segment evaluates PsA-related bony proliferation using the following grading: score 0 = normal, score 1 = bone proliferation of 1–2 mm or bone growth < 25 % of the original size (diameter), score 2 = bone proliferation 2–3 mm or bone growth with 25–50 %, score 3 = bone proliferation > 3 mm or bone growth > 50 % and score 4 = ankylosis.

The Destruction Score (0–200) and the Proliferation Score (0–160) are added together for a total score of between 0 and 360 points. The individual sum of scoring points is then divided by the number of evaluated joints [22].

SHS Score

The Erosion Score segment (total sum points: 280) and the Joint Space Narrowing Score segment (total sum points: 168) [23] of the hand and feet joints were determined using the SHS Score. To assess PsA-specific radiological damage, scores for the distal interphalangeal hand joints and pencil-in-cup/gross osteolysis deformities were added to the original SHS Score as published by Kavanaugh et al. [24]. The SHS Score thus ranged from 0 to 528 (total score sum) which is a composite of the erosion score (0–320) and the joint space narrowing score (0–208) [24]. Additionally, the individual sums of the scoring points were then divided by the number of evaluated joints.

Statistical analysis

The statistical analysis was performed using SPSS Version 21.0® (SPSS, Chicago, IL, USA), for Windows.

To evaluate reproducibility, 10 measurements of the same radiograph per score were repeated. The results were expressed as mean and standard deviation (SD) and reproducibility errors as a coefficient of variation (CV). The coefficients of variation are typically given on a percentage basis:

$$CV\,(\%) = (\text{standard deviation}/\text{mean}) \times 100\,\%.$$

The Pearson coefficient of correlation was used to investigate the association between the BX parameters, age, gender, the Psoriatic Arthritis Ratingen Score as well as the SHS Score.

Thodberg et al. [25] published reference curves for the MCI including healthy European adults. The peak MCI for males is determined at the age of 28 years (MCI 0.6055 ± 0.0509) and for females at the age of 36 years (0.60264 ± 0.0535) [25]. Based on the reference curves and the peak MCI, the T-score$_{MCI}$ of the MCI as a comparative measurement with healthy subjects could be determined. The T-score is calculated as follows [25]:

$$\textbf{T-Score}_{MCI} = \left(MCI_{patient} - MCI_{peak}\right)/SD_{peak}$$

The reduction of all BX parameters for the different scores was assessed using the Mann–Whitney *U* test.

The differences in BX parameters between patients with and without erosions were compared by the Mann–Whitney *U* test.

Sensitivity and specificity of MCI concerning the detection of erosions were based on receiver operating characteristic (ROC) curve analysis. The MCI mean value of the patients with erosions was used as the cut-off value.

The overall significance level was $p < 0.05$.

Results

Baseline characteristics

A total of 104 PsA patients (57 women and 47 men) were included in the analysis (see Table 1). The mean disease duration was 9.6 ± 6.7 years. The mean C-reactive protein was 9.8 mg/l and/or the mean erythrocyte sedimentation rate in the first hour was 16.3 mm. In this context, the mean tender joint count was 2.5 ± 2.5 joints and the mean swollen joint count was 2.3 ± 2.5 joints. Forty-nine patients (47.1 %) were treated with non-steroidal anti-inflammatory drugs, 42 patients (40.4 %) received synthetic disease-modifying antirheumatic drugs and 13 patients (12.5 %) received biological disease-modifying antirheumatic drugs.

Regarding the use of corticosteroids, 28 patients (26.9 %) were treated with corticosteroids (mean dose 5 mg/day) and 76 patients (73.1 %) received no corticosteroids.

Reproducibility

The CV was 0 % for BX parameters regarding the Destruction and Proliferation Scores (Psoriatic Arthritis Ratingen Score) and the Erosion and Joint Space Scores (SHS Score).

BX measurements for the PsA cohort

For the entire PsA study, the T-score of the MCI was −1.289 ± 1.313 SD. Regarding the association of age and BX parameters, a low significant correlation was evaluated (MCI: $r = -0.585$, $p < 0.001$; T-score$_{MCI}$: $r = -0.586$; $p < 0.001$; T: $r = -0.481$; $p < 0.001$). W revealed no significant correlation with age. A significant correlation between the BX parameters and gender was not observed.

BX measurements compared with standard scoring methods

Psoriatic Arthritis Ratingen Score

The BHI, MCI, T-score$_{MCI}$ and T presented significant negative coefficients of correlation with the different scores. The highest negative correlation was observed between the MCI ($r = -0.771$; $p < 0.001$) or the T-score$_{MCI}$ ($r = -0.775$; $p < 0.001$) and the Destruction Score. Similar results were detected between the Proliferation Score for the MCI ($r = -0.732$; $p < 0.001$) versus the T-score$_{MCI}$ ($r = -0.744$; $p < 0.001$). The BHI revealed a significant negative coefficient of correlation ($r = -0.682$; $p < 0.01$) for the Destruction Score and the Proliferation Score. W presented no significant coefficients of correlations to both scores.

SHS Score

Lower negative coefficients of correlation were observed between MCI, T-score$_{MCI}$ and BHI and the Joint Space Narrowing Score (MCI: $r = -0.558$, $p < 0.001$; T-score$_{MCI}$: $r = -0.552$, $p < 0.001$; BHI: $r = 0.522$, $p < 0.01$) or the Erosion Score (MCI: $r = -0.714$, $p < 0.001$; T-score$_{MCI}$: $r = -0.715$, $p < 0.001$; BHI: $r = 0.660$, $p < 0.01$). W also showed no significant coefficients of correlation regarding the SHS Score.

BX results show bone loss depending on severity of PsA

Psoriatic Arthritis Ratingen Score

Proliferation Score For the Proliferation Score, MCI (−28.3 %, $p < 0.01$) and T-score$_{MCI}$ significantly differed from 0.596 ± 0.052 (score 0) to 0.427 ± 0.045 (score 4) and from −0.427 ± 0.927 SD (score 0) to −3.616 ± 0.838, respectively (Table 2). The relative difference of T was −31.9 %. In this context, BHI presented a significant difference of −24.6 % ($p < 0.01$) from 5.85 ± 0.42 (score 0) to 4.41 ± 0.52 (score 4). W showed no significant changes between score 0 and score 4.

Destruction Score Using the Destruction Score, BHI presented a significant difference with −24.8 % ($p < 0.01$) from 5.88 ± 0.41 (score 0) to 4.42 ± 0.75 (score 5) (Table 2). MCI and T were also significantly differed between score 0 and score 5 with −30.8 % ($p < 0.01$) and −30.9 % ($p < 0.01$), respectively. The T-score$_{MCI}$ was significantly changed from −0.346 ± 0.926 (score 0) to −3.813 ± 1.035 (score 5). In accordance with the Proliferation Score for W, no significant differences were evaluated.

SHS Score

Erosion Score MCI revealed a significant difference of −28.5 % ($p < 0.01$) from 0.601 ± 0.059 (score 0) to 0.430 ± 0.046 (score 5) and T-score$_{MCI}$ showed a significant difference from −0.324 ± 1.039 (score 0) to −3.510 ± 0.912 (score 5) (Table 3). The T and BHI presented comparable differences with −31.3 % ($p < 0.01$) and −24.6 % ($p < 0.01$). W revealed no significant severity dependent change.

Joint Space Narrowing Score The Joint Space Narrowing Score presented a difference of the BHI (−21.1 %, $p < 0.01$) from 5.73 ± 0.57 (score 0) to 4.52 ± 0.52 (score 4) (Table 3). MCI (−24.9 %) and T-score$_{MCI}$ observed a significant difference from 0.582 ± 0.063 (score 0) to 0.437 ± 0.050 (score 4) and from −0.681 ± 1.163 (score 0) to −3.416 ± 0.952 (score 4) respectively. T revealed a significant difference of −26.8 % ($p < 0.01$). Finally, W presented a non-significant difference with 8.8 %.

BX parameters in dependence on the occurrence of erosions

PsA patients with erosions presented a significantly ($p < 0.01$) lower BHI (−10.2 %), MCI (−12.5 %) and T (−13.9 %) compared with patients without erosion (Table 4). In this context, the T-score$_{MCI}$ in PsA patients with erosions was significant lower (−1.722) than in patients without erosions (−0.324). W (4.4 %; p = NS) revealed no significant change between patients with and without erosions.

The sensitivity and specificity of the MCI regarding the detection of erosions was 88 % versus 49 % (accuracy 81 %, $p < 0.01$).

Discussion

The BX technique is a recently developed automated method for the measurement of the MCI based on the radiogeometrical analysis of metacarpal bones. The aim of this study was to evaluate the presence of periarticular cortical bone loss of the metacarpal bones in patients

Table 2 BoneXpert parameters in PsA patients stratified by Psoriatic Arthritis Ratingen Score Proliferation and Destruction Scores

Proliferation Score	BHI	MCI	T-score$_{MCI}$	T	W	Destruction Score	BHI	MCI	T-score$_{MCI}$	T	W
0 ($n = 34$)	5.85 (0.42)	0.596 (0.052)	−0.427 (0.927)	2.04 (0.26)	8.02 (1.05)	0 ($n = 41$)	5.88 (0.41)	0.600 (0.053)	−0.346 (0.926)	2.07 (0.25)	8.02 (1.02)
1 ($n = 28$)	5.74 (0.43)	0.576 (0.051)	−0.762 (0.911)	1.99 (0.25)	8.24 (1.05)	1 ($n = 14$)	5.73 (0.39)	0.575 (0.039)	−0.805 (0.710)	1.99 (0.23)	8.23 (1.07)
2 ($n = 17$)	5.32 (0.45)	0.531 (0.034)	−1.611 (0.648)	1.81 (0.30)	8.37 (1.13)	2 ($n = 12$)	5.44 (0.45)	0.551 (0.026)	−1.281 (0.547)	1.84 (0.29)	8.06 (1.14)
3 ($n = 14$)	5.19 (0.47)	0.505 (0.041)	−2.138 (0.819)	1.73 (0.26)	8.57 (0.84)	3 ($n = 16$)	5.17 (0.44)	0.513 (0.029)	−1.981 (0.627)	1.73 (0.24)	8.32 (0.80)
4 ($n = 11$)	4.41 (0.52)	0.427 (0.045)	−3.616 (0.838)	1.39 (0.23)	8.58 (1.20)	4 ($n = 13$)	5.10 (0.49)	0.494 (0.043)	−2.300 (0.839)	1.72 (0.27)	8.78 (1.03)
–	–	–	–	–	–	5 ($n = 8$)	4.42 (0.75)	0.415 (0.051)	−3.813 (1.035)	1.43 (0.39)	9.04 (1.20)
Absolute and relative changes between score 0 and score 4	−1.44 – 24.6 %	−0.169 – 28.3 %	3.189	−0.65 – 31.9 %	0.56 7.0 %	Absolute and relative changes between score 0 and score 5	−1.46 – 24.8 %	−0.185 – 30.8 %	3.467	−0.64 – 30.9 %	1.02 12.7 %
Significance	<0.01	<0.01	<0.01	<0.01	NS	Significance	<0.01	<0.01	<0.01	<0.01	NS

Data presented as mean (standard deviation)

BHI Bone Health Index, *MCI* Metacarpal Index, *NS* not significant, *PsA* psoriatic arthritis, *T* cortical thickness of the metacarpal bone, *W* width of the metacarpal bone

Table 3 BoneXpert parameters in PsA patients stratified by SHS Erosion and joint space narrowing scores

Erosion Score	BHI	MCI	T-score$_{MCI}$	T	W	Joint Space Narrowing Score	BHI	MCI	T-score$_{MCI}$	T	W
0 ($n = 33$)	5.90 (0.49)	0.601 (0.059)	−0.324 (1.039)	2.08 (0.28)	8.03 (0.95)	0 ($n = 35$)	5.73 (0.57)	0.582 (0.063)	−0.681 (1.163)	1.98 (0.32)	7.99 (0.89)
1 ($n = 13$)	5.80 (0.46)	0.593 (0.042)	−0.554 (0.845)	2.00 (0.28)	7.85 (0.89)	1 ($n = 26$)	5.65 (0.46)	0.568 (0.058)	−0.986 (1.055)	1.96 (0.25)	8.66 (0.94)
2 ($n = 13$)	5.59 (0.58)	0.553 (0.055)	−1.154 (1.104)	1.95 (0.33)	8.51 (1.09)	2 ($n = 16$)	5.57 (0.43)	0.547 (0.032)	−1.289 (0.591)	1.94 (0.26)	8.19 (1.20)
3 ($n = 19$)	5.28 (0.32)	0.523 (0.028)	−1.800 (0.536)	1.77 (0.21)	8.41 (1.20)	3 ($n = 15$)	5.34 (0.55)	0.537 (0.061)	−1.457 (1.153)	1.82 (0.32)	8.29 (1.16)
4 ($n = 16$)	5.22 (0.36)	0.515 (0.042)	−1.923 (0.754)	1.75 (0.22)	8.46 (1.16)	4 ($n = 12$)	4.52 (0.52)	0.437 (0.050)	−3.416 (0.952)	1.45 (0.23)	8.69 (1.04)
5 ($n = 10$)	4.45 (0.55)	0.430 (0.046)	−3.510 (0.912)	1.43 (0.25)	8.70 (0.95)	–	–	–	–	–	–
Absolute and relative changes between score 0 and score 5	−1.45 − 24.6 %	−0.171 − 28.5 %	−3.186	−0.65 − 31.3 %	0.67 8.3 %	Absolute and relative changes between score 0 and score 4	−1.21 − 21.1 %	−0.145 − 24.9 %	−2.735	−0.53 − 26.8 %	0.70 8.8 %
Significance	<0.01	<0.01	<0.01	<0.01	NS	Significance	<0.01	<0.01	<0.01	<0.01	NS

Data presented as mean (standard deviation)

BHI Bone Health Index, *MCI* Metacarpal Index, *NS* not significant, *PsA* psoriatic arthritis, *SHS Score* Psoriatic Arthritis modified van der Heijde Sharp Score, *T* cortical thickness of the metacarpal bone, *W* width of the metacarpal bone

Table 4 Changes of BX parameters dependent on the existence of bone erosions

BX parameter	Without erosions ($n = 33$)	Erosions ($n = 71$)	Difference
BHI mean (SD)	5.90 (0.49)	5.30 (0.60)	−10.2 % ($p < 0.01$)
MCI mean (SD)	0.601 (0.059)	0.526 (0.063)	−12.5 % ($p < 0.01$)
T-score$_{MCI}$ mean (SD)	−0.324 (1.039)	−1.722 (1.190)	1.398 ($p < 0.01$)
T mean (SD)	2.08 (0.28)	1.79 (0.31)	−13.9 % ($p < 0.01$)
W mean (SD)	8.03 (0.95)	8.38 (1.09)	4.4 (p = NS)

Data presented as mean (standard deviation)
BHI Bone Health Index, *BX* BoneXpert, *MCI* Metacarpal Index, *NS* not significant, *T* cortical thickness of the metacarpal bone, *W* width of the metacarpal bone

with PsA based on the BX method and to compare these findings with different scoring methods.

The MCI is an established measurement for the quantification of metacarpal bone loss, particularly in rheumatoid arthritis [26]. The T-score$_{MCI}$ of the MCI presented a significantly reduced negative value with −1.289 ± 1.313 in all PsA patients. The reduced T-score$_{MCI}$ was clearly associated with a reduced bone mineral density of the metacarpal bones in PsA. Kocijan et al. [27] also found a reduced trabecular bone mineral density of the distal radius and periarticular radius with −12.0 % versus −8.1 % using high-resolution peripheral quantitative computed tomography, in which the bone mineral density was measured proximal to the affected joints.

The comparison of the BX parameters (i.e. MCI) with the SHS Score presented equal coefficients of correlations as reported by Böttcher et al. [8] between the MCI as measured by the X-posure System (the traditional DXR system) and the Sharp Score in patients with rheumatoid arthritis. Focusing on the Proliferation Score and the Destruction Score of the Psoriatic Arthritis Ratingen Score [22], high coefficients of correlation were observed for MCI, precisely reflecting the radiographic changes in PsA by the Proliferation and Destruction Scores.

For all scores, the study found a severity-dependent reduction for the BX parameters (MCI, T-score$_{MCI}$, T and BHI) in PsA patients. The strongest reductions were observed for MCI and T using the Proliferation Score (MCI: −28.3 %; T: −31.9 %) and the Destruction Score (MCI: −30.8 %; T: −30.9 %). The reduced MCI and T is directly associated with cortical thinning and the periarticular demineralisation of the metacarpal bones. Such cortical thinning and periarticular demineralisation show direct association with bone destruction and bone proliferation in PsA. Different cross-sectional studies have reported a strong relationship between reduced metacarpal bone mineral density and MCI as measured by the X-posure System and radiographic joint destruction [8, 26]. For the Sharp Joint Space Narrowing Score and the Sharp Erosion Score a reduced MCI was found (−28.6 % versus −22.1 %) in RA patients [8].

The study also presented a lower MCI (−12.5 %, $p < 0.01$) and cortical thickness as detected by T (−13.9 %, $p < 0.01$) in patients with erosions compared with patients without erosions. These results indicate that the occurrence of erosions is associated with periarticular bone loss. Additionally, the BX technique presented a sensitivity and specificity of 88 % versus 49 % using MCI for the detection of erosions. In this context, the traditional DXR technique showed a sensitivity of 87 % and a specificity of 49 % (for the MCI) in the detection of rheumatoid arthritis [28].

The measurement of periarticular bone loss can be considered a complementary approach to verify PsA-related bony changes and a surrogate marker for PsA progression. The quantification of periarticular demineralisation based on the cortical indices is potentially influenced by the size of the patient. The BHI offers the advantage to quantify cortical thickness and periarticular demineralisation independent of the size of the patient, leading to a better understanding of cortical change.

One limitation of the study is the absence of healthy controls in the BX analysis. The healthy reference cohort data were published by Thodberg et al. [25] and the study used the T-score$_{MCI}$ to quantify the periarticular demineralisation in comparison with healthy subjects. Additionally, a limitation of the study is the absence of longitudinal data regarding therapeutic effects. Hoff et al. [9] presented data about the inhibition of periarticular demineralisation detected by the traditional DXR technique in PsA patients under anti-tumour necrosis factor treatment with infliximab. In this context, the quantification of periarticular demineralisation seems to be a marker for the response of therapy in PsA [9]. However, the data of the study should be used as a basis to compare different treatment strategies in PsA by the BX technique.

Conclusions

The development of digital imaging and computer-assisted diagnostic methods has enabled a more precise quantification of periarticular demineralisation by the new BX technique. Patients with PsA showed reduced periarticular mineralisation as measured by the MCI and the T-score$_{MCI}$. Additionally, the BX measurements revealed a strong association with the radiographic scoring methods. This new medical device offered the opportunity to quantify severity-dependent periarticular demineralisation in PsA patients with high reproducibility and can function as a surrogate marker of radiographic progression to consecutively optimise an appropriate individual therapeutic strategy.

Abbreviations

A: Cortical area (mm^2) estimated by BoneXpert; BHI: Bone Health Index estimated by BoneXpert; BX: BoneXpert; DXR: Digital X-ray radiogrammetry; L: Length of metacarpal bone (mm) measured by BoneXpert; MCI: Metacarpal Index measured by BoneXpert; PsA: Psoriatic arthritis; ROI: Region of interest; SD: Standard deviation; SHS Score: Psoriatic Arthritis modified van der Heijde Sharp Score; T: Cortical thickness of metacarpal bone (mm) measured by BoneXpert; V: Cortical bone volume (mm^2) estimated by BoneXpert; W: Width of metacarpal bone (mm) measured by BoneXpert

Acknowledgements

The authors thank Hans Henrik Thodberg (Director, Visiana, Holte, Denmark) for the use of the BoneXpert software. The authors also thank Thomas Lehmann (PhD) for the statistical advice.

Funding

There is no funding regarding the study.

Authors' contributions

AP designed the study, collected the data, analysed the radiographs, performed the statistical analysis, wrote the manuscript and revised the manuscript. LK collected the data, performed the BX measurements and participated in the statistical analysis as well as the study design. DMR performed the scoring of the radiographs, interpreted the scoring data and helped to draft the manuscript. LR performed the data collection and participated in the statistical analysis. MF performed the additional statistical analysis, interpreted the data and edited the manuscript after the revision. PO performed the clinical data collection, edited the manuscript and helped to revise the manuscript. GW interpreted the data, edited the manuscript and helped to revise the manuscript. JB participated on the study design, performed scoring of the hand X-ray images and wrote the manuscript. All authors read and approved the final manuscript.

Competing interests

The authors declare that they have no competing interests.

Author details

[1]Department of Internal Medicine III, Jena University Hospital—Friedrich Schiller University Jena, Erlanger Allee 101, Jena 07747, Germany. [2]Institute of Diagnostic and Interventional Radiology, Jena University Hospital—Friedrich Schiller University Jena, Erlanger Allee 101, Jena 07747, Germany. [3]Department of Internal Medicine I, Jena University Hospital—Friedrich Schiller University Jena, Erlanger Allee 101, Jena 07747, Germany. [4]Institute of Diagnostic and Interventional Radiology, SRH Wald-Klinikum Gera, Straße des Friedens 122, Gera 07548, Germany.

References

1. Gladman DD, Antoni C, Mease P, Clegg DO, Nash P. Psoriatic arthritis: epidemiology, clinical features, course and outcome. Ann Rheum Dis. 2005;64 Suppl 2:ii14–7.
2. Day MS, Nam D, Goodman S, Su EP, Figgie M. Psoriatic arthritis. J Am Acad Orthop Surg. 2012;20:28–37.
3. Wassenberg S. Radiographic scoring methods in psoriatic arthritis. Clin Exp Rheumatol. 2015;33 Suppl 93:S55–9.
4. Böttcher J, Pfeil A, Rosholm A, Malich A, Petrovitch A, Heinrich B, Lehmann G, Mentzel HJ, Hein G, Linss W, Kaiser WA. Influence of image-capturing parameters on digital X-ray radiogrammetry. J Clin Densitom. 2005;8:87–94.
5. Pfeil A, Renz DM, Fröber R, Hansch A, Lehmann G, Sommerfeld J, Malich A, Wolf G, Böttcher J. Influence of angulation on metacarpal bone mineral density measurements using digital X-ray radiogrammetry. Int J Comput Assist Radiol Surg. 2015;10:587–92.
6. Pfeil A, Haugeberg G, Hansch A, Renz DM, Lehmann G, Malich A, et al. The value of digital X-ray radiogrammetry in the assessment of inflammatory bone loss in rheumatoid arthritis. Arthritis Care Research (Hoboken). 2011;63:666–74.
7. Böttcher J, Pfeil A, Mentzel HJ, Kramer A, Schäfer ML, Lehmann G, Eidner T, Petrovitch A, Malich A, Hein G, Kaiser WA. Peripheral bone status in rheumatoid arthritis evaluated by digital X-ray radiogrammetry (DXR) and compared with multi-site quantitative ultrasound (QUS). Calcif Tiss Int. 2006;78:25–34.
8. Böttcher J, Pfeil A, Rosholm A, Petrovitch A, Seidl BE, Malich A, Kramer A, Lehmann G, Hein G, Kaiser WA. Digital X-ray radiogrammetry combined with semi-automated analysis of joint space distances as a new diagnostic approach in rheumatoid arthritis—a cross-sectional and longitudinal study. Arthritis Rheum. 2005;52:3850–9.
9. Hoff M, Kavanaugh A, Haugeberg G. Hand bone loss in patients with psoriatic arthritis: posthoc analysis of IMPACT II data comparing infliximab and placebo. J Rheumatol. 2013;40:1344–8.
10. Szentpetery A, Heffernan E, Haroon M, Kilbane M, Gallagher P, McKenna MJ, FitzGerald O. Striking difference of periarticular bone density change in early psoriatic arthritis and rheumatoid arthritis following anti-rheumatic treatment as measured by digital X-ray radiogrammetry. Rheumatology. 2016;55:891–6.
11. Thodberg HH, Kreiborg S, Juul A, Pedersen KD. The BoneXpert method for automated determination of skeletal maturity. IEEE Trans Med Imaging. 2009;28:52–66.
12. van Rijn RR, Lequin MH, Thodberg HH. Automatic determination of Greulich and Pyle bone age in healthy Dutch children. Pediatr Radiol. 2009;39:591–7.
13. Martin DD, Deusch D, Schweizer R, Binder G, Thodberg HH, Ranke MB. Clinical application of automated Greulich-Pyle bone age determination in children with short stature. Pediatr Radiol. 2009;39:598–607.
14. Thodberg HH, Jenni OG, Caflisch J, Ranke MB, Martin DD. Prediction of adult height based on automated determination of bone age. J Clin Endocrinol Metab. 2009;94:4868–74.
15. Martin DD, Sato K, Sato M, Thodberg HH, Tanaka T. Validation of a new method for automated determination of bone age in Japanese children. Horm Res Paediatr. 2010;73:398–404.
16. Thodberg HH, Neuhof J, Ranke MB, Jenni OG, Martin DD. Validation of bone age methods by their ability to predict adult height. Horm Res Paediatr. 2010;74:15–22.
17. Thodberg HH, Sävendahl L. Validation and reference values of automated bone age determination for four ethnicities. Acad Radiol. 2010;17:1425–32.
18. Thodberg HH, Jenni OG, Ranke MB, Martin DD. Standardization of the Tanner-Whitehouse bone age method in the context of automated image analysis. Ann Hum Biol. 2012;39:68–75.
19. Taylor W, Gladman D, Helliwell P, Marchesoni A, Mease P, Mielants H, CASPAR Study Group. Classification criteria for psoriatic arthritis: development of new criteria from a large international study. Arthritis Rheum. 2006;54:2665–73.
20. Thodberg HH, Olafsdottir H. Adding curvature to minimum description length shape models. Proc Br Mach Vision Conf. 2003;2:251–60.
21. Thodberg HH, van Rijn RR, Tanaka T, Martin DD, Kreiborg S. A paediatric bone index derived by automated radiogrammetry. Osteoporos Int. 2010;21:1391–400.
22. Wassenberg S, Fischer-Kahle V, Herborn G, Rau R. A method to score radiographic change in psoriatic arthritis. Z Rheumatol. 2001;60:156–66.
23. van der Heijde DM, van Leeuwen MA, van Riel PL, Koster AM, van 't Hof MA, van Rijswijk MH, van de Putte LB. Biannual radiographic assessments of hands and feet in a three-year prospective followup of patients with early rheumatoid arthritis. Arthritis Rheum. 1992;35:26–34.
24. Kavanaugh A, Ritchlin C, Rahman P, Puig L, Gottlieb AB, Li S, Wang Y, Noonan L, Brodmerkel C, Song M, Mendelsohn AM, McInnes IB. PSUMMIT-1 and 2 Study Groups. Ustekinumab, an anti-IL-12/23 p40 monoclonal antibody, inhibits radiographic progression in patients with active psoriatic arthritis: results of an integrated analysis of radiographic data from the phase 3, multicentre, randomised, double-blind, placebo-controlled PSUMMIT-1 and PSUMMIT-2 trials. Ann Rheum Dis. 2014;73:1000–6.
25. Thodberg HH, Böttcher J, Lomholt J, Kreiborg S, Wolf G, Pfeil A. A new implementation of digital X-ray radiogrammetry and reference curves of four indices of cortical bone for healthy European adults. Arch Osteoporos. 2016;11:17.
26. Böttcher J, Pfeil A, Rosholm A, Sörös P, Petrovitch A, Schaefer ML, Seidl BE, Malich A, Hansch A, Wolf G, Kaiser WA. Computerized quantification of joint space narrowing and periarticular demineralization in patients with rheumatoid arthritis based on digital X-ray radiogrammetry. Invest Radiol. 2006;41:36–44.
27. Kocijan R, Englbrecht M, Haschka J, Simon D, Kleyer A, Finzel S, Kraus S, Resch H, Muschitz C, Engelke K, Sticherling M, Rech J, Schett G. Quantitative and qualitative changes of bone in psoriasis and psoriatic arthritis patients. J Bone Miner Res. 2015;30:1775–83.

18

The impact of identifying carotid plaque on addressing cardiovascular risk in psoriatic arthritis

Michael Lucke[1], William Messner[2], Esther S. H. Kim[3] and M. Elaine Husni[4*]

Abstract

Background: Patients with psoriatic arthritis (PsA) are at an increased risk for cardiovascular (CV) disease. The aim of this study was to identify the frequency of carotid plaque in asymptomatic patients with psoriatic arthritis at baseline and follow-up screening, and to assess for the impact of demonstrating plaque on management of traditional cardiovascular risk factors.

Methods: Eighty-seven PsA patients underwent carotid duplex ultrasound screening. Repeat carotid duplex ultrasound was offered to all patients between 12 and 30 months. Preventive cardiology referrals were generated for all patients through the electronic health record. Traditional cardiovascular risk factors, medication use, and rates of utilization of preventive cardiology services were compared between patients with and without plaque.

Results: Carotid plaque was identified in 34/87 (39 %) of PsA patients. Age and triglyceride levels were predictors of plaque presence. Patients with plaque trended toward higher rates of smoking and diabetes, and higher low-density lipoprotein levels. Only 9/87 (10 %) patients completed at least one visit with preventive cardiology after enrollment despite referral. Low use of statin (21 %) and antiplatelet (27 %) medication was observed. Rates of biologic medication use for PsA were higher (75 %) than studies in similar cohorts of patients with carotid plaque. No association was seen between disease duration or activity and the presence of carotid plaque.

Conclusion: Despite demonstration of high cardiac risk by the presence of carotid plaque, implementation of preventive cardiovascular services and rates of statin and antiplatelet use remained low. Age and triglyceride levels were significant variables in predicting plaque presence. There is no evidence that demonstration of plaque resulted in further evaluation or changes in treatment regimens to address heightened cardiovascular risk.

Keywords: Psoriatic arthritis, Spondyloarthritis, Atherosclerosis, Carotid plaque

Background

Cardiovascular disease risk is elevated in psoriatic arthritis (PsA) compared with the general population and is a major source of morbidity and mortality [1, 2]. The prevalence of traditional risk factors is elevated in both cutaneous psoriasis and PsA compared with the general population [3, 4]. PsA patients suffer from more severe atherosclerosis compared with patients with cutaneous psoriasis [5]. Despite the elevated risk, there remains an unmet need in identifying and addressing CV risk in PsA. There is currently a lack of consensus guidelines in the United States on addressing CV risk in PsA. This study uniquely incorporates both serial carotid ultrasound (US) data in combination with automatic prompting for preventive cardiology referral to a rheumatology clinic population with the goal of assessing the impact of these interventions on CV risk factor modification.

Prior studies have demonstrated suboptimal evaluation and control of modifiable CV risk factors in patients with inflammatory arthritis by both rheumatologists and primary care physicians [6]. Additionally, subclinical atherosclerosis in PsA has been shown to be prevalent even without classic CV risk factors and current risk assessment tools such as the Framingham Risk Score underestimate CV risk in PsA [2, 7, 8], suggesting a role of

* Correspondence: Husnie@ccf.org
[4]Department of Rheumatic and Immunologic Diseases, Cleveland Clinic, 9500 Euclid Ave, desk A50, Cleveland, OH 44195, USA
Full list of author information is available at the end of the article

systemic inflammation in patients with psoriatic skin and joint disease [9, 10]. Prior investigations into the formation of combined cardiology and rheumatology clinics have identified that a high proportion of patients with inflammatory joint pain have indications for medical CV interventions [11], although there were low numbers of PsA patients in this cohort.

Carotid duplex ultrasound (CDU) is a noninvasive imaging technique which can identify the presence of carotid plaque, representing an unequivocal manifestation of atherosclerosis and serving as a surrogate for CV disease. Incorporation of CDU for patients at intermediate risk for CV disease has been used to further enhance CV risk stratification in the general population [12]. Several studies have supported the role of CDU in assessment of CV risk in rheumatoid arthritis, and patients with carotid plaque should be considered as having very high CV risk [13, 14]. In one series of rheumatoid arthritis patients, the presence of bilateral plaque on CDU screening quadrupled the incidence of new acute coronary syndromes independently of any other risk factors compared with patients without carotid plaque [14]. Subclinical atherosclerosis is elevated in patients with PsA compared with controls [1]; screening this population may help identify those patients who are optimal candidates for intensive medical treatment. Prior studies suggest that incorporation of CDU into treatment algorithms can impact progression of plaque and CV outcomes [15]. However, the general applicability of these findings in rheumatology or primary care clinic settings is not clear. Guidelines on the management of patients with identified carotid plaque and PsA have not been formulated.

This study investigates the impact of screening asymptomatic PsA patients for carotid plaque on CV risk factor control. PsA alone is not an indication for antiplatelet or lipid-lowering therapies but should be taken into consideration as part of comprehensive CV risk factor stratification.

Methods

Study patients and design

Eighty-seven patients with PsA enrolled in the COMPASS (Cardiometabolic Outcome Measures in Psoriatic ArthritiS Study) database underwent CDU and were screened for the presence of plaque. Patients were ≥18 years old and able to provide consent for enrollment. Patients with a diagnosis of PsA presenting for evaluation in a general rheumatology clinic at a tertiary academic medical center were identified for potential enrollment into the database. PsA was diagnosed after satisfying the criteria of the Classification of Psoriatic Arthritis Study Group with confirmation by a board-certified rheumatologist. Patients remained under the management of their clinical rheumatologist throughout the study.

Referral to preventive cardiology was automatically generated through the EPIC electronic health record as part of best practices management upon study enrollment for all patients. The preventive cardiology clinic at our institution provides complete CV risk assessment and management for both primary and secondary CV disease prevention by a multispecialty team of health care professionals who provide nutritional counseling, exercise instruction, lifestyle and behavioral counseling, smoking cessation programs, medical management of CV risk factors, psychological counseling, and referral to physicians or other health professionals as needed. Extensive assessment of patients' medical, family, and social history are incorporated with biomarkers and imaging data to risk stratify patients and provide appropriate prevention strategies. Recognizing the heightened CV risk associated with inflammatory arthritides, the preventive cardiology clinic utilizes a primary prevention consensus algorithm for inflammatory arthritis which includes lifestyle counseling for all patients, a goal low-density lipoprotein (LDL) of <100 mg/dl, as well as use of antiplatelet medications in patients with carotid plaque. Rates of completed preventive cardiology consults, defined as one recorded visit with preventive cardiology after enrollment in the COMPASS database, were assessed via electronic record chart review.

Data collection and assessment

Demographics, traditional CV risk factors, PsA duration, and medication use were recorded at baseline (Table 1) and yearly thereafter using a standardized protocol [16]. CV risk factors addressed included personal history of prior CV events, history of hypertension, history of hyperlipidemia, and history of diabetes. Smoking status was assessed by survey and chart review, and recorded as never, former, or current use, with any ongoing cigarette use defined as a current smoker. Hypertension control was assessed by a cross-sectional recording of last recorded blood pressure during chart review, with 140/90 mmHg used as a cutoff value in accessing control. Body mass index was recorded. Medications assessed included current or prior use of nonbiologic disease-modifying antirheumatic drugs (DMARDS), current or prior biologic DMARDs, nonsteroidal anti-inflammatory drugs (NSAIDS), and steroids. Patients were surveyed on prior dose and duration of prednisone use at enrollment and yearly thereafter. Medication use was confirmed by electronic record chart review at 12–30 months following enrollment. C-reactive protein (CRP), erythrocyte sedimentation rate (ESR), and lipid panels were assessed. When multiple laboratory tests

Table 1 Comparisons of variables between patients with and without plaque

		No plaque		Plaque		
Factor	Total *N* assessed	*N*	Statistics	*N*	Statistics	*p* value[a]
Age[b]	87	53	49.58 ± 10.56	34	58 ± 8.58	<0.001[T]
Male sex[c]	87	26	49.06	15	44.12	0.82[C]
History of hypertension[c]	86	17	32.69	23	67.65	0.003[C]
BP < 140/90 mmHg[c]	87	42	79.25	20	58.82	0.07[C]
Smoking status[c]	87					0.052[C]
No	44	29	54.72	15	44.12	
Former	26	18	33.96	8	23.53	
Current	17	6	11.32	11	32.35	
BMI[b]	79	47	30.87 ± 8.54	32	30.34 ± 6.16	0.75[T]
Diabetes[c]	87	7	13.21	9	26.47	0.20[C]
Total cholesterol[b]	75	44	184.5 ± 29.31	31	202.48 ± 45.16	0.057[T]
Triglyceride[d]	74	43	95 (70, 125)	31	144 (87.5, 177.5)	0.014[W]
HDL[b]	74	43	55.12 ± 15.49	31	56.16 ± 21.55	0.82[T]
LDL[b]	74	43	104.07 ± 26.35	31	118.74 ± 41.94	0.092[T]
Antiplatelet use[c]	87	14	26.42	10	29.41	0.95[C]
Statin use[c]	87	9	16.98	10	29.41	0.27[C]
Biologic use[c]	87					0.03[F]
No	17	14	26.42	3	8.82	
Former	5	1	1.89	4	11.76	
Current	65	38	71.7	27	79.41	
Traditional DMARD use[c]	87					0.75[F]
No	11	7	13.21	4	11.76	
Former	34	19	35.85	15	44.12	
Current	42	27	50.94	15	44.12	
History of CVD[c]	87	2	3.77	5	14.71	0.11[F]
ESR[d]	69	37	8 (4, 10)	32	8 (5.25, 12.25)	0.53[W]
CRP[d]	84	52	0.3 (0.1, 0.6)	32	0.3 (0.2, 1.22)	0.11[W]
PsO duration[b]	85	52	21.02 ± 14.79	33	22.58 ± 19.14	0.69[T]
PsA duration[b]	84	51	10.76 ± 8.32	33	12.76 ± 10.7	0.37[T]
Prednisone use > 1 month[c]	86	26	49.06	11	33.33	0.23[C]
Current NSAID use[c]	87	27	50.94	22	64.71	0.30[C]
Baseline SJC[d]	81	49	1 (0, 5)	32	0 (0, 4.5)	0.88[W]
Baseline TJC[d]	81	49	5 (0, 14)	32	5 (0.75, 16.25)	0.93[W]

[a]*C* Pearson's chi-squared test with Yates' continuity correction, *F* Fisher's exact test for count data, *T* Welch Two Sample T-test, *W* Wilcoxon rank sum test with continuity correction
[b]Mean ± SD
[c]Percentage
[d]Median (25th percentile, 75th percentile)
BP blood pressure, *CRP* C-reactive protein, *CVD* cardiovascular disease, *DMARD* disease-modifying antirheumatic drug, *ESR* erythrocyte sedimentation rate, *HDL* high-density lipoprotein, *LDL* low-density lipoprotein, *NSAID* nonsteroidal anti-inflammatory drug, *PsA* psoriatic arthritis, *SJC* swollen joint count, *TJC* tender joint count *PsO* psoriasis

were performed, the most recently performed test after entry into the cohort was used. Additional laboratory tests ordered by preventive cardiology clinics were recorded via electronic record chart review. A 68/66 tender/swollen joint count was performed by a physician, nurse practitioner, or physician assistant with training in performing joint counts.

The multivariate logistic regression model including age and triglycerides was performed (Table 2). When controlling for age and triglyceride levels in a

Table 2 Multivariate logistic regression model for identification of carotid plaque

Term	Coefficient	Standard error	*p* value	Odds ratio	95 % CI on odds ratio
Intercept	6.59	1.69	<0.001	–	–
Age	0.0936	0.0281	<0.001	1.098	1.043–1.166
Triglycerides	0.0087	0.00401	0.03	1.009	1.001–1.018

multivariate setting, hypertension is not significant ($p = 0.13$). However, age and triglycerides remain significant. The probability of observing carotid plaque increases with higher levels of both these variables.

Ultrasound imaging

A standardized protocol was performed by registered vascular sonographers who had been specifically trained in CDU imaging using the Philips iU22 US system with an 8–14 MHz linear transducer. A circumferential plaque screen including assessment of internal carotid, external carotid, and common carotid arteries was performed using both transverse and longitudinal views of the bilateral carotid arteries with plaque in any vessel recorded as a positive result. Carotid plaque was defined using the Mannheim consensus criteria [17]. Repeat CDU was offered to all 87 patients through telephone calls and was performed between 12 and 30 months in 50 patients (Fig. 1). Results of US imaging, reported as normal or abnormal, were sent to patients as per IRB protocol. All patients were also given an opportunity to allow release of results to their primary care physicians and rheumatologists.

Statistical analyses

Continuous variables were described using means and standard deviations or medians and interquartile ranges. Categorical variables were described using counts and percentages. Comparisons of continuous variables between groups were made using either Welch's two-sample *t* test or Wilcoxon's rank-sum test. Comparisons of categorical variables between groups were made using Pearson's chi-squared test or Fisher's exact test. Multivariate logistic regression modeling was used to measure relationships between patient CV risk factors and the presence of carotid plaque (Table 2). Where relevant in the multivariate modeling, missing values were handled by median imputation. All analyses were done using R software (version 3.0.2; Vienna, Austria). All testing was two-sided and considered significant at the 0.05 level.

Results

Carotid plaque was identified in 34/87 (39 %) of patients with PsA. Older age ($p < 0.001$), history of hypertension ($p < 0.003$), and triglyceride levels ($p < 0.014$) were statistically significant variables associated with the presence of carotid plaque (Table 1). A higher percentage of

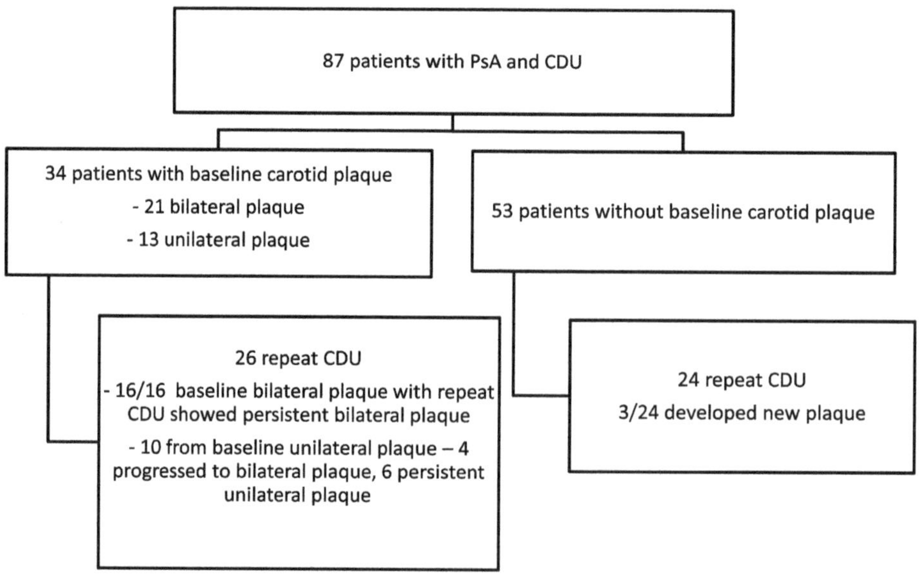

Fig. 1 Flow diagram. *CDU* carotid duplex ultrasound, *PsA* psoriatic arthritis

patients with plaque were current smokers (32 % versus 11 %). Patients with carotid plaque trended towards higher LDL levels compared with those without plaque (124 versus 102 mg/dl). Length of cutaneous psoriasis and PsA, as well as ESR and CRP, were not statistically significantly different between groups. Swollen joint count (SJC) and tender joint count (TJC) were comparable between groups, with a median of five tender joints in both groups and of zero and one swollen joint in the no plaque and plaque groups respectively.

Because the three significant CV risk factors (age, hypertension, and triglyceride levels) were intercorrelated, multivariate logistic regression modeling was implemented to limit possible confounding. Controlling for age and triglyceride levels, hypertension was not significant ($p = 0.13$). The multivariate logistic regression model including age and triglyceride as predictors demonstrates increased probability of observing carotid plaque with higher levels of these two variables.

Twenty-one patients had bilateral plaque present at baseline screening. Of the 16/21 patients with bilateral plaque and repeat carotid CDU screening, all demonstrated persistent plaque. Thirteen patients had unilateral plaque at baseline. Of the 10 patients with unilateral plaque who had a repeat CDU, 4/10 (40 %) showed progression from unilateral to bilateral plaque. A total 3/24 (12.5 %) of patients without plaque at baseline who had repeat CDU performed showed new plaque presence.

Only nine patients completed preventive cardiology appointments after enrollment in the COMPASS database. There was no evidence of a difference in the rates of utilization of preventive cardiology between patients with PsA without carotid plaque and those with plaque ($p = 0.73$). Four patients (11.7 %) with baseline plaque completed evaluations compared with five patients (9.4 %) without baseline plaque. Note that the 95 % confidence interval for the odds ratio between the groups is quite wide (0.234, 6.460), indicating that while there is no evidence of a difference, a meaningful difference cannot be ruled out. Routine interventions for these patients included a comprehensive assessment of diet, weight, and exercise. In addition to standard lipid profiles, a "preventive profile" consisting of lipoprotein (a), lipoprotein-associated phospholipase A2, fibrinogen, myeloperoxidase, NT-pro BNP, high-sensitivity CRP, and urine albumin:creatnine ratio was checked in 13/16 patients who saw preventive cardiology during or prior to study enrollment and were assessed to have elevated CV risk. Fourteen other patients were seen by a cardiologist for other reasons including hypertension, syncope, arrhythmias, and valvular heart disease.

High percentages (75 %) of our cohort were currently being treated with a biologic DMARD, the majority of which were on anti-TNF-α medications except for two patients on ustekinumab. Rates of biologic medication use in our cohort are significantly higher than in other studies on subclinical atherosclerosis in PsA; prior rates of biologic DMARD use range from 1% [7] to 51 % [9]. More patients with plaque were treated with biologic medications while more patients without plaque were taking a traditional DMARD. Methotrexate was the medication of choice in the vast majority of patients on a DMARD.

Only four patients with plaque had a prior history of CV disease, two of these patients were on maximum dose statins. No other patient in the study population was treated with maximum dose statins. Two patients without plaque had a history of CV disease (one cerebrovascular accident, one non-ST elevated myocardial infarction).

Discussion

Despite noninvasive screening demonstrating high rates of carotid plaque, few PsA patients completed consultations with the preventive cardiology service. There is no evidence that patients with carotid plaque utilized preventive cardiology visits more than those patients without plaque. This study incorporates multiple strategies to address CV risk in PsA through incorporation of both CDU and automatic referrals to preventive cardiology. Despite this, a minority of patients with and without carotid plaque met the stated LDL goals and few were on antiplatelet therapy.

A goal of electronic health records is to enhance meaningful use and allow identification of high-risk groups. In this study, incorporation of automatic "best practice" electronic referrals was not an effective strategy to increase rates of specialty CV screening, even with a preventive cardiology clinic available in the same institution. This additional optional electronic alert may have been perceived as too time consuming or not of high value in patient care by physicians, and may not be of high utility to improve outcomes as a general treatment strategy.

There was a high prevalence of traditional cardiac risk factors in our cohort; 8 % had a history of prior CV disease, 18 % were diabetic, 46 % had a history of hypertension, and 49 % had a history of smoking. Rates of referral completion were not changed by demonstrating high CV risk through detection of carotid plaque. Lack of appreciation of CV risk by patients, primary providers, and specialists may all contribute to the low referral rate. In addition to traditional risk factors, demonstration of carotid plaque can improve risk stratification but will only be impactful if incorporated into treatment plans by primary care physicians, rheumatologists, and/or cardiologists. The absence of guidelines on the use of this screening measure may have contributed to the lack of interventions in our group.

Identification of patients with PsA who may benefit most from the addition of CDU to traditional risk factor assessment is critical for meaningful implementation of this additional screening test. Early establishment of the level of CV risk has the potential to improve CV outcomes, but presently it is unclear how to best screen these patients with elevated baseline risk. Our results indicate that age and high triglyceride levels are associated with the presence of plaque, and smoking was more common in patients with plaque. As expected, the incidence of plaque increased with age. The 25th percentile for age in patients with plaque in our cohort was 51 with a median of 55. CDU may be a helpful risk stratification tool to assist in risk-prevention strategies in patients with PsA, particularly in patients over 50 years old requiring biologic use.

Prevalence of plaque in our PsA population is higher than in some PsA cohorts [7, 18], lower than other series [9], and similar to a rheumatoid arthritis cohort [19]. Rates of plaque in inflammatory arthritis have been shown to be increased compared with age-matched controls in the general population [20]. The high rates of plaque in PsA support a role for CDU in select PsA patients to identify high CV risk patients who lack traditional risk factors or overt CV disease. While an interval of 12–24 months may be too short to detect progression of atherosclerosis in some patients, new formation of plaque after 1–2 years of follow up in three patients suggests a potential role for serial monitoring of high-risk patients with CDU as well as early medical intervention. The 40 % (4/10 patients) rate of progression from unilateral plaque to bilateral plaque over 1–2 years suggests a role for medical interventions at the time of discovery of plaque but will require confirmation in a larger sample size. Lipid levels did not always correlate with plaque progression, as these three patients' LDL ranged from 73 to 187 mg/dl.

ESR and CRP levels have not been shown to be reliable measures of active disease in PsA and were not associated with plaque formation in our study, which did not use a high-sensitivity CRP assay and was limited by the use of a cross-sectional measurement. No significant difference in the prevalence of plaque and disease duration was found, which has also been noted in a recent publication [9]. Patients in our cohort had a high variability in the duration of disease. It is possible that anti-inflammatory treatments mitigated the effect of chronic inflammation associated with longer disease activity. Rates of biologic medication use in our cohort are significantly higher than other studies on subclinical atherosclerosis in PsA; prior rates of biologic DMARD use range from 1 % [7] to 51 % [9].

Although conflicting results have been reported, some studies have suggested that TNF-α antagonists may have a beneficial role in preventing progression of subclinical atherosclerosis [21]. A prior series of PsA patients showed a lower prevalence of carotid plaques in patients on TNF-α blockers compared with nonbiologic DMARDS [22]. In our cohort, there was a higher prevalence of biologic use in the carotid plaque group, which may be a reflection of higher disease activity and a tertiary center patient population.

The low sample size in this exploratory study of combining screening measures is a limitation. Another limitation of our cross-sectional study is an inability to access cardiac interventions performed outside our institution. As a retrospective chart review, some data including BMI and cholesterol panels were unavailable for analysis. In patients without plaque, 88 % had BMI data and 83 % had a cholesterol panel, versus 94 % and 91 % respectively of patients with plaque. The extent of cutaneous psoriasis was not measured between the groups.

The time frame of follow up may be too short to evaluate for changes in plaque formation. However, even over a short interval several patients demonstrated new plaque, suggesting an accelerated risk of CV events. The low total number of patients with new plaque limits the generalizability of this finding as well as further analysis of risks for progression. Likewise, there is limited power to analyze for efficacy of the preventive cardiology program in modifying CV risk factors between those who completed and did not complete an appointment. Low numbers of clinical CV events were seen, probably due to short duration of follow up. While the presence of plaque is a strong indicator of heightened CV risk, other variables such as plaque characteristics and change in plaque size were not assessed. Dose and duration of prednisone use and NSAID use were reliant upon patient survey and recollection. Dependence on patient survey responses were reduced by simultaneous medical record review to confirm medications and documented CV risk factors. The cross-sectional nature of the study did not allow for an assessment of the inflammatory burden of PsA over time.

The low rates of preventive cardiology clinic attendance despite automatic referral merits further investigation. It is possible that debate over the level of CV risk in PsA limited physician responses to electronic referral recommendations, which could be declined easily by the physician. Physicians may have been satisfied with control of the disease and did not perceive these patients to be at elevated risk. Lack of familiarity with CDU screening and the risk represented by carotid plaque may have also led to an under-appreciation of CV risk. While the results of the US scan were provided to the patient's primary rheumatologist and the patient, an interpretation of the findings regarding level of CV risk was not provided. Because the US examinations were conducted outside of a standard clinic visit, the results may not have been incorporated into the physician's assessment at the time of follow-up rheumatology visits. The distance required for return visits to a tertiary care center also likely impacted the percentage of patients completing preventive cardiology referrals. Physicians and patients, especially those with prior cardiology clinic visits, may not be aware of the multispecialty approach of the preventive cardiology clinic. It is possible that patients sought a cardiology opinion at a local facility; the study design did not collect additional information about interval visits with a local cardiologist.

Further evaluation into the barriers of addressing CV risk in PsA patients is required. CV risk stratification and management in PsA may be improved by incorporation of carotid CDU to assess for carotid plaque. The presence of a preventive cardiology program is not widely available, but even with the presence of this program at our institution it was underutilized by a high-risk population. Combined cardiology–rheumatology clinics have shown promise, with one study reporting successful treatment to lipid targets in 90 % of inflammatory joint pain patients referred to the combined clinic [11]. Translating identification of elevated CV risk in PsA patients into preventive interventions to reduce risk remains a challenge. With increasing evidence of this risk identified over recent years, development of further guidelines to address modifiable risk factors in this patient group is needed.

Conclusion

Interventions to aggressively assess and modify CV risk in PsA remain an unmet aspect of disease management despite the high morbidity and mortality of CV disease in this population. Rates of carotid plaque are high in PsA and patients with carotid plaque should be considered as having very high CV risk. In our cohort, patients aged over 50 with elevated triglyceride levels are at higher risk for development of carotid plaque. Despite demonstration of high cardiac risk by carotid plaque, implementation of preventive CV strategies in PsA patients remained poor. This study emphasizes the need for further consensus in establishing protocols for CV risk assessment in PsA.

Abbreviations

CDU, carotid duplex ultrasound; COMPASS, Cardiometabolic Outcome Measures in Psoriatic ArthritiS Study; CRP, C-reactive protein; CV, cardiovascular; DMARD, disease-modifying antirheumatic drug; ESR, erythrocyte sedimentation rate; LDL, low-density lipoprotein; NSAID, nonsteroidal anti-inflammatory drug; PsA, psoriatic arthritis; SJC, swollen joint count; TJC, tender joint count, US, ultrasound

Acknowledgments

The authors would like to thank Colin O'Rourke for statistical analysis and Alex Massiello for his technical assistance.

Funding

This study was supported by a grant from the National Psoriasis Foundation and the Arthritis National Research Foundation.

Authors' contributions

ML designed the study, gathered and interpreted data, and drafted the manuscript. MEH designed the study, interpreted data, and revised the manuscript critically. WM provided detailed statistical analysis and manuscript revision. ESHK provided expert guidance, interpretation of data, and critical review and revision of the manuscript. All authors read and approved the final manuscript.

Competing interests

ESHK serves as a consultant for Philips Ultrasound and has received $12,000 and < $10,000 support grant from General Electric. MEH has received $20,000 from the National Psoriasis Foundation and Arthritis National Research Foundation, and served on advisory boards for UCB, Amgen, Novartis, Eli lilly, Bristol Myers Squibb, and Abbvie (<10,000 each). The remaining authors declare that they have no competing interests.

Consent for publication

All authors read and reviewed the final manuscript and consent for publication.

Author details

[1]Department of Rheumatology, Allegheny Health Network, Pittsburgh, PA, USA. [2]Department of Quantitative Health Sciences, Cleveland Clinic, Cleveland, OH, USA. [3]Department of Cardiovascular Medicine, Cleveland Clinic, Cleveland, OH, USA. [4]Department of Rheumatic and Immunologic Diseases, Cleveland Clinic, 9500 Euclid Ave, desk A50, Cleveland, OH 44195, USA.

References

1. Janitski A, Symmons D, Peters MJ, Sattar N, McInnes I, Nurmohamed MT. Cardiovascular comorbidities in patients with psoriatic arthritis: a systematic review. Ann Rheum Dis. 2013;72(2):211–6.
2. Gladman DD, Ang M, Su L, Tom BD, Schentag CT, Farewell VT. Cardiovascular morbidity in psoriatic arthritis. Ann Rheum Dis. 2009;68(7):1131–5.
3. Husted JA, Thavaneswaran A, Chandran V, et al. Cardiovascular and other comorbidities in patients with psoriatic arthritis: a comparison with patients with psoriasis. Arthritis Care Res (Hoboken). 2011;63(12):1729–35.
4. Han C, Robinson Jr DW, Hackett MV, Paramore LC, Fraeman KH, Bala MV. Cardiovascular disease and risk factors in patients with rheumatoid arthritis, psoriatic arthritis, and ankylosing spondylitis. J Rheumatol. 2006;33(11):2167–72.
5. Eder L, Jayakar J, Shanmugarajah S, et al. The burden of carotid artery plaques is higher in patients with psoriatic arthritis compared with those with psoriasis alone. Ann Rheum Dis. 2013;72(5):715–20.
6. Desai SS, Myles JD, Kaplan MJ. Suboptimal cardiovascular risk factor identification and management in patients with rheumatoid arthritis: a cohort analysis. Arthritis Res Ther. 2012;14(6):R270.
7. Tam LS, Shang Q, Li EK, et al. Subclinical carotid atherosclerosis in patients with psoriatic arthritis. Arthritis Rheum. 2008;59(9):1322–31.
8. Eder L, Chandran V, Gladman DD. The framingham risk score underestimates the extent of subclinical atherosclerosis in patients with psoriatic disease. Ann Rheum Dis. 2014;73(11):1990-6.
9. Eder L, Thavaneswaran A, Chandran V, Cook R, Gladman DD. Increased burden of inflammation over time is associated with the extent of atherosclerotic plaques in patients with psoriatic arthritis. Ann Rheum Dis. 2015;74(10):1830-5.

10. Ramonda R, Lo Nigro A, Modesti V, et al. Atherosclerosis in psoriatic arthritis. Autoimmun Rev. 2011;10(12):773–8.
11. Rollefstad S, Kvien TK, Holme I, Eirheim AS, Pedersen TR, Semb AG. Treatment to lipid targets in patients with inflammatory joint diseases in a preventive cardio-rheuma clinic. Ann Rheum Dis. 2013;72(12):1968–74.
12. Peters SA, den Ruijter HM, Bots ML, Moons KG. Improvements in risk stratification for the occurrence of cardiovascular disease by imaging subclinical atherosclerosis: a systematic review. Heart. 2012;98(3):177–84.
13. Corrales A, Gonzalez-Juanatey C, Peiro ME, Blanco R, Llorca J, Gonzalez-Gay MA. Carotid ultrasound is useful for the cardiovascular risk stratification of patients with rheumatoid arthritis: results of a population-based study. Ann Rheum Dis. 2014;73(4):722–7.
14. Evans MR, Escalante A, Battafarano DF, Freeman GL, O'Leary DH, del Rincon I. Carotid atherosclerosis predicts incident acute coronary syndromes in rheumatoid arthritis. Arthritis Rheum. 2011;63(5):1211–20.
15. Spence JD, Hackam DG. Treating arteries instead of risk factors: a paradigm change in management of atherosclerosis. Stroke. 2010;41(6):1193–9.
16. Lin YC, Dalal D, Churton S, et al. Relationship between metabolic syndrome and carotid intima-media thickness: cross-sectional comparison between psoriasis and psoriatic arthritis. Arthritis Care Res (Hoboken). 2014;66(1):97–103.
17. Touboul PJ, Hennerici MG, Meairs S, et al. Mannheim carotid intima-media thickness and plaque consensus (2004-2006-2011). an update on behalf of the advisory board of the 3rd, 4th and 5th Watching the Risk Symposia, at the 13th, 15th and 20th European Stroke Conferences, Mannheim, Germany, 2004, Brussels, Belgium, 2006, and Hamburg, Germany, 2011. Cerebrovasc Dis. 2012;34(4):290–6.
18. Gonzalez-Juanatey C, Llorca J, Amigo-Diaz E, Dierssen T, Martin J, Gonzalez-Gay MA. High prevalence of subclinical atherosclerosis in psoriatic arthritis patients without clinically evident cardiovascular disease or classic atherosclerosis risk factors. Arthritis Rheum. 2007;57(6):1074–80.
19. Roman MJ, Moeller E, Davis A, et al. Preclinical carotid atherosclerosis in patients with rheumatoid arthritis. Ann Intern Med. 2006;144(4):249–56.
20. Salmon JE, Roman MJ. Subclinical atherosclerosis in rheumatoid arthritis and systemic lupus erythematosus. Am J Med. 2008;121(10 Suppl 1):S3–8.
21. Tam LS, Kitas GD, Gonzalez-Gay MA. Can suppression of inflammation by anti-TNF prevent progression of subclinical atherosclerosis in inflammatory arthritis? Rheumatology (Oxford). 2014;53(6):1108-19.
22. Di Minno MN, Iervolino S, Peluso R, Scarpa R, Di Minno G. CaRRDs study group. Carotid intima-media thickness in psoriatic arthritis: differences between tumor necrosis factor-alpha blockers and traditional disease-modifying antirheumatic drugs. Arterioscler Thromb Vasc Biol. 2011;31(3):705–12.

19

Concepts of pathogenesis in psoriatic arthritis: genotype determines clinical phenotype

Oliver FitzGerald[1], Muhammad Haroon[1], Jon T Giles[2] and Robert Winchester[2*]

Abstract

This review focuses on the genetic features of psoriatic arthritis (PsA) and their relationship to phenotypic heterogeneity in the disease, and addresses three questions: what do the recent studies on human leukocyte antigen (HLA) tell us about the genetic relationship between cutaneous psoriasis (PsO) and PsA – that is, is PsO a unitary phenotype; is PsA a genetically heterogeneous or homogeneous entity; and do the genetic factors implicated in determining susceptibility to PsA predict clinical phenotype? We first discuss the results from comparing the HLA typing of two PsO cohorts: one cohort providing the dermatologic perspective, consisting of patients with PsO without evidence of arthritic disease; and the second cohort providing the rheumatologic perspective, consisting of patients with PsA. We show that these two cohorts differ considerably in their predominant HLA alleles, indicating the heterogeneity of the overall PsO phenotype. Moreover, the genotype of patients in the PsA cohort was shown to be heterogeneous with significant elevations in the frequency of haplotypes containing *HLA-B*08*, *HLA-C*06:02*, *HLA-B*27*, *HLA-B*38* and *HLA-B*39*. Because different genetic susceptibility genes imply different disease mechanisms, and possibly different clinical courses and therapeutic responses, we then review the evidence for a phenotypic difference among patients with PsA who have inherited different HLA alleles. We provide evidence that different alleles and, more importantly, different haplotypes implicated in determining PsA susceptibility are associated with different phenotypic characteristics that appear to be subphenotypes. The implication of these findings for the overall pathophysiologic mechanisms involved in PsA is discussed with specific reference to their bearing on the discussion of whether PsA is conceptualised as an autoimmune process or one that is based on entheseal responses.

Introduction and concepts of pathogenesis

Psoriatic arthritis (PsA) is a heterogeneous disease with diverse clinical and radiographic manifestations. However, the specificity reported in development of the Classification Criteria for Psoriatic Arthritis [1] strongly implies that there are indeed common features which facilitate the diagnosis of PsA. Nonetheless, patients often differ considerably from one another in the type of their clinical manifestations, including whether or not they exhibit dactylitis, enthesitis, asymmetric or symmetric sacroiliitis, or joint deformity, but also in the presence and type of joint damage on plain radiography. For example, in a recent cohort study of patients with long-established PsA, 56% showed no evidence of erosive disease after a mean follow-up of 19 ± 9 years, while the balance had erosive disease [2]. Diverse other varied radiographic features were present, including features such as new bone formation, osteolysis and ankylosis (Table 1). The basis for this heterogeneity had not been adequately explained. In this review, the two major hypotheses relating to disease pathogenesis are discussed in light of recent data from studies of human leukocyte antigen (HLA) genotypes in PsA [3,4] and a study on the relationship of genotype to phenotype [2].

These hypotheses include the classical autoimmune basis of disease and the concept that PsA starts at the enthesis with microtrauma which then initiates innate immune events. While not being entirely mutually exclusive, these hypotheses present very different ideas about the initiation/causation of PsA.

* Correspondence: rjw8@columbia.edu
[2]Rheumatology Division, Department of Medicine, Columbia University College of Physicians and Surgeons, 630 West 168th Street, New York City, NY 10032, USA
Full list of author information is available at the end of the article

Psoriatic arthritis is an autoimmune disease

Several features in PsA suggest that an autoimmune process may drive the disease. Firstly, susceptibility to

Table 1 Phenotypic heterogeneity in a cohort of 282 cases of psoriatic arthritis

Age	55 ± 12
Male gender	134 (47)
Family history of psoriasis (*n* = 280)	175 (63)
Family history of PsA (*n* = 280)	45 (16)
Age of onset of psoriasis	28 ± 14
Psoriasis duration (years)	27 ± 14
Age of onset of PsA	35 ± 13
PsA duration (years)	19 ± 9
Years between psoriasis and PsA	6 (0 to 14)
Psoriasis before PsA	184 (65)
PsA before psoriasis	45 (16)
Psoriasis and PsA at same time	52 (18)
Nail disease	244 (79)
Pitting	96 (34)
Onycholysis	155 (55)
Peripheral arthritis	280 (99)
Polyarthritis	258 (91)
Oligoarthritis	21 (8)
Deformed joint count, if deformity	6 (4 to 12)
Enthesitis[a]	97 (34)
Dactylitis[a]	150 (53)
Sacroiliitis[a]	71 (25)
Asymmetric[a]	51 (18)
Symmetric[a]	18 (6)
Joint deformity[a]	183 (65)
Joint fusion[a]	83 (29)
Erosions[a] (*n* = 281)	123 (44)
Osteolysis[a] (*n* = 281)	41 (15)
Current PASI	1.2 (0.3 to 2.8)
Max PASI	3.8 (1.8 to 9.2)
Plaque psoriasis only	224 (79)
Psoriasis, nonplaque	59 (21)
Uveitis	9 (3)
Total on TNFi	176 (62)
Psoriasis requiring TNFi	32 (11)
PsA requiring TNFi	171 (60)
Number of TNFi, if on TNFi	1 (1 to 2; range 1 to 4)
Number of DMARDs	1 (1 to 2; range 0 to 5)

Data presented as mean ± standard deviation or *n* (%). DMARD, disease-modifying antirheumatic drug; PASI, Psoriasis Area Severity Index; PsA, psoriatic arthritis; TNFi, tumour necrosis factor inhibitor. [a]Variables used to construct the propensity score.

develop PsA is associated with class I major histocompatibility complex (MHC) genes [5]. Secondly, CD8$^+$ T cells, which present antigen to molecules encoded by HLA class 1 alleles, were shown to predominate in PsA synovial fluid with a reversal of the CD4:CD8 ratio found in rheumatoid arthritis (RA) [6]. Thirdly, CD8$^+$ T cells in synovial tissue and fluid obtained from PsA patients are clonally expanded with a reduction in nonspecific T-cell infiltration observed following methotrexate therapy [7,8]. Fourthly, the interesting observation in the setting of advanced HIV disease that both cutaneous psoriasis (PsO) and PsA can occur more frequently and more severely in the setting of CD4$^+$ T-cell depletion suggests that persisting memory-effector CD8$^+$ T cells (and not CD4$^+$ T cells as in RA) drive the disease. Fifthly, PsA developed for the first time after syngeneic bone marrow transplantation from a PsO donor [9]. Finally, there is the response to therapeutic agents directed at activated T cells (for example, cyclosporine, DAB389IL-2 or alefacept), as well as to effector pathways resulting from T-cell activation.

Given the above, one pathogenic hypothesis in PsA is that molecules encoded by certain HLA class 1 alleles bind self-peptides derived from proteins found in entheseal and synovial sites. CD8$^+$ T-cell clones specific for these self-peptide–MHC complexes are inappropriately activated, perhaps through the action of dendritic cells and the activated state perpetuated by the continual supply of self-peptides. This is the classic explanation for an autoimmune disease as a consequence of driver clones, and one would expect to recognise one or a few immunodominant T-cell receptor sequences in the inflammatory infiltrate. Clonally expanded T cells have indeed been demonstrated in PsA synovial fluid and tissue; however, despite extensive earlier analysis of the T-cell clonotypes, no evidence for an antigen driving this clonal expansion common to all cases has been identified [8].

Other components of the immune system have an active effector role in disease pathogenesis. Expression of MHC class I chain-related A (MICA) and interleukin (IL)-15 can lead to autoimmunity mediated by CD8$^+$ effector T cells, probably due to the capability of IL-15 to drive the expression of the natural killer group 2 member NKG2D [10]. A more recent study demonstrated that PsA patients had upregulated IL-15 and MHC class I chain-related A (MICA) in their affected synovial tissues [11]. This unique inflammatory environment enabled natural killer cell activation and killing via NKG2D and cytosolic phospholipase cPLA2, suggesting a destructive role for natural killer cells when activated by environmental stress signals during the initiation of PsA. Furthermore, as IL-15 could reproduce the phenotype of joint natural killer cells from blood natural killer cells, this study demonstrated that IL-15 is capable of priming resting natural killer cells in tissues to the effector phase. One additional possibility is that the clonally driven CD8$^+$ population contains an enriched population of IL-17$^+$CD8$^+$ T cells in PsA synovial fluid that is not found in RA synovial fluid, suggesting this population of T cells may be worthy of further study [12].

Psoriatic arthritis is an entheseal-based disease

Ever since the hypothesis published in 1998 [13] and through some elegant supporting anatomical and imaging studies [14], there has been growing support for the concept that the origin of inflammation in spondyloarthritis including PsA is at the enthesis. Enthesitis may be a prominent clinical feature at presentation in up to 38% of PsA patients [15]. Anatomical studies have shown that the enthesis is continuous with the joint structure [14] and that it also merges into the nail bed [16], allowing for the development of concepts that link entheseal involvement with prominent features of PsA, both synovitis and nail dystrophic change. Furthermore, magnetic resonance imaging (MRI) studies have highlighted bone marrow oedema at sites of entheseal attachment in PsA, leading to the hypothesis that it may be microtrauma at entheseal sites that in genetically susceptible individuals leads to inflammation, as evidenced by bone marrow oedema, which then spreads to secondarily involve structures such as the synovium or the nail. Immunohistologic studies that have demonstrated both $CD68^+$ macrophages [17] and $CD8^+$ T-cell infiltration [18] at sites of entheseal inflammation add further weight to these concepts.

Review: genetics of psoriatic arthritis

One of the striking features of PsA is that as many as 50% of PsA patients have a family history that includes one or sometimes multiple cases of PsA, PsO, or seronegative spondyloarthritis in their blood relatives, a likelihood 40-fold greater than that of their unaffected spouses [19-21]. Indeed, strong heritability has been demonstrated across four generations in an elegant study [22]. This, along with high twin concordance rates, establishes that germline genes importantly contribute to the definition of the predisposition to develop PsA. While the evidence that genetics plays a major role in who develops PsA has been present for many years, the identification of the genes responsible for conferring PsA has been a lengthy preoccupation for a number of investigators that was limited by the available technology, prevailing diagnostic criteria for PsA and the study size.

Background findings

Because the highly polymorphic MHC genes have an important role in regulating immune responsiveness and because PsA was considered an immune-mediated disease, MHC genes were the first candidates to be examined for a role in determining susceptibility to the development of PsA, and accordingly this review focuses on the contribution of HLA alleles. Association studies of PsA with MHC genes began with Brewerton's identification of a significantly increased frequency of *HLA-B*27* in individuals with PsA using serologic methods, where it was reported as strongly associated with axial disease [23]. Subsequently, the dominant HLA allele associated with susceptibility to PsO was identified as *HLA-C*06:02*, as it is now designated, although then it was termed *HLA-Cw6* and found to be present in approximately 60% of PsO cases. As anticipated from the presence of PsO in PsA, PsA was also associated with an elevated frequency of *HLA-C*06:02* as first reported in a study using serologic techniques by Murray and colleagues, where *C*06:02* was identified in 34.6% of PsA patients, 50% of PsO patients and 13.5% of controls [24]. In later studies, however, the proportion of serologically defined *HLA-C*06:02* varied from 60% to levels not significantly different from the frequency in healthy controls (15 to 20%). (For a more detailed summary of the divergent results among these earlier reports, see [25].) The earlier studies were notably limited by the imprecision of the earlier serologic method of determining HLA alleles, by comparing populations that varied in the frequencies of certain HLA alleles and, perhaps most importantly, by the classification criteria for PsA being incompletely delineated. The main alleles and haplotypes associated with PsO and PsA are summarised in Box 1.

New data concerning psoriatic arthritis genetics

Because of the importance of more precisely determining the role played by HLA alleles in PsA, using improved PsA case ascertainment based on the Classification Criteria for Psoriatic Arthritis (CASPAR) [1] and more accurate methods of allele determination, we set out to compare the similarities and differences in the frequency of HLA-B and HLA-C locus alleles between PsO and PsA. We were particularly interested in addressing the question of the genetic relationship between PsO and PsA and asking whether PsA is a genetically heterogeneous entity [4]. To achieve this, a PsO cohort of 214 patients was assembled from individuals presenting to a dermatologic clinic who were determined to be

Box 1. The most common human leukocyte antigen alleles and haplotypes implicated in psoriatic arthritis susceptibility and their location within the major histocompatibility complex

Alleles	Ancestral extended haplotypes
Increased susceptibility	
*HLA-C*06:02:01*	*B*37:01-C*06:02, B*57:01-C*06:02*
*HLA-B*27:05:02*	*B*27:05:02-C*01:02,B*27:05:02-C*02:02*
*HLA-B*08:01*	*B*08:01-C*07:01*
*HLA-B*38:01*	*B*38:01-C*12:03*
*HLA-B*39:01*	*B*39:01-C*12:03*
Increased susceptibility	
*HLA-B*44:02:01*	*B*44:02-C*05:02*
*HLA-B*44:03:02*	*B*44:03-C*16:01*

without features of arthritis, spondylitis or enthesitis through examination by a rheumatologist. This cohort was compared with a PsA cohort ($n = 359$) presenting to a rheumatology clinic, in effect comparing the dermatologist's perspective of the PsO phenotype with that of the rheumatologist, and asking whether the two perspectives were equivalent. All patients in both cohorts belonged to the relatively homogeneous Irish population and had Irish parents, which diminished the problem of ethnic differences between the cohorts.

The first point that emerged from the data analysis addressed the question of whether the distribution of the *HLA-C*06:02* alleles in the PsA cohort parallel that found in the PsO cohort (Table 2). As a highly significant difference in the frequency of *HLA-C*06:02* was found between PsA and PsO (57.5% vs. 28.7%), we rejected the hypothesis of genetic homogeneity of the PsO phenotype ($P = 9.94 \times 10^{-12}$), although *HLA-C*06:02* was moderately increased in frequency in PsA. Figure 1 shows the differences in distribution of *HLA-C*06:02:01* among the three cohorts of PsA, PsO and healthy controls.

Since the frequency of *HLA-C*06:02* was appreciably decreased in the PsA cohort compared with that in the PsO cohort, we then asked whether there are other HLA-B alleles that are significantly increased in the Irish PsA cohort. The data showed that *HLA-B*27:05:02* and *HLA-B*39:01:01* were susceptibility alleles for PsA, but are not high-risk alleles for PsO in the absence of arthritis, and *HLA-B*08:01* was associated with PsA susceptibility but appears protective for PsO, being significantly reduced in frequency in PsO (Table 3). This observation emphasised the role of *HLA-B* alleles in PsA susceptibility, a finding supported by the report from Okada and colleagues [26]. Taken together these findings demonstrate that PsA itself is much more genetically heterogeneous than PsO and provide further strong evidence for genetic heterogeneity of the general PsO phenotype. In parallel with our analysis, another group studied this question with similar methods and obtained almost identical results [3,4].

The number of different HLA alleles associated with PsA susceptibility, and their differing frequencies between PsA cases and those with isolated cutaneous-only PsO, are illustrated in Figure 2. These studies resolved several important points of divergence in the literature [25]. The genes associated with increased PsA susceptibility (*B*08:01*, *B*27:05*, *C*06:02*, *B*39:01* and *B*38:01* (not illustrated in the figure)) were almost exclusively present in seven classic ancestral haplotypes (for example, *B*08:01-C*07:01*, *B*27:05-C*02:02*, *B*27:05-C*01:02*, *B*37:01-C*06:02*, *B*57:01-C*06:02*, *B*39:01-C*12:03* and *B*38:01-C*12:03*). Apart from *C*06:02*, which is found on two ancestral haplotypes (*B*37:01-C*06:02* and *B*57:01-C*06:02*), none of the other HLA-B alleles were associated with *C*06:02*. Additionally, *B*44:02-C*05:01* and *B*44:03-C*16:01* were associated with significantly decreased susceptibility (not illustrated in the figure), which indicates a protective effect. Table 4 presents the contrasting molecular architecture and peptide binding properties between two HLA-B molecules associated with increased susceptibility and two that appear protective, being associated with significantly decreased susceptibility [4]. The two molecules encoded by *B*27:05:02* and *B*39:01:01* alleles have negatively charged glutamic acid in the B pocket that preferentially binds the second amino acid side chain (P2) of a peptide, as well as *B*08:01* and *B*38:01*, while the two molecules associated with decreased susceptibility have exactly the opposite charge properties. This interpretation was supported by the recent study from Okada and colleagues in a large cohort of PsA patients using imputed HLA typing of *HLA-B* alleles [26]. This suggests that the particular peptides bound by HLA molecules play an important role in influencing the development of the immune response underlying PsA. Intriguingly, the *B*39:06* allele, which differs by only a few amino acids from *B*39:01*, was not associated with PsA susceptibility, indicating a relatively precise molecular basis for susceptibility.

Different susceptibility genes imply different disease mechanisms, and possibly a different clinical course and therapeutic responses

While the genetic results have implications for who would develop PsA, they formed the basis for asking whether the different genotypes conferred different disease phenotypes. A precedent for an effect of susceptibility alleles on phenotype has been present since the initial study by Brewerton and colleagues where *HLA-B*27* was proposed as being linked to the presence of axial disease in PsA [23]. However, this association has been quite inconsistent in subsequent studies [27-31]. Analogously, *HLA-C*06:02* was reported to be associated with fewer involved or damaged joints [32].

Table 2 Distribution of the *HLA-C*06:02* and *HLA-B*57:01* alleles in psoriatic arthritis does not parallel that found in cutaneous psoriasis

HLA allele	PsA (%), $n = 359$	PsA versus control	PsO (%), $n = 214$	PsO versus control	Control (%), $n = 1,000$	PsA versus PsO
*B*57:01*	18.4	2.5 (1.6 to 3.8)	31.3	5.71 (3.9 to 8.3)	7.4	0.30 (0.17 to 0.53)
*C*06:02*	28.7	1.8 (1.3 to 2.5)	57.5	6.61 (4.18 to 9.1)	19.3	0.26 (0.16 to 0.42)

Data presented as percentage or odds ratio (95% confidence interval). HLA, human leukocyte antigen; PsA, psoriatic arthritis; PsO, cutaneous psoriasis.

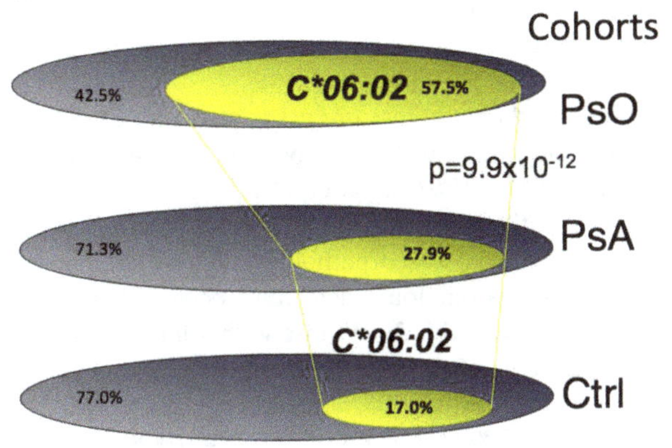

Figure 1 Distribution of *HLA-C*06:02:01* among psoriatic arthritis, psoriasis and healthy controls. Venn diagrams in each population illustrate the approximate proportion of individuals that bear the allele *HLA-C*06:02:01*. Ctrl, control; PsA, psoriatic arthritis; PsO, cutaneous psoriasis.

Genotype influences the duration between cutaneous and musculoskeletal involvement

The first clue in the present line of study that different clinical phenotypes may be determined by different genotypes was that the interval between the onset of PsO and the development of PsA was influenced by the patient's HLA type. The standard teaching is that PsA follows the onset of PsO by 10 to 15 years. We observed that arthritis develops much closer to the appearance of PsO in the HLA-*B*27:05:02* or *B*39:01:01* subset than in the *HLA-C*06:02* subset of PsA cases [4]. This indicated that susceptibility genes were involved in determining the time interval between PsO and PsA and that this time difference is a genetically determined quantitative trait. This suggested that the mechanism of genetic susceptibility in *B*27:05:02* individuals resulted in similar penetrance for musculoskeletal and skin disease, and that they were roughly contemporaneous in onset. Indeed nearly one-third of *B*27:05:02* patients had the onset of skin disease after the onset of musculoskeletal disease (that is, PsA *sine* PsO). Conversely for *HLA-C*06:02* patients, the interval between skin disease and musculoskeletal disease was the expected lag of over a decade and *HLA-C*06:02* appeared to specify an effect that included highly penetrant severe cutaneous disease and delayed milder musculoskeletal disease with greatly reduced penetrance.

Genetic influence on whether sacroiliitis is symmetrical or asymmetrical

In a follow up to the original genetic paper, 282 patients of the above described genetic study [4] who were available were extensively clinically and radiographically phenotyped, with the assessors completely blinded to the previously reported HLA typing results. We first explored univariate associations of HLA-B and HLA-C alleles and haplotypes with at least 10 occurrences in the cohort, previously associated with susceptibility with individual clinical characteristics using the asymmetric two-tailed Pearson chi-square method [2].

While ankylosing spondylitis is characterised by symmetrical sacroiliitis, in PsA sacroiliitis is more likely to be asymmetric [33]. Table 5 presents data on whether the finding of symmetric or asymmetric sacroiliitis by X-ray imaging is associated with an HLA genotype. The table shows that HLA-*B*27:05:02* and both of its haplotypes were strongly associated with symmetrical sacroiliitis. Symmetrical sacroiliitis and *B*27:05* was male preponderant (odds ratio = 11.91), resembling the findings in ankylosing spondylitis and supporting current endeavours to group the axial spondyloarthritis together. Both B*27 haplotypes (*B*27:05-C*01:02* and *B*27:05:02-C*02:02:01*) were equivalently associated with symmetric sacroiliitis (Table 6).

In contrast, asymmetric sacroiliitis, the more prevalent form of sacroiliitis in PsA, was not significantly associated with *B*27:05* but, rather, exhibited a strong association with the more prevalent *B*08:01-C*07:01* haplotype and its constituent alleles. As a rough estimate of the effect of these two haplotypes on the sacroiliitis phenotype, 24.4% of those bearing *B*27:05:02* developed symmetric sacroiliitis and 11.1% asymmetric sacroiliitis, while 2.9% of those with *B*08:01* developed symmetric sacroiliitis and 30.8% asymmetric sacroiliitis.

Human leukocyte antigen associations of enthesitis

Enthesitis is often a striking feature of PsA. McGonagle and colleagues, based on the finding of prominent bone marrow oedema at sites of ligamentous attachment on MRI scanning, proposed that PsA should be considered an entheseal-based disease with secondary involvement of synovial structures [13]. Subsequent studies confirmed the finding of marrow oedema changes but showed that it is non-PsA specific and is found in only a proportion of

Table 3 Additional HLA-B alleles that are significantly increased or decreased in the psoriatic arthritis cohort

HLA allele	PsA (%), *n* = 359	PsA versus control	PsO (%), *n* = 214	PsO versus control	Control (%), *n* = 1,000	PsA versus PsO
*B*27:05*	15.6	2.6 (1.7 to 4.2)	4.7	*P* = 0.23	5.5	3.77 (1.9 to 7.6)
*B*39:01*	6.4	3.5 (1.6 to 7.6)	1.4	*P* = 1	1.2	2.86 (1.1 to 7.6)
*B*08:01*	37.3	1.6 (1.2 to 2.0)	24.8	0.43 (0.25 to 0.76)	30.1	1.81 (1.6 to 6.5)
*B*44:02*	14.8	0.53 (0.36 to 0.80)	22.4	*P* = 0.7	24.6	0.60 (0.29 to 0.87)

Data presented as percentage or odds ratio (95% confidence interval). HLA, human leukocyte antigen; PsA, psoriatic arthritis; PsO, cutaneous psoriasis.

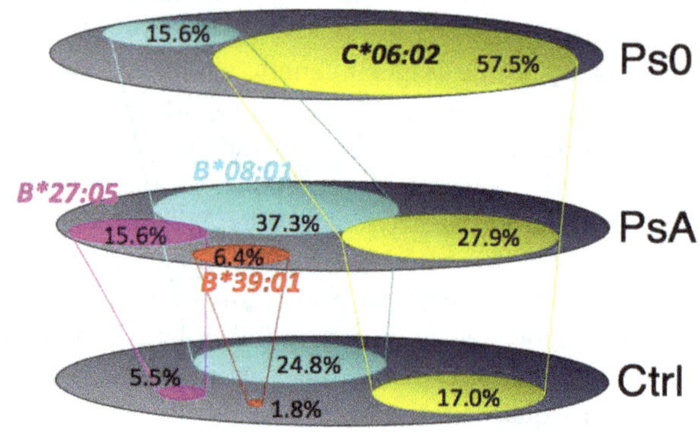

Figure 2 Certain HLA-B alleles in the psoriatic arthritis cohort are significantly increased in frequency compared with their frequency in cutaneous psoriasis and healthy controls. Venn diagrams in each population illustrate the approximate proportion of individuals that bear the alleles. Ctrl, control; PsA, psoriatic arthritis; PsO, psoriasis where there is no arthritis.

PsA patients [34]. We sought to investigate this aspect of PsA in greater depth using a genetic approach, and found that in univariate analysis the haplotype *B*27:05-C*01:02* and its two constituent alleles, *B*27:05* and *C*01:02*, were strongly associated with the development of clinically detectable enthesitis in PsA (Table 6). However, neither the associations with the *B*27:05:02-C*02:02:01* haplotype or its constituent alleles were similarly significant for the presence of enthesitis. This association suggests that a gene other than *HLA-B*27:05*, such as *C*01:02:01* that is present on the *B*27:05-C*01:02* haplotype, drives the association with enthesitis or that a combination of genes on that haplotype confers susceptibility to enthesitis. Furthermore, enthesitis was not significantly associated with the other major alleles implicated in PsA susceptibility. *B*08:01* was not associated with enthesitis while enthesitis was inversely associated with *C*06:02* (odds ratio = 0.45, $P = 0.045$), indicating that this susceptibility allele is protective for the presence of enthesitis. Accordingly, we conclude that the genetic factors contributing to enthesitis

Table 4 Amino acids in polymorphic sites of HLA-B molecules associated with increased or decreased psoriatic arthritis susceptibility and their contrasting effect on binding peptide P2 side chain anchor amino acids

HLA-B molecule	P2 pocket amino acid position		P2 amino acid binding preference	Allele risk estimate[a]
	45	67		
*B*27:05:02*	Glu	Cys	Arg	3.18 (2.14 to 4.71)
*B*39:01:01*	Glu	Cys	Arg	3.74 (1.99 to 7.01)
*B*44:02:01*	Lys	Ser	Glu	0.53 (0.38 to 0.74)
*B*44:03:01*	Lys	Ser	Glu	0.47 (0.24 to 0.92)

Arg, arginine; Cys, cysteine; Glu, glutamic acid; Lys, lysine; Ser, serine. [a]Data presented as odds ratio (95% confidence interval).

appear distinct from those operating in the development of other features of PsA.

Synovial-based phenotypes are associated with B*08:01

In contrast, we found in univariate analysis that the *B*08:01:01-C*07:01:01* haplotype and its alleles are not associated with enthesitis, but conversely were associated with more synovial-based pathology such as joint deformity and joint fusion. Joint deformity occurred in 46% of those with *B*08*, and 86% of those with joint deformity had *B*08* (odds ratio = 2.3, $P = 0.002$). Joint fusion was found in 48.8% of those with *B*08*, and 39% of those with joint deformity had *B*08* (odds ratio = 2.0, $P = 0.008$). There was no significant association of joint deformity or joint fusion with *B*27:05:02* or *C*06:02:01*.

Dactylitis exhibits a dual association with B*27:05 and B*08:01

Intriguingly, dactylitis was strongly associated with the presence of *B*27:05* and particularly the *B*27:05-C*01:02* haplotype (Table 7), but not the *B*27:05-C*02:02* haplotype, mirroring the haplotype association of enthesitis. However, alone among the phenotypic traits of severe PsA, dactylitis was also positively associated with the *B*08:01-C*07:01* haplotype, implying the possibility that a synovial-based process could also result in the phenotype of dactylitis, suggesting heterogeneity in the mechanism underlying this trait. This is fully compatible with the complexity of the process occurring in dactylitis [35-37], including varying contributions of flexor tenosynovitis, synovitis, enthesitis and more circumferential soft tissue oedema. It would be of interest to determine whether stratification of patients by either of these susceptibility alleles resulted in subgrouping patients with different types of digital processes (for example, tenosynovitis/synovitis vs. enthesitis).

Propensity to develop severe psoriatic arthritis

As an alternative approach to studying genotype–phenotype associations, we constructed a continuous variable severity score to order the cohort based on the presence of one or more of eight distinctive PsA phenotypic characteristics that we considered would denote a more severely involved patient, including enthesitis, symmetric or asymmetric sacroiliitis, dactylitis, joint deformity, joint erosion, joint fusion or osteolysis [2]. This score was used to group patients into three tertiles according to their rank in the severity score. As anticipated, the characteristics that formed the basis of the score, with the single exception of enthesitis, were significantly more prevalent in the group with a severity propensity score in the third tertile compared with those in the first tertile. We then determined the associations of HLA-B and HLA-C alleles and haplotypes with being in the top tertile of the PsA Severity

Table 5 Frequency of human leukocyte antigen allele or haplotype in forms of sacroiliitis

Marker	Sacroiliitis	Symmetrical sacroiliitis	Asymmetrical sacroiliitis
*B*08:01*	50.70%	16.70%	62.70%
P value	0.006	0.066	<0.000
OR (95% CI)	2.15 (1.06 to 1.77)	0.323 (0.91 to 1.143)	3.8 (1.9 to 7)
*B*27:05*	23.20%	61.10%	9.80%
P value	0.059	<0.000	0.185
OR (95% CI)	1.92 (0.97 to 3.79)	10.63 (3.86 to 29.3)	0.52 (0.19 to 1.39)
*C*01:02*	18.6%	36.80%	11.80%
P value	0.027	<0.000	0.9
OR (95% CI)	2.32 (1.08 to 5.00)	5.57 (2.02 to 15.5)	1.06 (0.41 to 2.76)
*C*02:02*	10%	26%	4%
P value	0.42	0.002	0.26
OR (95% CI)	1.47 (0.57 to 3.76)	5.19 (1.67 to 16.1)	0.43 (0.09 to 1.9)
*C*07:01*	48.60%	15.8%	60.80%
P value	0.119	0.022	0.001
OR (95% CI)	1.53 (0.89 to 2.62)	0.25 (0.07 to 0.89)	1.73 (1.47 to 5.1)
*B*08-C*07*	47%	16%	59%
P value	0.026	0.057	<0.000
OR (95% CI)	1.86 (1.07 to 3.23)	0.31 (0.089 to 1.1)	3.18 (1.7 to 5.92)
*B*27-C*01*	14.30%	31.60%	7.80%
P value	0.064	0.001	0.78
OR (95% CI)	2.2 (0.94 to 5.15)	5.9 (2.0 to 17)	0.85 (0.28 to 2.61)
*B*27-C*02*	8.6%	26.3%	2.00%
P value	0.474	<0.000	0.134
OR (95% CI)	1.44 (0.53 to 3.95)	6.4 (2.0 to 20)	2.4 (0.03 to 1.8)

CI, confidence interval; OR, odds ratio.

Table 6 Enthesitis is preferentially associated with the *B*27:05-C*01:02* haplotype

Marker	Enthesitis
*B*27:05*	28.10%
P value	<0.000
OR (95% CI)	3.65 (1.89 to 7.06)
*C*01:02*	21.60%
P value	<0.000
OR (95% CI)	4.39 (2.02 to 9.57)
*C*02:02*	10%
P value	0.25
OR (95% CI)	1.67 (0.69 to 4.01)
*B*27-C*01*	17.50%
P value	<0.000
OR (95% CI)	4.73 (1.96 to 11.41)
*B*27-C*02*	9.30%
P value	0.213
OR (95% CI)	1.80 (0.71 to 4.59)

CI, confidence interval; OR, odds ratio.

Propensity Score, developing an HLA risk score in which +1 was awarded to the haplotypes *B*27:05-C*02:02*, *B*37:01-C:06:02* and *B*08:01-C*07:01* while haplotypes including *B*44:02* or *C*07:02:01* were awarded −1 and *HLA_B*57:01-C*06:02* was awarded 0. Since the genotype of an individual contains two haplotypes, the risk score ranged from −2 to +2, allowing evaluation of the contribution of the alleles on both maternal and paternal chromosomes to disease phenotype. Each unit increase in this adjusted score, on average, was associated with a 168% higher odds of being in the most severe PsA tertile (odds ratio = 2.68, P <0.001). The additivity of the scores indicated that *B*27:05-C*02:02*, *B*37:01-C*06:02* and *B*08:01-C*07:01* were each equivalently associated together with a more severe phenotype, and this was counterpoised by the haplotypes associated with a zero or negative weight. Intriguingly, these findings appear to suggest that the presence of *B*37* on a haplotype containing *C*06:02* modifies the action of *C*06:02*, a point also raised by Okada and colleagues [26].

However, the haplotype *B*27:05-C*01:02*, which was associated with enthesitis in univariate analysis, was not

Table 7 Dactylitis is associated with both *HLA-B*27:05* and *B*08:01*, but not *HLA-C*06:02*

HLA allele or haplotype	Frequency (%) of HLA		Odds ratio (95% CI)	*P* value (two-sided)
	With trait	Without trait		
*B*27:05:02*	21.3	9.8	2.5 (1.2 to 5.0)	0.009
*B*27:05:02-C*01:02:01*	12.0	5.3	2.5 (1.0 to 6.1)	0.05
*B*27:05:02-C*02:02:02*	8.7	4.5	2.0 (0.7 to 5.4)	0.2
*B*08:01:01*	42.7	30.3	1.7 (1.1 to 2.8)	0.03
*B*08:01:01-C*07:01:01*	42.0	29.3	1.8 (1.1 to 2.9)	0.03
*C*06:02:01*	25.3	33.8	0.7 (0.4 to 1.1)	0.1
*B*44:02:01*	9.3	22.0	0.37 (0.2 to 0.7)	0.003
*B*44:02:01-C*05:01:01*	8.7	18.0	0.43 (0.2 to 0.89)	0.02
*B*44:03:01*	6.0	15.2	0.36 (0.2 to 0.8)	0.012
*B*44:03:01-C*16:01:01*	3.3	9.8	0.3 (0.1 to 0.9)	0.03

CI, confidence interval; HLA, human leukocyte antigen.

associated with an elevated severity propensity score. This indicates an unlinking of enthesitis with other elements that were studied in the PsA phenotype. Taken together, these findings suggest that there are distinct genetic factors contributing to enthesitis and these are different from those operating in the development of most other features associated with PsA.

Conclusions

Implications of newer findings on concepts of genotype–phenotype relationships

There are several implications for the finding that certain HLA alleles and, most strikingly, particular haplotypes that are implicated in the susceptibility to develop PsA contribute differentially and often additively to the magnitude of different traits comprising the phenotype of PsA [2]. Despite the relatively large size of this cohort, with 282 PsA cases clinically phenotyped and sequence-based HLA typed to at least four digits, the study must be considered exploratory and requires validation in different ethnic groups, especially those with a greater admixture of populations having different principal ancestral haplotypes. In this way, the association of a particular allele within the context of a given haplotype can be better determined. One anticipates that there will be different genotype–phenotype associations in a population that does not include the major Northern European haplotypes such as *B*08:01-C*07:01*, or those involving *B*27*. The disparate phenotypic associations of different alleles/haplotypes emphasise the distinct contribution of each different susceptibility allele; however, the overarching common features of all PsA patients may depend on the common molecular architecture of susceptibility molecules (Table 5), supported by the recent report of Okada and colleagues [26]. Apart from the general mechanistic interpretation of these genotype–phenotype associations that different HLA alleles bind different self-peptides and drive differing autoimmune responses directed to distinct target molecules, at this stage of knowledge it is not possible to speculate on the precise molecular mechanisms that may be operating to result in a different clinical phenotype. It is possible that some inflammatory pathways will be more analogous to those in PsO, while others may resemble those of ankylosing spondylitis.

It is interesting to note that the newer genetic findings are consistent with and appear to provide a molecular explanation for the long-held clinical observations of Moll and Wright [38], identifying entheseal predominant, synovial predominant and axial predominant as three of the major forms of PsA, with each now found to have differing HLA associations. The findings summarised in this review are also relevant to the discussion of pathogenic mechanisms in PsA.

First, since different HLA molecules bind different peptides, they probably imply the presence of distinct autoimmune responses that are driving each of the phenotypes separately associated with different HLA alleles. As a corollary, the different peptides suggest that different proteins, perhaps with a different cellular distribution, are targets of these responses. Indeed, the finding that several different HLA alleles confer susceptibility to PsA is an argument in favour of an autoimmune hypothesis, since it directs attention to the different peptide binding properties of the molecules encoded by the susceptibility alleles.

Secondly, one anticipates that these responses may be further distinguished by different predominant mechanisms that use one or another cytokine, and so forth, perhaps indicating that different drugs and biologics may be effective in different genetic subsets. These data also raise the possibility that there is a predominant type of target tissue involved in each separate process. For example, it may prove to be the case that whether you have *HLA-B*27:05* or *HLA-B*08:01* will determine whether you have symmetrical or asymmetrical sacroiliitis or whether you have a disease that is more axial or entheseal predominant, or perhaps more synovial predominant. The question of how these genotypes might result in a particular clinical phenotype is unclear, but the work of Sherlock and colleagues would suggest that in a mouse model the development of enthesitis may be linked to the presence of a particular subset of T cells (IL-23R$^+$, CD3$^+$CD4$^-$CD8$^-$). IL-23 elaborated at the enthesis through an effect of *HLA-B*27* on a haplotype encoding *C*01:02* acts on this entheseal cell population to elaborate inflammatory mediators including IL-6, IL-17 and IL-22 [39]. Furthermore, their data suggest that the presence of these entheseal resident cells and their production of IL-22, which activates signal transducer and activator of transcription 3-dependent osteoblast-mediated bone remodelling, explains why dysregulation of IL-23 results in inflammation at this precise anatomical site. This dysregulation of IL-23 is possibly determined at a genetic level as a result of the response of HLA-B*27 to microtrauma. Whether a similar model applies to human disease, or even a proportion thereof where there is prominent entheseal involvement (<30% of PsA cases), has yet to be demonstrated.

However, the present findings argue against the enthesitis hypothesis as a fundamental explanation for PsA in all cases. The data summarised in Table 7, showing that enthesitis is preferentially associated with the *B*27:05-C*01:02* haplotype, are not consistent with enthesitis being common to all PsA cases. Furthermore, in the development of the propensity score (Figure 3) the presence of enthesitis was not significantly associated with the other traits comprising the score measuring the propensity for severe PsA [2]. Furthermore, prominent entheseal involvement on MRI is seen in only a minority of patients. Indeed, one study found that MRI was not able to differentiate at the group level between early PsA and RA on the basis of entheseal-related disease [34]; however, a subgroup of PsA patients had diffuse extracapsular enhancement (30%) or diffuse bone oedema (20%). In addition and of interest [40], HLA-B27 positivity in PsA and in axial spondyloarthritis defined a group of patients with more severe axial bone marrow oedema on MRI that is probably related to the classic ankylosing spondylitis phenotype, while HLA-B27-negative PsA was likely to be reported as a negative MRI examination result.

For the two-thirds of PsA patients that appear to have a more synovial-predominant pattern of disease and who are likely to be *HLA-B*08:01*, a more conventional autoimmune basis of disease may apply. It is certainly possible in these subjects that molecules encoded by HLA class 1 alleles are recognising self-peptides derived from proteins found in synovial sites. CD8$^+$ T-cell clones specific for these self-peptides would be inappropriately activated, perhaps by dendritic cells, and the activated state perpetuated by the continual supply of self-peptides.

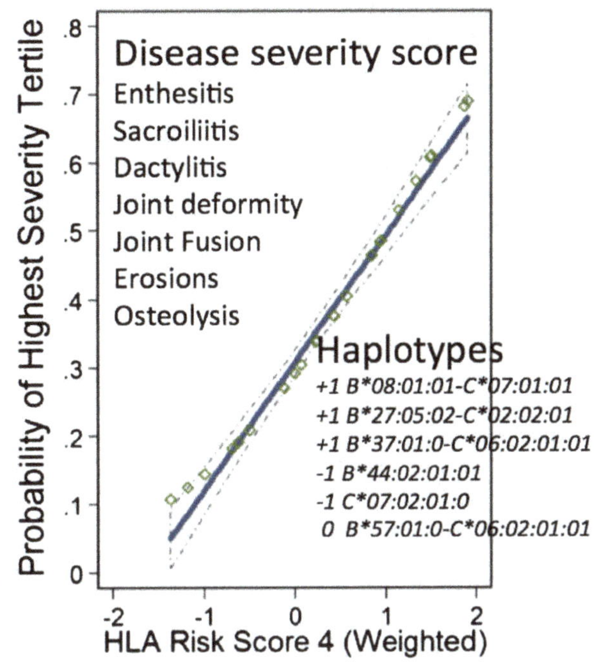

Figure 3 Contribution of positive and negative risk alleles on both chromosomes to psoriatic arthritis severity. An additive model including all genotypes positively or negatively associated with the propensity to develop severe psoriatic arthritis resulting in a composite human leukocyte antigen (HLA) risk score.

These interactions may result in the elaboration of cytokines such as interferon gamma or tumour necrosis factor alpha, which in turn drive the inflammatory cascade.

Such an explanation of disease pathogenesis goes some way to explain the consistent occurrence of dichotomous therapeutic responses whereby skin and articular structures, for example, respond with different magnitude or even direction to a given therapeutic agent (for example, cyclosporine, ustekinumab, IL-17 inhibition). Using the primary outcome measure of the American College of Rheumatology 20% (ACR20) improvement in clinical response, there is also a consistent degree of nonresponse to any therapeutic agent (30 to 50%) – suggesting that patients with certain clinical features will respond whereas other patients with other features will not. These observations are consistent with the hypothesis that discreet inflammatory pathways may operate across different tissue compartments.

Finally, we would propose a testable hypothesis whereby PsA can be considered to have at least four clinical phenotypes – synovitis predominant, entheseal predominant, axial predominant and mutilans – all determined by genotype. In each of these phenotypes and perhaps as a consequence of the inflammatory events that occur following the recognition of specific peptides presented by molecules encoded by susceptibility allotypes and recognised by specific T-cell clonotypes, a different pattern of inflammation involving diverse immunoreactant molecules and mediators such as cytokines may be unleashed that help to determine clinical disease expression. As mentioned, this is a testable hypothesis with RNA genome sequencing and protein and cytokine profiling of very well-characterised clinical phenotypic/genotypic groupings likely to reveal consistent differences between the genotypic groupings.

Abbreviations

HLA: human leukocyte antigen; IL: interleukin; MHC: major histocompatibility complex; MRI: magnetic resonance imaging; PsA: psoriatic arthritis; PsO: cutaneous psoriasis; RA: rheumatoid arthritis.

Competing interests

MH received an unrestricted educational grant from Abbvie. OF has received honoraria and grant support from and has been a member of advisory boards for Pfizer, Abbvie, MSD, Roche, UCB, Janssen and Cellgene. The remaining authors declare that they have no competing interests.

Author details

[1]Department of Rheumatology, St Vincent's University Hospital, Elm Park, Dublin 4, Ireland. [2]Rheumatology Division, Department of Medicine, Columbia University College of Physicians and Surgeons, 630 West 168th Street, New York City, NY 10032, USA.

References

1. Taylor W, Gladman D, Helliwell P, Marchesoni A, Mease P, Mielants H. Classification criteria for psoriatic arthritis: development of new criteria from a large international study. Arthritis Rheum. 2006;54:2665–73.
2. Haroon M, Winchester R, Giles JT, Heffernan E, FitzGerald O. Certain class I HLA alleles and haplotypes implicated in susceptibility play a role in determining specific features of the psoriatic arthritis phenotype. Annals Rheum Dis. 2014. Epub ahead of print (doi:10.1136/annrheumdis-2014-205461).
3. Eder L, Chandran V, Pellet F, Shanmugarajah S, Rosen CF, Bull SB, et al. Human leucocyte antigen risk alleles for psoriatic arthritis among patients with psoriasis. Annals Rheum Dis. 2012;71:50–5.
4. Winchester R, Minevich G, Steshenko V, Kirby B, Kane D, Greenberg DA, et al. HLA associations reveal genetic heterogeneity in psoriatic arthritis and in the psoriasis phenotype. Arthritis Rheum. 2012;64:1134–44.
5. Fitzgerald O, Winchester R. Psoriatic arthritis: from pathogenesis to therapy. Arthritis Res Ther. 2009;11:214.
6. Costello P, Bresnihan B, O'Farrelly C, FitzGerald O. Predominance of CD8+ T lymphocytes in psoriatic arthritis. J Rheumatol. 1999;26:1117–24.
7. Costello PJ, Winchester RJ, Curran SA, Peterson KS, Kane DJ, Bresnihan B, et al. Psoriatic arthritis joint fluids are characterized by CD8 and CD4 T cell clonal expansions appear antigen driven. J Immunol. 2001;166:2878–86.
8. Curran SA, FitzGerald OM, Costello PJ, Selby JM, Kane DJ, Bresnihan B, et al. Nucleotide sequencing of psoriatic arthritis tissue before and during methotrexate administration reveals a complex inflammatory T cell infiltrate with very few clones exhibiting features that suggest they drive the inflammatory process by recognizing autoantigens. J Immunol. 2004;172:1935–44.
9. Snowden JA, Kearney P, Kearney A, Cooley HM, Grigg A, Jacobs P, et al. Long-term outcome of autoimmune disease following allogeneic bone marrow transplantation. Arthritis Rheum. 1998;41:453–9.
10. Groh V, Bruhl A, El-Gabalawy H, Nelson JL, Spies T. Stimulation of T cell autoreactivity by anomalous expression of NKG2D and its MIC ligands in rheumatoid arthritis. Proc Natl Acad Sci U S A. 2003;100:9452–7.
11. Tang F, Sally B, Ciszewski C, Abadie V, Curran SA, Groh V, et al. Interleukin 15 primes natural killer cells to kill via NKG2D and cPLA2 and this pathway is active in psoriatic arthritis. PLoS One. 2013;8, e76292.
12. Menon B, Gullick NJ, Walter GJ, Rajasekhar M, Garrood T, Evans HG, et al. IL-17+CD8+ T-cells are enriched in the joints of patients with psoriatic arthritis and correlate with disease activity and joint damage progression. Arthritis Rheumatol. 2014;66:1272–81.
13. McGonagle D, Gibbon W, Emery P. Classification of inflammatory arthritis by enthesitis. Lancet. 1998;352:1137–40.
14. Benjamin M, McGonagle D. The anatomical basis for disease localisation in seronegative spondyloarthropathy at entheses and related sites. J Anat. 2001;199(Pt 5):503–26.
15. Kane D, Stafford L, Bresnihan B, FitzGerald O. A prospective, clinical and radiological study of early psoriatic arthritis: an early synovitis clinic experience. Rheumatology (Oxford). 2003;42:1460–8.
16. Tan AL, Benjamin M, Toumi H, Grainger AJ, Tanner SF, Emery P, et al. The relationship between the extensor tendon enthesis and the nail in distal interphalangeal joint disease in psoriatic arthritis – a high-resolution MRI and histological study. Rheumatology (Oxford). 2007;46:253–6.
17. McGonagle D, Marzo-Ortega H, O'Connor P, Gibbon W, Hawkey P, Henshaw K, et al. Histological assessment of the early enthesitis lesion in spondyloarthropathy. Ann Rheum Dis. 2002;61:534–7.
18. Laloux L, Voisin MC, Allain J, Martin N, Kerboull L, Chevalier X, et al. Immunohistological study of entheses in spondyloarthropathies: comparison in rheumatoid arthritis and osteoarthritis. Ann Rheum Dis. 2001;60:316–21.
19. Wright V. Psoriasis and arthritis. Ann Rheum Dis. 1956;15:348.
20. Moll JMH, Wright V. Familial occurrence of psoriatic arthritis. Ann Rheum Dis. 1973;32:181–201.
21. Kammer GM, Soter NA, Gibson DJ, Schur PH. Psoriatic arthritis: a clinical, immunologic and HLA study of 100 patients. Semin Arthritis Rheum. 1979;9:75.
22. Karason A, Love TJ, Gudbjornsson B. A strong heritability of psoriatic arthritis over four generations – the Reykjavik Psoriatic Arthritis Study. Rheumatology (Oxford). 2009;48:1424–8.
23. Brewerton DA, Caffrey M, Nicholls A, Walters D, James DC. HL-A 27 and arthropathies associated with ulcerative colitis and psoriasis. Lancet. 1974;1:956–8.
24. Murray C, Mann DL, Gerber LN, Barth W, Perlmann S, Decker JL, et al. Histocompatibility alloantigens in psoriasis and psoriatic arthritis. Evidence for the influence of multiple genes in the major histocompatibility complex. J Clin Invest. 1980;66:670–5.
25. Winchester R. Genetics of psoriasis and psoriatic arthritis. In: Ritchlin CT, FitzGerald O, editors. Psoriatic and reactive arthritis – a companion to rheumatology. Amsterdam: Elsevier; 2007. p. 65–80.
26. Okada Y, Han B, Tsoi LC, Stuart PE, Ellinghaus E, Tejasvi T, et al. Fine mapping major histocompatibility complex associations in psoriasis and its clinical subtypes. Am J Hum Genet. 2014;95:162–72.
27. Queiro R, Sarasqueta C, Belzunegui J, Gonzalez C, Figueroa M, Torre-Alonso JC. Psoriatic spondyloarthropathy: a comparative study between HLA-B27 positive and HLA-B27 negative disease. Semin Arthritis Rheum. 2002;31:413–8.
28. Gladman D, Anhorn K, Schachter R, Mervart H. HLA antigens in psoriatic arthritis. J Rheumatol. 1986;13:586.
29. Gladman DD, Farwell VT. The role of HLA antigens as indicators of disease progression in psoriatic arthritis. Multivariate relative risk model. Arthritis Rheum. 1995;38:845–50.
30. Queiro-Silva R, Torre-Alonso JC, Tinture-Eguren T, Lopez-Lagunas I. The effect of HLA-DR antigens on the susceptibility to, and clinical expression of psoriatic arthritis. Scand J Rheumatol. 2004;33:318–22.
31. Grubic Z, Peric P, Eeeuk-Jelicic E, Zunec R, Stingl K, Curkovic B, et al. The MICA-A4 triplet repeats polymorphism in the transmembrane region confers additional risk for development of psoriatic arthritis in the Croatian population. Eur J Immunogenet. 2004;31:93–8.
32. Ho PY, Barton A, Worthington J, Thomson W, Silman AJ, Bruce IN. HLA-Cw6 and HLA-DRB1*07 together are associated with less severe joint disease in psoriatic arthritis. Ann Rheum Dis. 2007;66:807–11.
33. McEwen C, DiTata D, Lingg C, Porini A, Good A, Rankin T. Ankylosing spondylitis and spondylitis accompanying ulcerative colitis, regional enteritis, psoriasis and Reiter's disease. A comparative study. Arthritis Rheum. 1971;14:291–318.
34. Marzo-Ortega H, Tanner SF, Rhodes LA, Tan AL, Conaghan PG, Hensor EM, et al. Magnetic resonance imaging in the assessment of metacarpophalangeal joint disease in early psoriatic and rheumatoid arthritis. Scand J Rheumatol. 2009;38:79–83.
35. Bakewell CJ, Olivieri I, Aydin SZ, Dejaco C, Ikeda K, Gutierrez M, et al. Ultrasound and magnetic resonance imaging in the evaluation of psoriatic dactylitis: status and perspectives. J Rheumatol. 2013;40:1951–7.

36. Healy PJ, Groves C, Chandramohan M, Helliwell PS. MRI changes in psoriatic dactylitis – extent of pathology, relationship to tenderness and correlation with clinical indices. Rheumatology (Oxford). 2008;47:92–5.
37. Olivieri I, D'Angelo S, Scarano E, Padula A. What is the primary lesion in SpA dactylitis? Rheumatology (Oxford). 2008;47:561–2.
38. Moll JM, Wright V. Psoriatic arthritis. Semin Arthritis Rheum. 1973;3:55–78.
39. Sherlock JP, Joyce-Shaikh B, Turner SP, Chao CC, Sathe M, Grein J, et al. IL-23 induces spondyloarthropathy by acting on ROR-gammat+CD3+CD4–CD8– entheseal resident T cells. Nat Med. 2012;18:1069–76.
40. Castillo-Gallego C, Aydin SZ, Emery P, McGonagle DG, Marzo-Ortega H. Magnetic resonance imaging assessment of axial psoriatic arthritis: extent of disease relates to HLA-B27. Arthritis Rheum. 2013;65:2274–8.

Ultrasound composite scores for the assessment of inflammatory and structural pathologies in Psoriatic Arthritis (PsASon-Score)

Anja Ficjan[1†], Rusmir Husic[1†], Judith Gretler[1], Angelika Lackner[1], Winfried B Graninger[1], Marwin Gutierrez[2], Christina Duftner[3], Josef Hermann[1] and Christian Dejaco[1*]

Abstract

Introduction: This study was performed to develop ultrasound composite scores for the assessment of inflammatory and structural lesions in Psoriatic Arthritis (PsA).

Methods: We performed a prospective study on 83 PsA patients undergoing two study visits scheduled 6 months apart. B-mode and Power Doppler (PD) findings were semi-quantitatively scored at 68 joints (evaluating synovia, perisynovial tissue, tendons and bone) and 14 entheses. We constructed bilateral and unilateral (focusing the dominant site) ultrasound composite scores selecting relevant sites by a hierarchical approach. We tested convergent construct validity, reliability and feasibility of inflammatory and structural elements of the scores as well as sensitivity to change for inflammatory items.

Results: The bilateral score (termed PsASon22) included 22 joints (6 metacarpophalangeal joints (MCPs), 4 proximal interphalangeal joints (PIPs) of hands (H-PIPs), 2 metatarsophalangeal joints (MTPs), 4 distal interphalangeal joints (DIPs) of hands (H-DIPs), 2 DIPs of feet (F-DIPs), 4 large joints) and 4 entheses (bilateral assessment of lateral epicondyle and distal patellar tendon). The unilateral score (PsASon13) compromised 13 joints (2 MCPs, 3 H-PIPs, 1 PIP of feet (F-PIP), 2 MTPs, 1 H-DIP and 2 F-DIPs and 2 large joints) and 2 entheses (unilateral lateral epicondyle and distal patellar tendon). Both composite scores revealed a moderate to high sensitivity (bilateral composite score 43% to 100%, unilateral 36% to 100%) to detect inflammatory and structural lesions compared to the 68-joint/14-entheses score. The inflammatory and structural components of the composite scores correlated weakly with clinical markers of disease activity ($corr_{coeffs}$ 0 to 0.40) and the health assessment questionnaire (HAQ, $corr_{coeffs}$ 0 to 0.39), respectively. Patients with active disease achieving remission at follow-up yielded greater reductions of ultrasound inflammatory scores than those with stable clinical activity (Cohen's d effect size ranging from 0 to 0.79). Inter-rater reliability of bi- and unilateral composite scores was moderate to good with ICCs ranging from 0.42 to 0.96 and from 0.36 to 0.71, respectively for inflammatory and structural sub-scores. The PsASon22 and PsASon13 required 16 to 26 and 9 to 13 minutes, respectively to be completed.

Conclusion: Both new PsA ultrasound composite scores (PsASon22 and PsASon13) revealed sufficient convergent construct validity, sensitivity to change, reliability and feasibility.

* Correspondence: christian.dejaco@gmx.net
†Equal contributors
[1]Department of Rheumatology and Immunology, Medical University Graz, Auenbruggerplatz 15, 8036 Graz, Austria
Full list of author information is available at the end of the article

Introduction

Current EULAR recommendations on the use of imaging techniques in rheumatoid arthritis (RA) recognize the high sensitivity of sonography to detect joint pathologies, suggesting the use of this technique for a more accurate assessment of patients' disease activity as compared to clinical examination alone [1]. In routine practice and clinical trials of psoriatic arthritis (PsA), disease activity is still monitored by RA-specific clinical composite scores [2]. These measures, however, are of questionable value for PsA because of the heterogeneous nature of the disease characterized by various articular and extra-articular manifestations [3].

We recently reported good performance of sonography for the assessment of disease activity in PsA as determined by the investigation of 68 synovial sites and periarticular structures, as well as 14 entheses [4]. A comprehensive ultrasound assessment as performed in this study, however, is not feasible in daily routine practice, whereas a reduced ultrasound composite score might enable sonographic scoring of PsA patients in interventional trials and clinical practice.

A single ultrasound composite score has been developed for the assessment of PsA patients so far: the Italian so-called five-targets score focuses on joints, tendons, entheses, skin and nails; however, as only one site is assessed for each item, this index is of limited value to determine overall disease activity [5]. The German U7 score, primarily developed for RA, has occasionally been used to monitor disease activity in PsA patients in interventional studies; however, this score does not include important PsA manifestations such as enthesitis or distal interphalangeal joint (DIP) arthritis [6,7].

The aim of this study was to develop ultrasound composite scores that (1) include all currently defined ultrasound pathologies of PsA, (2) are sensitive for detection of inflammation and structural damage as compared to the assessment of 68 joints and 14 entheses and (3) are feasible in clinical practice. We tested the construct validity, reliability and feasibility of inflammatory and structural elements of the new composite scores and investigated the sensitivity to change for the inflammatory items.

Materials and methods

Patients

We performed a prospective study on 83 consecutive PsA patients between July 2011 and May 2013. All patients fulfilled the classification for psoriatic arthritis (CASPAR) criteria and had peripheral articular manifestations [8]. The institutional review board of the Medical University Graz approved the study and written informed consent was obtained from each patient.

Two study visits were scheduled 6 months apart. At each visit, complete history and clinical assessments were performed by one of three rheumatologists (AF, JG and JH) unaware of the ultrasound results [4]. The following parameters were recorded: number of tender joints (TJ) and swollen joints (SJ) according to the 66/68 articular index, presence of enthesitis according to the Leeds enthesitis index (LEI) and a clinical counterpart of the Madrid sonographic enthesis index (MASEI) plus lateral epicondyle (cMASEI + E) [9,10]. Patients' global assessment of disease activity (PGA), patients' pain assessment (Ptpain) and the evaluator's global assessment of disease activity (EGA) were determined on visual analogue scales (range 0 to 100 mm). We also recorded patients' questionnaires as previously described [4]. Blood samples were routinely tested for erythrocyte sedimentation rate (ESR, range 0 to 10 mm/first hour) and C-reactive protein (CRP) (range 0 to 5 mg/L).

We calculated the following clinical composite scores: the disease activity index for psoriatic arthritis (DAPSA), the composite psoriatic disease activity index (CPDAI) and a modified psoriatic arthritis disease activity score (PASDAS) omitting the short form health survey 36 (SF-36) component, which was not available in our patients [11-13]. In addition, we applied the minimal disease activity (MDA) criteria (5 of the 7 following items: TJ ≤1, SJ ≤1, Psoriasis activity and severity index (PASI) ≤1, Ptpain ≤15 mm, PGA ≤20 mm, health assessment questionnaire (HAQ) ≤0.5, tender enthesal points ≤1]) [14] and asked the evaluating rheumatologist for an overall judgment of patients' clinical disease activity without using formal criteria or scores (two possible levels: active disease or remission).

Ultrasound protocol

Sonographic evaluations were performed by one of two rheumatologists (CDe, RH) at the same day of clinical investigation as previously described in detail [4]. Briefly, grey scale (GS) and power Doppler (PD) sonography were performed at 68 joints and 14 entheses using a MyLab Twice ultrasound device (Esaote, Genova, Italy) with two multifrequence linear transducers (6 to 18 MHz and 4 to 13 MHz). GS synovitis (GSS) and PD-signals at joints (PD-j) were subjectively graded from 0 to 3 [15-17]. Perisynovitis was investigated by dorsal scans of metacarpophalangeal joints (MCP) 2 to 5 and was graded in GS (GS-perisyn) and PD (PD-perisyn) with 0 = absent or 1 = present [18]. Tenosynovitis was identified in GS (GS-teno) and graded from 0 to 3 (wrists, ankles) or with 0 = absent or 1 = present at small joints. PD-signals related to tenosynovitis (PD-teno) were graded from 0 to 3. Erosions or osteophytes were also semiquantitatively graded from 0-3 [4].

Enthesitis was assessed according to the MASEI investigating the presence and/or extent of erosions, enthesophytes, PD-signals (PD-e) and GS-changes [9].

We considered GS-changes of enthesitis (GSE) as a combined feature including the loss of fibrillar pattern, hypoechoic aspect, bursitis (infrapatellar and/or retrocalcaneal bursa) and/or enthesal thickening. The following anatomical sites were scanned: the insertion of the common extensor tendon at the lateral epicondyle, the distal insertion of the triceps into the olecranon, the quadriceps insertion into the upper pole of the patella, the patellar tendon insertion into the lower pole of the patella and into the tibial anterior tuberosity, the insertion of the Achilles tendon as well as the insertion of plantar aponeurosis into the calcaneal bone [4]. GSS/GSE refers to GSS and GSE and PD-j/e combines PD-j and PD-e scores.

Construction of the ultrasound composite scores

Our aim was to develop ultrasound composite scores (1) that corroborate all currently defined ultrasound pathologies in PsA including GSS, GSE, PD-j, PD-e, GS-perisyn, PD-perisyn, GS-teno, PD-teno, erosions and ostheophytes/enthesophytes at small, middle/large and DIP joints as well as entheses (as appropriate); (2) that have a high sensitivity to detect these PsA characteristic ultrasound features as compared to the comprehensive assessment of 68 joints and 14 entheses; and (3) whose completion is feasible in clinical practice.

We used the 68-joints/14-entheses ultrasound score as a reference for the development of the new composite scores acknowledging that this instrument has not been validated for monitoring PsA patients yet. We constructed a bilateral and a unilateral composite score (focusing on the dominant site) using the Spanish 12-joint and the German 7-joint scores, respectively, as examples [6,19]. For the inclusion of relevant joints and entheses, we applied a hierarchical approach as exemplarily depicted in Additional file 1 and described in the following paragraph.

We conducted separate cycles of the procedure for each of the following anatomical regions and ultrasound pathologies: (1) small joints (defined as MCPs, metatarsophalangeal joints (MTP) as well as proximal interphalangeal joints (PIP) of hands (H-PIP) and feet (F-PIP)): GSS, PD-j, GS-perisyn (MCPs only), PD-perisyn (MCPs only), GS-teno, PD-teno, erosions and osteophytes; (2) DIP joints of the hand (H-DIP) and feet (F-DIP): GSS, PD-j, GS-teno, PD-teno, erosions and osteophytes; (3) large joints (defined as wrists, elbows, shoulders, hips, knees and ankles): GSS, PD-j, GS-teno (wrists and ankles only) and PD-teno (wrists and ankles only); and (4) entheses: GSE, PD-e, erosions and enthesophytes.

Each cycle started with the identification of the joint/enthesis most commonly revealing the ultrasound lesion of interest (for example, the joint that most frequently showed PD-positivity among small joints - MTP1). For the subsequent procedure, we excluded patients with a positive result at this step (in the example: patients with PD signals at MTP1). Among remaining cases, we identified the most frequently affected joint/enthesis again (in the example: cases with a positive PD result at MCP2). The rationale for excluding patients (and not simply searching for the second most commonly affected site among all cases) was to eliminate strong correlations between joint/enthesis, thus, maximizing the gain of sensitivity by any new site. We repeated this procedure n-times until a combination of sites reached ≥90% sensitivity to detect the corresponding ultrasound abnormality as compared to the 68-joint/14-entheses score. In case the gain of sensitivity by the inclusion of a new item was <20% or <10% for the bilateral or unilateral composite scores, respectively, or the overall prevalence of the finding at a given site was <5%, the selection process was terminated earlier. The rationale for premature termination was the prevention of mechanistic inclusion of sites with a negligible contribution to the overall performance of the composite scores potentially limiting the feasibility of the scores.

Next, we tested whether dorsal or palmar/plantar scans at H-PIPs, H-DIPs, MTPs, F-PIPs, F-DIPs and wrists, as well as medial/lateral or suprapatellar scans at knees, were dispensable for the composite scores. For this purpose, we analysed the proportion of ultrasound abnormalities exclusively detected by dorsal or palmar/plantar scans as well as by medial/lateral or suprapatellar scans of knees. Scans with a yield of <20% were omitted. MCPs were not subject to this analysis, because both palmar and dorsal scans are required to investigate the composite core elements peri- and tenosynovitis, respectively.

Statistical analysis and validation of the ultrasound composite scores

Statistical analysis was performed using SPSS (version 20.0). Descriptive statistics were used to summarize the data. For continuous non-parametric data, we show the median and range whereas for parametric data, the mean and standard deviation are depicted. Comparisons between independent groups were conducted using the Mann-Whitney *U*-test and paired data were analysed with the Wilcoxon test (non-parametric data) or Student's *t*-test (parametric data). Paired categorical data were analysed with the McNemar test.

For validation, we tested inflammatory (that is, GSS/GSE, PD-j/e, GS-Peri, PD-Peri, GS-Teno, PD-Teno) and structural elements (erosions, osteophytes/enthesophytes) of the new ultrasound scores separately. In addition, we constructed a global ultrasound inflammation subscore (GUIS) adding the results of GSS/GSE, PD-j/e, GS-perisyn, PD-perisyn, B-teno and PD-teno.

Convergent construct validity was investigated by the correlation (using Spearman's rank correlation test) of inflammatory items (including GUIS) with clinical parameters of disease activity, and by correlating structural components with the HAQ (analysing the total cohort as well as patients in clinical remission separately in order to adjust for the activity related component of disability [20]).

Sensitivity to change was determined for the inflammatory components (including GUIS) only, as for structural elements the 6-months follow-up period was considered to be too short for the detection of any alterations. We compared the changes of the inflammatory subscore from baseline to the 6-months follow-up visit between patients with stable clinical disease activity (that is, active or inactive disease at both visits) and those being active at baseline and achieving remission (as determined by the evaluating physician) or MDA at follow up. We also calculated Cohen's *d* effect-size statistic and the standardized response means (SRMs) of the total cohort versus patients in whom clinical disease activity improved [21]. Changes of the inflammatory elements were additionally correlated with alterations of clinical composite scores and its components. Inter-rater reliability of the ultrasound composite scores was determined by serial assessments of 10% of patients by two investigators (CDe, RH) and using the intraclass correlation coefficient (ICC).

Results

Clinical findings at baseline and follow-up visits

Patients' characteristics are summarized in Table 1. At baseline, 40 patients (48.2%) were in remission as judged by the evaluating physician and 28 patients (33.7%) fulfilled the MDA criteria. Of the 83 patients 13 (15.7%) did not complete 6-month follow up. At follow up, 41 patients (58.6%) had stable disease activity according to physician's evaluation (25 (35.7%) were inactive and 16 (22.9%) were active at both time points), 21 (30.0%) changed from active disease to remission and 3 (4.3%) from remission to active disease. Applying the MDA criteria, 15 of those (27.3%) being active at baseline reached MDA at follow up, 7 (25.0%) with MDA at baseline did not fulfill these criteria at the second visit, and 48 patients (68.6%) had stable disease (that is, were active (n =32) or had MDA (n =16) at both visits).

Synovial recesses and entheses selected for the ultrasound composite scores

Additional file 2 details the results of selection process for the ultrasound composite scores. We made a few manual selections to improve the feasibility of the scores: (1) we included the second H-PIP instead of the first H-PIP for the PsASon22 because H-PIP2 better fitted into the construct of MCP2, MCP3, H-PIP3, H-DIP2 and H-DIP3 (that was already gathered). Also, H-PIP1 emerged from the selection process because of a high prevalence of osteophytes; however, the sensitivity of H-PIP2 for the detection of osteophytes was only slightly lower than that of H-PIP1; (2) we omitted the insertion of the Achilles tendon from both the PsASon22 and the PsASon13 scores because this site was mainly relevant for the detection of enthesophytes; and (3) we omitted the distal insertion of the triceps into the olecranon from PsASon13 because this site was mainly relevant for the detection of enthesophytes. The combination of the insertion of the common extensor tendon at the lateral epicondyle and the patellar tendon insertion into the tibial anterior tuberosity already revealed a very high sensitivity to identify patients with enthesophytes.

Table 2 summarizes the proportion of ultrasound abnormalities exclusively detected by dorsal or palmar/plantar scans of H-PIPs, H-DIPs, MTPs, F-PIPs, F-DIPs and wrists as well as by medial/lateral or suprapatellar assessments of knees. We observed that ≥20% of structural and inflammatory pathologies at the H-PIP and H-DIP level were identified by palmar or dorsal scans only. At the knees, suprapatellar, medial/lateral scans are required not to miss patients with PD-signals. At the wrists and MTPs, palmar/plantar scans appeared to be less relevant given that only a minority of patients revealed ultrasound abnormalities at these sites. At F-PIPs and F-DIPs, the proportion of erosions detected by plantar scans was >20%; however, we decided to omit plantar scans from the composite scores due to the low absolute number of erosions at these sites.

The final composite scores are depicted in Figure 1 and detailed in Table 3. The bilateral score (PsASon22) includes 22 joints (6 MCPs, 4 H-PIPs, 2 MTPs, 4 H-DIPs, 2 F-DIPs, 4 large joints) and 4 entheses, whereas the unilateral score (PsASon13) compromises 13 joints (2 MCPs, 3 H-PIPs, 1 F-PIP, 2 MTPs, 1 H-DIP and 2 F-DIPs, 2 large joints) and 2 entheses.

Additional file 3 details the possible ranges of ultrasound composite scores and their components.

Sensitivity of the ultrasound composite scores for the detection of ultrasound pathologies

As detailed in Table 4, the bilateral composite score yielded sensitivity >80% for most lesions and sites using the 68-joints/14-entheses ultrasound score as the reference, whereas the unilateral score was less efficient revealing >80% sensitivity for GSS at small/large joints, GSE and osteophytes/enthesophytes only.

Both composite scores were more sensitive for the detection of PsA characteristic pathologies at small and large joints than at DIPs. Both composite scores were more efficient to identify osteophytes/enthesophytes than erosions, and among inflammatory lesions, GS-changes were more commonly detected than PD-signals.

Convergent construct validity of ultrasound composite scores

Tables 5 and 6 depict the association of inflammatory and structural components of the bilateral and unilateral

Table 1 Clinical findings at baseline and 6-month follow up in patients with psoriatic arthritis

	Baseline visit (n =83)	Follow up at 6 months (n =70)	*P*-value
Age at inclusion, years†	51.8 (11.7)	n.a.	n.a.
Female, n (%)	22 (26.2)	n.a.	n.a.
Body mass index, kg/m^2‡	27.2 (18.5 to 46.8)	n.a.	n.a.
Disease duration, years‡	7.5 (0 to 44.7)	n.a.	n.a.
Patients with a new diagnosis¥, n (%)	4 (4.8)	n.a.	n.a.
Axial involvement, n (%)	11 (13.3)	n.a.	n.a.
Smokers, n (%)			
Current	21 (25.3)	n.a.	n.a.
Previous	32 (38.6)		
PASDAS‡	5.9 (1.5)	5.2 (1.5)	<0.001
DAPSA‡	11.5 (0.1 to 70.2)	7.2 (0.1 to 73.5)	0.016
CPDAI‡	3.0 (0 to 9.0)	2.0 (0 to 11.0)	0.019
CRP, mg/L ‡	2.2 (0 to 49.5)	2.4 (0.2 to 35.0)	n.s.
ESR, mm/1st hour‡	9.5 (1 to 74)	10 (2 to 51)	n.s.
TJ, 68-joint count‡	4 (0 to 59)	1 (0 to 53)	0.012
SJ, 66-joint count‡	1 (0 to 15)	0 (0 to 17)	0.011
PGA, mm†	31.2 (22.7)	21.3 (23.5)	0.073
Ptpain, mm†	30.5 (24.5)	20.7 (21.0)	<0.001
EGA, mm†	22.0 (19.1)	11.5 (14.6)	0.009
HAQ†	0.7 (0.8)	0.6 (0.7)	<0.001
BASDAI‡	4.7 (0.9 to 5.5)	3.0 (0 to 6.0)	n.s.
ASQol‡	2.0 (0 to 11.0)	4.0 (0 to 8.0)	n.s.
Leeds enthesitis score‡	0 (0 to 4)	0 (0 to 2)	n.s.
Dactylitis score‡	0 (0 to 10)	0 (0 to 4)	n.s.
PASI‡	1.0 (0 to 23.2)	0.4 (0 to 36.3)	n.s.
DLQI‡	1.0 (0 to 20.0)	1.0 (0 to 18.0)	n.s.
DMARDs, n (%)			
MTX	33 (39.8)	30 (42.9)	
LFN	11 (13.3)	12 (17.1)	
MTX + LFN	3 (3.6)	3 (4.3)	n.s.
SSZ	2 (2.4)	2 (2.9)	
Anti-TNFα	31 (37.3)	30 (42.9)	
Corticosteroids, n (%)	6 (7.2)	4 (5.7)	n.s.
NSAIDs, n (%)			
On demand	56 (67.5)	57 (81.4)	n.s.
Regular intake	10 (12.0)	8 (11.4)	

‡Median (range); †mean (standard deviation); *P*-values are not adjusted for multiple testing; ¥diagnosis was established at the day of baseline study visit. ASQol, ankylosing spondylitis quality of life; BASDAI, Bath ankylosing spondylitis disease activity index; CPDAI, composite psoriatic disease activity index; CRP, C-reactive protein (normal values 0 to 5 mg/L); DAPSA, disease activity index for psoriatic arthritis; DLQI, dermatology life quality index; DMARDs, disease-modifying anti-rheumatic drugs; EGA, evaluator's global assessment of disease activity; ESR, erythrocyte sedimentation rate (normal values 1 to 10 mm/1st hour); HAQ, health assessment questionnaire; LFN, leflunomide; MTX, methotrexate; n, number; n.a., not applicable; n.s., not statistically significant; NSAIDs, non-steroidal anti-inflammatory drugs; PASDAS, psoriatic arthritis disease activity score; PASI, psoriasis area and severity index; PGA, patients' global assessment of disease activity; Ptpain, patients' pain assessment; SJ, swollen joint count; SSZ, sulfasalazine; TJ, tender joint count; TNF, tumour necrosis factor alpha. PGA, Ptpain and EGA were measured on visual analogue scales (range 0 to 100 mm) and are expressed in mm; BASDAI and ASQol values are shown for those 11 (13.3%) PsA patients with axial involvement.

Table 2 Ultrasound pathologies detected exclusively by dorsal or palmar/plantar scans of hand and foot joints and scans of different knee recesses

	Erosion					Osteophyte					GSS					PD-j				
	Dorsal only		Palmar/plantar only		Total	Dorsal only		Palmar/plantar only		Total	Dorsal only		Palmar/plantar only		Total	Dorsal only		Palmar/plantar only		Total
Grade (range 0 to 3)	1	2 to 3	1	2 to 3	1 to 3	1 to 3	2 to 3	1	1 to 3	1 to 3	1	1 to 3	1	2 to 3	1 to 3	1	2 to 3	1	2 to 3	1 to 3
	n (%)	n (%)	n (%)	n (%)	n (%)	n (%)	n (%)	n (%)	n (%)	n (%)	n (%)	n (%)	n (%)	n (%)	n (%)	n (%)	n (%)	n (%)	n (%)	n (%)
H-PIP + H-DIP	6 (13.0)	8 (17.4)	18 (39.1)	12 (26.1)	46 (100)	117 (19.5)	20 (3.3)	124 (20.6)	10 (1.7)	601 (100)	35 (17.3)	14 (6.9)	101 (50.0)	25 (12.4)	202 (100)	10 (22.2)	8 (17.8)	14 (31.1)	4 (8.9)	45 (100)
MTP	6 (8.3)	32 (44.4)	0	14 (19.4)	72 (100)	56 (26.4)	49 (23.1)	4 (1.9)	1 (0.5)	212 (100)	37 (42.1)	39 (44.3)	3 (3.5)	1 (1.1)	88 (100)	14 (50.0)	13 (46.4)	0	0	28 (100)
F-PIP + F-DIP	8 (34.8)	7 (30.4)	0	6 (26.1)	23 (100)	74 (27.8)	36 (13.5)	25 (9.4)	11 (4.1)	266 (100)	36 (53.7)	9 (13.4)	9 (13.4)	2 (3.0)	67 (100)	9 (37.5)	10 (41.7)	1 (4.2)	3 (12.5)	24 (100)
Wrist	-	-	-	-	-	-	-	-	-	-	47 (51.7)	15 (16.5)	1 (1.1)	4 (4.4)	91 (100)	21 (51.2)	11 (26.8)	2 (4.9)	0	41 (100)
											Medial/lat.		**Suprapat.**			**Medial/lat.**		**Suprapat.**		
Knees											20 (26.3)	9 (11.8)	15 (19.7)	0	76 (100)	10 (34.5)	9 (31.0)	10 (34.5)	2 (6.9)	29 (100)

The table depicts the number of joints at which the indicated ultrasound lesion [that is, erosions, osteophytes, grey scale synovitis (GSS) or Power Doppler signals (PD-j)] and the respective grading (1 or 2 to 3) were exclusively identified by dorsal (Dorsal only) or palmar/plantar (Palmar/plantar only) scans. Total refers to the overall number of joints positive for the specific ultrasound abnormality (irrespective of whether it was identified by dorsal, palmar/plantar or both scans). We conducted separate analyses for small finger joints except metacarpophalangeal joints (H-PIP + H-DIP), small joints of feet (MTP or F-PIP + F-DIP) and wrists. At the knees, we compared medial plus lateral (Medial/lat.) versus suprapatellar (Suprapat.) scans. Data in parenthesis reflect the percentage of positive joints out of the total number of joints revealing the indicated ultrasound finding. F-DIP, distal interphalangeal joint of the feet; F-PIP, proximal interphalangeal joint of the feet, GSS, grey scale synovitis; H-DIP, distal interphalangeal joint of hands; H-PIP, proximal interphalangeal joint of hands; MTP, metatarsophalangeal joint; PD-j, power Doppler at joints; T, total number of patients with the specific lesion; hyphens indicate "not assessed".

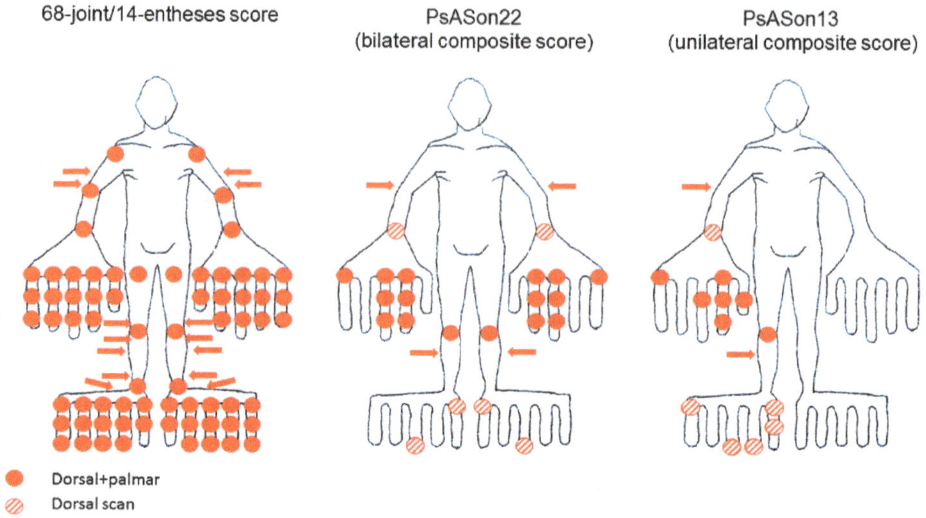

Figure 1 Joints and entheses included in ultrasound composite scores. Illustration depicts joints (circles) and entheses (arrows) included in the 68-joint/14-entheses score, and the bilateral 22-joint/4-entheses (PsASon22) and the unilateral 13-joint/2-entheses composite scores (PsASon13). For the unilateral score the dominant site is investigated (for example, the right site as shown in the figure). Solid circles indicate that both, palmar and dorsal sites (suprapatellar, medial and lateral scans for the knee) are assessed, whereas striped circles mark sites investigated by dorsal scans only.

composite scores, and the 68-joint/14-entheses score with clinical parameters of inflammation and disability (convergent construct validity). We observed weak to moderate correlations of the GSS/GSE, PD-j/e, and the GUIS scores with clinical composite scores, global assessments of pain/disease activity and acute phase reactants (Table 5). Importantly, the ultrasound composite scores yielded similar associations with clinical measures of disease activity to the 68-joint/14-entheses score (except for the component PD-teno that weakly correlated with clinical composite scores only when the sonographic 68-joint/14-entheses score was applied). Joint/enthesal erosions but not osteophytes correlated with HAQ, particularly in patients judged to be in remission in whom the activity related (that is, reversible) component of disability is assumed to be low (Table 6) [20].

Further subanalyses indicated that GSS and PD-j scores were associated with the number of SJ, the PD-j score with the number of TJ, and the GSE with the MASEI + epi (see Additional file 4).

Sensitivity to change in ultrasound composite scores

As detailed in Figure 2 and Additional file 5 we observed that patients changing from a clinical status of active disease to remission/MDA yielded greater reductions in the GUIS of the bilateral, the unilateral or the 68-joint/14-entheses scores compared to patients with unchanged clinical activity. The effect size (Cohen's *d* statistic) for the GUIS was low to moderate ranging from 0.40 (PsASon13) to 0.75 (68-joint/14-entheses score). SRM of patients changing from active disease to remission or MDA ranged from −1.04 to −0.09 (as compared to −0.53 to −0.04 in the entire cohort).

In subanalyses, we observed that the GSS/GSE was the most sensitive GUIS item to change (for details including effect size and SRM see Additional file 5). We also found weak to moderate correlations between ΔGUIS scores and ΔPASDAS, ΔDAPSA, ΔPtpain, ΔPGA and ΔEGA as depicted in Additional file 6.

Feasibility and inter-rater reliability

The median time to complete the bilateral and unilateral scores was 19 minutes (range 16 to 26) and 10 (9 to 13) minutes, respectively. Inter-rater reliability of components from bilateral and unilateral composite scores was moderate to good: ICCs for the GUIS were 0.84 and 0.54, respectively. ICCs of the GUIS components ranged from 0.42 (GS-teno) to 0.96 (PD-j) for the bilateral composite score and from 0.36 (GS-teno) to 0.71 (PD-j) for the unilateral score. The ICC for erosions was 0.75 and 0.64, respectively; and for the osteophyte/enthesophyte subscore, it was 0.92 and 0.41, respectively, for the bilateral and unilateral composite scores.

Discussion

In the present study, we propose two new ultrasound composite scores for the assessment of PsA specific inflammatory and structural lesions. Both composite scores had adequate convergent construct validity, yielded reliable results and the inflammatory elements revealed sufficient sensitivity to change. We found the bilateral score (PsASon22) more sensitive than the unilateral composite score

Table 3 Scans and anatomical sites of the bilateral (PsASon22) and unilateral ultrasound score (PsASon13)

	PsASon22	
Anatomical sites	**Scans (all bilateral)**	**Ultrasound findings**
Small finger joints:		
MCP2, MCP3, MCP5, H-PIP2,H-PIP3	Dorsal, palmar	GSS, PD-j, GS-Peri (MCP only), PD-Peri (MCP only), GS-Teno, PD-Teno, erosion, osteophyte
Distal interphalangeal finger joints:		
H-DIP2, H-DIP3	Dorsal, palmar	GSS, PD-j, GS-Teno, PD-Teno, erosion, osteophyte
Small joints of feet:		
MTP1	Dorsal	GSS, PD-j, erosion, osteophyte
Distal interphalangeal joints of feet:		
F-DIP3	Dorsal	GSS, PD-j, erosion, osteophyte
Large joints:		
Wrist	Dorsal	GSS, PD-j, GS-Teno (wrist only), PD-Teno (writs only)
Knee	Suppat., medial, lateral	
Entheses:		
Lateral epicondyle, distal patella	n.a.	GSE, PD-e, erosion, osteophyte
	PsASon13	
Anatomical sites	**Scans (all unilateral, dominant site)**	**Ultrasound findings**
Small finger joints:		
MCP2, MCP5, H-PIP1, H-PIP2,H-PIP3	Dorsal, palmar	GSS, PD-j, GS-Peri (MCP only), PD-Peri (MCP only), GS-Teno, PD-Teno, erosion, osteophyte
Distal interphalangeal finger joints:		
H-DIP3	Dorsal, palmar	GSS, PD-j, GS-Teno, PD-Teno, erosion, osteophyte
Small joints of feet:		GSS, PD-j, erosion, osteophyte
MTP1, MTP5, F-PIP1	Dorsal	
Distal interphalangeal joints of feet:		
F-DIP2, F-DIP3	Dorsal	GSS, PD-j, erosion, osteophyte
Large joints:		
Wrist	Dorsal	GSS, PD-j, GS-Teno (wrist only), PD-Teno (writs only)
Knee	Suppat., medial, lateral	
Entheses:		
Lateral epicondyle, distal patella	n.a.	GSE, PD-e, erosion, osteophyte

F-DIP, Distal interphalangeal joint of feet; F-PIP, proximal interphalangeal joints of feet; GS-Peri, grey scale perisynovitis; GS-Teno, grey scale tenosynovitis; GSE, grey scale changes at entheses; GSS, grey scale synovitis; H-DIP, distal interphalangeal joint of hands; H-PIP, proximal interphalangeal joint of hands; MCP, metacarpophalangeal joint; MTP, metatarsophalangeal joint; n.a.; not applicable; PD-e, power Doppler findings at entheses; PD-j, power Doppler findings at joints; PD-Peri, power Doppler Perisynovitis PD-Teno, power Doppler Tenosynovitis; suppat., suprapatellar.

(PsASon13) to detect PsA-specific pathologies whereas the latter was faster to accomplish.

The major strengths of our composite scores are the inclusion of all currently defined Ps-related ultrasound pathologies into the scores, and the data driven identification of joints, peri-articular structures and entheses, except for a few manual selections aimed at the improvement of the feasibility of the scores. The German U7 and the Italian five-targets scores, the two other ultrasound composite scores previously applied in PsA, were developed on a basis of clinical experience and focus on fewer sites and less PsA-specific pathologies than our instruments [5,6].

Our data demonstrate that palmar scans of wrists and plantar scans of feet are dispensable for the ultrasound composite scores, whereas the investigation of palmar and dorsal sites of fingers is required to achieve sufficient sensitivity to identify PsA-specific pathologies. Similar data were reported for the assessment of the rheumatoid hand, whereas a comparison between plantar and dorsal scans of feet has not been performed in other cohorts so far [22,23].

We did not include dactylitis into the composite scores, because of the lack of an established ultrasound definition. Earlier studies suggested that the combination of arthritis and tenosynovitis is the underlying pathology

Table 4 Sensitivity of the bilateral (PsASon22) (a) and unilateral (PsASon13) (b) ultrasound composite scores to detect PsA characteristic ultrasound findings

(a)	GSS/GSE	PD-j/e	GS-Teno	PD-Teno	GS-Peri	PD-Peri	Erosion	Osteop./enthesop.
Small joints	89.2	81.6			95.2	92.9	91.9	100
DIP joints	84.6	63.6	71.4	75.0	n.a.	n.a.	42.9	98.8
Large joints	93.3	97.7			n.a.	n.a.	n.a.	n.a.
entheses	100	87.8	n.a.	n.a.	n.a.	n.a.	71.9	94.0
(b)	**GSS/GSE**	**PD-j/e**	**GS-Teno**	**PD-Teno**	**GS-Peri**	**PD-Peri**	**Erosion**	**Osteop./enthesop.**
Small joints	92.8	73.5			57.1	50.0	79.7	100
DIPs	58.5	54.5	66.7	57.1	n.a.	n.a.	35.7	96.4
Large joints	81.3	72.1			n.a.	n.a.	n.a.	n.a.
entheses	100	67.3	n.a.	n.a.	n.a.	n.a.	50.0	88.0

Data indicate the sensitivity of the inflammatory and structural components of the bilateral (a) and unilateral (b) ultrasound composite scores to detect ultrasound pathologies using the 68-joints/14-entheses score as a reference. DIP, distal interphalangeal joints (of hands and feet); GS-Peri, grey scale Perisynovitis; GS-Teno, grey scale tenosynovitis; GSS/GSE, grey scale synovitis/grey scale changes of entheses; n.a., pathology not assessed at this site(s); osteop./entheop., osteophytes/enthesophytes; PD-j/e, power Doppler signals at joints/entheses; PD-Peri, power Doppler Perisynovitis; PD-Teno, power Doppler Tenosynovitis; Small joints compromise metacarpophalangeal joints, metatarsophalangeal joint and proximal interphalangeal joints of hands and feet.

of dactylitis, whereas recent ultrasound and magnetic resonance imaging data indicate that isolated tenosynovitis, soft tissue oedema and/or collateral tendon enthesitis are frequently observed in dactylitic fingers and toes [24-28]. An outcome measures in rheumatology (OMERACT) project aimed at the agreement on a new ultrasound definition of dactylitis is currently underway, and a revision of our composite scores may be considered once such a definition has been validated [27].

MTP1 was included into the composite scores because we frequently found GSS and PD-j changes at this site. Earlier studies in PsA and RA also reported a high prevalence of inflammatory changes at MTPs; however, we recognize potential overestimation of PsA-related synovitis at that site as MTP1 is also frequently affected by osteoarthritis and because there were some cases of concomitant gout mimicking PsA flares [29-34]. We did not systematically record ultrasound signs of crystal arthropathies in our patients, but emphasise that such a study should be performed in the future [35]. Similarly, PIP and DIP joints may be inflamed either due to PsA or (secondary or concomitant) symptomatic osteoarthritis, and it is currently impossible to reliably identify the true driver of inflammation by means of imaging methods alone [36,37]. This uncertainty also relates to RA-specific ultrasound scores, and we do currently not know whether ultrasound-verified synovitis caused by the primary disease or (secondary/concomitant) osteoarthritis has a different impact on clinical and structural outcomes in RA and PsA [6,38].

We observed a higher sensitivity of the bilateral versus the unilateral composite score for the detection of inflammatory and structural changes, but at the cost of time. In situations, where a high sensitivity is less relevant (for example, use of sonography to monitor treatment response) the unilateral score may be preferred, whereas for remission assessment the bilateral ultrasound score may produce more valuable results. In RA, subclinical arthritis was of high prognostic value regarding clinical relapses and progression of erosions, and we are currently investigating the relevance of ultrasound-verified inflammation for patients' related outcomes in PsA [39-41]. A further refinement of the ultrasound scores based on the results of this study (for example, by inclusion of sites with a high significance for the prediction of structural progression) cannot be excluded at this stage.

To test convergent construct validity, we correlated the inflammatory and structural components of the ultrasound scores with clinical measures of disease activity and disability, respectively. We applied the PASDAS, CPDAI and DAPSA as markers of clinical activity recognizing that none of these instruments have yet been established as the gold standard. HAQ better correlated with erosions than with osteophytes, whereas in RA the loss of cartilage was the most important factor contributing to patients' disability [20].

Among individual components of the GUIS, the GSS/GSE correlated best with clinical activity and revealed the highest sensitivity to change during follow up. This observation may be related to the facts that peripheral arthritis was present in the majority of patients (74.7% had active joint disease according to CPDAI at baseline), that joint disease highly impacts clinical composite scores and global measures of disease activity and that GSS/GEE had the largest variability among the GUIS components [4,42]. Also, we observed that both ultrasound scores were generally more sensitive to detect GS than PD changes at joints and entheses, possibly explained by a high prevalence of GS-abnormalities even in PsA patients with low or no clinical activity [4].

The major limitation of our study is the relatively low clinical disease activity of the cohort leading to a possible underestimation of the sensitivity to change of the

Table 5 Correlation of the inflammatory components of the bilateral (PsASon22) and unilateral (PsASon13) ultrasound composite scores, and the 68-joint/14-entheses score with clinical parameters

	Score	PASDAS	CPDAI	DAPSA	Ptpain	PGA	EGA	CRP	ESR
GSS/GSE	PsASon22	0.25*	NA	0.31**	NA	NA	0.29**	0.21†	0.32**
	PsASon13	0.22*	0.19†	0.28*	0.19†	NA	0.19†	0.21†	NA
	68joint/14enthes	0.33**	0.22†	0.41***	0.22*	0.24*	0.30**	0.28*	0.41***
PD-j/e	PsASon22	0.22*	NA	0.23*	NA	0.24*	0.22*	NA	0.37**
	PsASon13	NA	NA	NA	NA	NA	0.19†	NA	0.26*
	68joint/14enthes	0.28*	NA	0.26*	NA	0.24*	0.28*	NA	0.34**
GS-Teno	PsASon22	NA	NA	NA	NA	NA	NA	NA	NA
	PsASon13	NA	NA	NA	NA	NA	NA	NA	NA
	68joint/14enthes	NA	NA	NA	NA	NA	NA	NA	0.26*
PDNATeno	PsASon22	NA	NA	NA	NA	NA	NA	NA	0.40***
	PsASon13	NA	NA	NA	NA	NA	NA	NA	0.29**
	68joint/14enthes	0.31**	NA	0.28*	0.22*	0.28*	0.28*	0.30**	0.53***
GS-Perisyn	PsASon22	NA	NA	NA	NA	NA	NA	NA	NA
	PsASon13	NA	NA	NA	NA	NA	NA	NA	NA
	68joint/14enthes	NA	NA	NA	NA	NA	NA	NA	NA
PD-Perisyn	PsASon22	NA	NA	NA	NA	NA	NA	NA	NA
	PsASon13	NA	NA	NA	NA	NA	NA	NA	NA
	68joint/14enthes	NA	NA	NA	NA	NA	NA	NA	NA
GUIS	PsASon22	0.24*	NA	0.28*	NA	0.19†	0.25*	0.19†	0.35**
	PsASon13	NA	NA	0.22*	NA	NA	NA	NA	0.19†
	68joint/14enthes	0.36**	NA	0.39***	0.19†	0.28*	0.33**	0.26*	0.44***

Data indicate the correlation of the inflammatory components of the bilateral and unilateral ultrasound composite scores and the 68-joint/14-entheses score with clinical measures of disease activity. CPDAI, composite psoriatic disease activity index; CRP, C-reactive protein; DAPSA, disease activity index for psoriatic arthritis; EGA, evaluator's global assessment of disease activity; ESR, erythrocyte sedimentation rate; GS-Peri, grey scale perisynovitis; GS-Teno, grey scale tenosynovitis; GSS/GSE, grey scale synovitis/grey scale enthesitis ultrasound score; GUIS, global ultrasound inflammation subscore; PASDAS, modified psoriatic arthritis disease activity score; PD-j/e, power Doppler scores at joints/entheses; PD-Peri, power Doppler Perisynovitis; PD-Teno, power Doppler Tenosynovitis; PGA, patients' global assessment of disease activity; Ptpain, patients' pain assessment. ***P <0.001; **P <0.01; *P <0.05; †P <0.1; NA, no significant association found.

Table 6 Correlation of the structural components of the bilateral (PsASon22) and unilateral (PsASon13) ultrasound composite scores, and the 68-joint/14-entheses score with the health assessment questionnaire

	Score	HAQ	HAQ (clinical remission)
Erosion score (joint + entheses)	PsASon22	NA	0.35*
	PsASon13	0.22*	0.39*
	68joint/14enthes	0.20†	0.34*
Osteophyte/enthesophyte score	PsASon22	0.20†	NA
	PsASon13	NA	NA
	68joint/14enthes	NA	NA

Data indicate the correlation of erosion and osteophyte/enthesophyte scores from bilateral, unilateral and 68-joint scores with the health assessment questionnaire (HAQ) in the total cohort (n =83) and in patients in clinical remission according to the judgment of the evaluating rheumatologist (n =40). *P <0.05; †P <0.1; NA, no association found.

inflammatory elements. Previously proposed ultrasound scores in PsA and RA were validated in patients with high disease activity at baseline and subsequent treatment with biological agents [5,19,43]. Consequently, dramatic changes in disease scores were observed resulting in better sensitivity to change in the ultrasound composite scores by statistical means. The low disease activity in our cohort may also explain the relatively weak association between inflammatory items of the ultrasound composite scores and clinical factors. We previously concluded from an RA study that the strength of association between clinical and ultrasound measures diminishes as patients are in or close to remission [15]. Nevertheless, our ultrasound scores resulted in sufficient sensitivity to change and convergent construct validity, given that the comprehensive assessment of 68-joint/14-entheses did not produce better results than the reduced scores.

Other limitations of this study are the moderate size of the cohort, the relatively long disease duration, the single-centre design and the use of the as yet unvalidated 68-joint/14-entheses score as a reference for the development

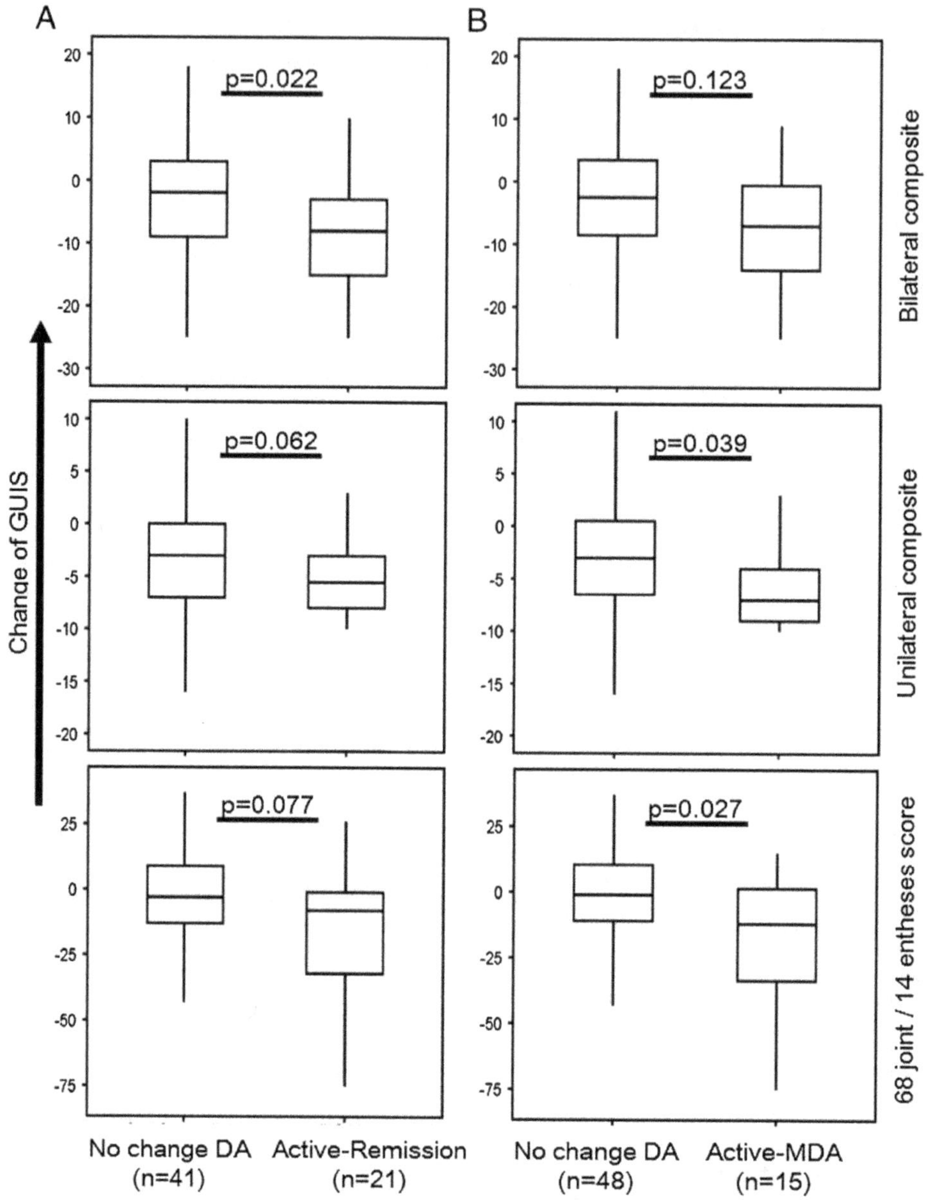

Figure 2 Sensitivity to change of ultrasound composite scores. Change (Δscore 6-month visit – score baseline) of global ultrasound inflammatory subscores (global ultrasound inflammation score (GUI-score)) in patients without a change in clinical disease activity (that is, active or remission at both baseline and follow-up visits) (no change DA) and patients who were active at baseline and achieved remission according to the evaluating physician **(A)**, active-remission) or minimal disease activity **(B)** (active-MDA) at 6 months follow-up. Whiskers box plots show the median and 50% of cases within the boxes and all data excluding mavericks between the end points of the whiskers. Differences were tested by the Mann-Whitney *U*-test.

of the composite scores. Also, we did not test the responsiveness of structural components of the scores because of the short follow-up period and the absence of paired results from other imaging methods. Future studies with a long-term (preferentially multicentre) design, the inclusion of various patients' subgroups (early disease, different clinical manifestations and new treatment with biologics) and the possibility to compare ultrasound data with other imaging methods are needed for external validation of our data.

Another interesting finding of this study is the better reliability of bilateral versus unilateral composite scores. This observation can be explained by the fact that scores with high variability of results (resulting from a larger number of sites included in the bilateral score) yield better statistical associations than scores with a narrow range [44]. The overall reproducibility of our composite scores, however, was comparable to that of previous RA- and PsA-specific scores [5,7,38].

Conclusion

We developed two new ultrasound composite scores for PsA. Both scores include most PsA-specific pathologies, are sensitive for the detection of inflammation, have adequate convergent construct validity, are reliable and feasible in clinical practice and inflammatory elements of the scores reveal sufficient sensitivity to change.

Additional files

Additional file 1: Flow chart illustrating exemplarily the identification of a combination of joints for the bilateral psoriatic arthritis score (PsASon22) that is sensitive for the detection of power Doppler (PD) signals among small joints. DIP, distal interphalangeal joints; GS-Peri, grey scale perisynovitis; GS-Teno, grey scale tenosynovitis; GSE, grey scale changes of entheses; GSS, grey scale synovitis; H-PIP, proximal interphalangeal joint of hands; MCP, metacarpophalangeal joint; MTP, metatarsophalangeal joint; osteo, osteophytes; PD-e, Power Doppler at entheses; pts, patients; step n, the procedure is repeated n-times.

Additional file 2: Results of the selection process of anatomical sites for (a) bilateral psoriatic arthritis (PsASon22) and (b) unilateral (PsASon13) ultrasound scores.

Additional file 3: Possible ranges in the (a) bilateral and (b) unilateral ultrasound composite scores, as well as (c) the 68-joint/ 14-entheses score, and their components.

Additional file 4: (a) Correlation of joint components from bilateral, unilateral and 68-joint scores with clinical parameters; (b) correlation of enthesal components from bilateral, unilateral and 14-entheses scores with clinical enthesis scores.

Additional file 5: (a) Sensitivity to change in ultrasound scores - change in clinical disease activity according to the evaluating rheumatologist; (b) sensitivity to change in ultrasound scores - change in clinical disease activity according to minimal disease activity criteria.

Additional file 6: Changes in ultrasound scores versus changes in clinical scores.

Abbreviations

CASPAR: classification for psoriatic arthritis; cMASEI + E: Madrid sonographic enthesitis index plus lateral epicondyle; CPDAI: composite psoriatic disease activity index; CRP: C-reactive protein; DAPSA: disease activitiy index for psoriatic arthritis; DIP: distal interphalangeal joint; EGA: evaluator's global assessment of disease activity; ESR: erythrocyte sedimentation rate; EULAR: European League Against Rheumatism; F-DIP: distal interphalangeal joint of the feet; F-PIP: proximal interphalangeal joint of the feet; GS: grey scale; GSE: grey scale changes of enthesitis; GS-perisyn: grey scale perisynovitis; GSS: grey scale synovitis; GS-teno: grey scale tenosynovitis; GUIS: global ultrasound inflammation subscore; HAQ: health assessment questionnaire; H-DIP: distal interphalangeal joint of the hands; H-PIP: proximal interphalangeal joint of the hands; ICC: intraclass correlation coefficient; LEI: Leeds enthesitis index; MASEI: Madrid sonographic enthesitis index; MCP: metacarpophalangeal joint; MDA: minimal disease activity; MTP: metatarsophalangeal joint; OMERACT: outcome measures in rheumatology; PASDAS: psoriatic arthritis disease activitiy score; PASI: psoriasis activity and severity index; PD: power Doppler; PD-e: power Doppler signals at enthesis; PD-j: power Doppler signals at joints; PD-perisyn: power Doppler signals related to perisynovitis; PD-teno: power Doppler signals related to tenosynovitis; PGA: patients' global assessment of disease activity; PIP: proximal interphalangeal joint; PsA: psoriatic Arthritis; Ptpain: patients' pain assessment; RA: rheumatoid arthritis; SF-36: short form health survey 36; SJ: swollen joints; SRM: standardized response means; TJ: tender joints.

Competing interests

The authors declare that they have no competing interests.

Authors' contributions

AF participated in clinical assessments, helped to analyse the data and to draft the manuscript, RH helped with ultrasound investigations, data analysis and manuscript drafting, JG participated in clinical assessments and critically revised the manuscript for important intellectual content, AL helped to analyse the data and critically revised the manuscript for important intellectual content, WBG helped to design the study and to draft the manuscript, MG helped to design the study data and critically revised the manuscript for important intellectual content, CDu participated in the design of the study and helped to draft the manuscript, JH participated in clinical assessments and manuscript drafting, CDe designed the study, participated in ultrasound investigations, helped to analyse the data and to draft the manuscript. All authors have given final approval of the version to be published and agree to be accountable for all aspects of the work in ensuring that questions related to the accuracy or integrity of any part of the work are appropriately investigated and resolved.

Acknowledgements

This study was supported by an unrestricted grant from Pfizer. The funding body was not involved in any part of the study.

Author details

[1]Department of Rheumatology and Immunology, Medical University Graz, Auenbruggerplatz 15, 8036 Graz, Austria. [2]Clinica Reumatologica, Università Politecnica delle Marche, Ospedale "Carlo Urbani", Via dei Colli 52, 60035 Jesi Ancona, Italy. [3]Department of Internal Medicine VI, Medical University Innsbruck, Anichstrasse 35, 6020 Innsbruck, Austria.

References

1. Colebatch AN, Edwards CJ, Ostergaard M, van der Heijde D, Balint PV, D'Agostino MA, Forslind K, Grassi W, Haavardsholm EA, Haugeberg G, Jurik AG, Landewe RB, Naredo E, O'Connor PJ, Ostendorf B, Potocki K, Schmidt WA, Smolen JS, Sokolovic S, Watt I, Conaghan PG: **EULAR recommendations for the use of imaging of the joints in the clinical management of rheumatoid arthritis.** *Ann Rheum Dis* 2013, **72:**804–814.
2. Smolen JS, Braun J, Dougados M, Emery P, Fitzgerald O, Helliwell P, Kavanaugh A, Kvien TK, Landewé R, Luger T, Mease P, Olivieri I, Reveille J, Ritchlin C, Rudwaleit M, Schoels M, Sieper J, de Wit M, Baraliakos X, Betteridge N, Burgos-Vargas R, Collantes-Estevez E, Deodhar A, Elewaut D, Gossec L, Jongkees M, Maccarone M, Redlich K, van den Bosch F, Wei JC-C, *et al*: **Treating spondyloarthritis, including ankylosing spondylitis and psoriatic arthritis, to target: recommendations of an international task force.** *Ann Rheum Dis* 2014, **73:**6–16.
3. Anandarajah AP, Ritchlin CT: **The diagnosis and treatment of early psoriatic arthritis.** *Nat Rev* 2009, **5:**634–641.
4. Husic R, Gretler J, Felber A, Graninger WB, Duftner C, Hermann J, Dejaco C: **Disparity between ultrasound and clinical findings in psoriatic arthritis.** *Ann Rheum Dis* 2013, **73:**1529–1536.
5. Gutierrez M, Di Geso L, Salaffi F, Bertolazzi C, Tardella M, Filosa G, Filippucci E, Grassi W: **Development of a preliminary US power Doppler composite score for monitoring treatment in PsA.** *Rheumatology (Oxford)* 2012, **51:**1261–1268.
6. Scheel AK, Hermann KG, Kahler E, Pasewaldt D, Fritz J, Hamm B, Brunner E, Muller GA, Burmester GR, Backhaus M: **A novel ultrasonographic synovitis scoring system suitable for analyzing finger joint inflammation in rheumatoid arthritis.** *Arthritis Rheum* 2005, **52:**733–743.
7. Backhaus M, Ohrndorf S, Kellner H, Strunk J, Backhaus TM, Hartung W, Sattler H, Albrecht K, Kaufmann J, Becker K, Sorensen H, Meier L, Burmester GR, Schmidt WA: **Evaluation of a novel 7-joint ultrasound score in daily rheumatologic practice: a pilot project.** *Arthritis Rheum* 2009, **61:**1194–1201.
8. Taylor W, Gladman D, Helliwell P, Marchesoni A, Mease P, Mielants H, CS Group: **Classification criteria for psoriatic arthritis: development of new criteria from a large international study.** *Arthritis Rheum* 2006, **54:**2665–2673.

9. De Miguel E, Cobo T, Munoz-Fernandez S, Naredo E, Uson J, Acebes JC, Andreu JL, Martin-Mola E: **Validity of enthesis ultrasound assessment in spondyloarthropathy.** *Ann Rheum Dis* 2009, **68:**169–174.
10. Healy PJ, Helliwell PS: **Measuring clinical enthesitis in psoriatic arthritis: assessment of existing measures and development of an instrument specific to psoriatic arthritis.** *Arthritis Rheum* 2008, **59:**686–691.
11. Schoels M, Aletaha D, Funovits J, Kavanaugh A, Baker D, Smolen JS: **Application of the DAREA/DAPSA score for assessment of disease activity in psoriatic arthritis.** *Ann Rheum Dis* 2010, **69:**1441–1447.
12. Mumtaz A, Gallagher P, Kirby B, Waxman R, Coates LC, Veale JD, Helliwell P, FitzGerald O: **Development of a preliminary composite disease activity index in psoriatic arthritis.** *Ann Rheum Dis* 2011, **70:**272–277.
13. Helliwell PS, FitzGerald O, Fransen J, Gladman DD, Kreuger GG, Callis-Duffin K, McHugh N, Mease PJ, Strand V, Waxman R, Azevedo VF, Beltran Ostos A, Carneiro S, Cauli A, Espinoza LR, Flynn JA, Hassan N, Healy P, Kerzberg EM, Lee YJ, Lubrano E, Marchesoni A, Marzo-Ortega H, Porru G, Moreta EG, Nash P, Raffayova H, Ranza R, Raychaudhuri SP, Roussou E, *et al*: **The development of candidate composite disease activity and responder indices for psoriatic arthritis (GRACE project).** *Ann Rheum Dis* 2013, **72:**986–991.
14. Coates LC, Fransen J, Helliwell PS: **Defining minimal disease activity in psoriatic arthritis: a proposed objective target for treatment.** *Ann Rheum Dis* 2010, **69:**48–53.
15. Dejaco C, Duftner C, Wipfler-Freissmuth E, Weiss H, Graninger WB, Schirmer M: **Ultrasound-defined remission and active disease in rheumatoid arthritis: association with clinical and serologic parameters.** *Semin Arthritis Rheum* 2012, **41:**761–767.
16. Dejaco C, Duftner C, Wipfler-Freissmuth E, Weiss H, Schneider T, Schirmer M: **Elderly versus young onset rheumatoid arthritis: Higher levels of ultrasound-detected inflammation despite comparable clinical disease activity.** *Arthritis Care Res (Hoboken)* 2013, **65:**304–308.
17. Hartung W, Kellner H, Strunk J, Sattler H, Schmidt WA, Ehrenstein B, Fleck M, Backhaus M: **Development and evaluation of a novel ultrasound score for large joints in rheumatoid arthritis: one year of experience in daily clinical practice.** *Arthritis Care Res (Hoboken)* 2012, **64:**675–682.
18. Gutierrez M, Filippucci E, Salaffi F, Di Geso L, Grassi W: **Differential diagnosis between rheumatoid arthritis and psoriatic arthritis: the value of ultrasound findings at metacarpophalangeal joints level.** *Ann Rheum Dis* 2011, **70:**1111–1114.
19. Naredo E, Rodriguez M, Campos C, Rodriguez-Heredia JM, Medina JA, Giner E, Martinez O, Toyos FJ, Ruiz T, Ros I, Pujol M, Miquel X, Garcia L, Aznar JJ, Chamizo E, Paez M, Morales P, Rueda A, Tuneu R, Corominas H, de Agustin JJ, Moragues C, Minguez D, Willisch A, Gonzalez-Cruz I, Aragon A, Iglesias G, Armas C, Pablo Valdazo J, Vargas C, *et al*: **Validity, reproducibility, and responsiveness of a twelve-joint simplified power doppler ultrasonographic assessment of joint inflammation in rheumatoid arthritis.** *Arthritis Rheum* 2008, **59:**515–522.
20. Aletaha D, Funovits J, Smolen JS: **Physical disability in rheumatoid arthritis is associated with cartilage damage rather than bone destruction.** *Ann Rheum Dis* 2011, **70:**733–739.
21. Altman D: *Practical Statistics for Medical Research.* 1st edition. London: Chapman and Hall; 1991.
22. Vlad V, Berghea F, Libianu S, Balanescu A, Bojinca V, Constantinescu C, Abobului M, Predeteanu D, Ionescu R: **Ultrasound in rheumatoid arthritis: volar versus dorsal synovitis evaluation and scoring.** *BMC Musculoskelet Disord* 2011, **12:**124.
23. Ohrndorf S, Halbauer B, Martus P, Reiche B, Backhaus TM, Burmester GR, Backhaus M: **Detailed joint region analysis of the 7-joint ultrasound score: evaluation of an arthritis patient cohort over one year.** *Int J Rheumatol* 2013, **2013:**493848.
24. Kane D, Greaney T, Bresnihan B, Gibney R, FitzGerald O: **Ultrasonography in the diagnosis and management of psoriatic dactylitis.** *J Rheumatol* 1999, **26:**1746–1751.
25. Olivieri I, Padula A, Scarano E, Scarpa R: **Dactylitis or "sausage-shaped" digit.** *J Rheumatol* 2007, **34:**1217–1222.
26. Wakefield RJ, Emery P, Veale D: **Ultrasonography and psoriatic arthritis.** *J Rheumatol* 2000, **27:**1564–1565.
27. Bakewell CJ, Olivieri I, Aydin SZ, Dejaco C, Ikeda K, Gutierrez M, Terslev L, Thiele R, D'Agostino MA, Kaeley GS: **Ultrasound and magnetic resonance imaging in the evaluation of psoriatic dactylitis: status and perspectives.** *J Rheumatol* 2013, **40:**1951–1957.
28. Healy PJ, Groves C, Chandramohan M, Helliwell PS: **MRI changes in psoriatic dactylitis–extent of pathology, relationship to tenderness and correlation with clinical indices.** *Rheumatology (Oxford)* 2008, **47:**92–95.
29. Szkudlarek M, Narvestad E, Klarlund M, Court-Payen M, Thomsen HS, Østergaard M: **Ultrasonography of the metatarsophalangeal joints in rheumatoid arthritis: comparison with magnetic resonance imaging, conventional radiography, and clinical examination.** *Arthritis Rheum* 2004, **50:**2103–2112.
30. Delle Sedie A, Riente L, Filippucci E, Scirè CA, Iagnocco A, Meenagh G, Gutierrez M, Valesini G, Montecucco C, Grassi W, Bombardieri S: **Ultrasound imaging for the rheumatologist. XXXII. Sonographic assessment of the foot in patients with psoriatic arthritis.** *Clin Exp Rheumatol* 2011, **29:**217–222.
31. Freeston J, Coates L, Nam J, Moverley A, Hensor E, Wakefield R, Emery P, Helliwell P, Conaghan P: **Is there sub-clinical synovitis in early psoriatic arthritis? A clinical comparison with grey scale and power Doppler ultrasound.** *Arthritis Care Res (Hoboken)* 2014, **66:**432–439.
32. Oliviero F, Scanu A, Galozzi P, Gava A, Frallonardo P, Ramonda R, Punzi L: **Prevalence of calcium pyrophosphate and monosodium urate crystals in synovial fluid of patients with previously diagnosed joint diseases.** *Joint Bone Spine* 2013, **80:**287–290.
33. Liu M, Li J-H, Li B, He C-D, Xiao T, Chen H-D: **Coexisting gout, erythrodermic psoriasis and psoriatic arthritis.** *Eur J Dermatol* 2009, **19:**184–185.
34. López-Reyes A, Hernández-Díaz C, Hofmann F, Pineda C: **Gout mimicking psoriatic arthritis flare.** *J Clin Rheumatol* 2012, **18:**220.
35. Grassi W, Meenagh G, Pascual E, Filippucci E: **"Crystal clear"-sonographic assessment of gout and calcium pyrophosphate deposition disease.** *Semin Arthritis Rheum* 2006, **36:**197–202.
36. Braum LS, McGonagle D, Bruns A, Philipp S, Hermann S, Aupperle K, Tan AL, Diekhoff T, Hamm B, Hermann K-GA: **Characterisation of hand small joints arthropathy using high-resolution MRI–limited discrimination between osteoarthritis and psoriatic arthritis.** *Eur Radiol* 2013, **23:**1686–1693.
37. Tan AL, Grainger AJ, Tanner SF, Emery P, McGonagle D: **A high-resolution magnetic resonance imaging study of distal interphalangeal joint arthropathy in psoriatic arthritis and osteoarthritis: are they the same?** *Arthritis Rheum* 2006, **54:**1328–1333.
38. Naredo E, Collado P, Cruz A, Palop MJ, Cabero F, Richi P, Carmona L, Crespo M: **Longitudinal power Doppler ultrasonographic assessment of joint inflammatory activity in early rheumatoid arthritis: predictive value in disease activity and radiologic progression.** *Arthritis Rheum* 2007, **57:**116–124.
39. Saleem B, Brown AK, Quinn M, Karim Z, Hensor EM, Conaghan P, Peterfy C, Wakefield RJ, Emery P: **Can flare be predicted in DMARD treated RA patients in remission, and is it important? A cohort study.** *Ann Rheum Dis* 2012, **71:**1316–1321.
40. Scire CA, Montecucco C, Codullo V, Epis O, Todoerti M, Caporali R: **Ultrasonographic evaluation of joint involvement in early rheumatoid arthritis in clinical remission: power Doppler signal predicts short-term relapse.** *Rheumatology (Oxford)* 2009, **48:**1092–1097.
41. Brown AK, Quinn MA, Karim Z, Conaghan PG, Peterfy CG, Hensor E, Wakefield RJ, O'Connor PJ, Emery P: **Presence of significant synovitis in rheumatoid arthritis patients with disease-modifying antirheumatic drug-induced clinical remission: evidence from an imaging study may explain structural progression.** *Arthritis Rheum* 2006, **54:**3761–3773.
42. Studenic P, Radner H, Smolen JS, Aletaha D: **Discrepancies between patients and physicians in their perceptions of rheumatoid arthritis disease activity.** *Arthritis Rheum* 2012, **64:**2814–2823.
43. Dougados M, Jousse-Joulin S, Mistretta F, d'Agostino M-A, Backhaus M, Bentin J, Chalès G, Chary-Valckenaere I, Conaghan P, Etchepare F, Gaudin P, Grassi W, van der Heijde D, Sellam J, Naredo E, Szkudlarek M, Wakefield R, Saraux A: **Evaluation of several ultrasonography scoring systems for synovitis and comparison to clinical examination: results from a prospective multicentre study of rheumatoid arthritis.** *Ann Rheum Dis* 2010, **69:**828–833.
44. Müller R, Büttner P: **A critical discussion of intraclass correlation coefficients.** *Stat Med* 1994, **13:**2465–2476.

21

Treatment patterns in psoriatic arthritis patients newly initiated on oral nonbiologic or biologic disease-modifying antirheumatic drugs

Huabin F Zhang[1], Geneviève Gauthier[2], Robert Hiscock[2] and Jeffrey R Curtis[3*]

Abstract

Introduction: This study aimed to describe treatment changes (discontinuation, switching, and therapy add-on) following the initiation of biologic or nonbiologic oral disease-modifying antirheumatic drugs (DMARDs) in psoriatic arthritis (PsA) patients.

Methods: Adult patients with ≥2 PsA diagnoses from physician office visits, initiated on a biologic or nonbiologic oral DMARD, were selected from the Truven Health Analytics MarketScan® Research Database (2005 to 2009). Patients were required to have continuous insurance coverage ≥6 months prior to and ≥12 months post index date (first prescription fill date). Treatment discontinuation, treatment switch, and therapy add-on were captured over the 1 year period following the index date. Treatment changes were described separately for patients initiated on nonbiologic and biologic DMARDs.

Results: A total of 1,698 and 3,263 patients were initiated on an oral nonbiologic DMARD and biologic DMARD respectively. For patients initiated on nonbiologic DMARDs, 69% had ≥1 therapy change over the 12 month study period (median time 85 days). Among patients who had a therapy change, 83% discontinued, 29% switched therapy (64% switched to a biologic DMARD), and 25% had a therapy add-on (76% added-on with a biologic DMARD). For patients initiated on a biologic DMARD, 46% had ≥1 therapy change (median time 110 days). Among patients who had a therapy change, 100% discontinued, 25% switched therapy (92% switched to another biologic DMARD), and 7% had a therapy add-on with a nonbiologic DMARD.

Conclusion: This study suggests that PsA patients newly initiated on a nonbiologic/biologic DMARD do not remain on the index treatment for a long period of time. A better understanding of factors related to these early treatment changes in PsA patients is needed.

Introduction

Psoriatic arthritis (PsA), an idiopathic, chronic, and often progressive immune-mediated autoinflammatory arthritis, affects peripheral and axial joints, nails and entheses, and is typically accompanied by psoriatic skin lesions [1,2]. Although phenotypically heterogeneous, PsA symptoms typically include joint pain, stiffness, swelling, nail psoriasis, dactylitis and generalized fatigue [1,3]. In the United States, the prevalence of PsA is estimated to be between 0.10% and 0.25% of the overall population [1].

* Correspondence: jcurtis@uab.edu
[3]University of Alabama at Birmingham, 510 20th St. South FOT 802D, Birmingham, AL 35294, USA
Full list of author information is available at the end of the article

The immediate treatment goals in PsA include mitigating joint pain and swelling, skin lesions, disease progression, and systemic sequelae [3,4]. The ultimate treatment goal - disease remission - is characterized by the absence of clinically discernible disease activity and the potential for joint healing [4,5]. Pharmacotherapy for PsA encompasses nonsteroidal anti-inflammatory drugs (NSAIDs) and intra-articular corticosteroid injections to manage musculoskeletal pain, stiffness, and swelling, as well as nonbiologic and biologic disease-modifying antirheumatic drugs (DMARDs), which have the potential to attenuate joint damage and promote disease remission [6].

American Academy of Dermatology (AAD) and the European League against Rheumatism (EULAR) recommended treatment guidelines for PsA advocate a stepwise approach to treatment based on symptom severity, joint involvement, and the extent of inflammation [6-8]. Mild PsA is typically treated with NSAIDs or intra-articular corticosteroid injections [6,9]. If a satisfactory response is not achieved after 3 months, or if there is evidence of persistent inflammation or of erosive or polyarticular disease, the guidelines suggest the option of using a traditional oral nonbiologic DMARD, such as methotrexate (MTX) [7-9]. Yet the clinical data supporting the use of MTX as a disease-modifying agent in PsA remain limited [10-13]. In a recent double-blind, randomized, placebo-controlled study in patients with active PsA, MTX treatment failed to improve objective assessments of synovitis or of tender and swollen joint counts, despite improvements in skin scores and patients' and assessors' global evaluations [13]. If traditional oral nonbiologic DMARDs cannot properly control the signs and symptoms of PsA, the guidelines suggest the use of biologics such as etanercept and adalimumab [7]. Biologics have demonstrated robust efficacy in PsA to date [2]. A recent study investigating potential effects of MTX co-medication with TNF inhibitor (TNFi) - a type of biologic - on treatment response and persistence in PsA patients found a benefit in terms of treatment persistence of using MTX concomitantly with another TNFi [14]. Despite the treatment guidelines and clinical studies that demonstrate the benefits and risks of oral DMARDs and biologics in PsA, it remains unclear how physicians generally approach the management of PsA. The main objective of this study was to describe treatment patterns (treatment discontinuation, treatment switches, and therapy add-ons) for PsA patients newly treated with oral nonbiologic or biologic DMARDs in a real-world setting.

Methods

Data source

This retrospective study used data from the US-based Truven Health Analytics MarketScan® Research Databases, acquired between the first quarter (Q1) of 2005 and Q4 of 2009. The database included approximately 25 million individuals, annually covered by 130 health plans and self-insured employers. The database covers all census regions in the US and contains information on patient demographics, enrollment history, claims for inpatient and outpatient medical services, and pharmacy claims. Patient data were de-identified and comply with the patient confidentiality requirements of the Health Insurance Portability and Accountability Act. Therefore, Institutional Review Board approval was not required.

Sample selection and construction

Adult PsA patients newly treated with oral nonbiologic DMARDs or biologic DMARDs were selected in this study. Patients initiated on nonbiologic DMARDs were required to be naïve to any biologic or nonbiologic DMARDs recommended for PsA before the first oral nonbiologic DMARD initiation date (index date). Biologic DMARD patients may have been pre-treated with a nonbiologic DMARD before the index date. Adult patients with active PsA were defined as those who were at least 18 years of age at the index date and had at least two physician PsA diagnoses (ICD-9-CM code: 696.0x) from two separate office visits over the 18-month observation period (that is, at least one diagnosis during the 6-month period before the index date (baseline period), and at least one during the 12-month period after the index date (study period)). Patients who did not have at least a 6-month baseline period or 12-month study period in the database were excluded from the study.

Oral nonbiologic DMARDs considered included MTX, cyclosporine, leflunomide, mycophenolate, gold compounds, antimalarials, minocycline, penicillamine, azathioprine, and sulfasalazine. Due to the wide use of MTX in PsA, a subgroup analysis was conducted for patients newly initiated on MTX. Biologic DMARDs in the study included etanercept, infliximab, golimumab, certolizumab pegol, adalimumab, anakinra, abatacept, and rituximab based on clinical use although some do not have indication in PsA. Patients were excluded if they had a diagnosis of ankylosing spondylitis (AS) (ICD-9-CM code: 720.0x) at any time before the index date.

Patients newly initiated on oral nonbiologic DMARDs and biologic DMARDs were analyzed separately during the baseline and study period. These two samples were not mutually exclusive. For example, a patient initiating therapy on an oral nonbiologic DMARD who later switched to a biologic DMARD could be included in both samples if the two initiation dates met all the aforementioned selection criteria. However, this had no impact on the study analyses and interpretation of the results, given that the two samples were analyzed independently, and no direct statistical analyses were performed between the two samples.

Outcome measures

Therapy change

As defined subsequently, therapy change was defined as the discontinuation of the index treatment (that is, the nonbiologic or biologic DMARD initiated at the index date), a switch from the index treatment to another treatment, or a therapy add-on. Patients may have had more than one therapy change over the study period.

Discontinuation

Treatment discontinuation was defined as the first occurrence of a treatment interruption of at least 60 consecutive days between the end of the drug supply for a prescription of the index treatment and the beginning of a next prescription for the index treatment, or the end of the one-year study period, whichever occurred first.

Treatment switch

A treatment switch was defined as the initiation of a treatment other than the index DMARD within 60 days of the interruption of the index treatment. For patients initiated on an oral nonbiologic or on a biologic DMARD, other nonbiologic (either oral or subcutaneous), or biologic DMARDs were considered as switch treatments. Additionally, as patients initiated on a biologic could have used nonbiologic DMARDs prior to the index date, the nonbiologic treatment (either oral or subcutaneous) to which the patient was being switched could not have been taken during the 60-day period prior to the switch date. For patients who initiated concomitant treatments on the index date, any treatments used at the index date were not considered potential switch treatments. Treatment switches were captured from the index date up to 60 days after the first discontinuation of the index treatment, or up to the end of the study period, whichever occurred first. All treatments initiated within the 60 days following treatment discontinuation were reported as a switch.

Therapy add-on

Therapy add-on was defined as the use of a DMARD treatment other than the treatment used at the index date for at least 28 consecutive days before the discontinuation of the index therapy. For patients initiated on an oral nonbiologic DMARD, the use of any other nonbiologic DMARDs (either oral or subcutaneous), or biologic DMARDs were considered potential therapy add-on treatments. For patients initiated on a biologic DMARD, nonbiologic DMARDs (either oral or subcutaneous) were considered potential therapy add-on treatment agents. Additionally, as patients who were initiated on a biologic DMARD may have used nonbiologic DMARDs prior to the index date, the DMARD used for add-on was required to have not been taken during the 60-day period prior to the start of therapy add-on. For patients who initiated concomitant treatments at the index date, any treatments used at the index date were not considered potential add-on treatments. Add-on rates were captured over the period spanning from the index date up to the discontinuation of the index treatment, or until the end of the study period, whichever occurred first.

Sensitivity analyses

It may be difficult in claims data to ensure that the selected PsA patients have been accurately diagnosed for PsA, particularly since some of the core symptoms of PsA are also present in AS or rheumatoid arthritis (RA). However, AS and RA may similarly lead to patient misclassification as a PsA diagnosis, or may have overlapping features with PsA. As a result, two sensitivity analyses were performed to test the robustness of our findings; (1) as AS patients were excluded in the main analysis, the first sensitivity analysis was conducted without excluding patients with AS, and (2) as RA patients were included in the main analysis, the second sensitivity analysis excluded patients diagnosed with RA.

Additionally, as a supplemental sensitivity analysis, discontinuation was defined as the first occurrence of a treatment interruption of at least 90 consecutive days between the end of the drug supply (for a prescription of the index treatment) and the beginning of a next prescription (for the index treatment), or the end of the one-year study period, whichever occurred first.

Statistical analyses

Baseline data were analyzed descriptively and reported separately for patients initiated on an oral nonbiologic DMARD, for patients initiated on a biologic DMARD, and for the subgroup of patients initiated on MTX. Reported characteristics included demographics (age, gender), treatment characteristics, specialist encounters, and comorbidities. The Charlson comorbidity index (CCI) adapted by Deyo for administrative databases was used to assess the level of comorbidity associated with each PsA cohort [15].

Treatment patterns were reported separately for patients initiated on an oral nonbiologic DMARD, on a biologic DMARD, and for patients from the MTX subgroup. The proportions of patients who discontinued the index treatment, switched to another DMARD, had a therapy add-on, or had any therapy changes over the 12-month study period were reported. Additionally, the proportion of patients who remained on the index treatment, and the proportion of patients using any nonbiologic or biologic DMARD at the end of each month during the 12-month study period were reported. No comparative analyses were performed between samples. As patients could have more than one type of treatment change, the percentage of all changes does not always add up to 100%.

The median time to the observed therapy change was also reported. Median time to therapy change was calculated among patients who incurred the studied therapy change as the number of days between the index date and the date of the studied therapy change.

Results

Overall, 1,698 patients met the sample selection criteria and initiated an oral nonbiologic DMARD on the index date, with the majority being initiated on MTX (71%, n = 1,217). Additionally, 3,263 patients met the sample selection criteria and initiated a biologic DMARD treatment on the index date (Figure 1).

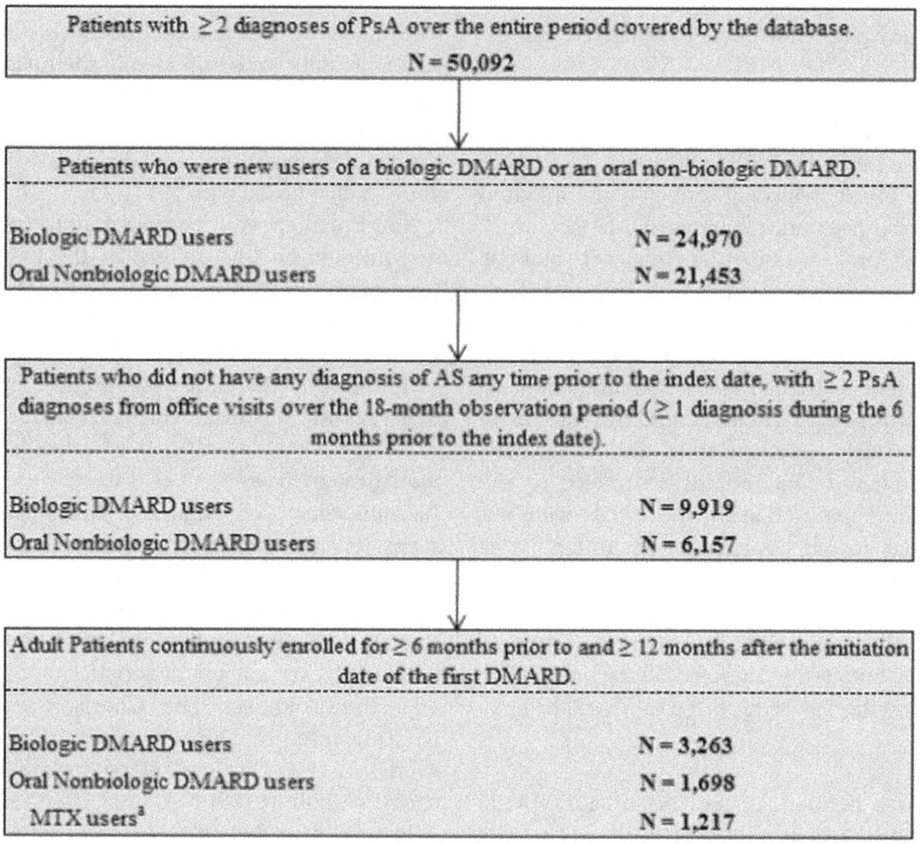

Figure 1 Sample selection criteria results. [a]MTX users are a subgroup of the oral nonbiologic DMARD users. DMARD, disease-modifying antirheumatic drug; MTX, methotrexate; NSAID, nonsteroidal anti-inflammatory drug; PsA, psoriatic arthritis.

Baseline characteristics

Patients' average age was approximately 50 years, and a slight majority (54%) was female (Table 1). Over 60% of patients were seen by a rheumatologist during the baseline period or at the index date, and approximately a quarter were seen by a dermatologist. Average CCI was 0.47, 0.44, and 0.52 for patients initiated on an oral nonbiologic DMARD, MTX, and biologic DMARD therapy, respectively. The most common comorbidities during the baseline period were psoriasis (approximately 35%), hypertension (approximately 20%), diabetes (approximately 11%), and hypothyroidism (approximately 6%) (Table 1).

During the baseline period, 58% of patients initiated on an oral nonbiologic DMARD were treated with an NSAID, and 32% received oral corticosteroids. For patients initiated on a biologic DMARD, 59% used a nonbiologic DMARD during the baseline period, 51% an NSAID, and 32% an oral corticosteroid. Approximately 10% of patients initiated on an oral nonbiologic DMARD used an oral corticosteroid at the index date, while approximately 46% of patients initiated on a biologic DMARD used a nonbiologic DMARD and/or an oral corticosteroid at the index date (35% used a biologic DMARD and a nonbiologic DMARD, 5% used a biologic DMARD and an oral corticosteroid, and 6% used a biologic DMARD, a nonbiologic DMARD, and an oral corticosteroid). These numbers included patients who initiated a nonbiologic DMARD and/or an oral corticosteroid at the index date or prior to the index date and whose prescription overlapped with the index date. For patients initiated on an oral nonbiologic DMARD, the average total healthcare cost per patient over the 6-month baseline period was $5,377, while the same period yielded an average cost of only $2,476 for patients initiated on a biologic DMARD.

Therapy changes

Oral nonbiologic DMARD users

Overall, 69% of patients initiated on an oral nonbiologic DMARD and 65% of patients in the MTX subgroup had at least one therapy change during the course of the 12-month study. The median time to the first therapy change was 85 days for patients initiated on an oral nonbiologic DMARD and 93 days for the MTX subgroup.

Among patients who had at least one therapy change, 47% of the oral nonbiologic DMARD users and 55% of the patients in the MTX subgroup used a biologic DMARD at some point during the 12-month study

Table 1 Baseline[a] characteristics

Characteristics	Oral nonbiologic DMARD patients N = 1,698	MTX patients N = 1,217	Biologic DMARD patients N = 3,263
Demographics			
Age, mean (SD)	49.8 (12.5)	49.8 (12.3)	49.4 (11.6)
Female, number (%)	927 (54.6)	657 (54.0)	1,736 (53.2)
Combination of treatment with another nonbiologic DMARD and/or oral corticosteriod at the index date	168 (9.9)	138 (11.3)	1,512 (46.3)
During the 6-month pre-index period, including the index date			
Specialist encounter, number (%)			
Rheumatologist or Dermatologist	1,175 (69.2)	841 (12.3)	2,347 (71.9)
Rheumatologist	1,055 (62.1)	755 (62.0)	2,008 (61.5)
Dermatologist	384 (22.6)	271 (22.3)	896 (27.5)
During the 6-month pre-index period			
Comorbidities[b,c], number (%)			
Hypertension	364 (21.4)	260 (21.4)	670 (20.5)
Diabetes	175 (10.3)	129 (10.6)	376 (11.5)
Hypothyroidism	114 (6.7)	81 (6.7)	200 (6.1)
Chronic pulmonary disease	111 (6.5)	72 (5.9)	176 (5.4)
Deficiency anemia	77 (4.5)	62 (5.1)	164 (5.0)
Psoriasis	545 (32.1)	420 (34.5)	1,194 (36.6)
Charlson comorbidity index, mean (SD)	0.47 (0.87)	0.44 (0.84)	0.52 (0.88)
Prior use of NSAID, oral corticosteriod, and nonbiologic DMARDs, number (%)			
NSAIDs	991 (58.4)	701 (57.6)	1,665 (51.0)
Oral corticosteriods	550 (32.4)	396 (32.5)	1,036 (31.7)
Nonbiologic DMARDs	0 (0.0)	0 (0.0)	1,938 (59.4)

[a]The baseline period consisted of the 6-month period prior to the index date. [b]Elixhauser A, Steiner C, Kruzikas D. Comorbidity Software. January 2004. HCUP Methods Series Report #2004-1. Online, February 6, 2004. US Agency for Healthcare Research and Quality: pp 12-15 [16]. [c] Only mental and physical comorbidities where at least one of the reported cohorts had a prevalence of ≥5% were reported in the table. DMARD, disease-modifying antirheumatic drugs; MTX, methotrexate; number, number of patients; NSAID, nonsteroidal anti-inflammatory drug.

period. The median time to the first biologic DMARD use was 138 days for oral nonbiologic DMARD users and 135 days for patients in the MTX subgroup (Figure 2).

Among patients who had at least one therapy change, 83% discontinued treatment (median time: 89 days), 29% switched (median time: 113 days), and 25% had a therapy add-on (median time: 116 days) (Figure 3). Among patients who switched therapies, 64% switched to a biologic DMARD (median time: 141 days), and 46% switched to another nonbiologic DMARD (median time: 111 days). Among patients who had a therapy add-on, 76% of patients added-on with a biologic DMARD (median time: 119 days), and 28% added-on with another nonbiologic DMARD (median time: 94 days).

Among the patients in the MTX subgroup who had at least one therapy change, 79% discontinued (median time: 96 days), 30% had a therapy add-on (median time: 122 days), and 25% switched (median time: 132 days) (Figure 3). Among the patients who switched therapies, 73% switched to a biologic DMARD (median time: 139 days), and 33% switched to another nonbiologic DMARD (median time: 161 days). Among the patients who had a therapy add-on, 84% had a biologic DMARD added (median time: 122 days), and 19% had another non-biologic DMARD added (median time: 125 days).

Among patients initiated on an oral nonbiologic DMARD, 80%, 62%, 43%, and 31% of the patients were still continuously treated with the index therapy by the end of the first, third, sixth, and twelfth month following the index date, respectively (Figure 4). Further, 88%, 77%, 66%, and 56% were still continuously treated with any nonbiologic or biologic DMARD at the end of the first, third, sixth, and twelfth month following the index date, respectively (Figure 5).

Biologic DMARD users

Overall, 46% of the patients had at least one therapy change during the course of the 12-month study period.

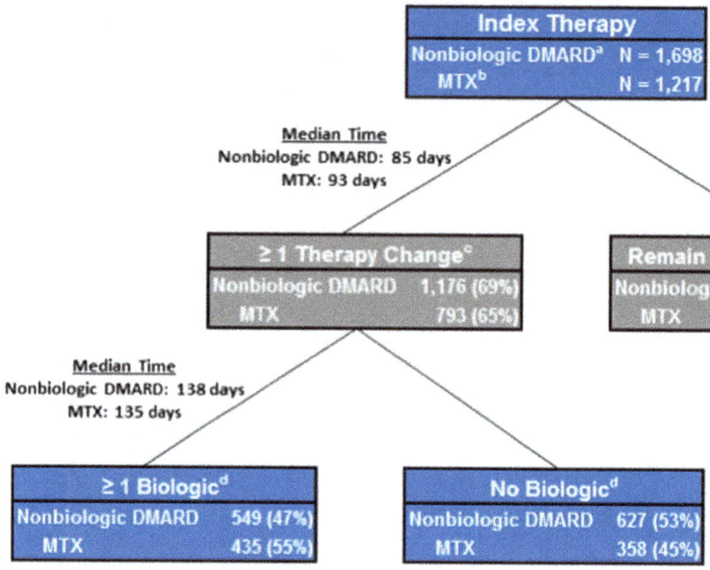

Figure 2 Biologic use in oral nonbiologic DMARD patients and in MTX patients. [a]This refers to oral nonbiologic DMARD users. [b]MTX users are a subgroup of the oral nonbiologic DMARD users. [c]These categories presented are mutually exclusive. [d]These categories presented are mutually exclusive. DMARD, disease-modifying antirheumatic drug; MTX, methotrexate.

The median time to the first therapy change was 110 days. All patients who had at least one therapy change discontinued the index biologic treatment at some point during the 12-month study period (median time: 122 days). Additionally, among patients who had at least one therapy change, 25% of patients switched (median time: 173 days), and 7% of patients had a therapy add-on with a nonbiologic DMARD (median time: 59 days). Among patients who switched therapies, 92% of the patients switched to another biologic DMARD (median time: 181 days), and 11% switched to a nonbiologic DMARD (median time: 92 days) (Figure 6). Moreover, 92%, 80%, 67%, and 54% of patients were still continuously treated with the index therapy by the end of the first, third, sixth, and twelfth month following the index date, respectively (Figure 4), and approximately

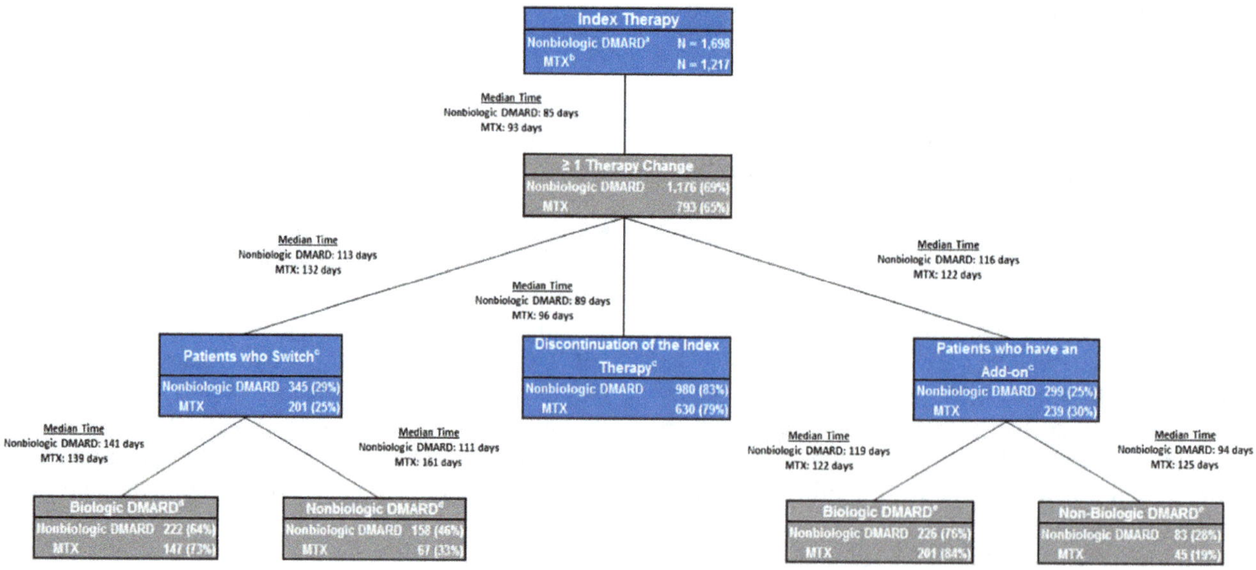

Figure 3 Detailed schematic of therapy changes in oral nonbiologic DMARD patients and in MTX. [a]This refers to oral nonbiologic DMARD users. [b]MTX users are a subgroup of the oral nonbiologic DMARD users. [c]These categories presented are not mutually exclusive. [d]These categories presented are not mutually exclusive. [e]These categories presented are not mutually exclusive. DMARD, disease-modifying antirheumatic drug; MTX, methotrexate.

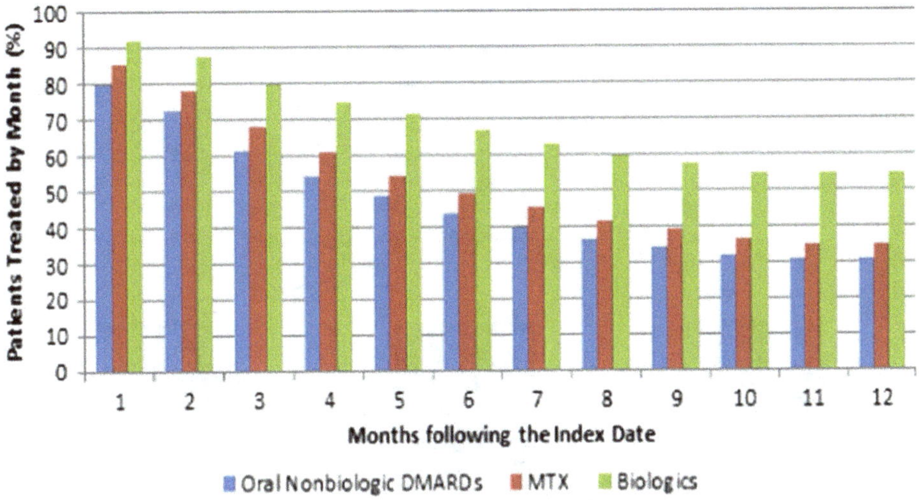

Figure 4 Patients remaining on the index therapy by month. DMARD, disease-modifying antirheumatic drug; MTX, methotrexate.

96%, 89%, 80%, and 69% were still continuously treated with a nonbiologic or biologic DMARD at the end of the first, third, sixth, and twelfth month following the index date, respectively (Figure 5).

Sensitivity analyses

Consistent results were found from the two sensitivity analyses performed on data subsets that (1) did not exclude patients with AS and (2) excluded patients with RA led to consistent findings (results not reported). Among all patients initiated on an oral nonbiologic DMARD, 51% were calculated to have discontinued their index therapy when using a 90-day treatment gap definition for discontinuation, as opposed to the 58% that discontinued in the study analysis with a 60-day treatment gap (results not reported). Additionally, among the entire subgroup of patients initiated on MTX, 44% discontinued their index therapy in the 90-day treatment gap analysis, as opposed to the 52% reported using a 60-day treatment gap. Further, among all patients that were initiated on a biologic DMARD, 36% discontinued their index therapy in the 90-day discontinuation gap analysis, as opposed to the 46% identified using a 60-day treatment gap (results not reported).

Discussion

This large, retrospective study described nonbiologic and biologic DMARD treatment patterns in patients

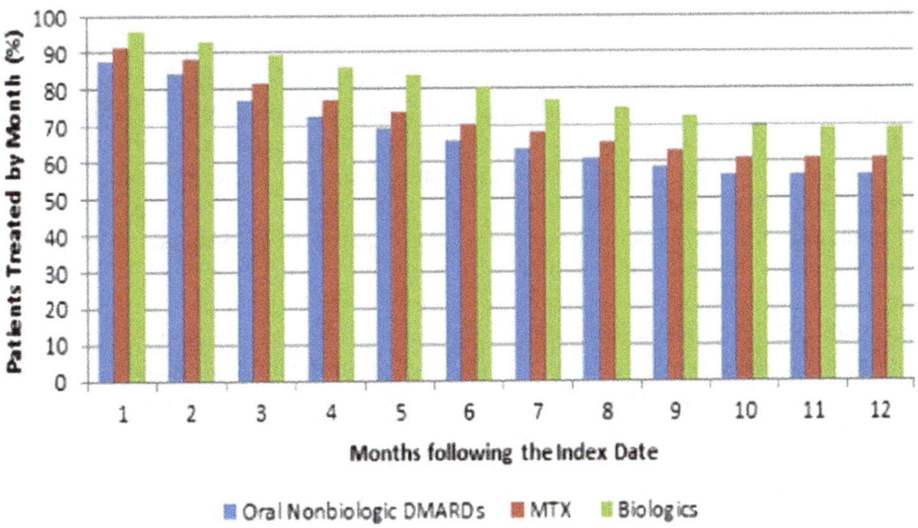

Figure 5 Patients remaining on any PsA-related therapy by month. In this figure, only nonbiologic DMARDs and biologic DMARDs are considered as any PsA-related therapy. DMARD, disease-modifying antirheumatic drug; MTX, methotrexate; PsA, psoriatic arthritis.

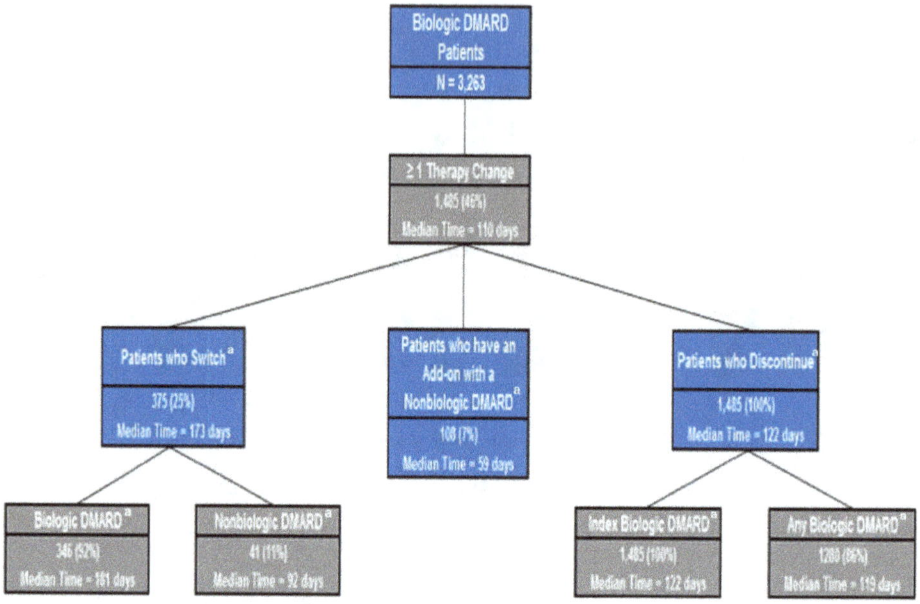

Figure 6 Detailed schematic of therapy changes in biologic DMARD patients. [a]These categories presented are not mutually exclusive.

with PsA based on real-world data gleaned from US-health plans and self-insured employers. Outcome measures included changes documented from the initial DMARD therapy over a 1-year period following treatment initiation, including treatment discontinuations, switches, and therapy add-ons. Recent studies have analyzed treatment patterns for specific biologic DMARDs (adalimumab, etanercept, and infliximab) in patients with RA, psoriasis, PsA, or AS, or in patients with PsA alone [17,18]. Other studies also examined treatment response to different patterns of treatments (for example, investigating the effectiveness of switching to a second TNFi) or the effect of concomitant MTX on treatment response and persistence. However, little is known about treatment patterns when patients are newly initiated on a DMARD, stratified by nonbiologic and biologic DMARDs. This study differs from those reported previously in the literature as it investigates treatment patterns in PsA patients following the initiation of nonbiologic and biologic DMARDs by separately grouping all patients initiated on various nonbiologic DMARDs together in one group, while pooling all patients initiated on various biologic DMARDs together in another study group.

The results revealed that in a sample of 1,698 commercially insured PsA patients newly initiated on an oral nonbiologic DMARD, mainly MTX, patient persistence with treatment was generally low and relatively brief. Almost 70% of these patients had at least one therapy change within the first year, with the initial change generally occurring within the first 3 months after the index date. Moreover, among patients who had at least one therapy change, the majority (83%) discontinued treatment after 3 months. Of those patients who switched treatment or had a therapy add-on, most switched to or added on a biologic DMARD. Similar to the findings in this study, investigators have shown that, in patients with RA, treatment persistence with nonbiologic DMARDs - mainly MTX, chloroquine, and sulfasalazine - erodes rapidly and progressively over time, with persistence rates declining from approximately 70% at one year to 34% at 2 years [19]. In the current analysis, only 31% of the patients persisted uninterruptedly with their initial nonbiologic DMARD therapy after one year, and slightly more than half (56%) persisted uninterruptedly with any nonbiologic or biologic DMARD after one year.

For the patients treated with a biologic DMARD, more than half (54%) persisted with their initial therapy throughout the entire 1-year study period and almost three-quarters (70%) remained on PsA therapy. Of the patients who switched therapy, the vast majority (92%) were treated with another biologic DMARD. These results suggest that patients initiated on a biologic DMARD tend to remain on this form of therapy and do not switch back to nonbiologic DMARDs. In addition, very few patients (7%) had a therapy add-on with a nonbiologic DMARD. Other investigators using retrospective data analyses have also found relatively robust treatment persistence with the use of biologic DMARDs in the treatment of PsA [17,18,20]. In these studies, one-year treatment persistence rates for biologic DMARDs ranged from approximately 50% to

70%, which are consistent with our findings. In one of the studies, relatively high rates of persistence after one year were associated with correspondingly high treatment-response rates [20].

In real-world clinical practice, patients may change therapies for different reasons. Although reasons for the low rate of persistence with the initial DMARD therapy were not available in the database, a potential reason for therapy change may include the lack of effectiveness of the DMARD at controlling patient symptoms and slowing disease progression. Patients might also switch or discontinue treatment due to tolerability or safety issues, or occurrence of adverse events, or discontinue treatment due to disease remission or pregnancy. PsA patients may also switch due to persistent activity of psoriasis rather than PsA Other potential reasons may also include changes in the reimbursement policy of healthcare plan or the involvement of multiple physicians in the management of PsA or other economic reasons. Moreover, many healthcare insurance plans require, for reimbursement purposes, that patients first use at least one to two nonbiologic DMARDs prior to using a biologic DMARD. This may also contribute to the high rates of therapy switch to/add-on of a biologic DMARD among patients initiated on a nonbiologic DMARD. However, further analyses would be warranted to confirm the main reasons for treatment changes in PsA patients.

Study limitations

Our study was subject to the common limitations of retrospective, observational studies based on healthcare claims data. For instance, the severity of PsA symptoms varied among individuals and could presumably affect a patient's treatment profile. However, claims databases record diagnostic and procedural codes only and do not reveal disease severity. Moreover, claim data typically report diagnoses/procedures associated with the healthcare services provided for reimbursement purposes and might underestimate patients' other comorbid conditions (not related to diagnoses received or procedures performed) that are not systematically reported by the physician. For example, in this study, there were only 32% of nonbiologic DMARD patients and 37% of biologic DMARD patients who had a recorded diagnosis for psoriasis. Similarly, only 1.6% of biologic DMARD patients and 2.3% of nonbiologic DMARD patients had a recorded diagnosis for obesity during the baseline period. This suggests an underestimation of the prevalence of these conditions. Further, claims databases do not provide any information regarding the underlying reasons for therapy changes. This study also was limited to a 12-month period following the initiation of a DMARD. Further analyses are warranted to observe treatment patterns over a longer period of time. In addition, the influence of corticosteroid use on treatment patterns was not assessed. Moreover, the study covered the period from 2005 to 2009, an interval when the use of biologic DMARDs for PsA was still relatively new. Patterns of biologic DMARD use may have changed in more recent years. Finally, when performing claims data analyses, it may be difficult to ensure that the selected PsA patients have been accurately diagnosed for PsA, especially as some of the core symptoms of PsA also are known to manifest in AS or RA. The two sensitivity analyses around these topics led to findings consistent with the main analysis.

Conclusion

This retrospective analysis, based on large and geographically broad US health plan data, provides real-world insight into nonbiologic and biologic DMARD treatment patterns in patients with PsA. The results suggest that the majority of patients treated with nonbiologic or biologic DMARDs change therapy early after treatment initiation, with many switching to a biologic DMARD therapy or, in nonbiologic users, adding on a biologic DMARD. Among the initial biologic DMARD patients who end up switching therapies, the majority do so with another biologic DMARD (as opposed to a non-biologic DMARD). These results suggest that a better understanding of factors related to early DMARD treatment changes in PsA patients are needed to optimize treatment.

Abbreviations

AAD: American Academy of Dermatology; AS: ankylosing spondylistis; CCI: Charlson comorbidity index; DMARD: disease-modifying antirheumatic drug; MTX: methotrexate; NSAID: nonsteroidal anti-inflamatory drug; PsA: psoriatic arthritis; RA: rheumatoid arthritis. TNFi, tumor necrosis factor inhibitor.

Competing interests

This study was funded by Celgene Corporation. Huabin Frank Zhang is an employee of Celgene Corporation and owns stock/stock options. Geneviève Gauthier and Robert Hiscock are employees of Analysis Group Inc., which has received consultancy fees from Celgene Corporation. Jeffrey R Curtis is an employee of the University of Alabama at Birmingham who has received consultancy fees from Celgene Corporation.

Authors' contributions

HFZ and JRC participated in the study design, interpretation of the results, and participated in the preparation and revision of the manuscript. GG and RH participated in the study design, data analysis, interpretation of the results, and participated in the preparation and revision of the manuscript. All authors read and approved the manuscript.

Author details

[1]Celgene Corporation, 86 Morris Ave, Summit, NJ 07901, USA. [2]Analysis Group Inc, 111 Huntington Ave #10, Boston, MA 02199, USA. [3]University of Alabama at Birmingham, 510 20th St. South FOT 802D, Birmingham, AL 35294, USA.

References

1. Lee S, Mendelsohn A, Sarnes E: **The burden of psoriatic arthritis: a literature review from a global health systems perspective.** *P T* 2010, 35:680–689.

2. Cantini F, Niccoli L, Nannini C, Kaloudi O, Bertoni M, Cassarà E: **Psoriatic arthritis: a systematic review.** *Int J Rheum Dis* 2010, **13:**300–317.
3. Arthritis Foundation: **Psoriatic arthritis.** [http://www.arthritis.org/conditions-treatments/disease-center/psoriatic-arthritis/]
4. Kavanaugh A, Fransen J: **Defining remission in psoriatic arthritis.** *Clin Exp Rheumatol* 2006, **24:**S83–S87.
5. Saber TP, Ng CT, Renard G, Lynch BM, Pontifex E, Walsh CA, Grier A, Molloy M, Bresnihan B, Fitzgerald O, Fearon U, Veale DJ: **Remission in psoriatic arthritis: is it possible and how can it be predicted?** *Arthritis Res Ther* 2010, **12:**R94.
6. Ritchlin CT, Kavanaugh A, Gladman DD, Mease PJ, Helliwell P, Boehncke WH, de Vlam K, Fiorentino D, Fitzgerald O, Gottlied AB, McHugh NJ, Nash P, Qureshi AA, Soriano ER, Taylor WJ: **Treatment recommendations for psoriatic arthritis.** *Ann Rheum Dis* 2009, **69:**1387–1394.
7. Day MS, Nam D, Goodman S, Su EP, Figgie M: **Psoriatic arthritis.** *J Am Acad Orthop Surg* 2012, **20:**28–37.
8. Gossec L, Smolen JS, Gaujoux-Viala C, Ash Z, Marzo-Ortega H, van der Heijde D, Fitzgerald O, Aletaha D, Balint P, Boumpas D, Braun J, Breedveld FC, Burmester G, Cañete JD, de Wit M, Dagfinrud H, de Vlam K, Dougados M, Helliwell P, Kavanaugh A, Kvien T, Landewé R, Luger T, Maccarone M, McGonagle D, McHugh N, McInnes IM, Ritchlin C, Sieper J, Tak PP, *et al*: **European League Against Rheumatism recommendations for the management of psoriatic arthritis with pharmacological therapies.** *Ann Rheum Dis* 2012, **71:**2–12.
9. Menter A, Korman NJ, Elmets CA, Feldman SR, Gelfand JM, Gordon KB, Gottlieb A, Koo JYM, Lebwohl M, Leonardi CL, Lim HW, Van Voorhees AS, Beutner KR, Ryan C, Bhushan R: **Guidelines of care for the management of psoriasis and psoriatic arthritis: Section 2. Overview and guidelines of care for treatment with an emphasis on the biologics.** *J Am Acad Dermatol* 2011, **58:**826–850.
10. Black RL, O'Brien WM, Vanscott EJ, Auerbach R, Eisen AZ, Bunim JJ: **Methotrexate Therapy in Psoriatic Arthritis; Double-Blind Study on 21 Patients.** *JAMA* 1964, **189:**743–747.
11. Willkens RF, Williams HJ, Ward JR, Egger MJ, Reading JC, Clements PJ, Cathcart ES, Samuelson CO Jr, Solsky MA, Kaplan SB, Guttadauria M, Halla JT, Weinstein A: **Randomized, double-blind, placebo controlled trial of low-dose pulse methotrexate in psoriatic arthritis.** *Arthritis Rheum* 1984, **27:**376–381.
12. Scarpa R, Peluso R, Atteno M, Manguso F, Spanò A, Iervolino S, Di Minno MN, Costa L, Del Puente A: **The effectiveness of a traditional therapeutical approach in early psoriatic arthritis: results of a pilot randomised 6-month trial with methotrexate.** *Clin Rheumatol* 2008, **27:**823–826.
13. Kingsley GH, Kowalczyk A, Taylor H, Ibrahim F, Packham JC, McHugh NJ, Mulherin DM, Kitas GD, Chakravarty K, Tom BD, O'Keeffe AG, Maddison PJ, Scott DL: **A randomized placebo-controlled trial of methotrexate in psoriatic arthritis.** *Rheumatology (Oxford)* 2012, **51:**1368–1377.
14. Fagerli KM, Lie E, van der Heijde D, van der Heijde D, Heiberg MS, Lexberg AS, Rødevand E, Kalstad S, Mikkelsen K, Kvien TK: **The role of methotrexate co-medication in TNF-inhibitor treatment in patients with psoriatic arthritis: results from 440 patients included in the NOR-DMARD study.** *Ann Rheum Dis* 2014, **73:**132–137.
15. Deyo RA, Cherkin DC, Ciol MA: **Adapting a clinical comorbidity index for use with ICD-9-CM administrative databases.** *J Clin Epidemiol* 1992, **45:**613–619.
16. Elixhauser A, Steiner C, Kruzikas D: **Comorbidity Software. HCUP Methods Series Report #2004-1.** [http://www.hcup-us.ahrq.gov/reports/ComorbiditySoftwareDocumentationFinal.pdf]
17. Bonafede M, Fox KM, Watson C, Princic N, Gandra SR: **Treatment patterns in the first year after initiating tumor necrosis factor blockers in real-world settings.** *Adv Ther* 2012, **29:**664–674.
18. Chastek B, Fox KM, Watson C, Gandra SR: **Etanercept and adalimumab treatment patterns in psoriatic arthritis patients enrolled in a commercial health plan.** *Adv Ther* 2012, **29:**691–697.
19. Pascual-Ramos V, Contreras-Yáñez I, Villa AR, Cabiedes J, Rull-Gabayet M: **Medication persistence over 2 years of follow-up in a cohort of early rheumatoid arthritis patients: associated factors and relationship with disease activity and with disability.** *Arthritis Res Ther* 2009, **11:**R26.
20. Glintborg B, Østergaard M, Dreyer L, Krogh NS, Tarp U, Hansen MS, Rifbjerg-Madsen S, Lorenzen T, Hetland ML: **Treatment response, drug survival, and predictors thereof in 764 patients with psoriatic arthritis treated with anti-tumor necrosis factor alpha therapy: results from the nationwide Danish DANBIO registry.** *Arthritis Rheum* 2011, **63:**382–390.

Progranulin antibodies entertain a proinflammatory environment in a subgroup of patients with psoriatic arthritis

Lorenz Thurner[1*], Marina Zaks[1], Klaus-Dieter Preuss[1], Natalie Fadle[1], Evi Regitz[1], Mei Fang Ong[2], Michael Pfreundschuh[1] and Gunter Assmann[1]

Abstract

Introduction: Psoriatic arthritis (PsA) is a distinctive inflammatory arthritis which may typically develop in a subgroup of individuals suffering from psoriasis. We recently described progranulin autoantibodies (PGRN-Abs) in the sera of patients with different autoimmune diseases including seronegative polyarthritis. In the present study we investigated the occurrence of PGRN-Abs in PsA.

Methods: PGRN-Abs were determined in 260 patients with PsA, 100 patients with psoriasis without arthritic manifestations (PsC) and 97 healthy controls using a recently described ELISA. PGRN plasma levels were determined from subgroups by a commercially available ELISA-kit. Possible functional effects of PGRN-antibodies were analysed *in vitro* by tumour necrosis factor (TNF)-α mediated cytotoxicity assays using WEHI-S and HT1080 cells.

Results: PGRN-Abs were detected with relevant titres in 50/260 (19.23%) patients with PsA, but in 0/100 patients with psoriasis without arthritic manifestations ($P = 0.0001$). All PGRN-Abs belonged to immunoglobulin G (IgG). PGRN-Abs were significantly more frequent in PsA patients with enthesitis or dactylitis. PGRN-Abs were also more frequent in PsA patients receiving treatment with TNF-α-blockers than in patients treated without TNF-α-blockers (20.8% versus 17.4%; $P = 0.016$). PGRN plasma levels were significantly lower in PGRN-Ab-positive patients with PsA than in healthy controls and patients with psoriasis without arthritic manifestations ($P < 0.001$), indicating a neutralizing effect of PGRN-Abs. Moreover cytotoxicity assays comparing PGRN-antibody positive with negative sera from matched patients with PsA, clearly showed a proinflammatory effect of PGRN antibodies.

Conclusion: Neutralizing PGRN-Abs occur with relevant titres in a subgroup of patients with PsA, but not in patients without arthritic manifestations (PsC). PGRN-Ab-positive patients had more frequent enthesitis or dactylitis. TNF-α-induced cytotoxicity assays demonstrated that the protective effects of progranulin were inhibited by serum containing PGRN-Abs. This suggests that PGRN-Ab might not only be useful as a diagnostic and prognostic marker, but may provide a proinflammatory environment in a subgroup of patients with PsA.

Introduction

Psoriatic arthritis (PsA) is a distinctive inflammatory form of arthritis that may develop in 20% to 25% of individuals with psoriasis [1]. In addition to manifestations of psoriasis in the skin, patients with PsA may present with mild to very severe development of oligoarthritis and/or polyarthritis, enthesitis, dactylitis or axial skeletal manifestations similar to spondyloarthritis. PsA has been considered a seronegative inflammatory arthritis according to the diagnostic criteria first published by Moll *et al.* in 1973 [2] and then redefined by the Classification *Criteria* for Psoriatic Arthritis (CASPAR) [3]. All definitions of PsA have in common the seronegative status of the disease because autoantibodies (Abs) such as rheumatoid factor (RF), anticyclic citrullinated autoantibodies and antinuclear autoantibodies are usually absent in PsA. Hence, in contrast to rheumatoid arthritis, autoreactive B

* Correspondence: Lorenz.Thurner@uks.eu
[1]Department of Internal Medicine I, José Carreras-Center for Immuno- and Gene Therapy, University of Saarland Medical School, Kirrbergerstr., D-66421 Homburg, Saar, Germany
Full list of author information is available at the end of the article

lymphocytes are believed to play only a minor role in PsA [4]. Regarding the occurrence of autoantibodies in PsA, increased frequencies of thyreoglobulin Abs (14.29%) and thyroid peroxidase Abs (23%) were reported in PsA, which was explained by a relatively high comorbidity rate, with 26% of patients with PsA having autoimmune thyroiditis [5]. In another study, 20S proteasome autoantibodies were more frequently detected in PsA patients (27.8%) than in in healthy controls (0%), as well as more frequently in systemic lupus erythematosus patients (42%) than in rheumatoid arthritis patients (5%) [6]. However, the numbers of patients were small in these studies (36 PsA patients and 30 healthy controls) [6], and, in both studies, no patients with psoriasis without arthritic manifestations (PsC) were included. To date, no specific serological markers discriminating patients with PsA from patients with PsC have been identified. Nevertheless, a small but significant occurrence of B lymphocytes was reported in the skin of patients with PsA, but not in patients with PsC [7].

Recently, we discovered progranulin autoantibodies (PGRN Abs) in a protein array-based screening of plasma from various primary vasculitides and found evidence that these PGRN Abs have a neutralizing effect on PGRN plasma levels [8]. PGRN is a secreted precursor protein that is cleaved at the linker regions between individual granulins by neutrophil elastase [9], proteinase 3 [10], matrix metalloproteinase 12 [11], matrix metalloproteinase 14 [9] and ADAMTS-7 (a disintegrin and metalloprotease with thrombospondin motif 7) [12]. Until recently, most research on PGRN had focused on its role in neurodegenerative diseases such as frontotemporal lobe dementia [13]. However, since Tang *et al.* [14] showed that PGRN is a high-affinity ligand of the tumour necrosis factor α (TNF-α) receptors 1 and 2 (TNFR1 and TNFR2) and that its anti-inflammatory effect is caused by direct inhibition of these receptors, PGRN has increasingly become the focus of research on autoimmune diseases.

Recently, Chen *et al.* [15] challenged the notion of this interaction of PGRN with TNFR1 and TNFR2 previously reported by Tang *et al.* [14], as they could not reproduce the interaction of PGRN with TNFR1 and TNFR2. However, they did not question the anti-inflammatory effect of PGRN [10]. Tang *et al.* responded in a letter to the editor that Chen *et al.* utilized PGRN, which might be folded improperly. Furthermore, Tang *et al.* stated that validation of recombinant PGRN's functionality based only on its C-terminal binding to sortilin would be insufficient to determine its quality regarding its other biological functions, which are not primarily mediated by PGRN's C-Terminus. Subsequently, Jian *et al.* showed in detail that PGRN binds as TNF-α to cysteine-rich domain 2 (CRD2) and CRD3 of TNFR and that proper folding of PGRN is essential for this binding. Furthermore, dithiothreitol treatment of PGRN, which had been performed by Chen *et al.*, abolishes the binding of PGRN to TNFR but enhances its binding to sortilin [16]. Recently, two other groups independently reproduced the binding of PGRN to TNFR1 and TNFR2, and inhibitory effect of this binding on TNF-α-induced effects [17,18]. Dramatic effects of PGRN deficiency have been shown *in vivo* in collagen-induced arthritis and collagen Ab-induced arthritis mouse models, resulting in fulminant courses of disease [14]. Furthermore, the administration of recombinant human PGRN or a recombinant PGRN derivative, antagonist of TNF/TNFR signalling via targeting to TNF receptors (ATSTTRIN), that consists of three modified granulin motifs and their accompanying linker regions [14] had strong anti-inflammatory effects comparable to, or even stronger than, the administration of etanercept [14]. Consequently, PGRN and ATSTTRIN have been regarded as promising next-generation TNF-α blockers [19]. In addition to this strong anti-inflammatory effect mediated by the inhibition of TNFR1 and TNFR2, several other functions of PGRN in humans have been reported [20].

Interestingly, the previously detected PGRN Abs showed neutralizing effects on PGRN plasma levels detected by enzyme-linked immunosorbent assay (ELISA) and Western blot analysis. This observation, given the anti-inflammatory properties of secreted PGRN, suggested a proinflammatory effect of PGRN Abs, which was supported by our observation that the presence of PGRN Abs is associated with active disease state in granulomatosis with polyangiitis [8]. Apart from primary systemic vasculitis, we also found neutralizing PGRN Abs in systemic lupus erythematosus as well as in rheumatoid arthritis [8]. Some of the rheumatoid arthritis patients with PGRN Abs were actually seronegative for RF or anticitrullinated protein Abs. Furthermore, PGRN Abs were detected in patients with spondyloarthritis. This observation led us to conduct the present study to investigate the presence of PGRN Abs in patients with the seronegative disorder PsA, compare it to patients with PsC and healthy controls and investigate possible functional effects of PGRN Abs *in vitro*.

Methods

Study participants

This study was approved by our regional ethical review committee (Ethikkommission der Ärztekammer des Saarlandes) and conducted according to the Declaration of Helsinki. Serum samples of patients with PsA were collected prospectively from patients attending three centres of rheumatology between October 2011 and July 2012: Saarland Rheumatology Centre, the Department of Internal Medicine I at University Hospital in Homburg/ 149 Saar, the Rheumatology Department of the University Hospital Frankfurt am Main and the Outpatient Center for Rheumatology in Berlin-Lichtenberg. Sera from patients with PsC were provided by the Department of Dermatology of

Saarland University Medical School. Serum samples taken from healthy controls were also obtained at Saarland University Medical School. All serum specimens were stored at −80°C at the Department of Internal Medicine I, José Carreras Research Centre, Saarland University Medical Centre. All patients were examined by a rheumatologist (PsA patients) and a dermatologist (PsC patients) to confirm the diagnosis of PsA according to the CASPAR criteria or to exclude PsA in PsC patients. All diagnoses of PsC were made by dermatologists and confirmed by a rheumatologist. All PsA patients were stratified into subgroups according to gender, age, presence or absence of manifestations of axial disease, enthesitis, dactylitis and therapeutic regimens such as TNF-α blocker–containing medication. Axial disease was defined by positive findings on X-rays or magnetic resonance imaging scans for spondyloarthritis and/or sacroiliitis. Patients were considered positive for enthesitis or dactylitis on the basis of a positive diagnosis during the course of disease; however, no imaging findings have been required. No subgroup stratification for patients with PsC was performed, because the PGRN Ab serostatus of all patients with PsC was negative. All patients and healthy controls gave their written informed consent to participate in the study.

Progranulin antibody enzyme-linked immunosorbent assay

The ELISA for PGRN Abs was performed as previously described [8]. In short, the *GRN* gene encoding PGRN was recombinantly expressed with a C-terminal FLAG-tag in HEK293 cells under the control of a cytomegalovirus promoter (pSFI). Total cell extracts were prepared and bound to Nunc MaxiSorp plates (eBioscience, Frankfurt, Germany) precoated with murine anti-FLAG mAb at a dilution of 1:2,500 (v/v; Sigma-Aldrich, Munich, Germany) at 4°C overnight. Blocking was performed with 1.5% (w/v) gelatin in Tris-buffered saline (TBS), and washing steps were performed with TBS with Triton X-100. The individual serum samples were diluted 1:100. ELISA was performed according to standard protocols with the following Abs: biotinylated goat antihuman heavy and light chain immunoglobulin G (IgG) at a dilution of 1:2,500 (Dianova, Hamburg, Germany); subclass-specific sheep antihuman IgG1, IgG2, IgG3 and IgG4 (Binding Site Group, Birmingham, UK) at dilutions of 1:5,000; goat antihuman IgM (Dianova) at a dilution of 1:2,500; or goat antihuman IgA (Dianova) at a dilution of 1:2,500. Following this step, corresponding biotinylated secondary Abs were used for immunoassays carried out to detect IgG subclasses and IgM. Peroxidase-labelled streptavidin (Roche Applied Science, Indianapolis, IN, USA) was used at a dilution of 1:50,000. As a cutoff for positivity, the average of the optical density (OD) of the negative samples plus three standard deviations was applied.

Progranulin plasma levels measured by enzyme-linked immunosorbent assay

PGRN plasma levels were determined with a commercially available ELISA kit (AdipoGen, Incheon, South Korea) according to the manufacturer's instructions. The median of the plasma PGRN level of the healthy control group was set at 100% [8].

Cytotoxicity assay

A nonradioactive cytotoxicity assay (EZ4U Cell Proliferation Assay; Biomedica, Vienna, Austria) was performed according to the manufacturer's instructions. For this TNF-α-induced cytotoxicity assay, we used the highly TNF-α-sensitive mouse fibrosarcoma WEHI-S cell line as the target cells [21]. The interaction of human recombinant PGRN with murine TNFR1 and TNFR2 was previously demonstrated *in vitro* and *in vivo* [14], and, moreover, human PGRN Abs bind murine PGRN (Additional file 1). As a human control target cell line, the TNF-α-sensitive HT-1080 fibrosarcoma cell line was used.

In short, 4×10^4 WEHI-S cells or 4×10^4 HT-1080 cells were seeded into 200 μl of cell culture at 37°C and 5% CO_2. To detect possible differences between added sera of patients with PsA with and without PGRN Abs, of patients with PsC, and of healthy controls, serum of a PGRN Ab-positive patient with PsA, serum of a matched PGRN Ab-negative patient with PsA, serum of a patient with PsC and serum of a healthy control were added in dilutions from 1:4 to 1:512 to cultured WEHI-S cells and HT-1080 cells, followed by administration of TNF-α (100 pg/ml). Serum samples from gender-, age-, disease- and therapy modality-matched patients were chosen. Serum samples from patients receiving TNF-α blockers or other biologicals were excluded. WEHI-S cells and HT-1080 cells without addition of TNF-α and serum, or solely with addition of TNF-α (100 pg/ml), were used as positive and negative controls. After 24-hour incubation at 37°C, 20 μl of chromophore substrate were added to each well. This chromophore substrate is converted only by vital cells. The adsorption of the product was measured at an OD of 450 nm.

Statistical analyses

Differences in age and gender between the populations of PsA patients, PsC patients and healthy controls were tested by Student's *t*-test. Different frequencies of PGRN Abs in the serum samples of patients with PsA and PsC were analysed by χ^2 test. Differences in the frequency of PGRN Abs between PsA patients after stratification into subgroups were also tested with the χ^2 test. For analysis of the differences in PGRN plasma levels between healthy controls, PGRN Ab-positive and PGRN Ab-negative patients with PsA and seronegative patients with PsC, the Mann–Whitney *U* test was applied. A two-sided test value less than 0.05 was considered statistically significant. All statistical analyses were performed in SPSS version 19.0 for Windows software (IBM SPSS, Chicago, IL, USA).

Results

Patient characteristics

The patients' characteristics are outlined in Table 1.

Frequency, titres and immunoglobulin G subclass of progranulin antibodies

Of 260 patients with PsA, 50 (19.23%) had PGRN Abs in their sera. No PGRN Abs were found in the sera of 100 patients with PsC (0%; P = 0.0001). Of 97 healthy controls, 1 (1.03%) had PGRN Abs (Figure 1a). PGRN Ab-positive patients had titres ranging from 1:400 to 1:1,600 (Figure 1b). The sera of the 50 PGRN Ab-positive PsA patients were tested for their Ig class. PGRN Abs belonged exclusively to IgG (50 of 50 patients). PGRN Abs were not detected for either IgA or IgM (Additional file 1). Subsequently, IgG subclasses of PGRN Abs were determined. The PGRN Abs in 44 patients (88%) belonged to the IgG1 subclass, 1 (2%) of 50 belonged to the IgG2 subclass, 5 (10%) 50 belonged to the IgG3 subclass and 0 (0.0%) of 50 belonged to the IgG4 subclass (Figure 1c).

Analysis of the progranulin-positive patients with psoriatic arthritis

All 260 PsA patients (210 PGRN Ab-negative, 50 PGRN Ab-positive) were stratified according to their clinical manifestations, such as enthesitis, dactylitis, axial manifestations and erosive-proliferative joint damage. Patients with PsA were also analysed in subgroups according to age at primary diagnosis, gender, human leucocyte antigen B27 status and treatment with TNF-α-blocking agents (Figure 2). Although there was no difference between PGRN Ab-positive and PGRN Ab-negative patients with respect to age at the time of PsA diagnosis, PGRN Ab-positive patients were significantly older (>50 years) than PGRN Ab-negative patients with PsA (21% vs. 15.4%; P = 0.016). PsA patients with either enthesitis or dactylitis had significantly higher frequencies of PGRN Abs (P = 0.001 and P = 0.026, respectively, compared to patients with PsA without enthesitis or dactylitis), whereas no statistically significant associations were found for axial manifestations or erosive joint destruction and PGRN Ab positivity. In addition, significantly more patients receiving TNF-α blocker treatment had PGRN Abs compared to patients receiving therapy without TNF-α blockers (20.8% vs. 17.4%; P = 0.016).

Table 1 Characteristics of patients with psoriatic arthritis and psoriasis without arthritis

Characteristics	PsA	PsC
Median age (min–max)	54 (24–81)	53 (16–80)
Gender, M/F (%)	43.5/56.4	64/36
Age at psoriasis diagnosis, years	35	33
Age at PsA diagnosis, years	46	
Enthesitis (%)[a]	39.5	
Dactylitis (%)	39.2	
Axial disease (%)	27.7	
Erosive (%)[b]	44.9	
HLA-B27-positive (%)	32.7	
DMARD (%)[c]	48.8	
TNF-α blockers (%)[d]	18.4	

DMARD: disease-modifying antirheumatic drug; HLA-B27: *human leucocyte antigen B27; PsA: psoriatic arthritis; PsC:* psoriasis without arthritic manifestations; *TNF-α:* tumour necrosis factor α. Missing data: [a]n = 69, [b]n = 24, [c]n = 29, [d]n = 9.

Progranulin plasma levels

PGRN plasma levels were significantly lower in PGRN Ab-positive patients with PsA (n = 10) compared to healthy controls (n = 10) (P < 0.001 by Mann-Whitney U test), patients with PsC (n = 10) (P < 0.001 by Mann-Whitney U test) and PGRN Ab-negative patients with PsA (n = 5) (P < 0.001 by Mann-Whitney U test). Furthermore, PGRN Ab-negative patients with PsA had significantly lower plasma levels of PGRN than healthy controls (P = 0.019 by Mann-Whitney U test). There was also a tendency toward lower PGRN plasma levels in PGRN Ab-negative patients with PsA than in patients with PsC (P = 0.055 by Mann-Whitney U test) (Figure 3).

Cytotoxicity assay

In the TNF-α-induced cytotoxicity assays, we analysed the protective effects of sera from healthy controls, patients with PsC and PGRN Ab-positive or PGRN Ab-negative patients with PsA. The addition of sera from healthy controls, patients with PsC and PGRN Ab-negative patients with PsA reduced TNF-α-induced cytotoxicity of WEHI-S and HT-1080 cells to a significantly higher degree than in the sera of PGRN Ab-positive patients with PsA. This difference was significant up to a serum dilution of 1:64 (Figures 4a and 4b).

Discussion

In the present study, we report the presence of PGRN Abs in relevant titres in a subgroup of patients with PsA (Figures 1a and b). These PGRN Abs had previously been found frequently in primary vasculitis, systemic lupus erythematosus and rheumatoid arthritis, but not at all or very infrequently in controls. Despite the obvious lack of specificity for PsA, PGRN Abs are of particular interest because they had a neutralizing effect on PGRN plasma levels detected by ELISA and Western blot analysis [8]. PGRN is known to be a strong secreted anti-inflammatory mediator [10] by direct inhibition

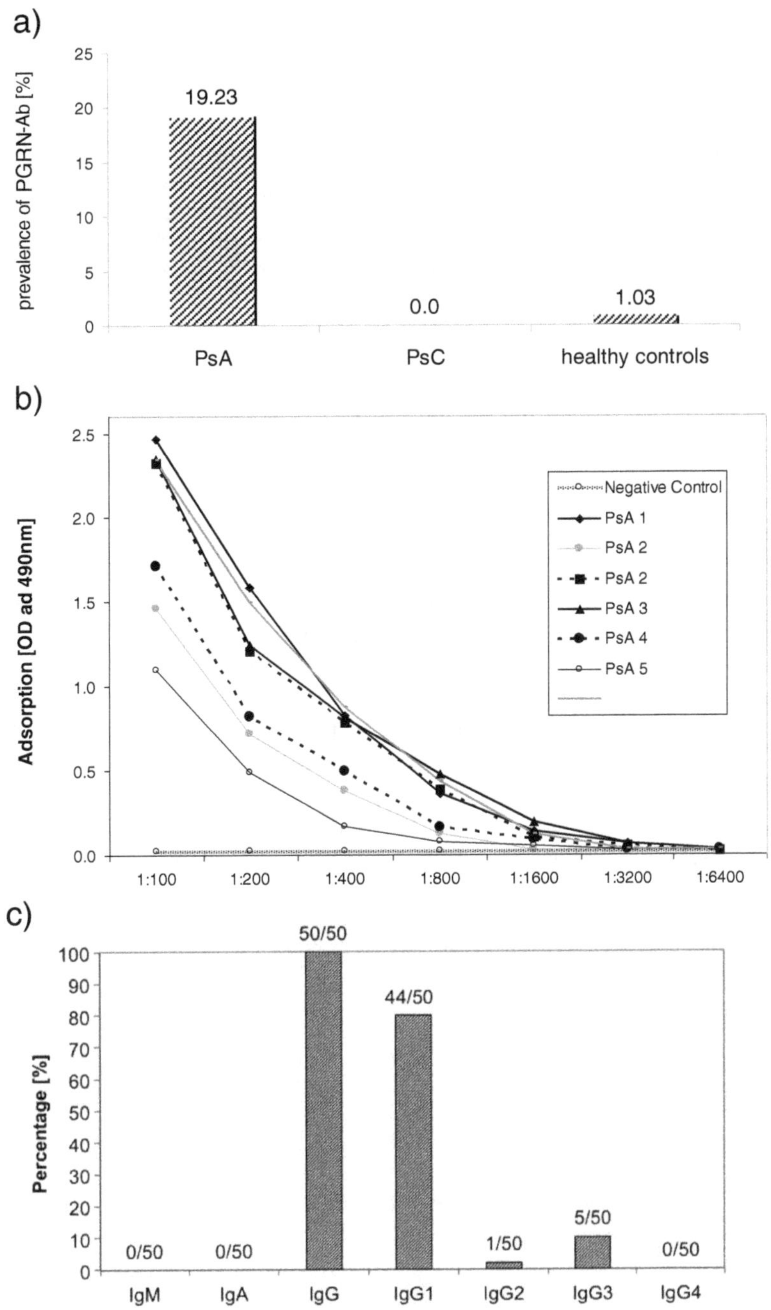

Figure 1 Occurrence of progranulin antibodies in psoriatic arthritis patients. (a) Prevalence of progranulin antibodies (PGRN Abs) in psoriatic arthritis (PsA) patients. **(b)** Titres of PGRN Abs in PsA patients. **(c)** Frequency of different immunoglobulin classes of PGRN Abs in PsA patients. Ig: immunoglobulin; OD, optical density; PsC: psoriasis without arthritic manifestations.

of TNFR1 and TNFR2 [14]. Our results support the hypothesis of a proinflammatory effect of PGRN Abs, as demonstrated by the loss of protective effects of PGRN in the presence of PGRN Abs containing PsA sera in TNF-α-mediated cytotoxicity assays (Figures 4a and 4b). Our results support the observation by Tang *et al.* of a direct inhibitory effect of PGRN on TNFR1 and TNFR2 and that administration of recombinant human PGRN protects cells from cytotoxic effects of TNF-α *in vitro* [14,16]. Given the fact that the half-life of PGRN is about 40 hours [14], in contrast to the short half-life of TNF-α (typical for cytokines) of 20 minutes [22], the effects of the intrinsic TNF-α in the serum of patients and controls is negligible. Our cytotoxicity assays revealed clear differences between the effects of serum from PGRN Ab-positive patients

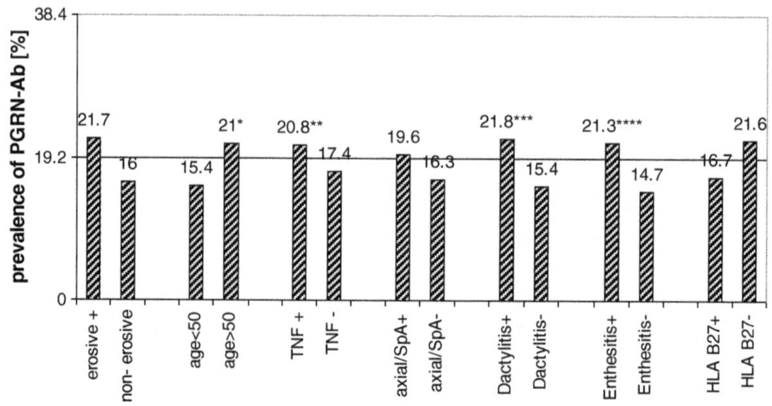

Figure 2 Progranulin antibodies in subpopulations of patients with psoriatic arthritis. The columns represent the percentage of progranulin antibody (PGRN Ab)-positive patients in different subgroups of psoriatic arthritis (PsA) compared to the average frequency of PGRN Abs in PsA patients (19.23%; horizontal line). HLA-B27: human leucocyte antigen B27; SpA: spondyloarthritis; TNF: tumour necrosis factor. **P* = 0.016, ***P* = 0.001, ****P* = 0.026, *****P* = 0.001.

with PsA on the one hand and serum from matched PGRN Ab-negative patients with PsA, patients with PsC or healthy controls on the other hand. The administration of serum samples of patients with PsA with neutralizing PGRN Abs, and thus with lower PGRN levels, protected the WEHI-S and HT-1080 cells from the cytotoxic effects of TNF-α far less than serum samples from patients with PsA without PGRN Abs, patients with PsC or healthy controls. This finding clearly proves the proinflammatory effect of neutralizing PGRN Abs *in vitro*.

The second important finding of the present study is that PGRN Abs were observed in patients with PsA, but not in patients with PsC (Figure 1). Interestingly, Veale *et al.* reported small but significant numbers of B cells in the skin of patients with PsA, but not in the skin of patients with PsC or in healthy controls [7]. In the present study, the occurrence of PGRN Abs in patients with PsA was associated with different clinical characteristics. PsA patients with dactylitis and enthesitis had PGRN Ab more frequently than PsA patients without such manifestations. Moreover, patients with PsA who

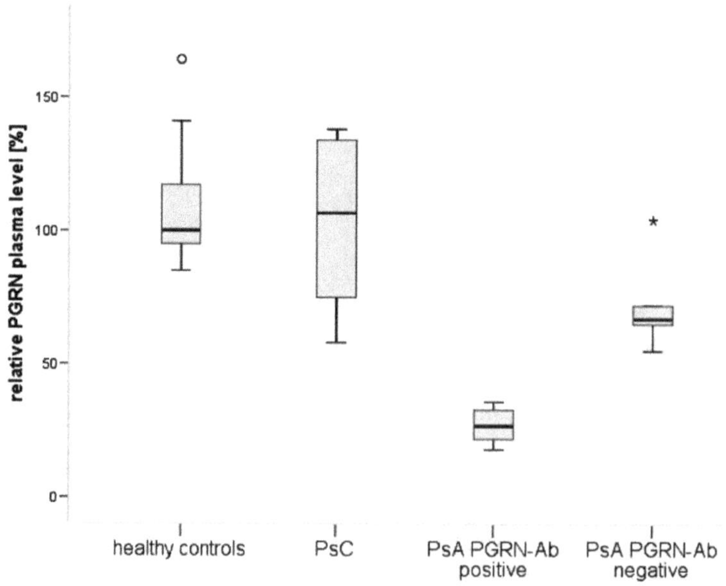

Figure 3 Association of progranulin antibody status and progranulin plasma levels in psoriasis patients. Progranulin (PGRN) plasma levels were determined in patients with psoriasis without arthritic manifestations (PsC) (*n* = 10), PGRN antibody (PGRN Ab)-positive patients with psoriatic arthritis (PsA) (*n* = 10), PGRN Ab-negative patients with PsA (*n* = 5) and in healthy controls (*n* = 10). Data are presented as 25% (box), 50% (median) and 75% (box) percentiles and the range (line). Median PGRN plasma level obtained from healthy controls was set at 100%.

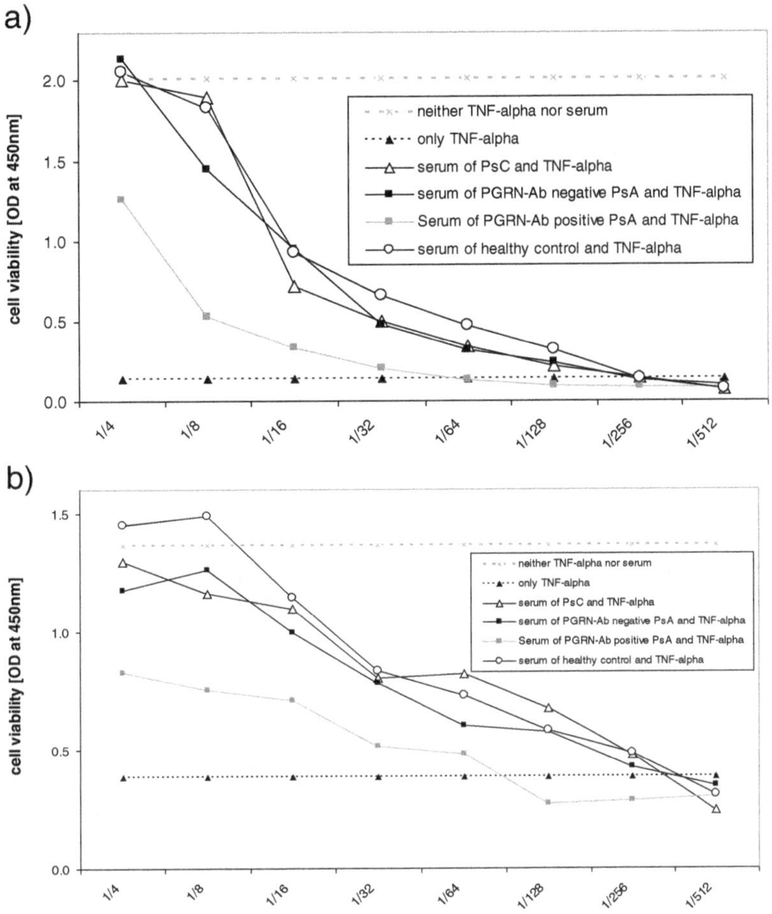

Figure 4 Tumour necrosis factor α-mediated cytotoxicity dependent on progranulin antibody status. (a) After administration of serum and TNF-α to WEHI-S cells, the adsorption of coloured formazan, which is a marker for cell viability, was detected at OD of 450 nm. **(b)** After administration of serum and TNF-α to HT-1080 cells, the adsorption of coloured formazan was detected at OD of 450 nm. Ab: antibody; PGRN: progranulin; PsA: psoriatic arthritis; PsC: psoriasis without arthritic manifestations.

received TNF-α blocker therapy for at least 3 months had PGRN Abs slightly more frequently (20.8% versus 17.4%), indirectly suggesting that PGRN Abs might be associated with a more aggressive course of disease, necessitating more intensive treatment. Generally, the grades of dactylitis and enthesitis in PsA patients have been suggested to be partly influenced, that is, enhanced, by TNF-α, which is supported by the efficacy of TNF-α blockers in PsA therapy [23-26]. Given the neutralizing effect of PGRN Abs on PGRN plasma levels in PsA patients (Figure 3), as well as in other autoimmune diseases [8], and, more important, given the results of the functional *in vitro* assays indicating a sensitizing effect of PGRN Abs for the effects of TNF-α in patients with PsA, a higher prevalence of PGRN Abs in patients with TNF-α-induced disease manifestations such as enthesitis and dactylitis could obviously be expected. Despite the statistical significance of our results, however, the relative differences in the frequency of PGRN Abs between the various subgroups were rather small (PGRN Ab-positive enthesitis 21.3% vs. PGRN Ab-negative enthesitis 14.7% and PGRN Ab-positive dactilytis 21.8% vs. PGRN Ab-negative enthesitis 15.4%). These results could be explained by the relatively small absolute numbers of patients with subentities and partly by missing data concerning dactylitis and enthesitis. Moreover, we observed a statistically nonsignificant trend between the occurrence of PGRN Abs and the presence of erosive joint disease (P = 0.061). In consideration of the suspected pathogenic proinflammatory effect of PGRN Abs disrupting the physiologic homeostasis of TNF-α/PGRN agonists and antagonists in a subgroup of patients with PsA, PGRN Abs might be of use as prognostic markers for the course of disease and/or as predictive markers for the effectiveness of TNF-α-blocking agents. Theoretically, the identification of neutralizing PGRN Abs in

PsA could eventually lead to a more individualized therapy because patients with PGRN Abs have lower physiologic TNF-α antagonist levels and might profit from dose intensification of TNF-α blockers. From this point of view, prospective studies of patients with PsA are needed to evaluate PGRN Abs as possible biomarkers for the diagnosis, risk stratification and choice of adequate treatment modality.

Conclusion

Neutralizing PGRN Abs occurred in relevant titres in a subgroup of patients with PsA, but not in PsC patients. PGRN Ab-positive patients with PsA had more frequently enthesitis and dactylitis than PGRN Ab-negative patients with PsA. Moreover in TNF-α-induced cytotoxicity assays using WEHI-S and HT-1080 cells, the protective effects of PGRN were inhibited by PGRN Ab-containing sera of patients with PsA. This suggests that PGRN Abs not only may be useful as a diagnostic and prognostic marker but also may be involved in the pathogenesis of the arthritic process in a subgroup of patients with PsA.

Abbreviations

Ab: Antibody; IgG: Immunoglobulin G; PGRN: Progranulin; PsA: Psoriatic arthritis; PsC: Psoriasis without arthritic manifestations; TNF-α: Tumour necrosis factor α; TNFR: Tumour necrosis factor receptor.

Competing interests

Saarland Universities Patent Marketing Agency, LT, KDP and MP filed 61/730,772, which covers means and methods for detecting autoimmune disorders in which progranulin may be involved.

Authors' contributions

MZ, NF and ER performed most of the experiments and were involved in data analysis. LT, MP and GA were involved in the study design and data analysis and drafted the manuscript. MFO was involved in data analysis. All authors read and approved the final manuscript.

Acknowledgments

We are grateful to Jutta Conigliaro, Christian Schorpp, Philipp Klemm, Alexandra Stark, Claudia Pföhler, Thomas Vogt, Boris Kubuschok, Niels Murawski, Carsten Zwick, Silke Zinke (Berlin) and Harald Burkhardt (Frankfurt am Main), who helped in the collection of blood samples from the respective patients, including clinical data. We are also grateful to Pierre Simon, Bernhard Thurner and Jan Voswinkel (Paris), who proofread the manuscript and gave helpful advice. LT received a Saarland University fellowship.

Author details

[1]Department of Internal Medicine I, José Carreras-Center for Immuno- and Gene Therapy, University of Saarland Medical School, Kirrbergerstr., D-66421 Homburg, Saar, Germany. [2]Institute of Medical Biostatistics, Saarland University, Kirrbergerstr., D-66421 Homburg, Saar, Germany.

References

1. Rahman P, Nguyen E, Cheung C, Schentag CT, Gladman DD: **Comparison of radiological severity in psoriatic arthritis and rheumatoid arthritis.** *J Rheumatol* 2001, **28**:1041–1044.
2. Moll JM, Wright V: **Psoriatic arthritis.** *Semin Arthritis Rheum* 1973, **3**:55–78.
3. Taylor W, Gladman D, Helliwell P, Marchesoni A, Mease P, Mielants H: **Classification criteria for psoriatic arthritis: development of new criteria from a large international study.** *Arthritis Rheum* 2006, **54**:2665–2673.
4. Nograles KE, Brasington RD, Bowcock AM: **New insights into the pathogenesis and genetics of psoriatic arthritis.** *Nat Clin Pract Rheumatol* 2009, **5**:83–91.
5. Peluso R, Lupoli GA, Del Puente A, Iervolino S, Bruner V, Lupoli R, Di Minno MN, Foglia F, Scarpa R, Lupoli G: **Prevalence of thyroid autoimmunity in patients with spondyloarthropathies.** *J Rheumatol* 2011, **38**:1371–1377.
6. Colmegna I, Sainz B Jr, Citera G, Maldonado-Cocco JA, Garry RF, Espinoza LR: **Anti-20S proteasome antibodies in psoriatic arthritis.** *J Rheumatol* 2008, **35**:674–676.
7. Veale DJ, Barnes L, Rogers S, Fitzgerald O: **Immunohistochemical markers for arthritis in psoriasis.** *Ann Rheum Dis* 1994, **53**:450–454.
8. Thurner L, Preuss KD, Fadle N, Regitz E, Klemm P, Zaks M, Kemele M, Hasenfus A, Csernok E, Gross WL, Pasquali JL, Martin T, Bohle RM, Pfreundschuh M: **Progranulin antibodies in autoimmune diseases.** *J Autoimmun* 2013, **42**:29–38.
9. Butler GS, Dean RA, Tam EM, Overall CM: **Pharmacoproteomics of a metalloproteinase hydroxamate inhibitor in breast cancer cells: dynamics of membrane type 1 matrix metalloproteinase-mediated membrane protein shedding.** *Mol Cell Biol* 2008, **28**:4896–4914.
10. Kessenbrock K, Fröhlich L, Sixt M, Lämmermann T, Pfister H, Bateman A, Belaaouaj A, Ring J, Ollert M, Fässler R, Jenne DE: **Proteinase 3 and neutrophil elastase enhance inflammation in mice by inactivating antiinflammatory progranulin.** *J Clin Invest* 2008, **118**:2438–2447.
11. Suh HS, Choi N, Tarassishin L, Lee SC: **Regulation of progranulin expression in human microglia and proteolysis of progranulin by matrix metalloproteinase-12 (MMP-12).** *PLoS One* 2012, **7**:e35115.
12. Bai XH, Wang DW, Kong L, Zhang Y, Luan Y, Kobayashi T, Kronenberg HM, Yu XP, Liu CJ: **ADAMTS-7, a direct target of PTHrP, adversely regulates endochondral bone growth by associating with and inactivating GEP growth factor.** *Mol Cell Biol* 2009, **29**:4201–4219.
13. Baker M, Mackenzie IR, Pickering-Brown SM, Gass J, Rademakers R, Lindholm C, Snowden J, Adamson J, Sadovnick AD, Rollinson S, Cannon A, Dwosh E, Neary D, Melquist S, Richardson A, Dickson D, Berger Z, Eriksen J, Robinson T, Zehr C, Dickey CA, Crook R, McGowan E, Mann D, Boeve B, Feldman H, Hutton M: **Mutations in progranulin cause τ-negative frontotemporal dementia linked to chromosome 17.** *Nature* 2006, **442**:916–919.
14. Tang W, Lu Y, Tian QY, Zhang Y, Guo FJ, Liu GY, Syed NM, Lai Y, Lin EA, Kong L, Su J, Yin F, Ding AH, Zanin-Zhorov A, Dustin ML, Tao J, Craft J, Yin Z, Feng JQ, Abramson SB, Yu XP, Liu CJ: **The growth factor progranulin binds to TNF receptors and is therapeutic against inflammatory arthritis in mice.** *Science* 2011, **332**:478–484.
15. Chen X, Chang J, Deng Q, Xu J, Nguyen TA, Martens LH, Cenik B, Taylor G, Hudson KF, Chung J, Yu K, Yu P, Herz J, Farese RV Jr, Kukar T, Tansey MG: **Progranulin does not bind tumor necrosis factor (TNF) receptors and is not a direct regulator of TNF-dependent signaling or bioactivity in immune or neuronal cells.** *J Neurosci* 2013, **33**:9202–9213.
16. Jian J, Zhao S, Tian Q, Gonzalez-Gugel E, Mundra JJ, Uddin SM, Liu B, Richbourgh B, Brunetti R, Liu CJ: **Progranulin directly binds to the CRD2 and CRD3 of TNFR extracellular domains.** *FEBS Lett* 2013, **587**:3428–3436.
17. Egashira Y, Suzuki Y, Azuma Y, Takagi T, Mishiro K, Sugitani S, Tsuruma K, Shimazawa M, Yoshimura S, Kashimata M, Iwama T, Hara H: **The growth factor progranulin attenuates neuronal injury induced by cerebral ischemia-reperfusion through the suppression of neutrophil recruitment.** *J Neuroinflammation* 2013, **10**:105.
18. Kawase R, Ohama T, Matsuyama A, Matsuwaki T, Okada T, Yamashita T, Yuasa-Kawase M, Nakaoka H, Nakatani K, Inagaki M, Tsubakio-Yamamoto K, Masuda D, Nakagawa-Toyama Y, Nishida M, Ohmoto Y, Nishihara M, Komuro I, Yamashita S: **Deletion of progranulin exacerbates atherosclerosis in ApoE knockout mice.** *Cardiovasc Res* 2013, **100**:125–133.
19. Sfikakis PP, Tsokos GC: **Towards the next generation of anti-TNF drugs.** *Clin Immunol* 2011, **141**:231–235.

20. Bateman A, Bennett HPJ: **The granulin gene family: from cancer to dementia.** *Bioessays* 2009, **31**:1245–1254.
21. Espevik T, Nissen-Meyer J: **A highly sensitive cell line, WEHI 164 clone 13, for measuring cytotoxic factor/tumor necrosis factor from human monocytes.** *J Immunol Methods* 1986, **95**:99–105.
22. Chapman PB, Lester TJ, Casper ES, Gabrilove JL, Wong GY, Kempin SJ, Gold PJ, Welt S, Warren RS, Starnes HF: **Clinical pharmacology of recombinant human tumor necrosis factor in patients with advanced cancer.** *J Clin Oncol* 1987, **5**:1942–1951.
23. Antoni C, Krueger GG, de Vlam K, Birbara C, Beutler A, Guzzo C, Zhou B, Dooley LT, Kavanaugh A, IMPACT 2 Trial Investigators: **Infliximab improves signs and symptoms of psoriatic arthritis: results of the IMPACT 2 trial.** *Ann Rheum Dis* 2005, **64**:1150–1157.
24. Mease PJ, Kivitz AJ, Burch FX, Siegel EL, Cohen SB, Ory P, Salonen D, Rubenstein J, Sharp JT, Tsuji W: **Etanercept treatment of psoriatic arthritis: safety, efficacy, and effect on disease progression.** *Arthritis Rheum* 2004, **50**:2264–2272.
25. Mease PJ, Gladman DD, Ritchlin CT, Ruderman EM, Steinfeld SD, Choy EH, Sharp JT, Ory PA, Perdok RJ, Weinberg MA, Adalimumab Effectiveness in Psoriatic Arthritis Trial Study Group: **Adalimumab for the treatment of patients with moderately to severely active psoriatic arthritis: results of a double-blind, randomized, placebo-controlled trial.** *Arthritis Rheum* 2005, **52**:3279–3289.
26. Ritchlin CT, Kavanaugh A, Gladman DD, Mease PJ, Helliwell P, Boehncke WH, de Vlam K, Fiorentino D, Fitzgerald O, Gottlieb AB, McHugh NJ, Nash P, Qureshi AA, Soriano ER, Taylor WJ, Group for Research and Assessment of Psoriasis and Psoriatic Arthritis (GRAPPA): **Treatment recommendations for psoriatic arthritis.** *Ann Rheum Dis* 2009, **68**:1387–1394.

23

Cumulative inflammatory burden is independently associated with increased arterial stiffness in patients with psoriatic arthritis

Jiayun Shen[1], Qing Shang[1], Edmund K Li[1], Ying-Ying Leung[2], Emily W Kun[3], Lai-Wa Kwok[1], Martin Li[1], Tena K Li[1], Tracy Y Zhu[1], Cheuk-Man Yu[1] and Lai-Shan Tam[1*]

Abstract

Introduction: The aim of this study was to examine whether the cumulative inflammatory burden is associated with an increase in arterial stiffness in a prospective cohort of psoriatic arthritis (PsA) patients.

Methods: In total, 72 PsA patients were followed for a median of 6.5 years. Cumulative inflammatory burden was represented by the cumulative averages of repeated measures of erythrocyte sedimentation rate (ca-ESR) and C-reactive protein (ca-CRP). Brachial-ankle pulse wave velocity (PWV) was measured at the last visit. We also included 47 healthy controls for PWV assessment.

Results: PWV was significantly higher in PsA patients compared with healthy controls after adjustment for age, gender and body weight (1466 ± 29 cm/s versus 1323 ± 38 cm/s, $P = 0.008$). PsA patients were divided into two groups based on whether their PWV value is ≥1450 cm/s (High PWV group, N = 38) or <1450 cm/s (Low PWV group, N = 34). The High PWV group had a significantly higher ca-ESR (29 (19 to 44) versus 18 (10 to 32) mm/1st hour, $P = 0.005$) and ca-CRP (0.7 (0.3 to 1.4) versus 0.4 (0.2 to 0.7) mg/dl, $P = 0.029$). Using regression analysis, high ca-ESR (defined as ≥75th percentile: 37 mm/1st hour) was associated with a higher likelihood of being in the High PWV group (odds ratio (OR): 9.455 (1.939 to 46.093), $P = 0.005$, adjusted for baseline clinical and cardiovascular risk factors; and 9.111 (1.875 to 44.275), $P = 0.006$, adjusted for last visit parameters).

Conclusions: Cumulative inflammatory burden, as reflected by ca-ESR, was associated with increased arterial stiffness in PsA patients even after adjustment for cardiovascular risk factors, emphasizing the important role of chronic inflammation in accelerating the development of cardiovascular risks in PsA patients.

Introduction

Psoriatic arthritis (PsA) is a chronic inflammatory arthritis associated with an increased risk of subclinical [1,2], clinical cardiovascular disease (CVD) [3] and early cardiovascular (CV) mortality [4]. Chronic inflammation plays a pivotal role in the pathogenesis of subclinical CVD in PsA patients [5,6]. Inflammation is involved in foam cell formation, endothelial dysfunction and Th1 cytokine production, which leads to the development of arterial dysfunction [7] and atherosclerotic plaque [8]. However, inflammatory markers including erythrocyte sedimentation rate (ESR) or C-reactive protein (CRP) failed to differentiate PsA patients with or without subclinical atherosclerosis in cross-sectional studies [1,9], most likely because PsA is a chronic relapsing condition in which inflammation may fluctuate over time. The chronic inflammatory burden may be better represented by the cumulative average of inflammatory markers than the measurement of these markers at a single time point. Eder and colleagues have recently reported that increased inflammatory burden over time, as reflected by cumulative average of ESR, is associated with the extent of atherosclerotic plaques in PsA patients from a prospective cohort [10]. This association is attenuated after adjustment for traditional CV risk factors. In patients with rheumatoid arthritis (RA), a prospectively study also demonstrated that higher average CRP levels are associated with incident or progressive plaque, but only in

* Correspondence: lstam@cuhk.edu.hk
[1]Department of Medicine & Therapeutics, The Prince of Wales Hospital, The Chinese University of Hong Kong, Shatin, Hong Kong, China
Full list of author information is available at the end of the article

patients with high CVD risk [11]. In RA, the average CRP correlates with the presence of subclinical atherosclerosis measured by carotid intima-media thickness (IMT) [12]. Also, the average CRP is associated with an increased risk of CV events and mortality in patients with long-standing RA [13]. Whether chronic inflammation can accelerate atherogenesis independently or mediate it via adverse modification of CV risk factors remains uncertain.

Arterial stiffness is an independent predictor of CV events and mortality [14]. Pulse wave velocity (PWV) is a measure of early structural vascular changes, which is determined by the elasticity and other properties of the artery, and is correlated with arterial distensibility and stiffness. An increase in brachial-ankle PWV by 100 cm/s corresponds to an age-, sex-, and risk factor-adjusted increase of 12% in total CV events, and 13% in CV mortality, respectively [15]. By applying a cutoff value of 1450 cm/s, brachial-ankle PWV was found to discriminate normal subjects from those with CVD or atherosclerotic risk factors with sensitivity of 62.1% and specificity of 69.5% in a large-scale population-based study involving 21,094 Chinese subjects [16]. Two previous case–control studies failed to find a correlation between ESR or CRP and PWV in PsA patients [17,18]. However, these studies were limited by small sample size and cross-sectional study design and were unable to assess the effect of cumulative inflammation over time. The effect of cumulative inflammatory burden in arterial stiffness in patients with RA is controversial [19,20]. Whether cumulative inflammatory burden over time may affect arterial stiffness as assessed by PWV in PsA has never been explored. We hypothesize that PsA patients with higher cumulative inflammatory burden (as measured by cumulative averages of the area under the curve (AUC) for ESR and CRP) would have increased arterial stiffness. In this study, we first compared the arterial stiffness between PsA patients and healthy controls. Second, we examined whether the cumulative inflammatory burden over time is associated with an increase in arterial stiffness in a prospective cohort of PsA patients.

Methods

Patients and healthy controls

Eighty-two PsA patients who participated in a prior subclinical study of atherosclerosis in PsA [1] were recruited for a PWV assessment between 2012 and 2013. Briefly, all participants fulfilled the Classification of Psoriatic Arthritis (CASPAR) criteria [21] and had been prospectively followed at the rheumatology clinic of two regional hospitals (The Prince of Wales Hospital and the Alice Ho Miu Ling Nethersole Hospital) since 2006 to 2007 (baseline visit). Exclusion criteria at baseline included overt CVD (including myocardial infarction, angina, stroke, and transient ischemic attack), inability to provide informed consent, clinically significant renal disease (serum creatinine level >270 mol/L), or pregnancy. Patients were assessed by rheumatologists every 4 to 6 months, which included a complete history, physical examination and laboratory evaluation: 72 patients who completed the last follow-up visit and had a successful brachial-ankle PWV assessment were included in the analysis.

We recruited 47 healthy controls from a broad spectrum of hospital staff. None of the controls had a known history of hypertension, diabetes, hyperlipidemia, or overt CVD (including myocardial infarction, angina, stroke, or transient ischemic attack), or family history of CVD.

Ethics approval was obtained from the Ethics Committee of The Chinese University of Hong Kong-New Territories East Cluster Hospitals, and written informed consent was obtained from all participants according to the Declaration of Helsinki.

Clinical interview at baseline and last follow-up visit

Pain and physicians' and patients' global assessments were evaluated using a 100-point visual analog scale, where 0 indicated excellent well-being and 100 indicated feeling extremely unwell. Physical examination included recording the number of tender and swollen joints using the 68 tender-joint/66 swollen-joint count, the presence of dactylitis, and the number of permanently deformed joints. The Health Assessment Questionnaire (HAQ) was used to evaluate physical function [22], and the Psoriasis Area and Severity Index (PASI) was used to assess the extent of skin involvement [23]. Overall disease activity was assessed using the Disease Activity in Psoriatic Arthritis (DAPSA) and Minimal Disease Activity (MDA) scores [24]. Anthropomorphic measurements including height, weight, and waist and hip circumference, and two consecutive blood pressure (BP) readings in the sitting position and heart rate were recorded. Other data obtained from PsA patients through the interview and chart review included smoking and drinking habits, history of diabetes, hypertension, hypercholesterolemia and overt CVD. Drug history was retrieved from case notes or elicited during the clinical assessment. All patients were interviewed and examined using standardized data collection instruments.

Laboratory tests

Complete blood count, liver and renal function tests, ESR and CRP were checked at every visit. Fasting blood glucose, and lipid profile (total cholesterol (TC), low-density lipoprotein-cholesterol (LDL), high-density lipoprotein-cholesterol (HDL), and triglycerides) were checked at baseline and the last visit. Cumulative inflammation over time was represented by the cumulative averages of ESR (ca-ESR) and CRP (ca-CRP).

Pulse wave velocity

Brachial-ankle PWV was assessed noninvasively in subjects in the supine position by a dedicated tonometry system (Non-Invasive Vascular Profile Device VP-2000; Omron Healthcare, Inc, Bannockburn, IL, USA) as described previously [25]. All PWV measurements were performed twice at each side of the body by a single skilled operator. The means of overall PWV measurements were recorded. The intra-class correlation coefficient (ICC) for intraobserver reliability was 0.84 [26].

Statistical analysis

Results are expressed as mean ± SD or median (interquartile range) as appropriate. Comparisons between two groups were assessed using the Student's *t*-test or Mann–Whitney *U*-test for continuous variables and the chi-square (χ^2) test for categorical variables. Analysis of covariance (ANCOVA) was used to compare means of PWV between PsA and control subjects by adjusting for parameters that were distributed differently between groups. Spearman's correlation was used to evaluate bivariate correlation. ca-ESR and ca-CRP were calculated from the AUC of all available measurements divided by the total number of months of follow-up. Univariate analysis was performed to ascertain the association between clinical parameters and PWV. The cutoff value for CV and atherosclerotic risk, which was derived from the large-scale Chinese population-based study [16], was used to divide the PsA patients into a high-PWV group (≥1,450 cm/s) or low-PWV group (<1,450 cm/s). Multivariable logistic regression analysis was used to determine the independent predictor(s) for being in the high-PWV group. All variables with P <0.1 in the univariate analysis were included in the multivariate analysis. All statistical analyses were conducted using IBM SPSS Statistics Version 22 (IBM, Armonk, NY, USA). A minimal level of significance of P <0.05 is used.

Results

Clinical features of PsA patients

A total of 72 (36 male and 36 female) PsA patients were included in the analysis. At baseline, the mean ± SD age was 49.6 ± 11.7 years and the median (IQR) disease duration was 9.2 (2.4 to 14.1) years. The median follow-up duration from baseline to the time of PWV assessment (last visit) was 6.5 (range: 4.8 to 7.7) years. Table 1 summarized the clinical features of the patients at baseline and last visit. Compared with baseline, significant improvement in disease activity parameters (number of tender and swollen joint counts, pain, DAPSA and CRP) and physical function (HAQ) were observed at the last visit, although the damaged joint count increased. CV risk factors remained stable except for systolic blood pressure (SBP) and HDL levels decreased. More patients were taking anti-hypertensive drugs, statins and biologic disease modifying anti-rheumatic drugs (DMARDs) at the last visit.

PWV in PsA patients and control subjects

The mean PWV in PsA patients and control subjects were 1,533 ± 307 cm/s and 1,219 ± 157 cm/s, respectively (P <0.001) (Figure 1A). The control subjects were significantly younger (43.1 ± 10.2 years versus 55.9 ± 11.6 years, P <0.001), had higher proportion of women (72.3% versus 50.0%, P = 0.015) and a lower body weight (58.2 ± 8.7 kg versus 65.7 ± 11.6 kg, P <0.001) at PWV assessment compared with the PsA patients. However, after adjustment for age, gender and body weight, the adjusted mean PWV was still significantly greater in PsA patients compared with control subjects (1,466 ± 29 cm/s versus 1,323 ± 38 cm/s, P = 0.008) (Figure 1B). If patients with hypertension, diabetes or hyperlipidemia were excluded, the age, gender, and body weight-adjusted mean for PsA patients (n = 20) and control subjects were 1,394 ± 46 and 1,248 ± 29 cm/s, respectively (P = 0.013) (Figure 1C).

Association between traditional cardiovascular risk factors and PWV

The associations between PWV and clinical features at both baseline and the last visit (PWV assessment visit) are shown in Table 2. At PWV assessment, patients in the high-PWV group (n = 38) were significantly older, had higher SBP and Framingham 10-year CVD risk score, were more likely to have diabetes and hypertension, and to be treated with anti-hypertensive drugs compared with the low-PWV group (n = 34) (all P <0.05).

Association between disease-related parameters and PWV

Disease-related variables were compared between the two PWV groups (Table 2). The high-PWV group had a trend of longer disease duration (P <0.1). At baseline, the high-PWV group had significantly higher ESR levels compared with patients in the low-PWV group (P = 0.048). At PWV assessment, the high-PWV group had significantly higher damaged joint count, ESR and CRP levels.

Association between cumulative inflammatory burden and PWV

The median ca-ESR was 24 (12 to 38) mm/1st h and the median ca-CRP was 0.6 (0.2 to 1.1) mg/dl in the PsA patients. There was a significant correlation between PWV and ca-ESR (Spearman's rho 0.390, P = 0.001) but not

Table 1 Clinical features at baseline and last visit in all PsA patients

	Baseline	Last visit	*P*-value
Male gender, n (%)	36 (50.0%)		
Age, years	49.6 ± 11.7	55.9 ± 11.6	
Psoriatic arthritis (PsA) characteristics			
PsA disease duration, years	9.2 (2.4 to 14.10)	15.7 (8.5 to 21.2)	
Tender joint count, 0 to 68	2 (0 to 8)	1 (0 to 4)	0.033
Swollen joint count, 0 to 66	0 (0 to 3)	0 (0 to 1)	0.032
Damaged joint count, 0 to 68	2 (0 to 5)	2 (0 to 6)	0.031
Visual analog scale pain, 0 to 100	50 (30 to 66)	30 (20 to 58)	0.001
Patients' global assessment, 0 to 100	50 (30 to 60)	40 (20 to 60)	0.298
Physicians' global assessment, 0 to 100	20 (0 to 30)	20 (5 to 35)	0.683
Psoriasis Area and Severity Index, 0 to 72	2.6 (0.9 to 7.5)	1.8 (0.4 to 6.3)	0.309
Health assessment questionnaire, 0 to 3	0.38 (0.12 to 0.94)	0.25 (0 to 0.69)	0.043
Minimal disease activity, n (%)	16 (22.2%)	14 (19.4%)	0.539
Disease Activity in Psoriatic Arthritis, 0 to 164	16 (8 to 21)	11 (6 to 16)	0.010
Erythrocyte sedimentation rate, mm/1st h	23 (10 to 37)	18 (8 to 34)	0.357
C-reactive protein, mg/dl	0.4 (0.2 to 1.3)	0.3 (0.1 to 0.7)	0.016
Cardiovascular risk factors			
Body weight, kg	65.2 ± 12.0	65.7 ± 11.6	0.436
Body height, cm	161 ± 8		
Systolic blood pressure, mmHg	136 ± 22	127 ± 15	<0.001
Hypertension, n (%)	36 (50.0%)	44 (61.1%)	0.555
Diabetes, n (%)	16 (44.4%)	16 (44.4%)	1.000
Framingham 10-year CVD risk >10%, n (%)	30 (41.7%)	36 (50.0%)	0.316
Total cholesterol, mmol/L	5.1 ± 0.9	4.9 ± 0.8	0.073
High-density lipoprotein cholesterol, mmol/L	1.6 ± 0.5	1.4 ± 0.4	<0.001
Triglycerides, mmol/L	1.5 ± 0.9	1.5 ± 0.9	0.558
Fasting glucose, mmol/L	5.5 ± 1.3	5.5 ± 1.6	0.861
Medications, n (%)			
Anti-hypertensive drugs	20 (27.8%)	42 (58.3%)	<0.001
Statins	1 (1.4%)	14 (19.4%)	<0.001
Nonsteroidal anti-inflammatory drugs	33 (45.8%)	31 (43.1%)	0.737
Steroids	4 (5.6%)	3 (4.2%)	0.999
Disease-modifying antirheumatic drugs	36 (50.0%)	40 (55.6%)	0.504
Biologics	0 (0%)	11 (15.4%)	0.001

Values are presented as number (percentage), median (interquatile range) or mean ± SD. CVD, cardiovascular disease.

ca-CRP (0.222, $P = 0.061$). The high-PWV group had significantly higher ca-ESR (31 (21 to 44) versus 17 (10 to 30) mm/1st h, $P < 0.001$) and ca-CRP (0.7 (0.3 to 1.4) versus 0.4 (0.2 to 0.7) mg/dl, $P = 0.029$) compared with the low-PWV group (Figure 2).

The association between the cumulative inflammatory burden and PWV was assessed by regression analysis (Table 3). High ca-ESR (defined as ≥75th percentile: 37 mm/1st h) was associated with a higher likelihood of being in the high-PWV group after adjustment for other clinical and CV risk factors at baseline (OR 9.455 (95% CI 1.939, 46.093), $P = 0.005$) or last visit (OR 9.111 (95% CI 1.875, 44.275), $P = 0.006$) (Table 3). In contrast, high ca-CRP (defined as ≥75th percentile 1.2 mg/dl) was not associated with a higher likelihood of being in the high-PWV group (Table 3).

Older age was the other independent risk factor associated with a higher likelihood of being in the high-PWV

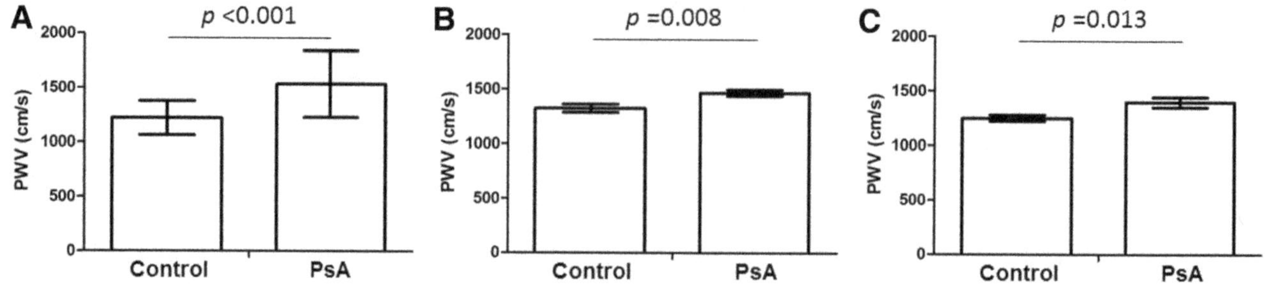

Figure 1 Pulse wave velocity (PWV) in control subjects and patients with psoriatic arthritis (PsA). (A) Unadjusted mean in control subjects (n = 47) and all PsA patients (n = 72). **(B)** Mean adjusted by age, gender and body weight in control subjects and all PsA patients. **(C)** Mean adjusted by age, gender and body weight in control subjects and PsA patients without hypertension, diabetes or hyperlipidemia (n = 20).

group (adjusted for baseline parameters: OR 1.137 (95% CI 1.058, 1.223), P <0.001; adjusted for last-visit parameters: OR 1.135 (95% CI 1.056, 1.219), P = 0.001).

Discussion

This is the first study to assess the association between cumulative inflammatory burden and arterial stiffness in PsA patients. High cumulative inflammatory burden as reflected by the ca-ESR was a predictor for higher PWV independently of traditional CV risk factors and other disease activity parameters. We also confirmed that PWV is increased in PsA patients compared with healthy control subjects in a larger cohort.

We have demonstrated a significant correlation between ca-ESR and PWV (P = 0.001) and a marginally significant correlation between ca-CRP and PWV (P = 0.061), suggesting that chronic inflammation may have a causative role in the development of arterial dysfunction in PsA patients. These results were consistent with previous findings that cumulative inflammatory burden (ca-ESR) was associated with increased aortic augmentation index in RA [19] and severity of carotid plaque in PsA [10]. One previous study reported that PWV associated with current CRP levels, but not with historical measures of cumulative ESR inflammatory burden in RA [20]. However, this study excluded patients with hypercholesterolemia and hypertension, and current smokers. In the current study ca-ESR, ca-CRP and single measurements of ESR and CRP at PWV assessment were associated with high PWV in the univariate analysis. Nonetheless, only ca-ESR was independently associated with high PWV in multivariate analysis after adjusting for other traditional CV risk factors and disease-related parameters, indicating that the cumulative inflammatory burden may better explain increased arterial stiffness than transient inflammatory status.

Different from ca-ESR, ca-CRP was not associated with PWV in multiple regression. A previous study from Eder *et al.* reported no association between ca-CRP and atherosclerosis in patients with PsA [10] while Giles *et al.* [11] reported that higher ca-CRP levels were associated with incident or progressive plaque, primarily in patients with elevated CVD risk in patients with RA. These seemingly contradictory findings may be explained by the relatively low levels of chronic inflammation that are commonly found in PsA compared with RA. A high-sensitivity (hs) CRP assay may be more informative, but was not available in our study. Serial monitoring of inflammatory markers including hsCRP should be considered in PsA patients.

Damaged joint count at the last visit was also associated with increased PWV in the univariate analysis. Indeed, damaged joint count could also represent the cumulative inflammatory burden and was found to be independently associated with atherosclerosis in RA [27]. However, the significance of damaged joint count was lost after adjusting for ca-ESR and other CV risk factors in PsA patients.

We also confirmed that arterial stiffness is increased in PsA patients. PWV was significantly higher in PsA patients after adjustment for age, gender and body weight, and even after PsA patients with hypertension, diabetes or hyperlipidemia were excluded. This is consistent with other studies with smaller case numbers that measured arterial stiffness by aortic PWV [17,18]. Costa *et al.* [17] reported increased PWV in 20 PsA patients compared with 20 controls. Soy *et al.* [18] also showed that PWV was higher in 9 PsA patients compared with 39 controls. In a previous study involving 73 PsA patients and 50 healthy controls, a significant increase in augmentation index was noticed, indicating impairment of both macrovascular and microvascular functions [28].

Although increased overall mortality in PsA patients has been reported in some [29-32] but not all [33,34] studies, previous data have consistently indicated an increased susceptibility to CVD and related mortality in PsA patients [3,35]. Our results indicated that the increased CVD and related mortalities may be partly mediated by increased arterial stiffness through persistent chronic inflammation. Inflammation accelerates subclinical

Table 2 Clinical features at baseline and last follow-up visit in patients in the high and low pulse-wave velocity (PWV) groups

	Baseline			Last visit		
	Low PWV	High PWV	*P*-value	Low PWV	High PWV	*P*-value
Male gender, n (%)	17 (50.0%)	19 (50.0%)	1.000	17 (50.0%)	19 (50.0%)	1.000
Age, years	**43.3 ± 10.2**	**55.2 ± 10.0**	**<0.001**	**49.6 ± 10.1**	**61.6 ± 9.9**	**<0.001**
Psoriatic arthritis (PsA) characteristics						
PsA disease duration, years	**7.6 ± 7.0**	**10.7 ± 7.5**	**0.073**	**13.9 ± 7.2**	**17.1 ± 7.8**	**0.075**
Tender joint count, 0 to 68	2 (0 to 6)	3 (0 to 8)	0.551	1 (0 to 3)	1 (0 to 5)	0.248
Swollen joint count, 0 to 66	0 (0 to 2)	1 (0 to 3)	0.827	0 (0 to 1)	0 (0 to 1)	0.376
Damaged joint count, 0 to 68	1 (0 to 3)	2 (0 to 6)	0.118	**0 (0 to 4)**	**4 (0 to 8)**	**0.010**
Visual analog scale pain, 0 to 100	40 (20 to 60)	50 (30 to 70)	0.212	30 (20 to 50)	30 (20 to 60)	0.964
Patients' global assessment, 0 to 100	50 (20 to 60)	50 (40 to 60)	0.258	50 (20 to 60)	33 (20 to 60)	0.654
Physicians' global assessment, 0 to 100	10 (0 to 20)	20 (5 to 30)	0.462	19 (6 to 35)	20 (7 to 30)	0.399
Psoriasis Area and Severity Index, 0 to 72	2.6 (1.0 to 7.3)	3.0 (0.7 to 7.7)	0.879	1.8 (0.6 to 5.4)	1.7 (0.3 to 7.4)	0.879
Health assessment questionnaire, 0 to 3	0.25 (0.13 to 0.63)	0.56 (0.13 to 1.00)	0.120	0.13 (0 to 0.50)	0.38 (0 to 1.13)	0.146
Minimal disease activity, n (%)	10 (29.4%)	6 (15.8%)	0.165	6 (17.6%)	8 (21.1%)	0.715
Disease Activity in Psoriatic Arthritis, 0 to 164	14 (7 to 19)	17 (12 to 22)	0.132	11 (7 to 15)	12 (5 to 18)	0.827
Erythrocyte sedimentation rate, mm/1st h	**16 (7 to 34)**	**27 (13 to 56)**	**0.048**	**11 (5 to 22)**	**29 (13 to 56)**	**<0.001**
C-reactive protein, mg/dl	0.3 (0.1 to 1.2)	0.5 (0.2 to 1.3)	0.527	**0.2 (0.1 to 0.5)**	**0.4 (0.2 to 0.8)**	**0.023**
Cardiovascular risk factors						
Body weight, kg	66.1 ± 12.4	64.4 ± 11.8	0.540	**68.1 ± 12.0**	**63.6 ± 11.0**	**0.099**
Body height, cm	161 ± 8	161 ± 9	0.891			
Systolic blood pressure, mmHg	132 ± 23	140 ± 21	0.113	**121 ± 13**	**132 ± 16**	**0.002**
Hypertension, n (%)	**10 (29.4%)**	**26 (68.4%)**	**0.001**	**15 (44.1%)**	**29 (76.3%)**	**0.005**
Diabetes, n (%)	**3 (8.8%)**	**13 (34.2%)**	**0.010**	**3 (8.8%)**	**13 (34.2%)**	**0.010**
Framingham 10-year CVD risk >10%, n (%)	**8 (23.5%)**	**22 (57.9%)**	**0.003**	**9 (26.5%)**	**27 (71.1%)**	**<0.001**
Total cholesterol, mmol/L	5.1 ± 0.9	5.1 ± 1.0	0.814	5.0 ± 1.0	4.8 ± 0.7	0.468
High-density lipoprotein cholesterol, mmol/L	1.6 ± 0.5	1.6 ± 0.5	0.782	1.5 ± 0.4	1.4 ± 0.4	0.467
Triglycerides, mmol/L	1.4 ± 0.7	1.6 ± 1.1	0.285	1.3 ± 0.8	1.5 ± 1.0	0.363
Fasting glucose, mmol/L	5.3 ± 1.6	5.7 ± 1.0	0.227	5.2 ± 1.0	5.6 ± 1.9	0.287
Medications, n (%)						
Anti-hypertensive drugs	**3 (8.8%)**	**17 (44.7%)**	**<0.001**	**14 (41.2%)**	**28 (73.7%)**	**0.005**
Statins	0 (0%)	1 (2.6%)	1.000	7 (20.6%)	7 (18.4%)	0.817
Nonsteroidal anti-inflammatory drugs	13 (38.2%)	20 (52.6%)	0.221	16 (47.1%)	15 (39.5%)	0.516
Steroids	2 (5.9%)	2 (5.3%)	0.999	1 (2.9%)	2 (5.3%)	0.999
Disease-modifying antirheumatic drugs	15 (44.1%)	21 (55.3%)	0.345	18 (52.9%)	22 (57.9%)	0.673
Biologics	0 (0%)	0 (0%)	N.S.	7 (20.6%)	4 (10.5%)	0.236

Variables with *P*-values <0.1 (values in bold text) were candidates for multivariate analysis. Values are presented as number (percentage), median (interquatile range), or mean ± SD.

atherosclerosis probably through adverse modification of the traditional CV risk factors [10]. In contrast, the association between cumulative inflammation and arterial stiffness was independent of traditional CV risk factors such as age, hypertension and diabetes. This may suggest that inflammation-induced arterial dysfunction is probably an early phase in the development of atherogenesis, and hence, PWV is a more sensitive marker reflecting changes in predominantly macrovascular functions in patients with rheumatic disease and chronic inflammation, compared to arterial remodeling as reflected by increased IMT and plaques.

PsA is associated with reduced levels of endothelial progenitor cells (EPCs) and impaired EPC function,

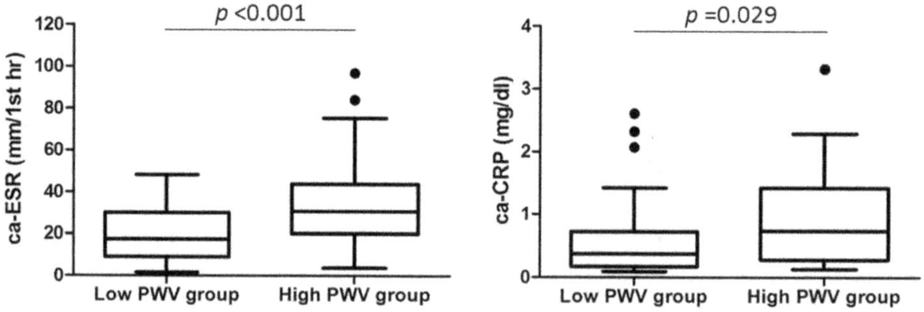

Figure 2 Cumulative inflammatory burden and pulse wave velocity (PWV). Cumulative average of erythrocyte sedimentation rate (ca-ESR) and C-reactive protein (CRP) in the low PWV group (PWV <1,450 cm/s, n = 34) and the high-PWV group (PWV ≥1,450 cm/s, n = 38).

leading to decreased release of nitric oxide (NO) [36]. Inflammatory cells such as macrophages and polymorphonuclear neutrophils produce a variety of matrix metalloproteinases (MMPs), which can alter the balance of elastin/collagen [37]. Chronic inflammation may also induce oxidative stress [7]. All these changes will lead to arterial stiffening. Inflammation also interacts with other important pathways such as advanced glycation end products (AGEs), which can irreversibly bind to collagens, resulting in stiffer AGE-linked collagen [38,39]. Moreover, AGEs can also promote inflammatory response through binding to the receptor (RAGE) and subsequently increase arterial stiffness [40,41]. TNF-α is a key cytokine involved in the pathogenesis of PsA [42], which can induce neutrophil chemotaxis, macrophage activation and superoxide production. This results in endothelial inflammation and dysfunction, and may contribute to the development of arterial damage [43]. Data from a non-randomized case–control study in patients with inflammatory arthritis (RA, PsA and ankylosing spondylitis) showed that long-term use of anti-TNF-α therapy may result in a significant improvement in PWV compared to the non-treated group [44]. Whether effective suppression of inflammation can improve arterial stiffness in PsA should be explored in future clinical trials.

Table 3 Association between cumulative inflammatory burden and high-PWV group by multivariable logistic regression

Model[a]	Factors	Odds ratio	95% CI	*P*-value
Baseline[b]	High cumulative ESR[d]	9.455	1.939, 46.093	0.005
	High cumulative CRP[e]	1.736	0.294, 10.268	0.543
Last visit[c]	High cumulative ESR[d]	9.111	1.875, 44.275	0.006
	High cumulative CRP[e]	0.888	0.088, 9.007	0.920

[a]Adjusted for parameters at baseline or last follow up. [b]Parameters entered: age, psoriatic arthritis (PsA) duration, hypertension, diabetes, Framingham risk score, use of anti-hypertension drugs, high erythrocyte sedimentation rate (ESR)[d], cumulative average (ca)-ESR[d] and ca-C-reactive protein (CRP)[e]. [c]Parameters entered: age, PsA duration, body weight, systolic blood pressure, hypertension, diabetes, damaged joints count, use of anti-hypertension drugs, Framingham risk score, high ESR[d] and CRP[e], high ca-ESR[d] and ca-CRP[e]. [d]Defined as ≥75th percentile: 37 mm/1st h. [e]Defined as ≥75th percentile: 1.2 mg/dl.

The strength of our study was the inclusion of a large prospective cohort with long-term follow up. Patients with CV risk factors were not excluded so that our results can be generalized to the usual PsA patient population. Our study also has a few limitations. First, our results may not be applicable to PsA patients from other ethnic backgrounds. Second, the outcome of this study (PWV) is only a surrogate of clinical CV events. In patients with PsA or RA, there are virtually no data to suggest whether PWV is a good surrogate of future CVD events. Third, arterial stiffness was assessed by brachial-ankle PWV but not the gold standard, carotid-femoral PWV. However, brachial-ankle PWV is highly correlated with carotid-femoral PWV and may provide qualitatively similar information [45]. Fourth, only baseline and last-visit clinical and traditional risk factors were adjusted for. With regards to the association between cumulative inflammatory burden and arterial stiffness, we have only addressed the role of cumulative averages of ESR and CRP. Unfortunately, we did not have data on other disease activity measures, for example, DAPSA and MDA during all the visits. It would be of interest for a future study to include a measure such as average mean DAPSA, or to determine whether achieving MDA for a prolonged period of time could be a potential predictor of arterial stiffness. Last but not least, baseline PWV measurement was not available to assess the relationship between cumulative inflammatory burden or the effect of treatment and the changes in arterial stiffness. Further prospective studies should be conducted to address this issue.

Conclusions

In conclusion, PsA patients have increased arterial stiffness compared with healthy control subjects. Cumulative inflammatory burden contributes to the increased arterial stiffness independent of traditional CV risk factors, suggesting that increasing arterial stiffness may be one of the mechanisms linking inflammation and CVD in PsA.

Abbreviations
AGEs: Advanced glycation end products; ANCOVA: analysis of covariance; AUC: area under the curve; BP: blood pressure; ca-CRP: cumulative averages of CRP; ca-ESR: cumulative averages of ESR; CASPAR: Classification of Psoriatic Arthritis; CRP: C-reactive protein; CV: cardiovascular; CVD: cardiovascular disease; DAPSA: Disease Activity in Psoriatic Arthritis; EPCs: endothelial progenitor cells; ESR: erythrocyte sedimentation rate; HAQ: Health Assessment Questionnaire; HDL: high-density lipoprotein cholesterol; Hs: high-sensitivity; ICC: intra-class correlation coefficient; IMT: intima-media thickness; LDL: low-density lipoprotein cholesterol; MDA: minimal disease activity; MMP: matrix metalloproteinase; NO: nitric oxide; PASI: Psoriasis Area and Severity Index; PsA: psoriatic arthritis; PWV: pulse wave velocity; RA: rheumatoid arthritis; RAGE: Receptor of AGEs; SBP: systolic blood pressure; TC: total cholesterol.

Competing interests
The authors declare that they have no competing interests.

Authors' contributions
JS participated in the design of the study, analysis and interpretation of data and manuscript drafting and revision. QS participated in data acquisition and manuscript revising. EL participated in study design, data acquisition and manuscript revision. YL, EK, LK, ML, TL and TZ participated in data acquisition and manuscript revision. CY participated in study design and manuscript revision. LT conceived of the study, and participated in its design, data acquisition, data analysis, manuscript drafting and revision. All authors read and approved the final manuscript.

Acknowledgement
This study is supported by a Chinese University research grant, a Hong Kong Arthritis & Rheumatism Foundation research grant, and an education grant from Janssen Pharmaceutical (Hong Kong). Janssen Pharmaceutical had no role in the study design, data collection, data analysis, or writing of the manuscript. The authors independently interpreted the results and made the final decision to submit the manuscript for publication.

Author details
[1]Department of Medicine & Therapeutics, The Prince of Wales Hospital, The Chinese University of Hong Kong, Shatin, Hong Kong, China. [2]Department of Rheumatology and Immunology, Singapore General Hospital, Outram Road, Singapore 169608, Singapore, Singapore. [3]Department of Medicine and Geriatrics, Taipo Hospital, Taipo, Hong Kong, China.

References
1. Tam LS, Shang Q, Li EK, Tomlinson B, Chu TT, Li M, et al. Subclinical carotid atherosclerosis in patients with psoriatic arthritis. Arthritis Rheum. 2008;59:1322–31.
2. Zhu TY, Li EK, Tam LS. Cardiovascular risk in patients with psoriatic arthritis. Int J Rheumatol. 2012;2012:714321.
3. Han C, Robinson Jr DW, Hackett MV, Paramore LC, Fraeman KH, Bala MV. Cardiovascular disease and risk factors in patients with rheumatoid arthritis, psoriatic arthritis, and ankylosing spondylitis. J Rheumatol. 2006;33:2167–72.
4. Gladman DD, Farewell VT, Wong K, Husted J. Mortality studies in psoriatic arthritis: results from a single outpatient center. II. Prognostic indicators for death. Arthritis Rheum. 1998;41:1103–10.
5. Tam LS, Tomlinson B, Chu TT, Li M, Leung YY, Kwok LW, et al. Cardiovascular risk profile of patients with psoriatic arthritis compared to controls–the role of inflammation. Rheumatology (Oxford). 2008;47:718–23.
6. Tam LS, Kitas GD, Gonzalez-Gay MA. Can suppression of inflammation by anti-TNF prevent progression of subclinical atherosclerosis in inflammatory arthritis? Rheumatology (Oxford). 2014;53:1108–19.
7. Park S, Lakatta EG. Role of inflammation in the pathogenesis of arterial stiffness. Yonsei Med J. 2012;53:258–61.
8. Hansson GK. Inflammation, atherosclerosis, and coronary artery disease. N Engl J Med. 2005;352:1685–95.
9. Eder L, Zisman D, Barzilai M, Laor A, Rahat M, Rozenbaum M, et al. Subclinical atherosclerosis in psoriatic arthritis: a case–control study. J Rheumatol. 2008;35:877–82.
10. Eder L, Thavaneswaran A, Chandran V, Cook R, Gladman DD. Increased burden of inflammation over time is associated with the extent of atherosclerotic plaques in patients with psoriatic arthritis. Ann Rheum Dis. 2014. doi: 10.1136/annrheumdis-2014-205267. [Epub ahead of print]
11. Giles JT, Post WS, Blumenthal RS, Polak J, Petri M, Gelber AC, et al. Longitudinal predictors of progression of carotid atherosclerosis in rheumatoid arthritis. Arthritis Rheum. 2011;63:3216–25.
12. Gonzalez-Gay MA, Gonzalez-Juanatey C, Pineiro A, Garcia-Porrua C, Testa A, Llorca J. High-grade C-reactive protein elevation correlates with accelerated atherogenesis in patients with rheumatoid arthritis. J Rheumatol. 2005;32:1219–23.
13. Gonzalez-Gay MA, Gonzalez-Juanatey C, Lopez-Diaz MJ, Pineiro A, Garcia-Porrua C, Miranda-Filloy JA, et al. HLA-DRB1 and persistent chronic inflammation contribute to cardiovascular events and cardiovascular mortality in patients with rheumatoid arthritis. Arthritis Rheum. 2007;57:125–32.
14. Cavalcante JL, Lima JA, Redheuil A, Al-Mallah MH. Aortic stiffness: current understanding and future directions. J Am Coll Cardiol. 2011;57:1511–22.
15. Vlachopoulos C, Aznaouridis K, Terentes-Printzios D, Ioakeimidis N, Stefanadis C. Prediction of cardiovascular events and all-cause mortality with brachial-ankle elasticity index: a systematic review and meta-analysis. Hypertension. 2012;60:556–62.
16. Wu L, Wang Y, Zheng L, Li J, Hu D, Xu Y, et al. Distribution of brachial-ankle pulse wave velocity values and optimal cut-off in distinguishing subjects with clinical condition in Chinese population. Int Angiol. 2012;31:252–9.
17. Costa L, Caso F, D'Elia L, Atteno M, Peluso R, Del Puente A, et al. Psoriatic arthritis is associated with increased arterial stiffness in the absence of known cardiovascular risk factors: a case control study. Clin Rheumatol. 2012;31:711–5.
18. Soy M, Yildiz M, Sevki Uyanik M, Karaka N, Gufer G, Piskin S. Susceptibility to atherosclerosis in patients with psoriasis and psoriatic arthritis as determined by carotid-femoral (aortic) pulse-wave velocity measurement. Rev Esp Cardiol (Engl Ed). 2009;62:96–9.
19. Crilly MA, Kumar V, Clark HJ, Scott NW, Macdonald AG, Williams DJ. Arterial stiffness and cumulative inflammatory burden in rheumatoid arthritis: a dose–response relationship independent of established cardiovascular risk factors. Rheumatology (Oxford). 2009;48:1606–12.
20. Maki-Petaja KM, Hall FC, Booth AD, Wallace SM, Yasmin, Bearcroft PW, et al. Rheumatoid arthritis is associated with increased aortic pulse-wave velocity, which is reduced by anti-tumor necrosis factor-alpha therapy. Circulation. 2006;114:1185–92.
21. Taylor W, Gladman D, Helliwell P, Marchesoni A, Mease P, Mielants H, et al. Classification criteria for psoriatic arthritis: development of new criteria from a large international study. Arthritis Rheum. 2006;54:2665–73.
22. Wong PC, Leung YY, Li EK, Tam LS. Measuring disease activity in psoriatic arthritis. Int J Rheumatol. 2012;2012:839425.
23. Fredriksson T, Pettersson U. Severe psoriasis–oral therapy with a new retinoid. Dermatologica. 1978;157:238–44.
24. Mease PJ. Measures of psoriatic arthritis: Tender and Swollen Joint Assessment, Psoriasis Area and Severity Index (PASI), Nail Psoriasis Severity Index (NAPSI), Modified Nail Psoriasis Severity Index (mNAPSI), Mander/Newcastle Enthesitis Index (MEI), Leeds Enthesitis Index (LEI), Spondyloarthritis Research Consortium of Canada (SPARCC), Maastricht Ankylosing Spondylitis Enthesis Score (MASES), Leeds Dactylitis Index (LDI), Patient Global for Psoriatic Arthritis, Dermatology Life Quality Index (DLQI), Psoriatic Arthritis Quality of Life (PsAQOL), Functional Assessment of Chronic Illness Therapy-Fatigue (FACIT-F), Psoriatic Arthritis Response Criteria (PsARC), Psoriatic Arthritis Joint Activity Index (PsAJAI), Disease Activity in Psoriatic Arthritis (DAPSA), and Composite Psoriatic Disease Activity Index (CPDAI). Arthritis Care Res (Hoboken). 2011;63:S64–85
25. Shang Q, Tam LS, Li EK, Yip GW, Yu CM. Increased arterial stiffness correlated with disease activity in systemic lupus erythematosus. Lupus. 2008;17:1096–102.
26. Tam LS, Shang Q, Li EK, Wong S, Li RJ, Lee KL, et al. Serum soluble receptor for advanced glycation end products levels and aortic augmentation index in early rheumatoid arthritis–a prospective study. Semin Arthritis Rheum. 2013;42:333–45.
27. Dessein PH, Joffe BI, Veller MG, Stevens BA, Tobias M, Reddi K, et al. Traditional and nontraditional cardiovascular risk factors are associated with atherosclerosis in rheumatoid arthritis. J Rheumatol. 2005;32:435–42.

28. Shang Q, Tam LS, Sanderson JE, Sun JP, Li EK, Yu CM. Increase in ventricular-arterial stiffness in patients with psoriatic arthritis. Rheumatology (Oxford). 2012;51:2215–23.
29. Ahlehoff O, Gislason GH, Charlot M, Jorgensen CH, Lindhardsen J, Olesen JB, et al. Psoriasis is associated with clinically significant cardiovascular risk: a Danish nationwide cohort study. J Intern Med. 2011;270:147–57.
30. Ali Y, Tom BD, Schentag CT, Farewell VT, Gladman DD. Improved survival in psoriatic arthritis with calendar time. Arthritis Rheum. 2007;56:2708–14.
31. Mok CC, Kwok CL, Ho LY, Chan PT, Yip SF. Life expectancy, standardized mortality ratios, and causes of death in six rheumatic diseases in Hong Kong. China Arthritis Rheum. 2011;63:1182–9.
32. Wong K, Gladman DD, Husted J, Long JA, Farewell VT. Mortality studies in psoriatic arthritis: results from a single outpatient clinic. I Causes and risk of death. Arthritis Rheum. 1997;40:1868–72.
33. Buckley C, Cavill C, Taylor G, Kay H, Waldron N, Korendowych E, et al. Mortality in psoriatic arthritis - a single-center study from the UK. J Rheumatol. 2010;37:2141–4.
34. Shbeeb M, Uramoto KM, Gibson LE, O'Fallon WM, Gabriel SE. The epidemiology of psoriatic arthritis in Olmsted County, Minnesota, USA, 1982–1991. J Rheumatol. 2000;27:1247–50.
35. Gladman DD, Ang M, Su L, Tom BD, Schentag CT, Farewell VT. Cardiovascular morbidity in psoriatic arthritis. Ann Rheum Dis. 2009;68:1131–5.
36. Westerweel PE, Verhaar MC. Endothelial progenitor cell dysfunction in rheumatic disease. Nat Rev Rheumatol. 2009;5:332–40.
37. Zieman SJ, Melenovsky V, Kass DA. Mechanisms, pathophysiology, and therapy of arterial stiffness. Arterioscler Thromb Vasc Biol. 2005;25:932–43.
38. Bailey AJ. Molecular mechanisms of ageing in connective tissues. Mech Ageing Dev. 2001;122:735–55.
39. Lee AT, Cerami A. Role of glycation in aging. Ann NY Acad Sci. 1992;663:63–70.
40. Throckmorton DC, Brogden AP, Min B, Rasmussen H, Kashgarian M. PDGF and TGF-beta mediate collagen production by mesangial cells exposed to advanced glycosylation end products. Kidney Int. 1995;48:111–7.
41. Yan SD, Schmidt AM, Anderson GM, Zhang J, Brett J, Zou YS, et al. Enhanced cellular oxidant stress by the interaction of advanced glycation end products with their receptors/binding proteins. J Biol Chem. 1994;269:9889–97.
42. Mease PJ. Tumour necrosis factor (TNF) in psoriatic arthritis: pathophysiology and treatment with TNF inhibitors. Ann Rheum Dis. 2002;61:298–304.
43. Gokce N, Vita JA. Clinical manifestations of endothelial dysfunction. In: Loscalzo J, Schafer AI, editors. Thrombosis and Hemorrhage. 3rd ed. Philadelphia, PA: Lippincott, Williams and Wilkins; 2002. p. 685–706.
44. Angel K, Provan SA, Fagerhol MK, Mowinckel P, Kvien TK, Atar D. Effect of 1-year anti-TNF-alpha therapy on aortic stiffness, carotid atherosclerosis, and calprotectin in inflammatory arthropathies: a controlled study. Am J Hypertens. 2012;25:644–50.
45. Sugawara J, Hayashi K, Yokoi T, Cortez-Cooper MY, DeVan AE, Anton MA, et al. Brachial-ankle pulse wave velocity: an index of central arterial stiffness? J Hum Hypertens. 2005;19:401–6.

24

Functional role of IL-22 in psoriatic arthritis

Anupam Mitra[1], Smriti K Raychaudhuri[2] and Siba P Raychaudhuri[2*]

Abstract

Introduction: Interleukin-22 (IL-22) is a cytokine of IL-10 family with significant proliferative effect on different cell lines. Immunopathological role of IL-22 has been studied in rheumatoid arthritis (RA) and psoriasis. Here we are reporting the functional role of IL-22 in the inflammatory and proliferative cascades of psoriatic arthritis (PsA).

Method: From peripheral blood and synovial fluid (SF) of PsA (n = 15), RA (n = 15) and osteoarthritis (OA, n = 15) patients, mononuclear cells were obtained and magnetically sorted for $CD3^+$ T cells. Fibroblast like synoviocytes (FLS) were isolated from the synovial tissue of PsA (n = 5), RA (n = 5) and OA (n = 5) patients. IL-22 levels in SF and serum were measured by enzyme linked immunosorbent assay (ELISA). Proliferative effect of human recombinant IL-22 (rIL-22) on FLS was assessed by MTT (3-(4, 5-Dimethylthiazol-2-yl)-2, 5-diphenyltetrazolium bromide, a yellow tetrazole) and CFSE dilution (Carboxyfluorescein succinimidyl ester) assays. Expression of IL-22Rα1 in FLS was determined by western blot.

Results: IL-22 levels were significantly elevated in SF of PsA patients (17.75 ± 3.46 pg/ml) compared to SF of OA (5.03 ± 0.39 pg/ml), $p < 0.001$. In MTT and CFSE dilution assays, rIL-22 (MTT, OD: 1.27 ± 0.06) induced significant proliferation of FLS derived from PsA patients compared to media (OD: 0.53 ± 0.02), $p < 0.001$. In addition, rIL-22 induced significantly more proliferation of FLS in presence of TNF-α. IL-22Rα1 was expressed in FLS of PsA, RA and OA patients. Anti IL-22R antibody significantly inhibited the proliferative effect of rIL-22. Further we demonstrated that activated synovial T cells of PsA and RA patients produced significantly more IL-22 than those of OA patients.

Conclusion: SF of PsA patients have higher concentration of IL-22 and rIL-22 induced marked proliferation of PsA derived FLS. Moreover combination of rIL-22 and TNF-α showed significantly more proliferative effect on FLS. IL-22Rα1 was expressed in FLS. Successful inhibition of IL-22 induced FLS proliferation by anti IL-22R antibody suggests that blocking of IL-22/IL-22R interaction may be considered as a novel therapeutic target for PsA.

Introduction

Psoriatic arthritis (PsA) is an inflammatory arthritis associated with psoriasis [1,2]. The role of genetic, immunological and environmental factors in the pathogenesis of PsA has been proposed, however the exact cause remains to be determined [3,4]. In the joint of PsA patients, there is hyperplasia of synovial lining cells and infiltration of mononuclear cells, which plays an important role in disease pathogenesis [5]. In PsA activated T cells produce increased amount of pro-inflammatory cytokines like IL-1β, IL-2, IFN-γ, TNF-α and IL-17 in the synovial fluid (SF) and thus contribute significantly to the disease pathogenesis [6-8]. Moreover fibroblasts isolated from skin and joints of patients with PsA showed increased proliferative activity and are capable of secreting IL-6, IL-1 and platelet derived growth factor [9]. It was reported previously that Th1 cytokines like IL-1β, TNF-α were higher in PsA compared to rheumatoid arthritis (RA) [6]. Recent findings suggest that there is hardly any difference in Th1 cytokines among these two groups [10]. The pro-inflammatory cytokine, TNF-α stimulates the proliferation of synovial fibroblasts leading to formation of pannus [11,12], as well as induces expression of chemokines and adhesion molecules which play important role in the pathogenesis of RA [13]. In most of the RA and PsA patients, neutralization of pro-inflammatory cytokines improve the disease condition but there are some patients who do not respond to this therapy [14,15]. This indicates that there are other cytokines and growth factors, which may play important roles in the disease process.

* Correspondence: sraychaudhuri@ucdavis.edu
[2]University of California, Davis, School of Medicine, Medicine/Rheumatology, Allergy & Clinical Immunology, Davis & VA Medical Center Sacramento, Mather, CA, USA
Full list of author information is available at the end of the article

IL-22, a newly discovered Th17 cytokine belongs to cytokine of IL-10 family, however differs from other cytokines of IL-10 family by being a potent proliferative and inflammatory agent for different cell lines [16-20]. Activated T cells of Th17 and Th22 subsets are the major source of IL-22 [21-24]. Apart from activated T cells, IL-22 can be produced by natural killer (NK) cells also [25]. IL-22 acts through IL-22 receptor, which is a complex of IL-22R1 and IL-10R2 [26]. IL-10R2 is ubiquitously expressed whereas IL-22R1 is expressed in liver, colon, small intestine, pancreas, kidney, skin and fibroblast like synoviocytes of joints [20,27]. In the pathogenesis of various autoimmune diseases such as psoriasis and RA, the role of IL-22 has been established [18-20,28]. Moreover, in collagen induced arthritis animal model, IL-22 has been found to play an important role in pannus formation as well as in osteoclastogenesis [29].

There is only one study which reported elevated levels of IL-22 in synovial fluid (SF) of PsA patients [30]. To our knowledge, there is no reported study on functional role of IL-22 in PsA. In this study we investigated the functional role of IL-22 in PsA. We measured IL-22 levels in serum and synovial fluid (SF) of PsA, RA and OA. To determine the functional significance, we evaluated the proliferative effect of human recombinant IL-22 (rIL-22) on fibroblast like synoviocytes (FLS) isolated from PsA synovial tissue. Expression of functional receptor of IL-22, IL-22Rα1 was determined at protein level in FLS. Further we examined the inhibitory effect of anti IL-22R antibody on IL-22 induced FLS proliferation in PsA.

Materials and methods

Study population

This study was approved by the Institutional Review Board (IRB) of Veterans Affairs Medical Centre (VAMC), Sacramento. After obtaining IRB approved informed consent form, specimens were collected from patients with active PsA, RA and OA. RA and OA patients were recruited according to the clinical, laboratory and radiographic classification criteria of the American College of Rheumatology (ACR). Patients with PsA had either oligoarthritis or symmetric polyarthritis as described by Moll and Wright [31]. All patients with PsA fulfilled the CASPAR classification criteria for PsA [32]. Before enrolling in this study, patients had undergone complete physical examination, evaluation of severity of psoriasis and arthritis, appropriate blood tests and radiological studies. Active PsA or RA was defined by the presence of at least 3 swollen and 3 tender joints. In patients with PsA, in addition to the above, presence of plaque psoriasis with a qualifying lesion of at least 2 cm in diameter was checked. All patients were evaluated for the swollen joint count, the tender joint count, patient's assessment of pain, ESR and CRP.

SF and blood were collected from patients with PsA (n = 15), RA (n = 15) and OA (n = 15). Synovial fluid mononuclear cells (SFMC) and peripheral blood mononuclear cells (PBMC) were isolated from SF and blood respectively. SF and synovial tissues were collected from one or both knees of PsA, RA and OA patients. Synovial tissues were studied from PsA (n = 5), RA (n = 5) and OA (n = 5) patients. These subjects had an arthroscopic procedure or joint replacement for treatment of their arthritis. All enrolled patients were on NSAID or Acetaminophen except two RA patients were on low dose oral steroid (≤ 7.5 mg/day), six RA patients were on hydroxychloroquine; six RA and five PsA patients were on low dose methotrexate (< 10 mg/week). None of the PsA patients was on steroid. None of the RA or PsA patients was on biologics for at least 3 months before the enrollment for this study.

ELISA of IL-22 in synovial fluid (SF) and serum of patients with PsA, RA and OA

Peripheral blood and SF from the knee joints of patients with PsA (n = 15), RA (n = 15) and OA (n = 15) were collected. The SF was immediately centrifuged at 1600 rpm for 20 min at 4°C to remove cells and debris. SF supernatants were carefully removed and stored at -20° C for ELISA of IL-22 (Human IL-22 ELISA Kit, eBioscience, San Diego, CA, USA). Serum was stored at -20°C for ELISA of IL-22. Sensitivity for IL-22 detection by this kit is 8-1000 pg/ml.

Functional role of human rIL-22 in FLS of patients with PsA

1. Isolation of FLS from synovial tissue

Fibroblast like synoviocytes (FLS) were isolated from synovial tissue biopsies of PsA (n = 5), RA (n = 5) and OA (n = 5) according to our standardized protocol [33,34]. FLS were cultured in DMEM (Mediatech, Manassas, VA, USA), supplemented with sodium pyruvate (Mediatech, Manassas, VA, USA), penicillin and streptomycin (Axenia BioLogix, Dixon, CA, USA) and 10% (v/v) fetal bovine serum (Axenia BioLogix, Dixon, CA, USA) (complete DMEM) at 37°C in a humidified atmosphere of 95% air and 5% CO2. After the third passage, all FLS were examined for the fibroblast specific markers ASO2 (EMD4Biosciences, San Diego, CA, USA) and CD55 (BD Pharmingen, San Diego, CA, USA). No expression of the macrophage specific marker CD68 (BD Pharmingen, San Diego, CA, USA) or pan endothelial cell adhesion molecule (PECAM), CD31 (BD Pharmingen, San Diego, CA, USA) were detected in FLS cultures, thus excluding possible contamination of synovial fibroblasts by synovial macrophages and endothelial cells. All experiments were performed with cells between 3rd and 6th passages.

2. Proliferative effect of human rIL-22 in FLS of PsA, RA and OA patients

The proliferative effect of human rIL-22 (eBioscience, San Diego, CA, USA) in FLS of PsA, RA and OA patients was assessed *in vitro* by MTT assay and Carboxy fluorescein succinimidyl ester (CFSE) dilution assay.

a. MTT assay- FLS from PsA (n = 5), RA (n = 5) and OA (n = 5) were used to determine the IL-22 induced proliferative effect. Human recombinant TNF-α (rTNF-α) was used as a positive control for proliferation assays [11,12]. We performed dose response curve and observed that human rIL-22 at 100 ng/ml, human anti IL-22R antibody (IL-22R Ab., R&D Systems, Minneapolis, MN, USA) at 1000 ng/ml and human rTNF-α (eBioscience, San Diego, CA, USA) at 20 ng/ml showed optimum response. We used these concentrations in subsequent experiments. Third to sixth passage FLS (20,000 cells/well) were cultured in triplicate in 24 well plate for 5 days with medium only, rIL-22 (100 ng/ml), IL-22R Ab (1000 ng/ml), IL-22R Ab (1000 ng/ml) + rIL-22 (100 ng/ml), rTNF-α (20 ng/ml) and rIL-22 (100 ng/ml) + rTNF-α (20 ng/ml). MTT assay was done as per our standardized protocol [34]. Briefly, MTT (Sigma, St. Louis, MO, USA) 5 mg/ml was added to each well followed by incubation for 4 hours. Acid-isopropanol (0.04 N HCl in isopropanol, 100 µl/well) was added and plates were maintained at room temperature for 5 minutes. The optical density was measured using a microtiter plate reader at 570/690 nm.

b. Carboxy fluorescein succinimidyl ester (CFSE) dilution assay- We used Cell Trace CFSE cell proliferation kit (Molecular Probes, Eugene, OR, USA). For this assay, we seeded 2×10^5 FLS in T25 flask and stained them with CFSE (2 µM) followed by incubation with media only, rIL-22 (100 ng/ml), rTNF-α (20 ng/ml) and rIL-22 (100 ng/ml) + rTNF-α (20 ng/ml) for 5 days. CFSE dilution was evaluated by flow cytometry (FACScalibur, BD Biosciences, San Jose, CA, USA). Data were analyzed using FlowJo software (Treestar, Ashland, OR, USA).

Western blot analysis of IL-22Rα1 expression in FLS of PsA, RA and OA

FLS of PsA, RA and OA were grown in T75 flask and upon 70-80% confluence, cells were scrapped with a cell scrapper, then centrifuged for 8 min at 1600 rpm, 22°C. Lysis buffer containing 150 mM NaCl (Fischer Scientific, Houston, TX, USA), 50 mM Tris-HCL of pH 7.2 (Sigma-Aldrich, St. Louis, MO, USA), 1% w/v Triton X-100 (Sigma-Aldrich, St. Louis, MO, USA), 1% w/v sodium deoxycholate (Sigma-Aldrich, MO, USA), 0.1% w/v SDS (Fischer Scientific, Houston, TX, USA) with protease inhibitor (Roche, Indianapolis, IN, USA) was added and incubated for 40 min at 4°C. Supernatants were collected after centrifugation at 4°C, 13000 rpm for 20 min and the protein concentration was estimated using BCA Protein Assay Reagent Kit (Thermo-Fisher scientific, Houston, TX, USA). Cell lysate protein (30 µg) was used for western blot analysis. Cell lysate was run in a 10% acrylamide gel (BIO-RAD, CA, USA). The Immuno-Blot PVDF membrane (BIO-RAD, Richmond, CA, USA) was blocked with 5% nonfat dried milk in TBST (50 ml of 1 M Tris, 30 ml of 3 M NaCl, 20 ml of 10% Tween, ddH2O, total volume 1L) for 2 hour at room temperature. Then blots were incubated overnight at 4°C with the primary antibody, IL-22Rα1 (R&D Sytems, Minneapolis, MN, USA) at 3 µg/ml concentrations; αtubulin (Cell signaling Technologies, Danvers, MA, USA), 1:250 concentrations. Blots were washed 5x in TBST and secondary antibody (Jackson Immunoresearch Labs, PA, USA) was added at 1:5000 dilution. After keeping the blot in secondary antibody for 1 hr, it was washed 5x in TBST and then developed using ECL western blotting detection reagents solution (Thermo-Fisher Scientific, Houston, TX, USA) for chemiluminescent detection. Band density was measured using Image J software (NIH, Bethesda, MD, USA).

Inhibitory effect of human anti IL-22R antibody (IL-22R Ab) on rIL-22 induced FLS proliferation

FLS (20,000/well) were seeded in a 24-well plate with 1 ml of complete DMEM (DMEM, 10%FBS, antibiotics). Cells were pre-treated with IL-22R Ab (1000 ng/ml) for 1 hr at 37°C then human rIL-22 (100 ng/ml) was added and incubated at 37°C in CO2 incubator for 5 days. MTT assay was done to determine the inhibitory effect of IL-22R Ab on IL-22 induced FLS proliferation.

Source of IL-22

To determine the source of IL-22, SFMC and PBMC isolated from SF and peripheral blood of PsA (n = 15), RA (n = 15) and OA (n = 15) were examined. PBMCs were isolated by Ficoll-hypaque gradient (GE Healthcare, Piscataway, NJ, USA) centrifugation of peripheral blood. Synovial fluid was treated with hyaluronidase enzyme (Sigma-Aldrich, MO, USA) at 1 mg/ml concentration for 5 mins at room temperature, then centrifuged at 2000 rpm for 20 min at 4°C. Cell pellet were resuspended in 1 ml of RPMI 1640 (Mediatech, Manassas, VA, USA) complete media (RPMI-1640 containing 10% FBS, antibiotics). Then the $CD3^+$ T cells were separated magnetically from SFMC and PBMC using Easy Sep negative selection human T cell enrichment kit (Stem

Cell Technology, Vancouver, BC, Canada) according to manufacturer's protocol and the purity was determined by flow cytometry using human anti CD3 antibody (BD pharmingen, San Diego, CA, USA). In a 24-well tissue culture plate, 1×10^6 synovial $CD3^+$ T cells and peripheral blood $CD3^+$ T cells were seeded separately and stimulated with 50 ng/ml of phorbol myristate acetate (PMA) and 1 µg/ml of ionomycin (Sigma-Aldrich, MO, USA) for 24 hrs and 10 µg/ml of phytoheamagglutinin (PHA, Invitrogen, CA, USA) for 48 hrs. For mimicking physiological stimulation, FLS were cultured in 24-well plates coated with human anti CD3 and anti CD28 (5 µg/ml each) (BD Biosciences, San Diego, CA, USA) at 37°C. After 24 and 48 hrs, supernatant was collected and IL-22 was measured in the supernatant by ELISA.

Statistical analysis

All experiments were done in triplicate. Results were expressed as Mean ± SEM. For analysis of flow cytometric data, we considered the % of divided cells of each treatment group using the FlowJo software (TreeStar Inc, Ashland, OR, USA). All data were analyzed statistically using the GraphPad Prism software version 5.0 (GraphPad Software Inc, La Jolla, CA, USA). Non-parametric tests (Wilcoxon matched pairs signed rank test, Mann Whitney test, Friedman's ANOVA, Kruskal Wallis ANOVA with Dunn's multiple comparison test) were used to determine the statistical significance. A p value < 0.05 was considered statistically significant.

Results

Synovial fluid IL-22 levels were elevated in PsA

IL-22 levels in SF of PsA (17.75 ± 3.46 pg/ml) were significantly higher compared to that in OA (5.03 ± 0.39 pg/ml, $p < 0.001$, Kruskal-Wallis ANOVA with Dunn's multiple comparison test) (Figure 1). In SF of RA, highest concentration of IL-22 (21.06 ± 3.55 pg/ml) was observed. However, there was no significant difference of IL-22 levels between SF of PsA (17.75 ± 3.46 pg/ml) and RA (21.06 ± 3.55 pg/ml). Serum IL-22 levels in PsA, RA and OA were 9.22 ± 0.54 pg/ml, 9.64 ± 1.20 pg/ml and 4.45 ± 0.25 pg/ml respectively, p = ns, Kruskal Wallis ANOVA with Dunn's multiple comparison test (Figure 1). We found significantly higher levels of IL-22 in SF of PsA (17.75 ± 3.46 pg/ml) and RA (21.06 ± 3.55 pg/ml) compared to that in serum of PsA (9.22 ± 0.54 pg/ml) and RA (9.64 ± 1.20 pg/ml) ($p < 0.01$, Mann Whitney test). In OA, there was no significant difference of IL-22 levels between SF (5.03 ± 0.39 pg/ml) and serum (4.45 ± 0.25 pg/ml).

Human rIL-22 induced marked proliferation of FLS

MTT and CFSE dilution assay were done to determine the proliferative effect of human rIL-22 in FLS of PsA, RA and OA. In MTT assay, significantly higher proliferation of PsA derived FLS were observed with rIL-22 (OD: 1.27 ± 0.06) compared to media (OD: 0.53 ± 0.02, $p < 0.001$, Friedman's ANOVA with Dunn's multiple comparison test) (Figure 2A). In this experiment we used rTNF-α as a positive control [11,12] and significant proliferation were found with rTNF-α (OD: 1.53 ± 0.05) compared to media (OD: 0.53 ± 0.02, $p < 0.001$, Friedman's ANOVA with Dunn's multiple comparison test). There was no significant difference of proliferation between the rIL-22 (OD: 1.27 ± 0.06) and rTNF-α (OD: 1.53 ± 0.05) treated FLS. Here we observed a novel finding that rIL-22 induced significantly more proliferation in presence of rTNF-α (OD: 2.06 ± 0.11) than rIL-22 alone (OD: 1.27 ± 0.06, $p < 0.01$) (Figure 2A).

We also did this experiment in RA FLS and observed similar results; human rIL-22 (OD: 1.58 ± 0.05) and rTNF-α (OD: 1.96 ± 0.04) induced significant proliferation compared to media (OD: 0.65 ± 0.04, $p < 0.001$, Friedman's ANOVA with Dunn's multiple comparison test). In RA also, rIL-22 in presence of rTNF-α (OD: 2.37 ± 0.11) induced significantly more proliferation than rIL-22 alone (OD: 1.58 ± 0.05, $p < 0.01$). In OA FLS, rIL-22 (OD: 0.73 ± 0.12) as well rTNF-α (OD: 0.90 ± 0.16) induced significant proliferation compared to media (OD: 0.38 ± 0.05, $p < 0.05$, Friedman's ANOVA with Dunn's multiple comparison test).

We further confirmed the proliferative effect of human rIL-22 on FLS by CFSE dilution assay. In this assay, similar results were found regarding proliferation of FLS with rIL-22. In FLS of PsA, human rIL-22 (19.64 ± 3.13%) and human rTNF-α (24.60 ± 4.95%) induced significantly more proliferation compared to that in media only (5.58 ± 0.98%, $p < 0.01$, Friedman's ANOVA with Dunn's multiple comparison test) (Figure 2B and 2C). Here also, rTNF-α (24.60 ± 4.95%) showed more proliferation of FLS than rIL-22 (19.64 ± 3.13%), but there was no significant difference in proliferation of FLS between these two groups. In this assay also, rIL22 in presence of rTNF-α (30.76 ± 4.17%) showed more proliferation than rIL-22 alone (19.64 ± 3.13%, $p < 0.05$) (Figure 2B and 2C).

In RA patients also, rIL-22 (21.57 ± 3.33%) and rTNF-α (27.45 ± 3.29%) induced significant proliferation compared to that in media (6.43 ± 1.61%, $p < 0.01$, Friedman's ANOVA with Dunn's multiple comparison test). There was no significant difference of proliferation between rIL-22 and rTNF-α treated FLS. In RA also, we observed that rIL-22 induced significantly more proliferation of FLS in presence of rTNF-α (33.11 ± 2.42%) compared to rIL-22 alone (21.57 ± 3.33, $p < 0.05$).

IL-22Rα1 was expressed in FLS

IL-22Rα1 expression at protein level was done by western blotting. Expressions of IL-22Rα1 were found in

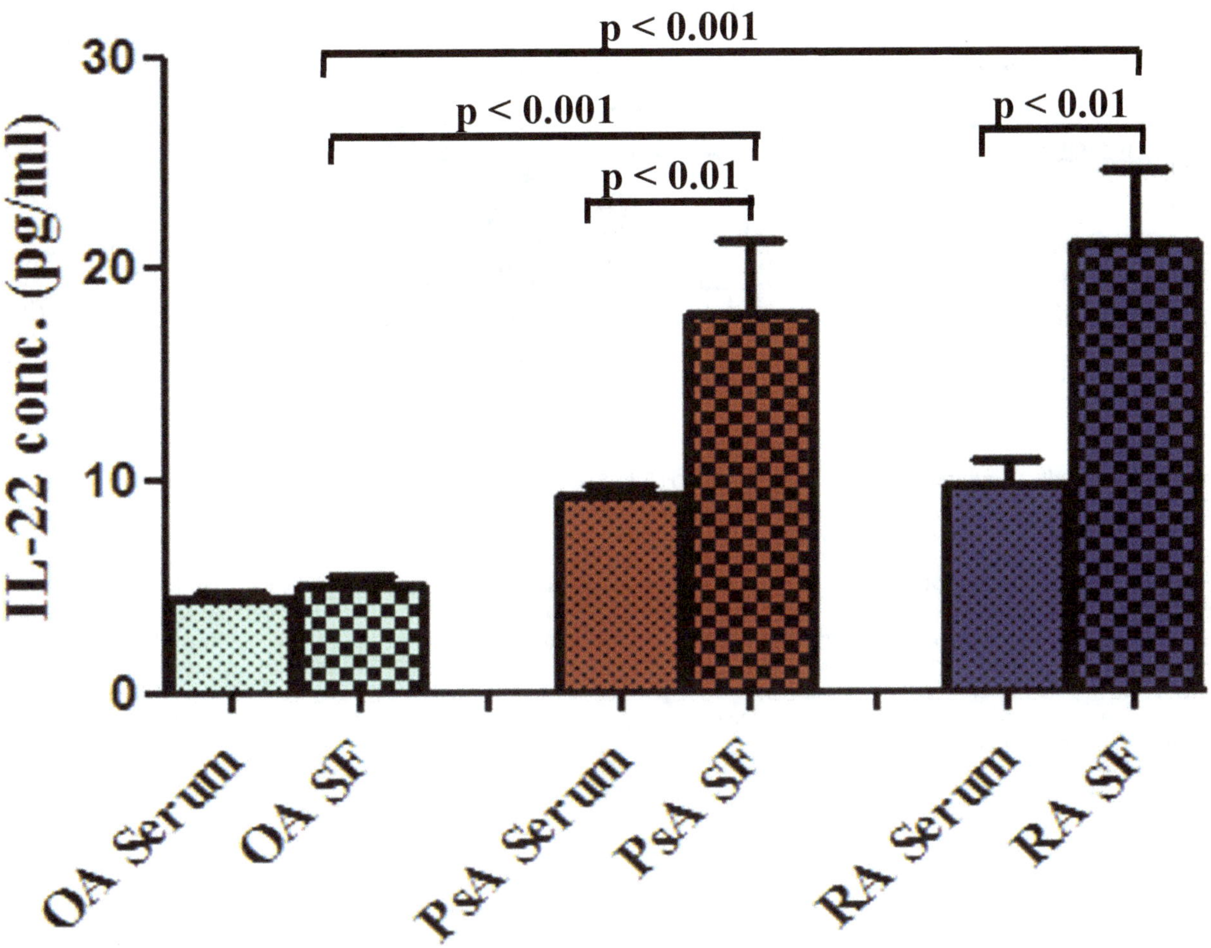

Figure 1 IL-22 in SF and serum of PsA and RA were elevated compared to OA patients. Synovial fluid (SF) and peripheral blood (PB) were collected from psoriatic arthritis (PsA, $n = 15$), rheumatoid arthritis (RA, $n = 15$) and osteoarthritis (OA, $n = 15$) patients. IL-22 levels were measured in SF and serum samples by ELISA. All experiments were done in triplicate. Results were expressed as Mean ± SEM. Nonparametric tests; Mann Whitney and Kruskal Wallis ANOVA with Dunn's multiple comparison tests were used to determine statistical significance.

FLS of PsA, RA and OA patients (Figure 3A). The relative intensity (R.I) of IL-22Rα1 in FLS of PsA, RA and OA patients was 0.92 ± 0.07, 0.94 ± 0.16 and 0.69 ± 0.18 respectively. There was no significant difference (Kruskal Wallis ANOVA with Dunn's multiple comparison test) in expressions of IL-22Rα1 between FLS of PsA, RA and OA patients (Figure 3B).

Inhibitory effect of anti IL-22R antibody on rIL-22 induced FLS proliferation

In MTT assay, there was a significant difference of proliferation between media (OD: 0.53 ± 0.02) and IL-22 + IL-22R Ab (OD: 0.76 ± 0.03, $p < 0.05$) treated FLS (Figure 4). Anti IL-22R (IL-22R Ab) antibody (OD: 0.76 ± 0.03) significantly inhibited the rIL-22 induced FLS proliferation in PsA (1.27 ± 0.06, $p < 0.01$, Friedman's ANOVA with Dunn's multiple comparison test) (Figure 4). There was no significant difference of proliferation between media (OD: 0.53 ± 0.02) and only IL-22R Ab (OD: 0.63 ± 0.03) treated FLS.

In FLS of RA also, IL-22R Ab (OD: 0.71 ± 0.03) significantly inhibited rIL-22 induced FLS proliferation (OD: 1.58 ± 0.05, $p < 0.001$, Friedman's ANOVA with Dunn's multiple comparison test. There was no significant difference of proliferation between media (OD: 0.65 ± 0.04) and only IL-22R Ab. (OD: 0.71 ± 0.03) treated FLS. In OA FLS, IL-22R Ab (OD: 0.49 ± 0.02) inhibited the rIL-22 induced proliferation (OD: 0.73 ± 0.12, p = ns), but there was no significant difference.

Synovial fluid of PsA and RA patients are enriched with IL-22 producing $CD3^+$ T cells

$CD3^+$ T cells were obtained from synovial fluid and peripheral blood of PsA, RA and OA by magnetic bead

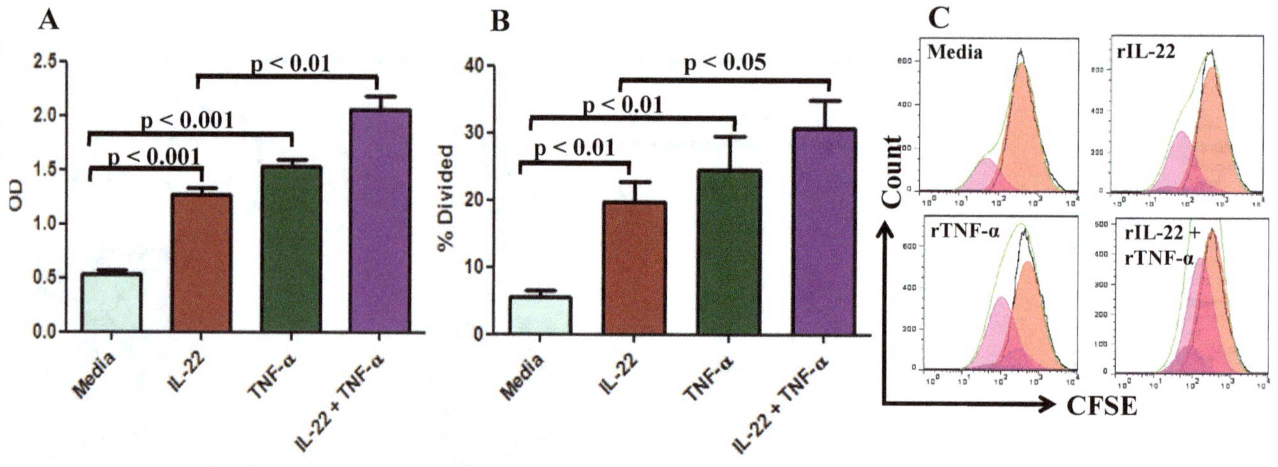

Figure 2 Human rIL-22 induced marked proliferation of FLS in PsA patients. FLS were isolated from synovial tissue of patients with psoriatic arthritis (PsA, $n = 5$). **(A)** FLS (20,000 cells/well) of PsA patients were seeded in a 24-well plate in triplicate and incubated for 5 days at 37°C in presence or absence of human rIL-22 (100 ng/ml), human rTNF-α (20 ng/ml) and combination of rIL-22 (100 ng/ml) + rTNF-α (20 ng/ml). FLS used in these experiments were between 3rd and 6th passage. MTT assay was done to determine FLS proliferation and results were expressed as Mean ± SEM of OD. **(B)** FLS (2×10^5 cells) of PsA patients were seeded in T25 flask in triplicate, stained with CFSE (2 μM) and incubated for 5 days at 37°C in presence or absence of human rIL-22 (100 ng/ml), human rTNF-α (20 ng/ml) and combination of rIL-22 (100 ng/ ml) + rTNF-α (20 ng/ml). Data were acquired in FACScalibur flow cytometer and analysis was done using FlowJo software. Proliferation was measured in terms of percent of divided cells and data were expressed as Mean ± SEM. The bar diagram represents the percent divided cells of FLS in PsA patients. **(C)** A representative histogram showing the proliferative effect of different treatments (rIL-22, rTNF-α, rIL-22 + rTNF-α) compared to media in FLS obtained from PsA patients. Non parametric test, Friedman's ANOVA with Dunn's multiple comparison test was done to determine statistical significance.

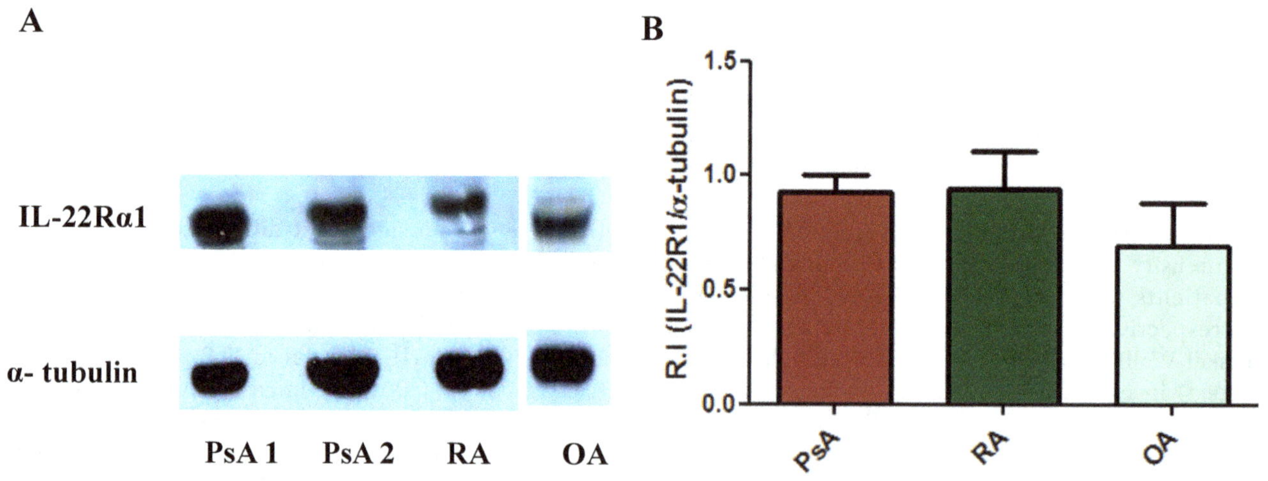

Figure 3 Western blot analysis of IL-22Rα1 expression in FLS of PsA, RA and OA patients. Expression of IL-22Rα1 in FLS isolated from PsA ($n = 5$), RA ($n = 5$) and OA ($n = 5$) patients was assessed. **(A)** A representative western blot showing expression of IL-22Rα1 in PsA, RA and OA patients. **(B)** A bar diagram showing relative intensity (R.I) of IL-22Rα1 expression in FLS obtained from PsA, RA and OA patients. Results were expressed as Mean ± SEM. Non parametric test, Kruskal Wallis with Dunn's multiple comparison test was done to determine the statistical significance.

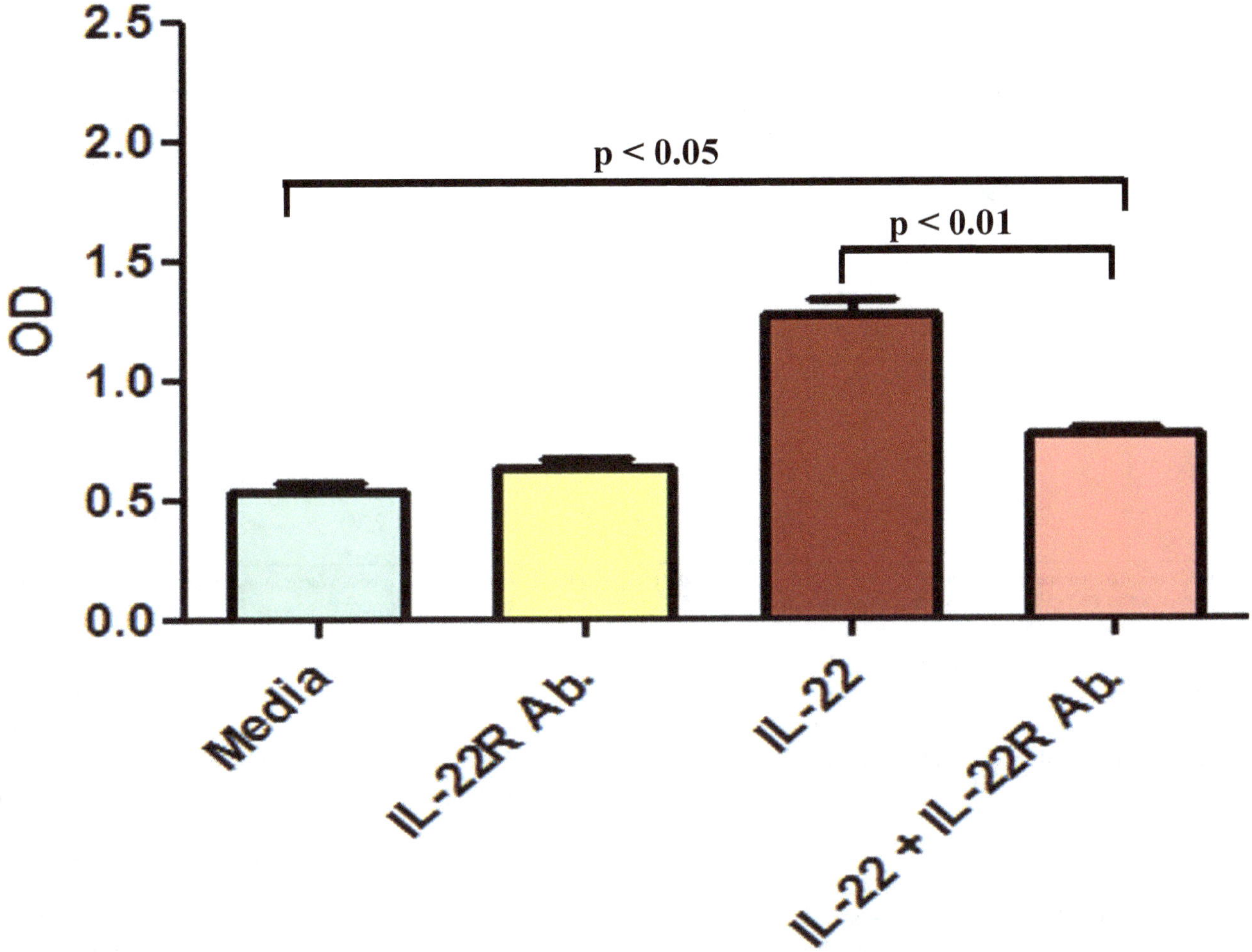

Figure 4 Human anti IL-22R antibody significantly inhibited rIL-22 induced FLS proliferation in PsA. FLS were pretreated with anti IL-22R antibody (1000 ng/ml) for 1 hr then incubated with rIL-22 (100 ng/ml) at 37°C for 5 days. MTT assay was done to evaluate the inhibitory effect of anti IL-22R antibody (IL-22R Ab). Each experiment was done in triplicate. Results were expressed as Mean ± SEM of OD. Non parametric test, Friedman's ANOVA with Dunn's multiple comparison test was done to determine statistical significance.

sorting. The purity of enriched T cells was > 90% by flow cytometric analysis. Activated synovial T cells of PsA and RA produced significantly more IL-22 than that of OA. Moreover in PsA and RA, activated synovial T cells produced significantly more IL-22 than peripheral blood T cells of same patients [Table 1].

Discussion

Several reports suggest that IL-22, a relatively new Th17 cytokine plays a critical role in the inflammation and proliferation cascade of various autoimmune diseases like rheumatoid arthritis and psoriasis [16-20,35,36]. In psoriasis, a correlation between serum IL-22 level and psoriasis area and severity index (PASI) score has been observed [28]. Higher levels of IL-22 were found in synovial fluid of PsA and RA patients [30,37]. Moreover systemic as well as intra-articular anti-TNF therapy showed reduction of increased IL-22 level in serum and synovial fluid of psoriasis and PsA patients respectively [30,38]. To our knowledge, there is no report available on the role of IL-22 in PsA. In this study we demonstrated the functional significance of IL-22 in PsA.

We observed significantly elevated levels of IL-22 in SF of PsA (17.75 ± 3.46 pg/ml) compared to OA (5.03 ± 0.39 pg/ml). We found highest concentration of IL-22 in SF of RA (21.06 ± 3.55 pg/ml), but it was not significantly different from PsA (17.75 ± 3.46 pg/ml) (Figure 1).

Most of the reports demonstrated T cells as a major source of IL-22 [18,21,22]. In addition NK cells have been reported to produce IL-22 [25] and there is one report where IL-22 was identified in FLS of RA synovial tissues [20]. Here we showed that activated synovial $CD3^+$ T cells of PsA and RA produced more IL-22 than those of OA [Table 1]. Synovial fluid from healthy

Table 1 IL-22 production by activated synovial fluid (SF) and peripheral blood (PB) CD3⁺ T cells.

		IL-22 concentration (pg/ml)				
		24 hr. Incubation			48 hr. Incubation	
		Unstimulated (Mean ± SEM)	CD3/CD28 Stimulated (Mean ± SEM)	PMA/ Ionomycin Stimulated (Mean ± SEM)	Unstimulated (Mean ± SEM)	PHA Stimulated (Mean ± SEM)
PsA (*n* = 10)	SF-T cells	3.85 ± 0.51	14.57 ± 0.80*$	18.92 ± 0.89**#$	4.21 ± 0.5	95.55 ± 7.81***#$
	PB-T cells	3.65 ± 0.23	10.44 ± 0.66*	12.83 ± 0.79*	4.28 ± 0.44	48.13 ± 6.38***$
RA (*n* = 10)	SF-T cells	4.22 ± 0.31	14.32 ± 0.96*$	18.91 ± 1.97**#$	4.63 ± 0.37	81.63 ± 5.90***#$
	PB-T cells	4 ± 0.16	10.56 ± 0.48*	11.88 ± 0.18*	4.1 ± 0.26	53.08 ± 4.58***$
OA (*n* = 8)	SF-T cells	4.63 ± 0.57	8.61 ± 0.79	13.59 ± 0.81*	4.79 ± 0.12	39.06 ± 3.92***
	PB-T cells	3.94 ± 0.22	6.88 ± 0.34	11.44 ± 0.78*	4.04 ± 0.18	32.78 ± 2.56***

* $p < 0.05$, ** $p < 0.01$, compared to 24 hr unstimulated media; *** $p < 0.001$, compared to 48 hr unstimulated media, Wilcoxon matched pairs signed rank test. # $p < 0.05$, compared to PB-T cells; $ $p < 0.05$, $$ $p < 0.01$, compared to that of OA, Mann Whitney test.

volunteers could not be obtained. We chose osteoarthritis patients (OA), a non-inflammatory arthritis as a negative control. Moreover we observed that activated synovial T cells produced significantly more IL-22 compared to activated peripheral blood T cells of same patients [Table 1].

In RA, it had been shown that rIL-22 induced marked proliferation of FLS and IL-22 receptors (IL-22R1) were present in those FLS [20]. In this study, we demonstrated that human rIL-22 induced significant proliferation of FLS of PsA and IL-22Rα1 were expressed in PsA FLS (Figure 2A, B and 3A). We also confirmed the expression of IL-22Rα1 in FLS of RA and OA [20]. There was no significant difference in IL-22Rα1 expressions among PsA, RA and OA FLS (Figure 3B). We observed more proliferation of FLS with rTNF-α in comparison to rIL-22, however there was no significant difference (Figure 2A and 2B). We also showed that the rIL-22 induced proliferation of FLS is inhibited by IL-22R antibody in PsA (Figure 4). These observations suggest that functionally active IL-22 is present in increased amount in the SF of PsA.

We observed a novel finding in PsA and RA that combination of rTNF-α and rIL-22 induced significantly more proliferation of FLS than rIL-22 alone (Figure 2A and 2B). In few studies on human keratinocytes, it have been shown that IL-22 together with TNF-α produce synergistic effect in terms of secretion of antimicrobial peptides and chemokines [39,40] however to our knowledge there is no study showing the combined effect of IL-22 and TNF-α on the proliferation of FLS. In this study we did not elucidate the mechanism responsible for this combined effect of IL-22 with TNF-α in FLS proliferation. Both TNF-α and IL-22 exert proliferative effect by inducing phosphorylation of extracellular signal regulated kinases (ERK)/p38 MAPK [20,41]. In a study on keratinocytes, Eyerich *et al* showed the synergistic effect of IL-22 and TNF-α on induction of immune genes by phosphorylation of different MAPK specially p38 [39]. Thus it is possible that combination of IL-22 and TNF-α induce more phosphorylation of Erk/MAPK pathway than either of IL-22 or TNF-α alone resulting in more proliferation of FLS.

Conclusions

To summarize, in this study we observed significantly elevated levels of IL-22 in synovial fluid of PsA compared to OA patients and activated synovial T cells produced more IL-22 than activated peripheral blood T cells in PsA. IL-22 is functionally active since it induced significant proliferation of FLS. Thus IL-22 has the potential to contribute in the pannus formation. Moreover, IL-22 in combination with TNF-α induced significantly more proliferation of FLS than IL-22 or TNF-α alone which provides a new insight in the pathogenesis of PsA. Here we have also shown that the IL-22 induced FLS proliferation can be blocked significantly by anti IL-22R antibody. Thus, IL-22/IL-22R system may be a potential novel target of drug development for psoriatic arthritis.

Abbreviations

CFSE: carboxy fluorescein succinimidyl ester; ELISA: enzyme-linked immunosorbent assay; FLS: fibroblast like synoviocytes; MTT: [3-(4,5-

Dimethylthiazol-2-yl)-2,5-Diphenyltetrazolium Bromide]; ns: not significant; OA: osteoarthritis; OD: optical density; PB: peripheral blood; PBMC: peripheral blood mononuclear cells; PHA: phytohaemagglutinin; PMA: phorbol myristate acetate; PsA: psoriatic arthritis; RA: rheumatoid arthritis; rIL-22: recombinant interleukin 22; rTNF-α: recombinant tumor necrosis factor alpha; SF: synovial fluid; SFMC: synovial fluid mononuclear cells.

Acknowledgements
This work was supported by VA Merit grant awarded to Dr. Siba P Raychaudhuri. The authors greatly appreciate technical support from C. Abria, A. Datta Mitra, D. Schrock, K. Ohata, S. Pathak, and S. Sharma.

Author details
[1]University of California, Davis, School of Medicine, Dermatology, Davis & VA Medical Center Sacramento, Mather, CA, USA. [2]University of California, Davis, School of Medicine, Medicine/Rheumatology, Allergy & Clinical Immunology, Davis & VA Medical Center Sacramento, Mather, CA, USA.

Authors' contributions
AM performed all experiments with help from others and did the statistical analysis. SKR designed experiments, supervised statistical analysis. SPR conceived the study and helped in designing experiments. All authors have contributed to the conception and/or acquisition of data and analysis for this project and to either drafting or revising the manuscript. All authors read and approved the final manuscript.

Competing interests
The authors declare that they have no competing interests.

References

1. Wright V, Moll JMH: **Psoriatic arthritis.** In *Seronegative Polyarthritis.* Edited by: Wright V, Moll JMH. Amsterdam: North Holland Publishing Co; 1976:169-223.
2. Gladman DD, Antoni C, Mease P, Clegg DO, Nash P: **Psoriatic arthritis: epidemiology, clinical features, course, and outcome.** *Ann Rheum Dis* 2005, **64**:ii14-17.
3. Rahman P, Elder JT: **Genetic epidemiology of psoriasis and psoriatic arthritis.** *Ann Rheum Dis* 2005, **64**:ii37-39.
4. Gladman DD: **Psoriatic arthritis.** *Dermatol Ther* 2004, **17**:350-363.
5. Veale D, Yanni G, Rogers S, Barnes L, Bresnihan B, Fitzgerald O: **Reduced synovial membrane macrophage numbers, ELAM1 expression, and lining layer hyperplasia in psoriatic arthritis as compared with rheumatoid arthritis.** *Arthritis Rheum* 1993, **36**:893-900.
6. Ritchlin C, Haas-Smith SA, Hicks D, Cappuccio J, Osterland CK, Looney RJ: **Patterns of cytokine production in psoriatic synovium.** *J Rheumatol* 1998, **25**:1544-1552.
7. Raychaudhuri SP, Raychaudhuri SK, Genovese MC: **IL-17 receptor and its functional significance in psoriatic arthritis.** *Mol Cell Biochem* 2012, **359**:419-429.
8. Veale DJ, Ritchlin C, FitzGerald O: **Immunopathology of psoriasis and psoriatic arthritis.** *Ann Rheum Dis* 2005, **64**:ii26-29.
9. Espinoza LR, Espinoza CG, Cuéllar ML, Scopelitis E, Silveira LH, Grotendorst GR: **Fibroblast function in psoriatic arthritis. II: increased expression of PDGF receptors and increased production of GF and cytokines.** *J Rheumatol* 1994, **21**:1507-1511.
10. van Kuijk AW, Reinders-Blankert P, Smeets TJ, Dijkmans BA, Tak PP: **Detailed analysis of the cell infiltrate and the expression of mediators of synovial inflammation and joint destruction in the synovium of patients with psoriatic arthritis: implications for treatment.** *Ann Rheum Dis* 2006, **65**:1551-1557.
11. Gitter BD, Labus JM, Lees SL, Scheetz ME: **Characteristics of human synovial fibroblast activation by IL-1β and TNF-α.** *Immunology* 1989, **66**:196-200.
12. Yokota K, Miyazaki T, Hirano M, Akiyama Y, Mimura T: **Simvastatin inhibits production of interleukin 6 (IL-6) and IL-8 and cell proliferation induced by tumor necrosis factor-alpha in fibroblast-like synoviocytes from patients with rheumatoid arthritis.** *J Rheumatol* 2006, **33**:463-471.
13. Choy EH, Panayi GS: **Cytokine pathways and joint inflammation in rheumatoid arthritis.** *N Engl J Med* 2001, **344**:907-9 16.
14. Ritchlin CT: **Therapeutic considerations in spondyloarthritis patients who fail tumour necrosis factor antagonists.** *Best Pract Res Clin Rheumatol* 2010, **24**:683-692.
15. Mease P: **TNF alpha therapy in psoriatic arthritis and psoriasis.** *Ann Rheum Dis* 2004, **63**:755-758.
16. Dumoutier L, Louahed J, Renauld JC: **Cloning and characterization of IL-10-related T cell-derived inducible factor (IL-TIF), a novel cytokine structurally related to IL-10 and inducible by IL-9.** *J Immunol* 2000, **164**:1814-1819.
17. Dumoutier L, Van Roost E, Colau D, Renauld JC: **Human interleukin-10-related T cell-derived inducible factor: molecular cloning and functional characterization as an hepatocytestimulating factor.** *Proc Natl Acad Sci USA* 2000, **97**:10144-10149.
18. Wolk K, Witte E, Wallace E, Döcke WD, Kunz S, Asadullah K, Volk HD, Sterry W, Sabat R: **IL-22 regulates the expression of genes responsible for antimicrobial defense, cellular differentiation, and mobility in keratinocytes: a potential role in psoriasis.** *Eur J Immunol* 2006, **36**:1309-1323.
19. Boniface K, Bernard F-X, Garcia M, Gurney AL, Lecron J-C, Morel F: **IL-22 inhibits epidermal differentiation and induces proinflammatory gene expression and migration of human keratinocytes.** *J Immunol* 2005, **174**:3695-3702.
20. Ikeuchi H, Kuroiwa T, Hiramatsu N, Kaneko Y, Hiromura K, Ueki K, Nojima Y: **Expression of interleukin-22 in rheumatoid arthritis: potential role as a proinflammatory cytokine.** *Arthritis Rheum* 2005, **52**:1037-1046.
21. Zenewicz LA, Flavell RA: **Recent advances in IL-22 biology.** *Int Immunol* 2011, **23**:159-163.
22. Kotenko SV, Langer JA: **Full house: 12 receptors for 27 cytokines.** *Int Immunopharmacol* 2004, **4**:593-608.
23. Pestka S, Krause CD, Sarkar D, Walter MR, Shi Y, Fisher PB: **Interleukin-10 and related cytokines and receptors.** *Annu Rev Immunol* 2004, **22**:929-979.
24. Renauld JC: **Class II cytokine receptors and their ligands: key antiviral and inflammatory modulators.** *Nat Rev Immunol* 2003, **3**:667-676.
25. Ren J, Feng Z, Lv Z, Chen X, Li J: **Natural killer-22 cells in the synovial fluid of patients with rheumatoid arthritis are an innate source of interleukin 22 and tumor necrosis factor-α.** *J Rheumatol* 2011, **38**:2112-2118.
26. Kotenko SV, Izotova LS, Mirochnitchenko OV, Esterova E, Dickensheets H, Donnelly RP, Pestka S: **Identification of the functional interleukin-22 (IL-22) receptor complex: the IL-10R2 chain (IL-10Rbeta) is a common chain of both the IL-10 and IL-22 (IL-10-related T cell-derived inducible factor, IL-TIF) receptor complexes.** *J Biol Chem* 2001, **276**:2725-2732.
27. Wolk K, Kunz S, Witte E, Friedrich M, Asadullah K, Sabat R: **IL-22 increases the innate immunity of tissues.** *Immunity* 2004, **21**:241-254.
28. Meephansan J, Ruchusatsawat K, Sindhupak W, Thorner PS, Wongpiyabovorn J: **Effect of methotrexate on serum levels of IL-22 in patients with psoriasis.** *Eur J Dermatol* 2011, **21**:501-504.
29. Geboes L, Dumoutier L, Kelchtermans H, Schurgers E, Mitera T, Renauld JC, Matthys P: **Proinflammatory role of the Th17 cytokine interleukin-22 in collagen-induced arthritis in C57BL/6 mice.** *Arthritis Rheum* 2009, **60**:390-395.
30. Fiocco U, Sfriso P, Oliviero F, Roux-Lombard P, Scagliori E, Cozzi L, Lunardi F, Calabrese F, Vezzù M, Dainese S, Molena B, Scanu A, Nardacchione R, Rubaltelli L, Dayer JM, Punzi L: **Synovial effusion and synovial fluid biomarkers in psoriatic arthritis to assess intraarticular tumor necrosis factor-α blockade in the knee joint.** *Arthritis Res Ther* 2010, **12**:R148.
31. Wright V, Moll JM: **Psoriatic arthritis.** *Bull Rheum Dis* 1971, **21**:627-632.
32. Taylor W, Gladman D, Helliwell P, Marchesoni A, Mease P, Mielants H, CASPAR Study Group: **Classification criteria for psoriatic arthritis: development of new criteria from a large international study.** *Arthritis Rheum* 2006, **54**:2665-2673.
33. Raychaudhuri SP, Raychaudhuri SK: **The regulatory role of nerve growth factor and its receptor system in fibroblast-like synovial cells.** *Scand J Rheumatol* 2009, **38**:207-215.
34. Raychaudhuri SK, Raychaudhuri SP: **Functional significance of nerve growth factor and its receptor (TrkA) in inflammatory arthritis.** *Arthritis Res Ther* 2010, **12**:404.

35. Fitch E, Harper E, Skorcheva I, Kurtz SE, Blauvelt A: **Pathophysiology of psoriasis: recent advances on IL-23 and Th17 cytokines.** *Curr Rheumatol Rep* 2007, **9**:461-417.
36. Zheng Y, Danilenko DM, Valdez P, Kasman I, Eastham-Anderson J, Wu J, Ouyang W: **Interleukin-22, a T(H)17 cytokine, mediates IL-23 induced dermal inflammation and acanthosis.** *Nature* 2007, **445**:648-651.
37. Kim KW, Kim HR, Park JY, Park JS, Oh HJ, Woo YJ, Park MK, Cho ML, Lee SH: **IL-22 promotes osteoclastogenesis in rheumatoid arthritis through induction of RANKL in human synovial fibroblasts.** *Arthritis Rheum* 2011, doi: 10.1002/art.33446.
38. Caproni M, Antiga E, Melani L, Volpi W, Del Bianco E, Fabbri P: **Serum levels of IL-17 and IL-22 are reduced by etanercept, but not by acitretin, in patients with psoriasis: a randomized-controlled trial.** *J Clin Immunol* 2009, **29**:210-214.
39. Eyerich S, Wagener J, Wenzel V, Scarponi C, Pennino D, Albanesi C, Schaller M, Behrendt H, Ring J, Schmidt-Weber CB, Cavani A, Mempel M, Traidl-Hoffmann C, Eyerich K: **IL-22 and TNF-α represent a key cytokine combination for epidermal integrity during infection with candida albicans.** *Eur J Immunol* 2011, **41**:1894-1901.
40. Guilloteau K, Paris I, Pedretti N, Boniface K, Juchaux F, Huguier V, Guillet G, Bernard FX, Lecron JC, Morel F: **Skin Inflammation Induced by the Synergistic Action of IL-17A, IL-22, Oncostatin M, IL1{alpha}, and TNF-{alpha} Recapitulates Some Features of Psoriasis.** *J Immunol* 2010.
41. Zhang Y, Dong J, He P, Li W, Zhang Q, Li N, Sun T: **Genistein Inhibit Cytokines or Growth Factor-Induced Proliferation and Transformation Phenotype in Fibroblast-Like Synoviocytes of Rheumatoid Arthritis.** *Inflammation* 2012, **35**:377-387.

25

Psoriatic arthritis: recent progress in pathophysiology and drug development

Douglas James Veale[1,2]

Abstract

Psoriatic arthritis (PsA) is the second most common inflammatory arthropathy, after rheumatoid arthritis diagnosis, in early arthritis clinics. Most patients have established psoriasis, often for years, prior to the onset of joint pain and swelling; in addition, associated features of nail disease, dactylitis, enthesitis, spondylitis or uveitis may be present. Psoriasis may not be immediately apparent, as small or patchy lesions may occur in the scalp or perineum. PsA presents as a symmetrical polyarthritis, similar to rheumatoid arthritis, or an asymmetrical oligoarthritis with a predilection for the distal interphalangeal joints. Spinal involvement is similar, although not identical, to ankylosing spondylitis. Joint damage occurs early; up to 50% of PsA patients have an 11% annual erosion rate in the first 2 years of disease duration, suggesting it is not a benign condition. There have been significant advances in our understanding of PsA pathogenesis in recent years, in the areas of genetics and molecular biology, implicating both the innate and the adaptive immune systems. This has lead to the introduction of evidence-based targeted therapy, primarily with tumour necrosis factor inhibitor (TNFi) agents. Therapy with disease-modifying anti-rheumatic drugs, such as methotrexate and leflunomide, remains the first-choice therapeutic intervention, even though there are few randomised controlled trials with these agents. In contrast, a number of successful studies of TNFi agents demonstrate excellent efficacy, in combination with methotrexate, and several novel agents are currently in development for the treatment of PsA.

Introduction

Psoriasis (PsO) is a common dermatosis characterised by thickened, red and scaly plaques [1]. PsO affects up to 2% of the population, often presenting in adolescence, on the scalp, and the extensor surfaces of the elbows and knees, although covert lesions may occur in the natal cleft, the navel or in the perineum. Psoriatic arthritis (PsA) develops in 10 to 40% of PsO patients depending on the source of the study population, as in an academic teaching hospital or in the community. In 80% of patients the arthritis manifests after the development of PsO, often by 10 years or more [2].

PsA may appear in a very similar clinical pattern to rheumatoid arthritis (RA), as a symmetrical small joint arthropathy involving the wrists, metacarpophalangeal joints and the proximal interphalangeal joints. In contrast, patients may develop asymmetric joint involvement, including a characteristic inflammatory arthritis of the distal interphalangeal joints, often colocalised with trophic changes in the associated nail. Patients are now defined as negative for circulating rheumatoid factor. In addition to PsO, PsA has a number of long-recognised associated clinical features including dactylitis, enthesitis, spondylitis and uveitis, the latter three resulting in grouping of PsA in the classification of seronegative spondyloarthropathies. The nail dystrophy includes features such as pitting and onycholysis that are present in up to 60% of patients with PsO, and equally may affect the fingernails and the toenails [3]. The association of the nail dystrophy with arthritis at the distal interphalangeal joint has recently led to the proposal of a common pathophysiologic mechanism [4]. A polyarticular or oligoarticular peripheral arthritis will account for 75% of new cases of PsA, but patients may present with a pure spondylitis on a clinical background of PsO [2].

Many different clinical classifications have been proposed for PsA since the original subtypes were described in 1973; however, the most recent was developed by an international multicentre study resulting in the CASPAR criteria and has now been widely adopted [5]. Five hundred

Correspondence: douglas.veale@ucd.ie
[1]Dublin Academic Medical Centre, Centre for Arthritis and Rheumatic Diseases, St Vincent's University Hospital, Elm Park, Dublin 4, Ireland
[2]The Conway Institute of Biomolecular and Biomedical Research, University College Dublin, Dublin 4, Ireland

and eighty-eight PsA patients were compared with 536 consecutive controls in a prospective clinical study examining these diagnostic criteria in relation to existing classification criteria in defining PsA. The CASPAR criteria have 98% specificity and 91% sensitivity.

There are reports suggesting that PsA is a benign arthropathy and erosive bone damage is uncommon [6], but Kane and Pathare examined an early arthritis clinic cohort followed up over 2 years and reported significant bone erosions in as many as 50% of PsA patients despite apparently good disease control with disease-modifying anti-rheumatic drugs such as methotrexate [7]. The primary objective in the management of PsA is to relieve signs and symptoms of the arthritis, but increasingly treatment strategies also aim to preserve function, prevent disability and maintain quality of life. These therapeutic strategies have targeted both the skin and joint features of disease, and more recently have set out to prove efficacy in the associated features of nail dystrophy, dactylitis, enthesitis, uveitis and spondylitis. As in the management strategies for RA, early diagnosis and introduction of effective treatment is pivotal to control inflammation, and prevent damage and disability. Over the last 12 years the use of targeted biologic therapies, namely tumour necrosis factor inhibitor (TNFi) agents, has revolutionised the therapy of both PsO and PsA, such that the combination therapy of methotrexate plus a TNFi is a widely used therapeutic intervention in PsA [8]. The spectrum of targeted therapies using specific biologic agents to block the inflammatory cascade has further been expanded to include IL-17 and IL-12/23. In addition, there is evidence to support using the CD80/86 receptor costimulatory molecule abatacept to treat PsA [9]. More recently, several small molecular inhibitors are in development and will undoubtedly be developed for the treatment of PsO and PsA.

Pathophysiology of psoriatic arthritis

In PsO and PsA, as in many autoimmune and autoinflammatory diseases, there is a complex interaction of genetic and environmental factors leading to a self-sustained and persistent immune response. What is not clear, however, is the relationship between skin disease and joint disease, because it now appears they may have independent rather than shared genetic associations. In addition, the evidence for environmental influences is limited due to the heterogeneous clinical phenotypes. As a result, the debate continues in relation to PsO and PsA being different manifestations of the same disease [10].

The broad clinical spectrum in PsA disease probably reflects a significant genetic heterogeneity, evident from the results of the numerous early human leukocyte antigen (HLA) association studies [11,12]. The more recent genome-wide association studies provide further evidence of genetic heterogeneity; although modest in size, they do suggest links between key factors in the immune responses both locally in the skin and also systemically, implicating both innate and adaptive immunity [13,14]. Genes identified in relation to specific networks of signalling molecules implicated in the barrier function of skin include *LCE3*, *DEFB4*, and *GJB2*, while *TNFAIP3*, *TNIP1*, *NFKBIA*, *REL*, *FBXL19*, *TYK2*, and *NOS2* involved in nuclear factor-κB and interferon signalling are implicated in the innate immune system, and *HLA-C*, *IL-12B*, *IL-23R*, *IL-23A*, *TRAF3IP2*, and *ERAP1* relate to CD8 T-lymphocyte and IL-23/IL-17-mediated lymphocyte signalling in the adaptive immune response [13-15]. In another recent report, the *RUNX3* gene has been reported to be overexpressed in patients with PsO and PsA. *RUNX3* is an important transcriptional regulator of CD8 T-cell differentiation, so this observation provides further evidence for the potential role of CD8 T-cell-dependent pathways in PsA [16].

In a review of the genome-wide association study data, Bluett and Barton highlight that, of all the genetic associations, many are in fact shared between PsO and PsA, except for HLA B27 and the IL-13 gene locus [17]. In addition to the HLA B27 link between PsA and ankylosing spondylitis, a number of other shared genetic associations have been confirmed including those implicated in lymphocyte signalling, notably ERAP1, IL-23R and IL-12B [18]. An interesting functional link has been described in an animal model of enthesitis, in which a unique IL-23R$^+$, RAR-related orphan receptor γt$^+$CD3$^+$CD4$^-$CD8$^-$, stem cell antigen 1$^+$ T-cell subset is resident at the entheseal insertion [19]. This is evidence that IL-23 is essential for the development of enthesitis by acting on this unique resident T-cell subset. The importance of these observations in novel drug development is clear because the IL-17/IL-23 axis is now being targeted with new monoclonal antibody therapies in PsO and is under investigation (phase II studies) for the treatment of PsA. The association with HLA B27 and CD8 T-lymphocyte function also supports a potential pathogenic role as the major histocompatibility complex class I molecules may present arthritogenic peptides to CD8$^+$ T lymphocytes or select an autoreactive T-cell repertoire.

There is some evidence that trauma or infection may be a potentially important environmental trigger in genetically susceptible individuals for both PsO and PsA. One early study did report an association between trauma and the later development of PsA in a digit, which was known as the deep Koebner response after the well-described Koebner response phenomenon in PsO [1]. Although the mechanism of the Koebner phenomenon is poorly understood, stimulation of sensory nerve endings and release of proinflammatory neuropeptides, as a result of trauma, probably trigger an immune response [20]. Neuropeptides, including substance P and vasoactive intestinal peptide, are reported as overexpressed in lesional skin of PsO patients and in synovial tissue of PsA [21,22]. A role for psychological stress has also been proposed, although it is difficult to elucidate a mechanistic pathway for stress – it may also be linked to neuropeptide release within the central nervous system. A small number of studies and case reports provide some evidence of a temporal link between physical trauma and the onset of PsA [23,24].

A close relationship has been reported between streptococcal infections and the onset of a subset of skin disease, guttate PsO, which appears to be linked to the HLA-Cw*06 genotype [25]. The presence of bacteria or related antigens, however, has not been described in the synovial tissue from joints of PsA patients. HIV has also been associated with an increased incidence of developing PsO and PsA, which raises the possibility that specific $CD8^+$ T cells play a pathophysiological role in the skin and joint disease [26].

Innate and adaptive immunity appears to be dysregulated in patients with PsO and PsA. As mentioned above, the recent genome-wide association studies provide evidence that nuclear factor-κB and interferon signalling, key regulators in the innate immune system, are associated with both PsO and PsA. In addition, there is evidence that genes associated with the adaptive immune response, in particular T-helper type (Th)1 and Th17 cells, are also associated with these diseases. In PsO skin lesions, the genomic data implicate T cells but also dendritic cells as key in the inflammatory process, while interferon-gamma and tumour necrosis factor (TNF)α appear to be the key cytokines. In early PsO skin lesions, the plasmacytoid dendritic cells appear to be increased in number – these may be activated in a Toll-like receptor-9-dependent mechanism by trauma, as suggested above, or infection, for example antimicrobial peptide LL-37 cathelicidin [27]. In PsO skin the plasmacytoid dendritic cell has an important inducer role by release of interferon-alpha [1]. At the same time, keratinocytes in the expanded PsO epidermis are a rich source of proinflammatory trigger molecules including antimicrobial peptides such as LL-37, β defensins and S100A7 (psoriasin) that appear to be regulated by IL-23 [28]. Th1 differentiation appears to be dependent in particular on IL-12, the main source of which is the dendritic cells. Th1 cells secrete mainly interferon-gamma, TNFα and IL-1, but the importance of IL-17, produced mainly by Th17 cells but also possibly by neutrophils and mast cells, has increasingly been recognised in the past few years [29]. The Th17 cell may be especially important in the immune responses and barrier function of the skin, because it also secretes IL-22, a key cytokine driving adaptive immune cell function and keratinocyte proliferation. The production of IL-17 by Th17 cells appears to be largely under the influence of IL-21, a mechanism that involves activation of the signal transducer and activator of transcription (STAT) signalling pathway [30], and is an important observation in relation to kinase inhibitors that may soon be available for the treatment of PsO and PsA.

Braverman and Yen described morphological vascular changes in PsO skin in the early 1970s [31]. The subsequent revelation that T cells undergo clonal expansion only after they migrate across the vascular endothelium suggests a key primary role for these cells in the evolution of the inflammatory lesion in PsO and PsA.

Many angiogenic cytokines including TNF, transforming growth factor beta, platelet-derived growth factor, and vascular endothelial growth factor are overexpressed in PsO skin and may be responsible for inducing changes in effector cell function as well as in endothelial cell function and growth. Similar morphological changes have been described in the synovial blood vessels in the PsA joint, and recently we have described associations with significant functional changes in infiltrating immune cells at a molecular level [32]. This further suggests that vascular endothelial cells participate actively in the immune response rather than act as a passive conduit for lymphocytes and monocytes entering inflamed tissues. Indeed, there is a close link between angiogenesis, inflammation, tissue hypoxia and the production of cytokines and matrix-degrading enzymes such as the metalloproteinases that facilitate effector cell activation and migration in the synovial tissue *in vivo* [33].

The chronic inflammatory lesion in PsO and in PsA appears fundamentally reliant on the presence of a brisk and persistent vascular response, which in turn is directly related to joint damage and possibly bone erosion. Many of the destructive matrix metalloproteinase enzymes are upregulated in the synovium, usually in response to cytokines (for example, IL-1 and TNFα). Bone erosion and severe osteolysis in a subgroup of PsA patients has led to a focus on the role of the osteoclast. Increased osteoclast activity at the cartilage–pannus junction also appears to be associated with increased receptor activator of nuclear factor-κB ligand expression and reduced osteoprotegerin. In a recent report, we have shown that the receptor activator of nuclear factor-κB ligand/osteoprotegerin can be altered via histamine acting through an orphan receptor in human chondrocytes. [34]. Osteoclast precursor cells have recently been described circulating in increased numbers in peripheral blood of PsA patients but may be suppressed following treatment with TNFi agents [35].

Drug development for psoriatic arthritis

The aim of treatment for PsA patients is to provide symptom relief, to prevent disability, to maintain function and to improve quality of life. In this respect, the introduction of biologic agents – mostly in combination with conventional disease-modifying anti-rheumatic drugs methotrexate, leflunomide, and salazopyrine – has revolutionised PsA therapy. In particular, the TNFi drugs appear to effectively inhibit the inflammatory response, while also preventing bone erosion, thereby preserving function and quality of life. New targeted biologic therapies have recently been reported as effective, including anti-cytokine drugs against TNFα, IL-17 and IL-12/23, while the co-stimulatory molecule CTLA4Ig has also been shown to be effective in PsA. Small molecule inhibitors targeting kinases, which are delivered per oral, may be developed for the treatment of PsO and PsA.

Tumour necrosis factor inhibitor therapy for psoriatic arthritis

TNF targeted therapy appears to be highly effective for the symptoms and signs of peripheral joint arthritis; however, in contrast to conventional disease-modifying anti-rheumatic drug agents, TNFi drugs also appear highly effective in treating spinal symptoms [8]. There are now five TNFi agents available, all showing apparently equivalent efficacy in the skin and joint manifestations of PsO and PsA [36,37]. TNFi agents are cost-effective and inhibit radiological progression of bone erosions in peripheral joints, maintain function and improve quality of life [38]. The results from the British Society for Rheumatology Biologics Register observational cohort study highlight the effectiveness of TNFi therapy in the treatment of patients with PsA [39]. The more recently developed TNFi agents golimumab and certolizumab pegol have also been shown effective in the treatment of PsA [40,41]. Golimumab is a next-generation TNF-targeting monoclonal antibody with high affinity, greater TNF-binding capacity and therefore a dosing interval extended to once a month – the reduced frequency of self-injection may be attractive to patients. Certolizumab pegol is a polyethylene glycolylated Fab′ fragment of a humanised monoclonal antibody, the polyethylene glycol moiety markedly increasing the half-life of the drug. In contrast to other TNFi agents, certolizumab pegol did not mediate increased levels of apoptosis, suggesting that these mechanisms are not essential for the TNFi effect [42].

Novel biologic therapies for psoriatic arthritis

In recent years, a number of biologic agents have been developed against candidate targets identified by studies of the pathophysiology of PsA. T-cell receptor activation follows interaction and binding of the T-cell surface-expressed CD28 molecule with the CD80/86 molecule on the surface of the antigen-presenting cell, producing a second costimulatory signal. Abatacept is a soluble, fully human fusion protein consisting of the extracellular domain of CTLA-4 linked to a modified Fc portion of human IgG1. Expression of CTLA-4 after activation competes with CD28 binding to CD80/86, which in turn leads to homeostatic downmodulation of activated T cells. Abatacept therefore selectively inhibits T-cell activation via competitive binding to CD80/86 and subsequent reduction in the levels of proinflammatory cytokines [43]. At higher doses, abatacept has been shown effective in the treatment of a significant subgroup of PsA patients [9].

Probably the most significant advances in our understanding of the pathophysiology of PsO and PsA, as outlined above, are around the IL-17 and IL-12/IL-23 pathway and the characterisation of the Th17 cell. Several monoclonal antibodies have been developed and shown to be effective in targeting this key regulatory pathway in patients with PsO and/or PsA. A first study shows the effects of secukinumab, a fully human anti-IL-17A monoclonal antibody, in a small proof-of-concept study; the second demonstrates efficacy of a fully human anti-IL-12/IL-23 monoclonal antibody, ustekinumab, in a large, phase III randomised controlled trial [44,45]. The secukinumab study included 42 patients for 24 weeks and failed to meet the primary endpoint; however, significant improvements in secondary measures were observed. Ustekinumab, recently approved for use in PsA by the US Food and Drug Administration, was studied in over 600 active PsA patients and showed significant responses compared with placebo over 52 weeks and may offer an alternative therapeutic mechanism of action to currently approved biological treatments. Finally, the two anti-IL-17 receptor antibodies brodalimumab and ixekizumab have been shown in short phase II studies to be significantly beneficial in plaque PsO, but studies in PsA are awaited [46,47].

Small molecule inhibitors for psoriatic arthritis

Biologic therapies have offered a major advance in the treatment of PsA over the past decade. In our experience, a remission rate of 60% may be achieved in routine clinical practice, but some patients demonstrate an inadequate or poor response [48].

The most recent advances in drug development have focused on small molecule inhibitors, including the phosphodiesterase 4 inhibitor apremilast, in PsO, PsA and RA, and the kinase inhibitors in RA and PsO. Some long-term results of a large phase III randomised controlled trial (PALACE 1 study) of apremilast in PsA were presented at the recent European League Against Rheumatism meeting [49]. Over 60% of patients receiving 20 mg twice daily and completing 52 weeks of the study demonstrated an American College of Rheumatology 20% improvement response. There were no new safety concerns, although tolerability due to gastrointestinal disturbances can be an issue in the short term. There are a number of kinase inhibitors targeting Jak1/2, Jak3, and Syk in development, and tofacitinib targeting primarily Jak3 is now licensed for use in RA patients in the USA, Japan and Switzerland. Tofacitinib has been the subject of detailed and extensive clinical trials in RA patients, demonstrating significant benefit for the signs and symptoms of RA, and inhibits radiological progression [50]. Furthermore, a phase IIb study of tofacitinib has shown significant improvement in moderate-to-severe PsO [51]. There are clinical trials ongoing with tofacitinib in patients with PsO and/or PsA; in addition, trials are registered at clinicaltrials.gov, but have not yet commenced, of tofacitinib in patients with PsA.

Conclusion

There have been significant advances in the detailed genetic and immunologic factors implicated in the pathophysiology of PsA in recent years. Many of these advances have been informed by rapid improvement in technologies, with respect to genomics and molecular biology, and by our increased knowledge of the immunology of inflammatory autoimmune diseases including RA and PsO. The exciting progress of drug development outlined in this article is, in part, directly related to the translational research and implementation of knowledge gained and to advanced technology in the past two decades. The challenges for clinicians and rheumatologists remain complex: how can patients be identified at the earliest timepoint; can we develop useful new biomarkers for early diagnosis and prognosis; and, finally, can we personalise the growing number of therapeutic interventions to individuals or groups of patients?

Abbreviations

HLA: Human leukocyte antigen; IL: Interleukin; PsA: Psoriatic arthritis; PsO: Psoriasis; RA: Rheumatoid arthritis; Th: T-helper type; TNF: Tumour necrosis factor; TNFi: Tumour necrosis factor inhibitor.

Competing interests

DJV received unrestricted educational funding from Abbvie, Actelion, MSD, Opsona, Pfizer, Roche and UCB; is on the speaker bureau for Actelion, MSD, Pfizer, Janssen, and UCB; and is advisor to Abbvie, Actelion, MSD, Pfizer, Roche and UCB.

References

1. Nestle FO, Kaplan DH, Barker J: **Psoriasis.** *N Engl J Med* 2009, **361**:496–509.
2. Veale D, Rogers S, Fitzgerald O: **Classification of clinical subsets in psoriatic arthritis.** *Br J Rheumatol* 1994, **33**:133–138.
3. Klaassen KM, van de Kerkhof PC, Pasch MC: **Nail psoriasis: a questionnaire-based survey.** *Br J Dermatol* 2013, **169**:314–319.
4. McGonagle DG, Helliwell P, Veale D: **Enthesitis in psoriatic disease.** *Dermatology* 2012, **225**:100–109.
5. Taylor W, Gladman D, Helliwell P, Marchesoni A, Mease P, Mielants H, CASPAR Study Group: **Classification criteria for psoriatic arthritis: development of new criteria from a large international study.** *Arthritis Rheum* 2006, **54**:2665–2673.
6. Shbeeb M, Uramoto KM, Gibson LE, O'Fallon WM, Gabriel SE: **The epidemiology of psoriatic arthritis in Olmsted County, Minnesota, USA, 1982–1991.** *J Rheumatol* 2000, **27**:1247–1250.
7. Kane D, Pathare S: **Early psoriatic arthritis.** *Rheum Dis Clin North Am* 2005, **31**:641–657.
8. Gossec L, Smolen JS, Gaujoux-Viala C, Ash Z, Marzo-Ortega H, van der Heijde D, FitzGerald O, Aletaha D, Balint P, Boumpas D, Braun J, Breedveld FC, Burmester G, Canete JD, de Wit M, Dagfinrud H, de Vlam K, Dougados M, Helliwell P, Kavanaugh A, Kvien TK, Landewe R, Luger T, Maccarone M, McGonagle D, McHugh N, McInnes IB, Ritchlin C, Sieper J, Tak PP, *et al*: **European League Against Rheumatism recommendations for the management of psoriatic arthritis with pharmacological therapies.** *Ann Rheum Dis* 2012, **71**:4–12.
9. Mease P, Genovese MC, Gladstein G, Kivitz AJ, Ritchlin C, Tak PP, Wollenhaupt J, Bahary O, Becker JC, Kelly S, Sigal L, Teng J, Gladman D: **Abatacept in the treatment of patients with psoriatic arthritis: results of a six-month, multicenter, randomized, double-blind, placebo-controlled, phase II trial.** *Arthritis Rheum* 2011, **63**:939–948.
10. Ciocon DH, Kimball AB: **PsO and psoriatic arthritis: separate or one and the same?** *Br J Dermatol* 2007, **157**:850–860.
11. Lambert JR, Wright V, Rajah SM, Moll JM: **Histocompatibility antigens in psoriatic arthritis.** *Ann Rheum Dis* 1976, **35**:526–530.
12. Gladman DD, Anhorn KA, Schachter RK, Mervart H: **HLA antigens in psoriatic arthritis.** *J Rheumatol* 1986, **13**:586–592.
13. Apel M, Uebe S, Bowes J, Giardina E, Korendowych E, Juneblad K, Pasutto F, Ekici AB, McManus R, Ho P, Bruce IN, Ryan AW, Behrens F, Böhm B, Traupe H, Lohmann J, Gieger C, Wichmann HE, Padyukov L, Fitzgerald O, Alenius GM, McHugh NJ, Novelli G, Burkhardt H, Barton A, Reis A, Hüffmeier U: **Variants in RUNX3 contribute to susceptibility to psoriatic arthritis, exhibiting further common ground with ankylosing spondylitis.** *Arthritis Rheum* 2013, **65**:1224–1231.
14. Hüffmeier U, Uebe S, Ekici AB, Bowes J, Giardina E, Korendowych E, Juneblad K, Apel M, McManus R, Ho P, Bruce IN, Ryan AW, Behrens F, Lascorz J, Böhm B, Traupe H, Lohmann J, Gieger C, Wichmann HE, Herold C, Steffens M, Klareskog L, Wienker TF, Fitzgerald O, Alenius GM, McHugh NJ, Novelli G, Burkhardt H, Barton A, Reis A: **Common variants at TRAF3IP2 are associated with susceptibility to psoriatic arthritis and PsO.** *Nat Genet* 2010, **42**:996–999.
15. Ellinghaus E, Stuart PE, Ellinghaus D, Nair RP, Debrus S, Raelson JV, Belouchi M, Tejasvi T, Li Y, Tsoi LC, Onken AT, Esko T, Metspalu A, Rahman P, Gladman DD, Bowcock AM, Helms C, Krueger GG, Koks S, Kingo K, Gieger C, Wichmann HE, Mrowietz U, Weidinger S, Schreiber S, Abecasis GR, Elder JT, Weichenthal M, Franke A: **Genome-wide meta-analysis of psoriatic arthritis identifies susceptibility locus at REL.** *J Invest Dermatol* 2012, **132**:1133–1140.
16. Nair RP, Duffin KC, Helms C, Ding J, Stuart PE, Goldgar D, Gudjonsson JE, Li Y, Tejasvi T, Feng BJ, Ruether A, Schreiber S, Weichenthal M, Gladman D, Rahman P, Schrodi SJ, Prahalad S, Guthery SL, Fischer J, Liao W, Kwok PY, Menter A, Lathrop GM, Wise CA, Begovich AB, Voorhees JJ, Elder JT, Krueger GG, Bowcock AM, Abecasis GR: **Collaborative Association Study of PsO. Genome-wide scan reveals association of PsO with IL-23 and NF-κB pathways.** *Nat Genet* 2009, **41**:199–204.
17. Bluett J, Barton A: **What have genome-wide studies told us about psoriatic arthritis?** *Curr Rheumatol Rep* 2012, **14**:364–368.
18. Jadon D, Tillett W, Wallis D, Cavill C, Bowes J, Waldron N, Dixon A, Sengupta R, Barton A, Korendowych E, McHugh NJ: **Exploring ankylosing spondylitis-associated ERAP1, IL23R and IL12B gene polymorphisms in subphenotypes of psoriatic arthritis.** *Rheumatology (Oxford)* 2013, **52**:261–266.
19. Sherlock JP, Joyce-Shaikh B, Turner SP, Chao CC, Sathe M, Grein J, Gorman DM, Bowman EP, McClanahan TK, Yearley JH, Eberl G, Buckley CD, Kastelein RA, Pierce RH, Laface DM, Cua DJ: **IL-23 induces spondyloarthropathy by acting on ROR-γt$^+$CD3$^+$CD4$^-$CD8$^-$ entheseal resident T cells.** *Nat Med* 2012, **18**:1069–1076.
20. Fearon U, Veale DJ: **Pathogenesis of psoriatic arthritis.** *Clin Exp Dermatol* 2001, **26**:333–337.
21. Eedy DJ, Johnston CF, Shaw C, Buchanan KD: **Neuropeptides in PsO: an immunohistochemical and radioimmunoassay study.** *J Invest Dermatol* 1991, **96**:434–438.
22. Veale D, Farrell M, FitzGerald O: **Mechanisms of joint sparing in a patient with unilateral psoriatic arthritis and a long-standing hemiplegia.** *Br J Rheumatol* 1993, **32**:413–416.
23. Punzi L, Pianon M, Bertazzolo N, Fagiolo U, Rizzi E, Rossini P, Todesco S: **Clinical, laboratory and immunogenetic aspects of post-traumatic psoriatic arthritis: a study of 25 patients.** *Clin Exp Rheumatol* 1998, **16**:277–281.
24. Langevitz P, Baskila D, Gladman DD: **Arthritis precipitated by physical trauma.** *J Rheumatol* 1990, **17**:695–697.
25. Mallbris L, Wolk K, Sánchez F, Ståhle M: **HLA-Cw*06 associates with a twofold higher prevalence of positive streptococcal throat swab at the onset of PsO: a case control study.** *BMC Dermatol* 2009, **9**:5.

26. Espinoza LR, Berman A, Vasey FB, Cahalin C, Nelson R, Germain EF: **Psoriatic arthritis and acquired immuno-deficiency syndrome.** *Arthritis Rheum* 1988, **31:**1034–1040.
27. Reinholz M, Ruzicka T, Schauber J: **Cathelicidin LL-37: an antimicrobial peptide with a role in inflammatory skin disease.** *Ann Dermatol* 2012, **24:**126–135.
28. Nakajima K, Kanda T, Takaishi M, Shiga T, Miyoshi K, Nakajima H, Kamijima R, Tarutani M, Benson JM, Elloso MM, Gutshall LL, Naso MF, Iwakura Y, DiGiovanni J, Sano S: **Distinct roles of IL-23 and IL-17 in the development of PsO-like lesions in a mouse model.** *J Immunol* 2011, **186:**4481–4489.
29. Moran EM, Heydrich R, Ng CT, Saber TP, McCormick J, Sieper J, Appel H, Fearon U, Veale DJ: **IL-17A expression is localised to both mononuclear and polymorphonuclear synovial cell infiltrates.** *PLoS One* 2011, **6:**e24048.
30. Wei L, Laurence A, Elias KM, O'Shea JJ: **IL-21 is produced by Th17 cells and drives IL-17 production in a STAT3-dependent manner.** *J Biol Chem* 2007, **282:**34605–34610.
31. Braverman IM, Yen A: **Microcirculation in psoriatic skin.** *J Invest Dermatol* 1974, **62:**493–502.
32. Gao W, Sweeney C, Walsh C, Rooney P, McCormick J, Veale DJ, Fearon U: **Notch signalling pathways mediate synovial angiogenesis in response to vascular endothelial growth factor and angiopoietin 2.** *Ann Rheum Dis* 2013, **72:**1080–1088.
33. Ng CT, Biniecka M, Kennedy A, McCormick J, Fitzgerald O, Bresnihan B, Buggy D, Taylor CT, O'Sullivan J, Fearon U, Veale DJ: **Synovial tissue hypoxia and inflammation in vivo.** *Ann Rheum Dis* 2010, **69:**1389–1395.
34. Marzaioli V, McMorrow JP, Angerer H, Gilmore A, Crean D, Zocco D, Rooney P, Veale D, Fearon U, Gogarty M, McEvoy AN, Stradner MH, Murphy EP: **Histamine contributes to increased RANKL to osteoprotegerin ratio through altered nuclear receptor 4A activity in human chondrocytes.** *Arthritis Rheum* 2012, **64:**3290–3301.
35. Anandarajah AP, Schwarz EM, Totterman S, Monu J, Feng CY, Shao T, Haas-Smith SA, Ritchlin CT: **The effect of etanercept on osteoclast precursor frequency and enhancing bone marrow oedema in patients with psoriatic arthritis.** *Ann Rheum Dis* 2008, **67:**296–301.
36. Ritchlin CT, Kavanaugh A, Gladman DD, Mease PJ, Helliwell P, Boehncke WH, de Vlam K, Fiorentino D, Fitzgerald O, Gottlieb AB, McHugh NJ, Nash P, Qureshi AA, Soriano ER, Taylor WJ, Group for Research and Assessment of PsO and Psoriatic Arthritis (GRAPPA): **Treatment recommendations for psoriatic arthritis.** *Ann Rheum Dis* 2009, **68:**1387–1394.
37. Mease P: **Update on treatment of psoriatic arthritis.** *Bull NYU Hosp Jt Dis* 2012, **70:**167–171.
38. Rodgers M, Epstein D, Bojke L, Yang H, Craig D, Fonseca T, Myers L, Bruce I, Chalmers R, Bujkiewicz S, Lai M, Cooper N, Abrams K, Spiegelhalter D, Sutton A, Sculpher M, Woolacott N: **Etanercept, infliximab and adalimumab for the treatment of psoriatic arthritis: a systematic review and economic evaluation.** *Health Technol Assess* 2011, **15:i-xxi:**1–329.
39. Saad AA, Ashcroft DM, Watson KD, Symmons DP, Noyce PR, Hyrich KL, BSRBR: **Efficacy and safety of anti-TNF therapies in psoriatic arthritis: an observational study from the British Society for Rheumatology Biologics Register.** *Rheumatology (Oxford)* 2010, **49:**697–705.
40. Kavanaugh A, van der Heijde D, McInnes IB, Mease P, Krueger GG, Gladman DD, Gomez-Reino J, Papp K, Baratelle A, Xu W, Mudivarthy S, Mack M, Rahman MU, Xu Z, Zrubek J, Beutler A: **Golimumab in psoriatic arthritis: one-year clinical efficacy, radiographic, and safety results from a phase III, randomized, placebo-controlled trial.** *Arthritis Rheum* 2012, **64:**2504–2517.
41. Gladman D, Fleischmann R, Coteur G, Woltering F, Mease PJ: **Effect of certolizumab pegol on the multiple facets of psoriatic arthritis as reported by patients with and without prior anti-TNF exposure: 24-week patient-reported outcome results of Rapid-PSA study.** *Ann Rheum Dis* 2013, **72**(Suppl):s260.
42. Chimenti MS, Saraceno R, Chiricozzi A, Giunta A, Chimenti S, Perricone R: **Profile of certolizumab and its potential in the treatment of psoriatic arthritis.** *Drug Des Devel Ther* 2013, **7:**339–348.
43. Veale DJ: **New therapies and new goals for psoriatic arthritis.** *Arthritis Rheum* 2011, **63:**874–876.
44. McInnes IB, Sieper J, Braun J, Emery P, van der Heijde D, Isaacs JD, Dahmen G, Wollenhaupt J, Schulze-Koops H, Kogan J, Ma S, Schumacher MM, Bertolino AP, Hueber W, Tak PP: **Efficacy and safety of secukinumab, a fully human anti-interleukin-17A monoclonal antibody, in patients with moderate-to-severe psoriatic arthritis: a 24-week, randomised, double-blind, placebo-controlled, phase II proof-of-concept trial.** *Ann Rheum Dis* 2013. [Epub ahead of print].
45. McInnes IB, Kavanaugh A, Gottlieb AB, Puig L, Rahman P, Ritchlin C, Brodmerkel C, Li S, Wang Y, Mendelsohn AM, Doyle MK, PSUMMIT 1 Study Group: **Efficacy and safety of ustekinumab in patients with active psoriatic arthritis: 1 year results of the phase 3, multicentre, double-blind, placebo-controlled PSUMMIT 1 trial.** *Lancet* 2013, **382:**780–789.
46. Papp KA, Leonardi C, Menter A, Ortonne JP, Krueger JG, Kricorian G, Aras G, Li J, Russell CB, Thompson EH, Baumgartner S: **Brodalumab, an anti-interleukin-17-receptor antibody for PsO.** *N Engl J Med* 2012, **366:**1181–1189.
47. Leonardi C, Matheson R, Zachariae C, Cameron G, Li L, Edson-Heredia E, Braun D, Banerjee S: **Anti-interleukin-17 monoclonal antibody ixekizumab in chronic plaque PsO.** *N Engl J Med* 2012, **366:**1190–1199.
48. Saber TP, Ng CT, Renard G, Lynch BM, Pontifex E, Walsh CA, Grier A, Molloy M, Bresnihan B, Fitzgerald O, Fearon U, Veale DJ: **Remission in psoriatic arthritis: is it possible and how can it be predicted?** *Arthritis Res Ther* 2010, **12:**R94.
49. Kavanaugh A, Mease PJ, Adebajo AO, Wollenhaupt J, Hu C, Shah K, Stevens RM, Gomez-Reino JJ: **Long-term (52-week) results of a phase 3, randomized, controlled trial of apremilast, an oral phosphodiesterase 4 inhibitor, in patients with psoriatic arthritis.** *Ann Rheum Dis* 2013, **72**(Suppl):s0001.
50. van der Heijde D, Tanaka Y, Fleischmann R, Keystone E, Kremer J, Zerbini C, Cardiel MH, Cohen S, Nash P, Song YW, Tegzova D, Wyman BT, Gruben D, Benda B, Wallenstein G, Krishnaswami S, Zwillich SH, Bradley JD, Connell CA, ORAL Scan Investigators: **Tofacitinib (CP-690,550) in patients with rheumatoid arthritis receiving methotrexate: twelve-month data from a twenty-four-month phase III randomized radiographic study.** *Arthritis Rheum* 2013, **65:**559–570.
51. Mamolo C, Harness J, Tan H, Menter A: **Tofacitinib (CP-690,550), an oral Janus kinase inhibitor, improves patient-reported outcomes in a phase 2b, randomized, double-blind, placebo-controlled study in patients with moderate-to-severe PsO.** *J Eur Acad Dermatol Venereol* 2013. [Epub ahead of print].

Permissions

All chapters in this book were first published in AR&T, by BioMed Central; hereby published with permission under the Creative Commons Attribution License or equivalent. Every chapter published in this book has been scrutinized by our experts. Their significance has been extensively debated. The topics covered herein carry significant findings which will fuel the growth of the discipline. They may even be implemented as practical applications or may be referred to as a beginning point for another development.

The contributors of this book come from diverse backgrounds, making this book a truly international effort. This book will bring forth new frontiers with its revolutionizing research information and detailed analysis of the nascent developments around the world.

We would like to thank all the contributing authors for lending their expertise to make the book truly unique. They have played a crucial role in the development of this book. Without their invaluable contributions this book wouldn't have been possible. They have made vital efforts to compile up to date information on the varied aspects of this subject to make this book a valuable addition to the collection of many professionals and students.

This book was conceptualized with the vision of imparting up-to-date information and advanced data in this field. To ensure the same, a matchless editorial board was set up. Every individual on the board went through rigorous rounds of assessment to prove their worth. After which they invested a large part of their time researching and compiling the most relevant data for our readers.

The editorial board has been involved in producing this book since its inception. They have spent rigorous hours researching and exploring the diverse topics which have resulted in the successful publishing of this book. They have passed on their knowledge of decades through this book. To expedite this challenging task, the publisher supported the team at every step. A small team of assistant editors was also appointed to further simplify the editing procedure and attain best results for the readers.

Apart from the editorial board, the designing team has also invested a significant amount of their time in understanding the subject and creating the most relevant covers. They scrutinized every image to scout for the most suitable representation of the subject and create an appropriate cover for the book.

The publishing team has been an ardent support to the editorial, designing and production team. Their endless efforts to recruit the best for this project, has resulted in the accomplishment of this book. They are a veteran in the field of academics and their pool of knowledge is as vast as their experience in printing. Their expertise and guidance has proved useful at every step. Their uncompromising quality standards have made this book an exceptional effort. Their encouragement from time to time has been an inspiration for everyone.

The publisher and the editorial board hope that this book will prove to be a valuable piece of knowledge for researchers, students, practitioners and scholars across the globe.

List of Contributors

Beate Böhm, Harald Burkhardt and Frank Behrens
Divisions of Rheumatology, Department of Internal Medicine II, Johann Wolfgang Goethe University, Theodor-Stern-Kai 7, 60590 Frankfurt am Main, Germany

Steffen Uebe, Maria Apel, André Reis and Ulrike Hüffmeier
Institute of Human Genetics, University of Erlangen-Nuremberg, Schwabachanlage 10, 91054 Erlangen, Germany

Anupam Mitra
University of California, Davis, School of Medicine, Dermatology, Davis & VA Medical Center Sacramento, Mather, CA, USA

Smriti K Raychaudhuri and Siba P Raychaudhuri
University of California, Davis, School of Medicine, Medicine/Rheumatology, Allergy & Clinical Immunology, Davis & VA Medical Center Sacramento, Mather, CA, USA

Lorenz Thurner, Marina Zaks, Klaus-Dieter Preuss, Natalie Fadle, Evi Regitz, Michael Pfreundschuh and Gunter Assmann
Department of Internal Medicine I, José Carreras-Center for Immuno- and Gene Therapy, University of Saarland Medical School, Kirrbergerstr., D-66421 Homburg, Saar, Germany

Mei Fang Ong
Institute of Medical Biostatistics, Saarl and University, Kirrbergerstr., D-66421 Homburg, Saar, Germany

Geneviève Gauthier and Robert Hiscock
Analysis Group Inc, 111 Huntington Ave #10, Boston, MA 02199, USA

Jeffrey R Curtis
University of Alabama at Birmingham, 510 20th St. South FOT 802D, Birmingham, AL 35294, USA

Anja Ficjan, Rusmir Husic, Judith Gretler, Angelika Lackner, Winfried B Graninger, Josef Hermann and Christian Dejaco
Department of Rheumatology and Immunology, Medical University Graz, Auenbruggerplatz 15, 8036 Graz, Austria

Marwin Gutierrez
Clinica Reumatologica, Università Politecnica delle Marche, Ospedale "Carlo Urbani", Via dei Colli 52, 60035 Jesi Ancona, Italy

Christina Duftner
Department of Internal Medicine VI, Medical University Innsbruck, Anichstrasse 35, 6020 Innsbruck, Austria

Jiayun Shen, Qing Shang, Edmund K Li, Lai-Wa Kwok, Martin Li, Tena K Li, Tracy Y Zhu, Cheuk-Man Yu and Lai-Shan Tam
Department of Medicine & Therapeutics, The Prince of Wales Hospital, The Chinese University of Hong Kong, Shatin, Hong Kong, China

Ying-Ying Leung
Department of Rheumatology and Immunology, Singapore General Hospital, Outram Road, Singapore 169608, Singapore, Singapore

Emily W Kun
Department of Medicine and Geriatrics, Taipo Hospital, Taipo, Hong Kong, China

Oliver FitzGerald and Muhammad Haroon
Department of Rheumatology, St Vincent's University Hospital, Elm Park, Dublin 4, Ireland

Jon T Giles and Robert Winchester
Rheumatology Division, Department of Medicine, Columbia University College of Physicians and Surgeons, 630 West 168th Street, New York City, NY 10032, USA

Michael Lucke
Department of Rheumatology, Allegheny Health Network, Pittsburgh, PA, USA

William Messner
Department of Quantitative Health Sciences, Cleveland Clinic, Cleveland, OH, USA

Esther S. H. Kim
Department of Cardiovascular Medicine, Cleveland Clinic, Cleveland, OH, USA

Huabin F Zhang
Celgene Corporation, 86 Morris Ave, Summit, NJ 07901, USA

M. Elaine Husni
Department of Rheumatic and Immunologic Diseases, Cleveland Clinic, 9500 Euclid Ave, desk A50, Cleveland, OH 44195, USA

Alexander Pfeil, Laura Krojniak, Lisa Reinhardt, Peter Oelzner and Gunter Wolf
Department of Internal Medicine III, Jena University Hospital—Friedrich Schiller University Jena, Erlanger Allee 101, Jena 07747, Germany

Diane M. Renz
Institute of Diagnostic and Interventional Radiology, Jena University Hospital—Friedrich Schiller University Jena, Erlanger Allee 101, Jena 07747, Germany

Marcus Franz
Department of Internal Medicine I, Jena University Hospital—Friedrich Schiller University Jena, Erlanger Allee 101, Jena 07747, Germany

Joachim Böttcher
Institute of Diagnostic and Interventional Radiology, SRH Wald-Klinikum Gera, Straße des Friedens 122, Gera 07548, Germany

Martin Bergman
Taylor Hospital, 8 Morton Avenue, Suite 304, Ridley Park, PA 19078, USA

Amy Lundholm
Lankenau Medical Center, Wynnewood, PA, USA

Rubén Queiro
Department of Rheumatology, HU, Central de Asturias, Av. Roma, s/n, 33011 Oviedo, Asturias, Spain

Juan D. Cañete
Department of Rheumatology, HU, Clinic and IDIBAPS, C/Villarroel, 170-08036 Barcelona, Spain

Carlos Montilla
Department of Rheumatology, HU, Parque Natural de las Batuecas 17, Cabrerizos, Salamanca Cp 37193, Spain

Miguel Abad
Department of Rheumatology HU, Virgen del Puerto, Paraje Valcorchero s/n, 10600 Plasencia, Spain

María Montoro, Susana Gómez and Ana Cábez
Medical Department, Pfizer, Avenida de Europa, 20 B, 28108 Alcobendas, Madrid, Spain

Agnes Szentpetery, Muhammad Haroon, Musaab Elmamoun, Phil Gallagher and Oliver FitzGerald
Department of Rheumatology, St. Vincent's University Hospital, Dublin,I reland

Eric Heffernan
Department of Radiology, St. Vincent's University Hospital, Dublin, Ireland

Martina Gogarty
School of Biochemistry and Immunology, TCD, Dublin, Ireland

Lisa Mellerick
Department of Histopathology, St. Vincent's University Hospital, Dublin, Ireland

Aurelie Fabre
Department of Histopathology, St. Vincent's University Hospital, Dublin, Ireland
Research Pathology, Immunohistochemistry Core Facility, UCD Conway Institute, UCD School of Medicine, Dublin, Ireland

Janet McCormack
Research Pathology, Immunohistochemistry Core Facility, UCD Conway Institute, UCD School of Medicine, Dublin, Ireland

Genevieve Kelly and Brian Kirby
Department of Dermatology, St. Vincent's University Hospital, Dublin, Ireland

Ari Polachek
Centre for Prognostic Studies in the Rheumatic Diseases, Toronto Western Hospital, University of Toronto, 1-412, 399 Bathurst Street, Toronto, ON M5T 2S8, Canada

Richard Cook
Department of Statistics and Actuarial Science, University of Waterloo, Waterloo, ON, Canada

Vinod Chandran
Department of Medicine and Laboratory Medicine, Institute of Medical Science, University of Toronto, Toronto, ON, Canada
Department of Pathobiology, Institute of Medical Science, University of Toronto, Toronto, ON, Canada
Centre for Prognosis Studies in the Rheumatic Diseases, Krembil Research Institute, Toronto Western Hospital, Toronto, ON, Canada

Dafna D. Gladman
Center for Prognostic Studies in the Rheumatic Diseases, Toronto Western Hospital, University of Toronto, Toronto, ON, Canada

Lihi Eder
Department of Medicine, University of Toronto, Women's College Research Institute, Women's College Hospital, Room 6326, 76 Grenville Street, Toronto, ON M5S 1B2, Canada

Leonieke J. J. van Mens, Marleen G. H. van de Sande, Inka A. Fluri, Sadaf Atiqi and Dominique L. P. Baeten
Department of Clinical Immunology & Rheumatology, Amsterdam Rheumatology and immunology Center, Academic Medical Center/ University of Amsterdam, Meibergdreef 9, 1105 AZ Amsterdam, The Netherlands

Arno W. R. van Kuijk
Rheumatology, Amsterdam Rheumatology and immunology Center Reade, Amsterdam, The Netherlands

Lihi Eder
Women's College Research Institute, Women's College Hospital, Suite 6326, 76 Grenville St, Toronto, Ontario M5S 1B2, Canada
Department of Medicine, University of Toronto, Toronto, ON, Canada

Ilan Feldhamer, Sari Greenberg-Dotan and Erez Batat
Chief Physician's Office, Central Headquarters, Clalit Health Services, Tel Aviv, Israel

Arnon Dov Cohen
Chief Physician's Office, Central Headquarters, Clalit Health Services, Tel Aviv, Israel
Siaal Research Center for Family Medicine and Primary Care, Faculty of Health Sciences, Ben-Gurion University of the Negev, Be'er-Sheva, Israel

Devy Zisman
Department of Rheumatology, Carmel Medical Center, Haifa, Israel
The Ruth and Bruce Rappaport Faculty of Medicine, Technion—Israel Institute of Technology, Haifa, Israel

Peter Nash
Department of Medicine, University of Queensland, Brisbane, Australia

Philip J. Mease
Swedish Medical Centre and University of Washington, Seattle, WA, USA

Iain B. McInnes
University of Glasgow, Glasgow, UK

Proton Rahman
Memorial University of Newfoundland, St. John's, NL, Canada

Christopher T. Ritchlin
Allergy/Immunology and Rheumatology Division, University of Rochester, Rochester, NY, USA

Ricardo Blanco
Hospital Universitario Marqués de Valdecilla, IDIVAL, Santander, Spain

Eva Dokoupilova
Medical Plus, s.r.o., Uherské Hradiště, and University of Veterinary and Pharmaceutical Sciences, Faculty of Pharmacy, Brno, Czech Republic

Mats Andersson and Shephard Mpofu
Novartis Pharma AG, Basel, Switzerland

Radhika Kajekar and Luminita Pricop
Novartis Pharmaceuticals Corporation, East Hanover, NJ, USA

Muhammad Haroon and Muddassar Ahmad
Division of Rheumatology, Department of Medicine, University Hospital Kerry, Tralee, Ireland

Muhammad Nouman Baig and John Rice
Department of Orthopaedics, University Hospital Kerry, Tralee, Ireland

Olivia Mason
CSTAR (Centre for Support and Training in Analysis and Research), University College Dublin, Dublin, Ireland

Oliver Fitz Gerald
Department of Rheumatology, St Vincent's University Hospital, Dublin, Ireland

Iain B. McInnes
Institute of Infection, Immunity & Inflammation, College of Medical, Veterinary and Life Sciences, University of Glasgow, 120 University Place, Glasgow G12 8TA, UK

Philip J. Mease
Swedish Medical Center and University of Washington, Seattle, WA, USA

Georg Schett
Friedrich-Alexander University of Erlangen-Nuremberg and Universitatsklinikum Erlangen, Erlangen, Germany

Bruce Kirkham
Guy's & St Thomas' NHS Foundation Trust, London, UK

Vibeke Strand
Stanford University School of Medicine, Palo Alto, CA, USA

Nicole Williams
RTI Health Solutions, Durham, NC, USA

Todd Fox and Steffen M. Jugl
Novartis Pharma AG, Basel, Switzerland

Luminita Pricop and Kunal K. Gandhi
Novartis Pharmaceuticals Corporation, East Hanover, NJ, USA

José Inciarte-Mundo, Julio Ramirez, Maria Victoria Hernández, Virginia Ruiz-Esquide, Andrea Cuervo, Sonia Raquel Cabrera-Villalba, Juan D. Cañete and Raimon Sanmarti
Department of Rheumatology, Hospital Clinic, University of Barcelona, Carrer Villarroel 170, 08036 Barcelona, Spain

Mariona Pascal and Jordi Yagüe
Department of Immunology, Hospital Clinic, University of Barcelona, Barcelona, Spain

Vibeke Strand
Division of Immunology/Rheumatology, Stanford University School of Medicine, Palo Alto, CA, USA

Evo Alemao, Thomas Lehman, Alyssa Johnsen, Subhashis Banerjee and Harris A. Ahmad
Bristol-Myers Squibb, Princeton, NJ, USA

Philip J. Mease
Swedish Medical Center and University of Washington, Seattle, WA, USA

L. C. Coates
Nuffield Department of Orthopaedics, Rheumatology and Musculoskeletal Sciences, University of Oxford, Botnar Research Centre, Windmill Road, Oxford OX3 7LD, UK

D. Gladman
Department of Medicine, Rheumatology, University of Toronto, Toronto Western Hospital, Toronto, Ontario, Canada

DP. Nash
Department of Medicine, University of Queensland, Brisbane, Australia

O. FitzGerald
Department of Rheumatology, St Vincent's University Hospital and Conway Institute for Biomolecular Research, University College Dublin, Dublin, Ireland

A. Kavanaugh
UC San Diego School of Medicine, La Jolla, CA, USA

T. K. Kvien
Department of Rheumatology, Diakonhjemmet Hospital, Oslo, Norway

L. Gossec
Sorbonne Universités, UPMC Université Paris 06, Paris, France
Rheumatology Department, Hôpital Pitié Salpêtrière, AP-HP, Paris, France

V. Strand
Division of Immunology/Rheumatology, Stanford University School of Medicine, Palo Alto, CA, USA

L. Rasouliyan
RTI Health Solutions, Barcelona, Spain

L. Pricop and K. Ding
Novartis Pharmaceuticals Corporation, East Hanover, NJ, USA

S. M. Jugl and C. Gaillez
Novartis Pharma AG, Basel, Switzerland

Raquel Celis, Raimon Sanmartí, Julio Ramírez and Juan D Cañete
Arthritis Unit, Rheumatology Department, Hospital Clinic de Barcelona and IDIBAPS, c/Villarroel, 170, 08036 Barcelona, Spain

Núria Planell
Plataforma de Bioinformática, Centro de Investigación Biomédica en Red de Enfermedades Hepáticas y Digestivas (CIBERehd), c/Córcega 180, 08036 Barcelona, Spain

José L Fernández-Sueiro
Rheumatology Division, Complejo Hospitalario Universitario, c/Xubias, 84, 15006 La Coruña, Spain

Isidoro González-Álvaro
Rheumatology Department, Hospital Universitario de la Princesa, IIS Princesa. c/Diego de León, 62, 28006 Madrid, Spain

José L Pablos
Instituto de Investigación, Hospital 12 de Octubre (I+12), Avda Córdoba s/n° 28041 Madrid, Spain

Arno WR van Kuijk, Danielle M Gerlag and Christina L Jonckheere
Division of Clinical Immunology and Rheumatology, Academic Medical Center/University of Amsterdam, Amsterdam, The Netherlands

Maria C Lebre
Division of Clinical Immunology and Rheumatology, Academic Medical Center/University of Amsterdam, Amsterdam, The Netherlands
Department of Experimental Immunology, Academic Medical Center/University of Amsterdam, Amsterdam, The Netherlands

Maarten C Kraan
Division of Clinical Immunology and Rheumatology, Academic Medical Center/University of Amsterdam, Amsterdam, The Netherlands
AstraZeneca, Mölndal, Sweden

Paul P Tak
Division of Clinical Immunology and Rheumatology, Academic Medical Center/University of Amsterdam, Amsterdam, The Netherlands
Academic Medical Center/University of Amsterdam and GlaxoSmithKline, Stevenage, UK

Jan D Bos
Department of Dermatology, Academic Medical Center/University of Amsterdam, Amsterdam, The Netherlands

Menno de Rie
Department of Dermatology, Academic Medical Center/University of Amsterdam, Amsterdam, The Netherlands
Department of Dermatology, Erasmus Medical Center, Rotterdam, The Netherlands

Matteo Nicola Dario Di Minno, Roberta Lupoli, Anna Russolillo and Giovanni Tarantino
Department of Clinical and Experimental Medicine, Reference Centre for Coagulation Disorders, Federico II University, Via Sergio Pansini 5, Naples, 80129 Italy

Rosario Peluso and Raffaele Scarpa
Department of Clinical and Experimental Medicine, Rheumatology Research Unit, Psoriatic Arthritis Clinic, Federico II University, Via Sergio Pansini 5, Naples, 80129 Italy

Salvatore Iervolino
Rheumatology and Rehabilitation Research Unit, I.R.C.C.S. "Salvatore Maugeri" Via Bagni Vecchi 1, Telese Terme (BN), 82037 Italy

Douglas James Veale
Dublin Academic Medical Centre, Centre for Arthritis and Rheumatic Diseases, St Vincent's University Hospital, Elm Park, Dublin 4, Ireland
The Conway Institute of Biomolecular and Biomedical Research, University College Dublin, Dublin 4, Ireland

Index

www.ingramcontent.com/pod-product-compliance
Lightning Source LLC
LaVergne TN
LVHW080727210926
848485LV00003B/533
* 9 7 8 1 6 3 9 2 7 3 9 5 9 *